Infectious Diseases of Hu

Infectious Diseases of Humans

Dynamics and Control

ROY M. ANDERSON

Linacre Professor,
Univesity of oxford

and

ROBERT M. MAY

Royal Society Research Professor,
University of Oxford

Oxford New York Tokyo
OXFORD UNIVERSITY PRESS

Oxford University Press, Great Clarendon Street, Oxford OX2 6DP
Oxford New York
Athens Auckland Bangkok Bogota Buenos Aires Calcutta
Cape Town Chennai Dar es Salaam Delhi Florence Hong Kong Istanbul
Karachi Kuala Lumpur Madrid Melbourne Mexico City Mumbai
Nairobi Paris São Paolo Singapore Taipei Tokyo Toronto Warsaw
and associated companies in
Berlin Ibadan

Oxford is a registered trade mark of Oxford University Press

Published in the United States by
Oxford University Press Inc., New York

First published 1991
First published in paperback 1992.
Reprinted 1993, 1995, 1998

British Library Cataloguing in Publication Data
Anderson, Roy M. (Robert Malcolm) 1947–
Infectious diseases of humans.
1. Man. Communicable diseases. Epidemiology
I. Title II. May, Robert M. (Roy McCredie) 1936–
614.4
ISBN 0-19-854599-1
ISBN 0-19-854040-X (Pbk)

Library of Congress Cataloging in Publication Data
Anderson, Roy M.
Infectious diseases of humans: dynamics and control / Roy M.
Anderson and Robert M. May.
Includes bibliographical references.
Includes indexes.
1. Communicable diseases—Epidemiology—Mathematical models.
2. Microbial ecology—Mathematical models. I. May, Robert M.
(Robert McCredie), 1936– . II. Title.
[DNLM: 1. Communicable Disease Control. 2. Communicable Diseases—
parasitology. 3. Epidemiologic Methods. 4. Host-Parasite
Relations. 5. Models, Theoretical. WA 110 A549i]
RA643.A56 1991 614.5—dc20 90-14312
ISBN 0-19-854599-1
ISBN 0-19-854040-X (Pbk)

Printed in Great Britain by
J. W. Arrowsmith Ltd., Bristol, Avon

Preface

We first met in 1974. It was, however, not until 1977 that we were drawn into collaboration by our separately developing interests in the possibility that viral, bacterial, protozoan, fungal, and helminth infections may play an important part in regulating the numerical abundance and geographical distribution of many animal populations.

As we began systematically to pursue these interests, the search for good, long-term runs of appropriate data on which to ground the mathematical models, and against which to test their predictions, led us more and more to focus on the population biology of infectious diseases of humans. Given the original ecological motivation of much of our work, a lot of it has been published in primarily ecological journals. But as the work has come increasingly to deal with detailed analysis of specific problems of human health—the evaluation of immunization programmes against viral and bacterial infections, or programmes of chemotherapy or vector control against protozoan or helminth infections—there are many publications in parasitological and public health journals. In the mid-1980s we began to feel we should draw this scattered body of work together, integrating it with advances made by other people, into a synoptic account of how the models can be combined with epidemiological data from field and laboratory, to give keener insights into population-level consequences of the dynamic interplay between infections and their host populations.

In 1986 the Rockefeller Foundation generously provided us with the chance to spend a month at their study centre at Bellagio, isolated from the cares of the everyday world. In this month we began to realize the magnitude of the task we had so lightly set ourselves. Nevertheless we did manage to write the greater part of the text (literally writing it: we both still write first drafts by hand, RMM with many scratchings-out and RMA with liberal use of "white-out/Tipp-Ex" so that he emerges from a writing session with face and hands speckled with white spots). Finishing and revising the text, completing confrontations between theory and data that were only sketched in draft (and which comprise the bulk of the several hundred figures in the book), and including new work, has taken time. In early 1990 we realized we were dealing with a diverging task, and called a halt to continual up-dating. We believe the book realizes our initial aim, in that—as explained more fully in the introductory chapter—it synthesizes a scattered literature, while presenting a substantial amount of new work (much of it prompted by such synthesis).

Many patrons have supported our work generously. These include the Wellcome Trust, the Rockefeller Foundation, the U.S. National Science

Foundation (through both its mathematics and its ecology programmes), the UK Medical Research Council, Natural Environment Research Council, and Overseas Development Agency. We thank these institutions, and particularly the programme officers (especially Bridget Ogilvie at the Wellcome Trust and Ken Warren at the Rockefeller Foundation) who have taken a close interest in the work. Our universities (Imperial College, London, for RMA, Princeton University up to 1988 and then the University of Oxford and Imperial College for RMM) have been extremely supportive, providing facilities, good administration, and a steady stream of enthusiastic undergraduates, graduate students, and postdoctoral researchers.

Neither this book nor the work in it would have existed without the stimulus and advice provided by a host of scientific colleagues. We are enormously grateful to each and every one of them. Once we start listing names, there is really no natural stopping-place. But we must single out those at our home institutions whose inputs have shaped this book: Sally Blower, Don Bundy, Andy Dobson, Bryan Grenfell, Sunetra Gupta, Michael Hassell, Anne Keymer, Angela McLean, Graham Medley, James Nokes, Jon Seger, and Helen Udy. Our editor at Oxford University Press, Judith May, has been unfailingly helpful and encouraging. Last, but by no means least, we acknowledge the emotional support and understanding provided by Jane Anderson and Perri May.

London   R.M.A.
August 1990   R.M.M.

Contents

Appendices

1

Introduction

'Policy is of course based on theory, though not always on the
best theory.'

Hobsbawm, 1969

1.1 Historical background

The historical and epidemiological literature abound with accounts of infectious
diseases invading human communities and of the concomitant effects on
population abundance, social organization, and the unfolding patterns of
historical events. A catalogue of the number of deaths induced by the major
epidemics of historical times is staggering, and dwarfs the total deaths on all
past battlefields.

In Europe in the fourteenth century, for example, there were around
25 million deaths, out of a population of roughly 100 million, from bubonic
plague alone. In the 1665 plague epidemic in London, more than 68 000 people
are thought to have died. The emotions triggered by this particular episode are
dramatically captured in Daniel Defoe's journal. 'It was then indeed, that man
withered like the grass and that his brief earthly existence became a fleeting
shadow. Contagion was rife in all our streets and so baleful were its effects,
that the church yards were not sufficiently capacious to receive the dead. It
seemed for a while as though the brand of an avenging angel had been unloosed
in judgement . . .' (cited in Brayley 1722). In his *History of Epidemics in Britain*
Creighton described the outbreak of plague in 1665 at Eyam, a small village
in Derbyshire, as 'the most famous of all English plagues . . . the whole of the
drama conveniently centred within a circuit of half a mile in a cup of healthy
hills' (Creighton 1894). The Rector of Eyam, William Mompesson, fearing that
fleeing inhabitants would carry the 'invisible seeds of the disease' and so spread
the infection to neighbouring villages and towns, persuaded the inhabitants of
the village to confine themselves within a circle of about half a mile around the
village. Out of a total population of around 350 no fewer than 258 persons died
(Figure 1.1).

Apart from the plague, many other infectious diseases created a fearful toll
in human life. In 1520 the Aztecs lost about half of their population of three
and a half million from smallpox. McNeill has put forward compelling
arguments that this particular infection was of central importance in determining
the success of Cortez's invasion of Mexico (McNeill 1976). On the night when
the Aztecs drove Cortez and his men out of Mexico City, killing many of them,
an epidemic of smallpox was raging in the city. McNeill argues that the

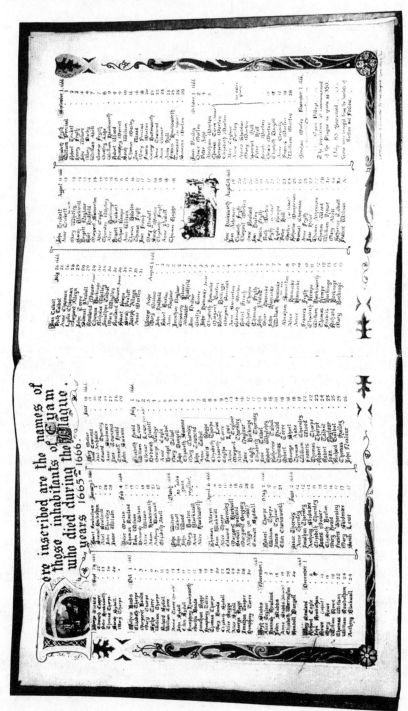

Fig. 1.1. The church register of deaths caused by the 1665 plague epidemic in the village of Eyam in Derbyshire.

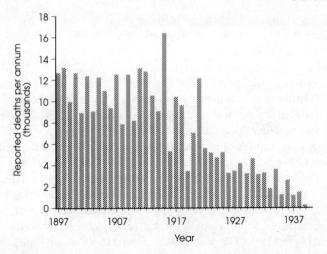

Fig. 1.2. Yearly numbers of deaths attributed to measles in England and Wales over the period 1897 to 1939 (based on information from the Registrar General's Statistical Review of England and Wales).

paralysing effect of this lethal epidemic goes far in explaining why the Aztecs did not pursue the defeated Spanish, thus giving them time to rest, regroup, gather Indian allies, and so achieve their eventual victory via a further siege of the city. The differential impact of smallpox on the Spanish invaders and the Amerindian nations of Mexico illustrates certain key dimensions of epidemiological investigation; namely, the genetic basis for resistance to infection, the selective pressures applied by disease agents on human communities, and the notion of acquired immunity to infection.

In more recent times infections other than plague and smallpox have had a major influence. It has been estimated that Russia suffered about two and a half million deaths from typhus in the war years from 1918 to 1921, and in the world epidemics of influenza in 1919, 20 million people are thought to have died over a brief span of 12 months.

The observed improvement in human mortality rates within Europe and North America over the past three centuries, with life expectancy at birth increasing from around 25–30 years in 1700 to around 70–75 years in 1970, comes mainly from a decline in deaths induced by directly transmitted viral and bacterial infections. A combination of nature and nurture is implicated: higher standards of hygiene and nutrition have combined with probable changes in the genetic structure of human and parasite populations to decrease the pathogenicities of many childhood infections (McNeill 1976; McKeown 1979). An illustration of this trend is displayed in Fig. 1.2, where the number of deaths in England and Wales attributed to measles is recorded for the period 1897 to 1939 (well before the introduction of mass immunization). Changes may have taken place largely as a consequence of the selective pressures exerted by infections that induced mortality prior to the host's attainment of reproductive maturity (Haldane 1949). A number of published studies suggest how infectious diseases such as malaria and smallpox can influence the genetic structure of human populations as measured, for example, by the frequencies of different blood group genes (Flint *et al.* 1986; Hirayami *et al.* 1987).

Despite the observed decline in overall mortality in Europe, the frequency and magnitude of epidemics of disease paradoxically increased during the eighteenth and nineteenth centuries, as a result of changing social patterns and the growth of large centres of population in increasingly industrialized societies. Similar trends have been apparent in certain developing countries in Africa and Southeast Asia in recent years with the rapid growth of large urban centres of population. The reversal of this trend in the developed world during the present century is largely due to the development and widespread use of vaccines to immunize susceptible populations against a variety of directly transmitted viral and bacterial infections. The world-wide eradication of smallpox in the late 1970s and the decline in the incidence of diphtheria and paralytic poliomyelitis in Europe are testimony to the effectiveness of this method of control.

Currently, of course, the human immunodeficiency virus (HIV), the aetiological agent of acquired immunodeficiency syndrome (AIDS), is beginning to have a significant impact on patterns of mortality in both developed and developing countries. In the United States alone, AIDS is reported to have caused tens of thousands of deaths over the period from the start of the epidemic in the late 1970s to the end of June 1987, and many hundreds of thousands more are likely to die of AIDS from HIV infection acquired over the same period. With the current focus of medical, scientific, and public attention on AIDS, however, it is easy to forget that many viral and bacterial infections of childhood, such as measles and pertussis, that are primarily a cause of morbidity in the well nourished developed world, remain a major cause of mortality in developing countries (Fig. 1.3). These infections in conjunction with others,

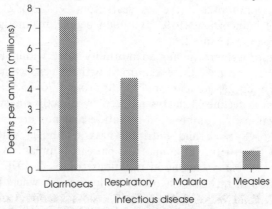

Fig. 1.3. Annual deaths from various infectious diseases in Africa in 1978 as compiled by Walsh and Warren (1979).

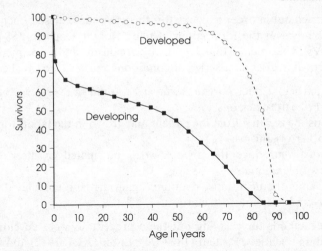

Fig. 1.4. Typical age-specific survival curves for human populations in developed and developing countries (from Bradley 1972).

such as malaria and the viral and bacterial diarrhoeal diseases, still play a dominant role in shaping age-specific patterns of human mortality in many regions of the world (Fig. 1.4).

Human fascination with epidemics of infectious diseases and their associated human mortality has a long history. The lists of epidemics compiled by the Chinese scholar Ssu Kuang, who lived during the Sung Dynasty (AD 960–1279) in China, the 'Epidemics' of the Greek scholar Hippocrates (458–377 BC), and the rudimentary medical statistics of John Grant (1620–74) and William Rethy (1623–87), who studied the London Bills of Mortality in the seventeenth century, well illustrate this point. However, the scientific study of the epidemiology of infectious diseases did not begin in earnest until the development of the 'germ theory of disease'.

In the earliest medical literature there are vague expressions of the idea that invisible living creatures might be responsible for disease. Such references are found, for example, in the writings of Aristotle (384–22 BC) and of the Arabian physician Rhazes (AD 860–932). In the sixteenth century, the 'germ theory' began to emerge in more definite form. Frascastorius (1475–1503), a celebrated physician of Verona, published an article in which he clearly expressed the belief that invisible living organisms are able to cause disease and transmit illness by direct or indirect contact from person to person. With the development of simple magnifying lenses, and the construction of the first microscopes, the Dutchman Leeuwenhoek (1632–1723) demonstrated that micro-organisms really do exist, and ideas concerning their relation to disease began to crystallize. In 1840, Jacob Henle (1809–85), a German scientist and an immediate predecessor of Pasteur and Koch, expressed the germ theory of disease as it is known today and, furthermore, laid down a set of necessary procedures which would have to be carried out in order to prove this theory. Today, these principles are more widely known, in the form enunciated by Robert Koch in 1884, as 'Koch's postulates'. They dictate that, before any organism can be accepted as the cause of a particular disease, a series of conditions must all be satisfied. These are:

(1) the particular micro-organism must be found in every case of disease and not in healthy persons;
(2) it must be isolated from the patient and grown in the laboratory apart from all other organisms;
(3) it must reproduce the disease when inoculated by itself into healthy susceptible animals;
(4) the same organism must be found again in these inoculated animals and recovered in laboratory cultures.

Reliable methods for carrying out these procedures were developed by three outstanding scientists, Pasteur (1827–75), Lister (1827–1912) and Koch (1843–1910), in the latter half of the nineteenth century and the early part of the twentieth century.

The discoveries and developments of Henle, Pasteur, and Koch had an enormous impact, leading the biomedical sciences away from the notions of miasmas and humours, towards more rigorous and testable concepts of specific aetiologies, quantitative epidemiological study, and appropriate preventive and therapeutic measures both at the level of the individual patient and at the level of the community. This new direction was also spurred by the work of a number of epidemiologists, notably Panum and Snow, whose detailed studies of population patterns of disease seriously challenged the idea of miasmas and helped resurrect Fracastorius's ideal of 'contagium vivum' (Fine 1979). The discipline of epidemiology has progressed a long way since these early beginnings, and the growth of knowledge in the fields of immunology and of cellular and molecular biology has provided many tools to help in the quantification of patterns of infection within human populations. Despite this progress, however, in much of medical teaching and research today there still remains a reluctance to turn to the disciplines of population ecology, mathematics, and statistics to aid in the interpretation of observed patterns of infection within human communities and in the design of programmes for the control of infection and disease. A possible explanation of this trend may be found in the history of the development of mathematical epidemiology.

1.2 Mathematical epidemiology

The application of mathematics to the study of infectious disease appears to have been initiated by Daniel Bernoulli in 1760. He used a mathematical method to evaluate the effectiveness of the techniques of variolation against smallpox, with the aim of influencing public health policy (Bernoulli 1760). There then followed a long gap until the middle of the nineteenth century when, in 1840, William Farr effectively fitted a normal curve to smoothed quarterly data on deaths from smallpox in England and Wales over the period 1837–9 (Farr 1840). This descriptive approach was developed further by John Brownlee who published a paper entitled 'Statistical studies in immunity; the theory of an epidemic' in 1906, in which he fitted Pearsonian frequency distribution curves to a large series of epidemics (Brownlee 1906). The empirical approaches adopted by Farr and Brownlee were in great contrast to the work of two other scientists of the same period, Hamer and Ross. Their contribution was to apply post-germ-theory thinking towards the solution of two specific quantitative problems: the regular recurrence of measles epidemics and the relationship between numbers of mosquitoes and the incidence of malaria (Hamer 1906; Ross 1908; Moshkovskii 1950). They were the first to formulate specific theories about the transmission of infectious disease in simple but precise mathematical statements and to investigate the properties of the resulting models. Their work, in conjunction with the studies of Ross and Hudson (1917), Soper (1929), and Kermack and McKendrick (1927), began to provide a firm theoretical framework for the investigation of observed patterns.

Hamer (1906) postulated that the course of an epidemic depends on the rate of contact between susceptible and infectious individuals. This notion has become one of the most important concepts in mathematical epidemiology; it is the so-called 'mass action principle' in which the net rate of spread of infection is assumed to be proportional to the product of the density of susceptible people times the density of infectious individuals. The principle was originally formulated in a discrete-time model, but in 1908 Ronald Ross (celebrated as the discoverer of malarial transmission by mosquitoes) translated the problem into a continuous-time framework in his pioneering work on the dynamics of malaria (Ross 1911, 1915, 1916, 1917).

The ideas of Hamer and Ross were extended and explored in more detail by Soper (1929) who deduced the underlying mechanisms responsible for the often-observed periodicity of epidemics, and by Kermack and McKendrick (1927) who established the celebrated threshold theory. This theory, according to which the introduction of a few infectious individuals into a community of susceptibles will not give rise to an epidemic outbreak unless the density or number of susceptibles is above a certain critical value, is, in conjunction with the mass action principle, a cornerstone of modern theoretical epidemiology.

Since this early beginning, the growth in the literature concerned with mathematical epidemiology has been very rapid indeed (Fig. 1.5). Recent reviews of the literature have been published by Dietz (1988), Bailey (1975), Becker (1979), and Dietz and Schenzle (1985). From an early stage it became apparent that variation and the elements of chance were important determinants of the spread and persistence of infection and this led to the development of stochastic theories. Much of the literature over the past three decades has been concerned with probabilistic models (see Bartlett 1955, 1960; Bailey 1975).

In recent work there has been an emphasis on the application of control

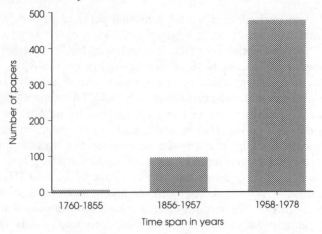

Fig. 1.5. The mathematical epidemiological literature, as reflected in the bibliographies of Bailey's (1975) and Becker's (1979) reviews. Though not a catalogue of all publications on this subject, these represent the most comprehensive available bibliographies and they give a good impression of the growth of the literature.

theory to epidemic models (Wickwire 1977), the study of the spatial spread of diseases (Mollison 1977; Cliff *et al.* 1983; Källén *et al.* 1985), the investigation of the mechanisms underlying recurrent epidemic behaviour (Hethcote *et al.* 1981; Aron and Schwartz 1984), the importance of heterogeneity in transmission (Anderson and May 1986), and the extension of the threshold theory to encompass more complex deterministic and stochastic models (Whittle 1955; Becker 1979; Anderson and May 1978, 1979*b*; May and Anderson 1979; Ball 1983; Anderson 1990).

Surprisingly, however, despite the current sophistication of this literature, the insights gained from theoretical work have, in general, had little impact on empirical approaches to epidemiological study and the design of public health policy. In part this is a consequence of the abstractly mathematical nature of the literature, which has tended to become rather detached from its empirical base. Becker (1979), for example, notes that of 75 papers on epidemiological models published over the period 1974–8, only five contained any reference to empirical observations. It hardly needs stressing that, if theoretical work is to play a role in the solution of practical problems in disease control and in the interpretation of observed trends, a much greater emphasis must be placed on data-oriented studies. This observation brings us to the major aim of this book.

1.3 Aims of the book

The primary aim of this book is to show how simple mathematical models of the transmission of infectious agents within human communities can help to interpret observed epidemiological trends, to guide the collection of data towards further understanding, and to design programmes for the control of infection and disease.

Our major goal is further understanding of the interplay between the variables that determine the course of infection within an individual, and the variables that control the pattern of infection within communities of people. Quite properly, the medical epidemiologist's main concern is often with the recondite biological and medical details that make each infection unique. In contrast, our aim is to understand the basic similarities and differences in terms of such factors as: the number of population variables (and consequent equations) needed for a sensible characterization of the system; the typical relations among the various rate parameters (such as birth, death, recovery, and transmission rates); and the form of the mathematical expression that captures the essence of the transmission process. In the absence of such a unified framework each infection tends to develop its own, often arcane, literature.

In view of the successes achieved by combining empirical and theoretical work in the physical sciences, it is surprising that many people still question the potential usefulness of mathematical models in epidemiology. Of course, as we have just noted, a great deal of recent mathematical epidemiology has taken flight from its original moorings, and soars free from the constraints of data or relevance. But to go from observation of this fact to the belief that mathematical models have, in principle, nothing to contribute to the design of public health programmes is a mistake. Sensibly used, mathematical models are no more, and no less, than tools for thinking about things in a precise way. Primary health care by its nature deals with population-level aspects of the transmission and persistence of infections, and the relation between infection in *individuals* and infection in *populations* often has aspects that the most experienced medical practitioner would find hard to intuit.

Those who do acknowledge the case for using mathematical studies as a tool for understanding epidemiological processes may nevertheless have reservations about the very simple models that we often use, particularly at the beginning of both Part I and Part II. To those familiar with the manifold complexities of real infections in real populations, our 'basic models' may seem oversimplified to the point of lunacy. We see these models as having many uses: they provide insight into essential aspects of host–parasite interactions; they serve as a point of departure for adding realistic complications step by step, in an understandable way (so that we do not lose our way in a snowstorm of parameters); and, most important of all, they help to suggest what kinds of data need to be sought in order effectively to design and monitor programmes of control. In just such a way Newton's First Law ('a body remains in its state of rest or uniform motion in a straight line, unless acted on by external forces') serves as a point of departure for exploring what happens when forces do act; before the First Law was enunciated clearly, intuitive attempts to understand how things moved were rather muddled. Notice, incidentally, that this law may well have seemed abstract or 'unrealistic' to many, because (until the dawn of the space age) objects were never seen moving uniformly in straight lines, since frictional or other forces were always acting on them. By the same token, the Hardy–Weinberg theorem in population genetics is useful in telling us what happens—gene frequencies do not change—in the absence of selection, migration, drift, or mutation. As all four of these processes are usually acting, the theorem might seem daft; its important role is as a yardstick against which to assess the effects of the above mentioned complications.

Against this background we offer the simple models in this book as illuminating caricatures, as foundations to build on, and as analytic tools for thinking about the information needed for improving epidemiological understanding and in planning programmes of control. The real world is undeniably replete with many complications—economic and social as well as biological—and it is easy to lose sight of general principles when grappling with the complex details that ultimately make each association between host and parasite unique. This defence of simple models is ironically summed up by the science-fiction writer Poul Anderson: 'I have yet to see any problem, however complicated, which, when you look at it in the right way, did not become still more complicated'.

In summary, therefore, the book aims to fill a useful niche intermediate between mathematical texts on infectious disease dynamics and texts on epidemiological statistics. Mathematical details are kept to a minimum, and the book is directed towards epidemiologists, public health workers, parasitologists, and ecologists. It is hoped, however, that sufficient details of the models are included to stimulate interest amongst applied mathematicians and statisticians. Although primarily aimed at review and synthesis, the book does contain much new material. It does not contain an exhaustive bibliography of all past work in mathematical epidemiology but is more a personal (and perhaps idiosyncratic) view of what we regard as interesting and important, in a practical sense, for improving understanding of the epidemiology, transmission dynamics, and control of infectious diseases of humans. Particular attention is paid to melding theory with observation and the estimation of parameter values from empirical data.

1.4 Organization of the book

The book is divided into two parts (I and II) which deal, respectively, with microparasites (broadly speaking, viruses, bacteria, and protozoa) and macroparasites (helminths and arthropods). Before Part I begins, Chapter 2 outlines the rationale for this broad division into two parts and discusses certain definitions and basic concepts in epidemiology.

Part I on microparasites begins with Chapter 3 which presents a summary of the biological characteristics of host–microparasitic associations. It introduces topics such as acquired and herd immunity, the course of infection in an individual host, and ideas and some new models for network or antigen-driven immune systems. An outline is also presented of the different types of epidemiological data that are commonly recorded in studies of infectious diseases. The chapter ends with the formulation of a basic model of transmission.

The static or equilibrium properties of the model are examined in Chapter 4. This chapter develops around basic concepts, introducing summary epidemiological parameters—such as the basic reproductive rate of the infection and the average age at infection—to show how they can aid in the interpretation of observed trends. Chapter 5 turns to static or equilibrium aspects of control by mass vaccination, and shows how the basic model may be adapted to provide specific guidelines for the design of control programs. Chapter 6 considers dynamic aspects of the basic model, paying attention both to the dynamics of epidemic infections and to the non-seasonal oscillations that are often observed in the incidence of endemic infection. This chapter presents a new and systematic approach to the relation between epidemic and endemic dynamics; the two situations are not usually thought of within a common framework. Chapter 7 then explains how these dynamic phenomena are affected by immunization or other programmes of control.

Chapter 8 discusses tests of the assumption of homogeneous mixing, which is made throughout Chapters 4–7. A variety of refinements and complications, mainly having to do with inhomogeneities of one kind and another, are then discussed and developed further in the next chapters. Chapter 9 deals with heterogeneities introduced by age dependence in transmission rates. This long chapter shows how such age-related complications can affect vaccination programmes and estimates of the critical level of immunization coverage needed to eradicate an infection. In particular, a new model is presented in which the steady state (before the advent of immunization) can be a curious mixture of endemic and epidemic infection; the infection sweeps as a mini-epidemic through successive age cohorts of school-enterers, against an endemic background without which the infection would not persist. Chapter 10 considers genetic factors, and outlines a general approach for evaluating the effects of these and other heterogeneities. The lengthy Chapter 11 takes up sexually transmitted diseases (STDs) (where heterogeneity in degrees of sexual activity within the population at risk plays an important part in explaining observed trends). Chapter 11 deals first with endemic STDs (with gonorrhoea as an illustration), and then gives detailed attention to the transmission dynamics of the epidemic of HIV/AIDS in developed and developing countries. Chapter 12 explores the effects of other heterogeneities, mainly having to do with geographical variations in population density or with variations in family size. Throughout Chapters 9–12 the general ideas are illustrated by applications to specific examples (vaccination against measles, rubella, polio, hepatitis B, and other infections; transmission dynamics and potential demographic impact of HIV/AIDS in Africa, etc.). Some of these applications have been published in the relevant technical literature, while others are presented here for the first time.

Part I ends with two chapters dealing with the dynamics of transmission within growing human populations in developing countries (Chapter 13) and with infections that are indirectly transmitted by arthropod vectors (Chapter 14). Both these chapters contain a significant amount of new material.

Macroparasitic infections are examined in Part II. This section starts with Chapter 15, a discussion of life cycles, general biology, and observed epidemiological patterns. This is followed by the development of a basic model to describe the transmission of macroparasitic infection in Chapter 16 (statics) and Chapter 17 (dynamics). Various summary statistics are introduced, and—extending previous analyses—the problems of control by chemotherapy and vaccination are discussed in these two chapters. The topic of acquired immunity is developed in Chapter 18, with a review of experimental facts and pertinent models. In particular, Chapter 18 presents some new ideas about the balance between age-related exposure to infection and the acquisition of immunity, and how this balance may determine the patterns of infection observed in human communities. Chapter 19 analyses a variety of refinements and complications introduced by heterogeneities in transmission. Problems associated with indirect transmission of infection via intermediate host species are addressed in Chapter 20, which combines reviews of existing work with some new ideas and analysis. Chapter 21 gives an evangelical account of the contributions to our understanding of the population dynamics of macroparasites that have been, and can be, made by experimental studies of host models in the laboratory. Chapter 22 deals with the evolution of drug resistance by macroparasitic populations, presenting some new work bearing on this important practical problem. This chapter also develops some interesting parallels between the evolution of drug resistance and the selective effects exerted on parasites by the host's immune system.

The book ends with a discussion in Chapter 23 of broader issues. These include the role of infectious disease agents as regulators of the abundance of their host population, coevolution amongst host and parasite populations, the importance of an ecological approach to epidemiological study, and future research needs and directions.

2

A framework for discussing the population biology of infectious diseases

By focusing on the overall population biology of associations between hosts and parasites, and emphasizing broad themes that are common to most systems, we seek to provide a framework within which a vast amount of information about parasitic infections may be organized in an orderly way. We aim to codify similarities and differences among the various viral, bacterial, protozoan, fungal, and helminth parasites, identifying the ecologically based patterns of relationships among epidemiological parameters such as transmission rates, virulence, life span of the parasite within the host, and so on.

To this end, the present chapter outlines some basic concepts. We begin by making a distinction between 'microparasites' and 'macroparasites'; this rough dichotomy cuts across conventional taxonomic lines to focus on the population biology of the parasite. Next we discuss the idea of the basic reproductive rate of the parasite, and then go on to outline some ideas about threshold host densities and about modes of transmission.

2.1 Microparasites and macroparasites

Microparasites may be thought of as those parasites which have direct reproduction—usually at very high rates—within the host (Anderson and May 1979b). They tend to be characterized by small size and a short generation time. Hosts that recover from infection usually acquire immunity against reinfection for some time, and often for life. Although there are important exceptions, the duration of infection is typically short relative to the expected life span of the host. This feature, combined with acquired immunity, means that for individual hosts microparasitic infections are typically of a transient nature. Most viral and bacterial parasites, and (in a more equivocal way) many protozoan and fungal parasites, fall broadly into the microparasitic category.

For such infective agents, it makes sense to divide the host population into relatively few classes of individuals: susceptible, infected, recovered-and-immune. Such a *compartmental model* for the dynamic interaction between parasitic and host populations is depicted schematically in Fig. 2.1. Our operational definition of a microparasite is, indeed, an organism whose population biology can to a sensible first approximation be described by some such compartmental model.

Greater detail and realism can be achieved by adding more compartments or categories to the model (for example, a class of latent, but not yet infectious, individuals). The essential feature of these compartmental models, however, is

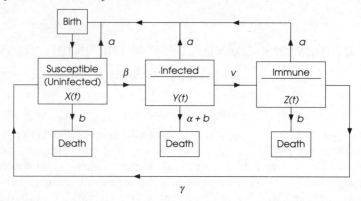

Fig. 2.1. Schematic representation of the flow of hosts between susceptible ($X(t)$), infected ($Y(t)$) and immune ($Z(t)$) classes, which records the dynamic interaction between a directly transmitted microparasite and its host population. In this diagram hosts reproduce at a per capita rate a and die at a per capita rate b. The infected hosts experience an additional death rate α, induced by microparasitic infection. The average durations of stay in the infected and immune classes are denoted by $1/v$ and $1/\gamma$, respectively. The transmission coefficient which determines the rate at which new infections arise as a consequence of mixing between the susceptible and infected individuals is defined by β.

that little or no account is taken of the degree of severity of the infection (i.e. the abundance of the parasite within the host); individuals either 'have measles' or they do not. In other words, the reality of infected individuals with differing nutritional, environmental, or genetic status is replaced by the simplified abstraction of some average 'infected' or 'immune' individual.

In addition to the distinction between infected and immune hosts, it is often desirable to distinguish between infection and disease. Thus, for example, in the literature concerned with microparasitic infections of humans, the period from the point of infection to the appearance of symptoms of disease is termed the incubation period. The duration of symptoms of disease, as illustrated diagrammatically in Fig. 2.2, is not necessarily synchronous with the period during which an infected host is infectious to susceptible individuals. Furthermore, a host may be infected but not yet infectious. The period from the point of infection to the beginning of the state of infectiousness is termed the latent period. With respect to the ecology of parasite transmission the sum of the average latent and average infectious periods is referred to as the average generation time of the infection (Fig. 2.2).

Most of the epidemiological and demographic parameters in Fig. 2.1—host birth and death rates, disease-induced death rates, recovery rates, rates of loss of immunity—can be measured directly by appropriate studies. The transmission rate, however, combines many biological, social, and environmental factors, and (as discussed in the next chapter) is thus rarely amenable to direct

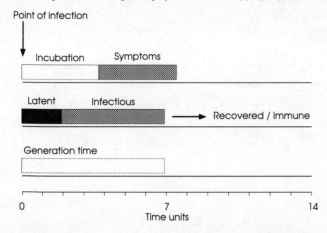

Fig. 2.2. Diagrammatic illustration of the relationship between the incubation, latent, and infectious periods for a hypothetical microparasitic infection. Note that the infectious period and the duration of symptoms of disease are not necessarily synchronous.

measurement. Indeed, it will often be that the best way to assess transmission rates is to infer them indirectly from data on population-level processes, as discussed below.

Macroparasites may be thought of as those having no direct reproduction within the definitive host (Anderson and May 1979b). This category embraces most parasitic helminths and arthropods. Macroparasites are typically larger and have much longer generation times than microparasites, with the generation time often being an appreciable fraction of the host life span. When an immune response is elicited, it usually depends on the past and present number of parasites harboured by the host, and it tends to be of a relatively short duration once parasites are removed (for example, by chemotherapy) from the host. Thus macroparasitic infections are typically of a persistent nature, with hosts being continually reinfected.

For macroparasites, the various factors characterizing the interaction—egg output per female parasite, pathogenic effects on the host, evocation of an immune response in the host, parasite death rates, and so on—can all depend on the number of parasites in a given host. Mathematically, this means that the relatively simple compartmental models must be replaced by more complicated models which take full account of the distribution of parasites among the hosts. Such a *distributional model* is shown schematically in Fig. 2.3. Operationally, our definition of a macroparasite is one whose population biology requires such a full description of the distribution of parasites among hosts.

Macroparasites are rarely, if ever, distributed in an independently random way among their hosts, but rather show an aggregated or 'clumped' distribution with often a minority of the host population harbouring the majority of the

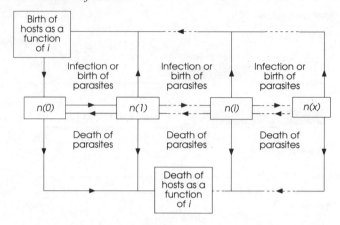

Fig. 2.3. Diagrammatic flow chart for a directly transmitted macroparasitic infection, based on a model with compartments for the number of hosts, $n(i)$, harbouring i parasites $(i = 0, 1, 2, \ldots)$. The birth and death rates of the host population are denoted as functions of parasite burden.

parasite population. It is not uncommon to find 80 per cent or more of the macroparasites contained in 20 per cent or fewer of their human hosts.

From a public health viewpoint, it is significant that for many macroparasites a distinction can be made between infection (harbouring one or more parasites) and disease (harbouring a parasite burden large enough to produce pathogenic symptoms, or even host death). For a canonical microparasitic infection, such as smallpox, it is reasonable to assume that a given host does, or does not, 'have smallpox'; for a macroparasitic infection, such as hookworm or *Ascaris* or schistosomiasis, there is a real distinction between being infected with one or two worms, and carrying a worm burden large enough to cause illness.

The division into microparasites and macroparasites, whether made on biological or mathematical grounds, is necessarily a rough one. The distinction essentially corresponds to the extremes of a continuum, Many parasites are not easily forced into this dichotomous scheme. A lot of protozoan parasites, for instance, may to a good approximation have their epidemiology described by the compartmental models characteristic of microparasites, while on the other hand their patterns of persistence within the host population (with hosts continually being reinfected) are characteristic of macroparasites. Thus, as discussed later, an account of the degree of immunity that can naturally be elicited against malaria requires a model intermediate between the two extremes.

In short, the paradigmatic notions of microparasite and macroparasite are deliberate oversimplifications, which aim to emphasize the population dynamics of host–parasite associations and to de-emphasize conventional taxonomic categorizations. Realistic refinements can be grafted on, layer by layer, as we proceed from basic understanding to detailed application.

2.2 Basic reproductive rate of a parasite

The basic reproductive rate, R_0, is essentially the average number of successful offspring that a parasite is intrinsically capable of producing (Macdonald 1952; Dietz 1975, 1976; Yorke *et al.* 1979; May and Anderson 1979; Anderson 1981*b*; Anderson and May 1982*d*). It is, in effect, Fisher's (1930) 'net reproductive value' for the parasite. This concept is central to any discussion of the overall population biology of an organism. Clearly a parasitic species must have $R_0 > 1$ if it is to be capable of invading, and establishing itself within, a host population.

For a microparasite (represented by a compartmental model), R_0 is more precisely defined as the average number of secondary infections produced when one infected individual is introduced into a host population where everyone is susceptible.

When such a microparasitic infection becomes established in a host population, the fraction remaining susceptible decreases. Eventually an equilibrium may be attained, with the rate at which susceptible individuals are infected being balanced against a rate at which newly susceptible individuals appear (usually by birth, but possibly also by immigration or by loss of immunity). At equilibrium, each infection will on average produce exactly one secondary infection; that is, at equilibrium the effective reproductive rate of the parasite is $R = 1$. If we assume the host population is homogeneously mixed, in the sense that, on average, all hosts have intrinsically similar epidemiological properties (independent of age, genetic make-up, social habits, geographical location, etc.), then the number of secondary infections produced by an infected individual will be linearly proportional to the probability that any one random contact is with a susceptible individual. In this event, the effective reproductive rate, R, is equal to the basic rate, R_0, discounted by x, the fraction of the host population that is susceptible: $R = R_0 x$. Thus, under the rough approximation of treating the host population as homogeneously mixed, for a microparasite the equilibrium condition $R = 1$ leads to an important relation between R_0 and the fraction, x^*, of the host population that is susceptible at equilibrium:

$$R_0 x^* = 1. \tag{2.1}$$

Equation (2.1) has applications which will be discussed later. Beyond this, it has general interest for ecologists. For one thing, it is notoriously difficult to assess the intrinsic reproductive capacity, R_0, of any species of organism (even humans). It is also a problem for ecologists to determine exactly what density-dependent mechanisms operate to hold the reproductive rates of natural populations below their intrinsic capacities—capacities which could, if realized, blanket the world with that species. Equation (2.1) resolves both these problems for microparasites: because x^* can be found from serological or other data on age-specific susceptibility, the elusive quantity R_0 can be calculated (see Table 4.1, p. 70); and the density-dependent process holding R below R_0 is simply the removal of susceptibles by immunity, following infection (which corresponds, in essence, to a very simple form of predation upon hosts by the parasite). Thus eqn (2.1) and the surrounding discussion illustrate the concepts of basic reproductive rates and density-dependent regulation of populations more clearly and quantitatively than the examples conventionally used in introductory biology textbooks and courses.

Unfortunately, eqn (2.1) depends on the assumption of homogeneous mixing. When age-related differences in transmission rate, and other inhomogeneities are acknowledged, some of the simplicity of eqn (2.1), and possibly also of the definition of R_0, can be lost. But the ideas presented here still underpin the more detailed discussion of such complications in Chapters 8–12.

For a macroparasite (represented by a distributional model), R_0 is the average number of female offspring produced throughout the lifetime of a mature female parasite, which themselves achieve reproductive maturity in the absence of density-dependent constraints.

The factors governing equilibrium in a host–macroparasite system are more complex than those in host–microparasite systems. In the absence of any density-dependent constraints, a macroparasite with $R_0 > 1$ could attain arbitrarily high population levels, as hosts with high parasite burdens continued to put out large numbers of eggs, leading to yet higher parasite burdens per host. In reality, various kinds of density-dependent processes intervene to halt such an exponential run-away: egg output per parasite declines as the number of parasites in a host increases; hosts with high burdens may be less likely to acquire further infections, for a diversity of possible reasons; parasite death rates may increase as the number of parasites in a host increases; the overall transmission rate may saturate to some upper limit when the parasite population is large; and a high burden may simply kill the host. Precisely which of these density-dependent factors, individually or in combination, will be primarily responsible for establishing equilibrium is likely to vary from one host–parasite association to the next. Examples are pursued in detail in Part II.

So far, we have dealt with the differing details of the definition of R_0 for microparasites and macroparasites, with the way density-dependent effects keep effective reproductive rates below R_0, and with ways of inferring the magnitude of R_0 from observations around equilibrium. There are, however, situations where we can observe a parasite in the initial phases of population growth, where density-dependent limitations have not yet come to be significant. Such situations arise, for instance, when a measles epidemic starts to spread among an island population who have not experienced measles for a generation or more (so that essentially all are susceptible), or when a new infection such as the human immunodeficiency virus (HIV, the aetiological agent of AIDS) begins its exponential rise among the population at risk, or when hookworm, *Ascaris*, or other helminths begin to re-establish themselves after being removed from a population by chemotherapy.

The initial, exponential rise in the proportion of hosts who are infected,

$P(t)$, depends on the rate at which new infectives are being produced, Λ:

$$P(t) = P(0) \exp(\Lambda t). \tag{2.2}$$

For both microparasites and macroparasites, Λ depends on R_0 and on the parasite lifespan, D:

$$\Lambda = (R_0 - 1)/D. \tag{2.3}$$

For microparasites D is essentially the duration of infectiousness, while for macroparasites it is the average life expectancy of adult parasites. The result (2.3) is established in detail for microparasites and macroparasites, separately in Chapters 6 and 16, respectively. The result, however, may be explained intuitively: each infection produces R_0 new infections in its lifetime, of duration D, and then dies; thus $R_0 - 1$ net infections are added in an interval D, corresponding to $(R_0 - 1)/D$ per unit time. As for eqn (2.1), eqn (2.3) depends on the assumption of homogeneous mixing and more complicated expressions are obtained once various kinds of inhomogeneities are taken into account. Nevertheless, the above discussion indicates how those rare instances where parasite populations are growing free from density-dependent checks can be used to estimate R_0, provided D is known.

2.3 Threshold host densities

In many simple circumstances, R_0 may be taken to be linearly proportional to the total number or density of hosts that are candidates for infection, whence

$$R_0 = N/N_T. \tag{2.4}$$

Here N is the host population size, and the proportionality constant (which subsumes all manner of biological, social, and environmental aspects of transmission) has been written as $1/N_T$. The condition $R_0 > 1$ for establishment of the parasite thus translates into the requirement that the host population, N, exceeds a certain threshold magnitude, N_T:

$$N > N_T. \tag{2.5}$$

More generally, R_0 is likely to be some non-linear function of N, $R_0 = f(N)$. As discussed in Chapter 9, data for measles and pertussis in Britain, for example, can be seen to obey a power-law relation $R_0 = (N/N_T)^\nu$, with $\nu < 1$. Likewise for macroparasites various effects can lead to R_0 increasing less fast than linearly with increasing host density. The criterion $R_0 > 1$, however, will still usually lead to a threshold condition, eqn (2.5); the essential idea of a threshold host density retains its validity.

An important class of exceptions are those infections that are transmitted by intimate contact with a defined group of people, as happens for sexually transmitted diseases, infections associated with sharing of needles by drug abusers, and the like. Here R_0 depends on the average rate at which new partners are acquired, which usually has no direct dependence on N; doubling the population size does not affect sexual habits, except perhaps indirectly through social changes precipitated by greater crowding. Sexually transmitted parasites, which often produce long-lasting infections and do not induce acquired immunity in recovered hosts, can be admirably adapted to persist in low-density populations of promiscuous hosts; here a threshold average number of sexual partners replaces the threshold host density of eqn (2.5).

So far, our discussion of threshold densities has focused on the condition $R_0 > 1$. If populations were always large enough for us to ignore stochastic and other effects associated with the inconvenient fact that humans are born, infected, and die in integer units (rather than in a continuous and deterministic fashion), we would need go no further. But there are at least two effects that can lead to threshold densities in practice being higher than estimated from $R_0 > 1$ alone.

The first such effect has to do with the necessity for the equilibrium number of infected individuals to be, on average, large enough that statistical fluctuations are unlikely to break the chain that maintains the infection. In the simple case of a microparasitic infection in a homogeneously mixed population of susceptibles, infecteds, and immunes, the number of latent plus infected hosts at equilibrium, $H^* + Y^*$, is roughly (see Chapter 6)

$$H^* + Y^* = (1 - 1/R_0)[(D + D')/L]N. \qquad (2.6)$$

Here, as before, D is the average duration of infectiousness, D' is the average duration of latency, L is the average life expectancy of a host, and N is the total number of hosts. We require that $H^* + Y^*$ should be significantly greater than unity, so that statistical fluctuations are not likely to carry the number of infected hosts to zero and extinguish the infection from the population. This means that N must be significantly greater than $L/(D + D')$. As L is measured in decades, and D and D' typically in days or weeks, this can require N to be of order 10^5 or more (which in some cases may be larger than the N_T of eqn (2.5)). We think it is useful to call the above effect *endemic fade-out*.

Even more severe constraints can be put on population size by the severe oscillations in numbers of susceptibles and infectives that characterize the introduction of a microparasite into a previously unexposed population. As discussed more fully in Chapter 6, the number of infected individuals falls to very low levels in the wake of the first epidemic. Stochastic effects may well lead to 'fade-out' of the infection during this epidemic phase of parasite establishment, thus preventing the infection from damping to the more easily maintained endemic state. We call this phenomenon *epidemic fade-out*. On the one hand, the number of infections in the trough following the epidemic introduction will be substantially less than given by eqn (2.6). On the other hand, the parasite need only survive in a few such troughs, and in this respect needs a narrower margin to cushion it against stochastic extinction during these relatively short episodes than it does over the long haul in the endemic state.

Whether such stochastic fade-out in the epidemic phase puts more, or less, stringent requirements on N than does stochastic extinction in the endemic state (via eqn (2.6)) will depend on the details for a specific microparasite.

In short, the threshold density may be governed by deterministic factors ($R_0 > 1$), or by one or other of a variety of stochastic considerations. Whatever the determining factor, a direct assessment of the threshold density is usually difficult. Some useful generalizations can nevertheless be made. Many microparasitic infections, such as smallpox or measles, are of very short duration and have relatively low transmission efficiencies; that is, the transmission stages are short-lived in the external environment and fairly direct contact is required to produce infection. In this event, a large population of hosts will be needed before R_0 can exceed unity, and thus the threshold density for the host population, N_T, will be large. In other words, such infections require a large population of hosts in order to give birth to new susceptibles at a rate that keeps pace with their loss by infection. Specifically, it has been estimated that N_T for maintaining measles in human communities is around 300 000 individuals or more (Bartlett 1957; Black 1966).

Conversely, the reproductive life span of many macroparasites within a host is an appreciable fraction of the host's life, and transmission pathways are often quite efficient, involving intermediate vector hosts or long-lived transmission stages. Threshold host densities for the maintenance of macroparasitic populations can thus be small.

These notions have some general implications that may be of interest to animal ecologists. In so far as directly transmitted microparasites typically require high host densities in order to persist, they should more commonly be associated with animals which exhibit herd or schooling behaviour, or which breed in large colonies. A certain amount of anecdotal support for these ideas comes form the observed abundance of such infections within modern human societies, large herds of ungulates, breeding colonies of seabirds, and communities of social insects. Humans get microparasitic infections, such as colds, while relatively solitary carnivores such as tigers are afflicted more by macroparasites, such as intestinal worms. But there is a need for comparative studies in which data are compiled systematically to test these ecological ideas.

2.4 Direct and indirect transmission

The above ideas about the essential character of the parasite and about its overall reproductive rate are valid, independent of the details of the transmission process. We conclude this chapter by considering some of the different ways parasites may be transmitted, which are summarized schematically in Fig. 2.4.

For *direct* transmission, depicted in Fig. 2.4(a), the transmission stages of the parasite pass directly from one host to the next. Some parasites, including many viruses and bacteria, pass by direct contact between hosts or in vapour droplets.

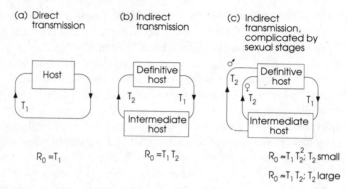

Fig. 2.4. Diagrammatic representation of direct and indirect transmission and the complications introduced by the sexual stages of macroparasitic organisms. The quantities T_1 and T_2 denote summary transmission parameters for the flow of parasites from definitive host to intermediate host (T_1) and intermediate host to definitive host (T_2). (See text for details.).

Other parasites, such as hookworm and many other helminths, have free-living transmission stages. These transmission stages may be capable of surviving for a long time in the external environment, as is the case, for example, for anthrax and the nematode *Ascaris*; in this event, the transmission rate depends not simply on the number of current infections, but rather on a summation over past infections (appropriately discounted as one goes further back in time).

As indicated in Fig. 2.4(a), for direct transmission the various factors are concatenated into an overall transmission factor T_1, which gives R_0.

When transmission is *indirect*, as illustrated in Fig. 2.4(b) and (c), the parasite (micro or macro) passes through one or more species of intermediate host in order to complete its life cycle. In simple cases, as indicated in Fig. 2.4(b), the basic reproductive rate will be a product of the factors involved in transmission from the definitive to the intermediate host, T_1, and those from the intermediate back to the definitive host, T_2: $R_0 = T_1 T_2$.

The dynamics of such indirect transmission systems can be messier than comparable systems with direct transmission, because changes in the levels of infection in the definitive host population can lead to changes in the levels of infection among intermediate hosts, and so on. Often, however, the characteristic time-scales for population change in intermediate host populations (typically arthropods) are significantly shorter than those for definitive, human host populations, so that intermediate vectors may be regarded as effectively at the equilibrium appropriate to the prevailing host state.

The buffering effect of a reservoir of intermediate hosts can often mean that $R_0 > 1$ even though the definitive host population is relatively small; the intermediate host population can compensate for the relative paucity of definitive hosts in the overall combination $T_1 T_2$ that gives R_0.

Figure 2.4(c) illustrates an additional complication that arises for the many macroparasites with a sexual stage in the definitive host. In this case, as first emphasized by Macdonald (1965) for the schistosome flukes, it is necessary to have a mated pair of adult macroparasites in the definitive host. If the average level of transmission from intermediate to definitive host, T_2, is low, then the probability of having one mated pair scales approximately as T_2^2, and $R_0 \simeq T_1 T_2^2$. Conversely, at high transmission levels, a host is likely to acquire several parasites, in which case these complications are not important and $R_0 \simeq T_1 T_2$. These effects, and their possible implications for control strategies, are discussed more fully in Chapter 20.

2.5 Summary

A framework for studying host–parasite associations is outlined, placing emphasis on population biology rather than on taxonomy. The broad categories of microparasites and macroparasites are distinguished on biological grounds, and defined in terms of the structure of the mathematical models used to study them (compartmental and distributional, respectively). The basic reproductive rate, R_0, of a parasite is defined, and some of the density-dependent processes which in practice constrain reproductive rates below R_0 are sketched. We show how threshold host densities for maintenance of infection may arise deterministically (from $R_0 > 1$) or stochastically (from either epidemic or endemic fade-out) and we speculate on some possible ecological implications. The chapter ends with a brief review of various kinds of direct and indirect transmission of infection, noting the implications for R_0 and threshold densities.

Part I

Microparasites

3

Biology of host–microparasite associations

Our operational definition of a microparasite encompasses a wide variety of different organisms ranging from simple viruses to ontogenetically complex organisms such as the malarial parasites. Their life cycles may be simple with transmission from person to person being direct, through contact with infective stages that are free-living in the environment, or through intimate contact between hosts such that no free-living phase occurs (e.g. the sexually transmitted infections), or through vectors or intermediate hosts within which parasite development or reproduction may or may not occur. Development during the life cycle may again be simple, as in the case of viral replication within a host cell and transmission between cells, or highly complex as in the alternate phases of asexual and sexual reproduction in the life cycles of the malarial or trypanosome protozoan parasites. We do not discuss here the recondite details that make each parasite life cycle distinct since this approach is well covered by other texts (see Fenner and White 1975; Cox 1982). Instead we focus on two areas: the first concerns immune responses to microparasitic infection and their consequences for population growth of a parasite within an individual host; and the second concerns the epidemiological data that are available (or can in practice be acquired) both to estimate model parameters and to test theoretical predictions.

3.1 Immunity to viruses, bacteria, and protozoa

We consider host responses to infection separately for viruses, bacteria, and protozoa, because differences in antigenic complexity lead to important complications in the study and interpretation of observed epidemiological patterns for the different types of parasite.

3.1.1 *Viruses*

Viruses must enter a host cell to proliferate since they lack the necessary machinery to manufacture proteins and metabolize sugars. Some viruses also lack the enzymes required for nucleic acid replication and are dependent on the host cell for these functions also. The number of genes carried by different viruses may be as few as 3 or as many as 250, but this is still much fewer than even the simplest bacteria. The illnesses produced by virus infections vary from acute (death or recovery from infection), recurrent (repeated growth and decay in the virus population within an individual), inapparent (dormant infections where the virus is not readily detectable), or subclinical (symptomless infection where the virus can be detected). The immune responses may range from apparently non-existent to lifelong immunity, or even to chronic immuno-pathology (i.e. disease induced directly by the host's immune response).

Most is understood about those viruses that induce acute infections. We will concentrate on these since the majority of the work that is to follow in Part I is concerned with the interpretation of their transmission and persistence within human communities. Little is understood at present of the immunological mechanisms underlying the recurrent, inapparent, or subclinical virus infections.

A typical virus infection starts with local invasion of an epithelial surface and then, after one or more phases of replication and population growth (i.e. viraemic phases), results in infection of the target organ (e.g. skin, lungs, nervous system, etc.). The relevance of any particular immunological defence mechanism (i.e. antibody or cell mediated immunity) depends on the way the viral antigens (largely proteins or glycoproteins) and virion (a single infective virus unit) are encountered by the host's defence system (see Roitt *et al.* 1985). Antibody is only capable of directly bonding to extracellular viruses: IgG and IgM antibodies are limited in their actions to plasma and tissue fluids, whereas secretory IgA is thought to protect epithelial surfaces.

The elements of the adaptive immune response of the host recognize specific antigens on the virus and virally infected cells. It is important to make the distinction between viral antigens, which are coded for, at least in part, by the viral genome, and those antigens induced in the cell by the presence of the virus and coded for by the host genome. Although these 'host-coded' antigens are potentially useful as markers of infected cells, or indeed virus infection, they are of little use in producing protective immunity. Antibody specific to viral antigens (produced as a response to infection) may directly kill the virus, upset the virus–cell interaction (i.e. inhibit viral replication), or lyse (kill) cells infected with the virus. Antibody to some components of the virus surface (critical sites, e.g. haemaglutin of the influenza virus) kills (or neutralizes) more effectively than antibody to other components (non-critical sites, e.g. neuraminidase of the influenza virus). The interferons, a family of cell-regulatory glycoproteins produced by many cell types in response to infection, act in a protective capacity. They induce a state of cell resistance to viral penetration and replication in cells not already infected (an altruistic act, since interferon produced by an infected cell only helps to protect uninfected cells). Apart from the protection induced by antibody and the release of interferon, cell mediated action (e.g. cytotoxic activity) may also be important but it is less well understood at present. There is evidence for K (killer) and cytotoxic T cell activity in inducing protection and host recovery (Mimms and White 1984).

What typically happens during an acute viral infection in humans is illustrated schematically in Fig. 3.1. Following a phase of population growth and transport to the target organ, there follows a period of rapid replication resulting in an exponential increase in viral abundance. The rate of increase will depend in part on the efficacy of the host's immunological response. If the response is effective, antibody and cellular responses will eventually restrict viral

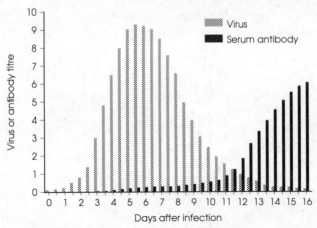

Fig. 3.1. Schematic illustration of the rise in viraemia and serum antibodies specific to viral antigens following first exposure of the host to infection.

population growth causing the intrinsic growth rate of the infectious agent to become negative, such that population size decays either to extinction or to very low levels. Viral persistence at very low population levels may occur for some infections such as those caused by the retroviruses and the herpes viruses (Kaplan 1973; Weiss 1982). Alternatively, the host's immunological response may fail to limit viral population growth and host death may result. An empirical example of the different phases of an acute viral infection and host recovery is presented in Fig. 3.2. The example is for parvovirus infection in humans (human parvovirus; HPV) and it shows both the trajectory of viral population growth and the pattern of antibody production (Anderson *et al.* 1985). Following infection there is an initial lag phase when no antibody can be detected. Production of IgM rises more rapidly initially than that of IgG. In a typical immune response the antibody level following secondary exposure to infection rises more rapidly, attains a higher titre and consists predominantly of IgG (IgM dominates during initial infection).

Broadly speaking, we can identify three distinct phases in the process of infection. First, there is the *latent period* during which the host is infected but non-infectious, corresponding to the period when viral abundance is low following initial infection. The second segment is the *infectious period* during which viral abundance is high and virus is either being excreted (via the saliva, respiratory tract excretions, faeces or urine, or other host secretions or excretions) or is present in damaged epithelial cells such that transmission can occur via physical contacts between individuals. There is usually a rough correspondence between the infectious period and the period during which symptoms of infection are apparent. The time period between initial infection and the appearance of symptoms of disease is called the *incubation period*

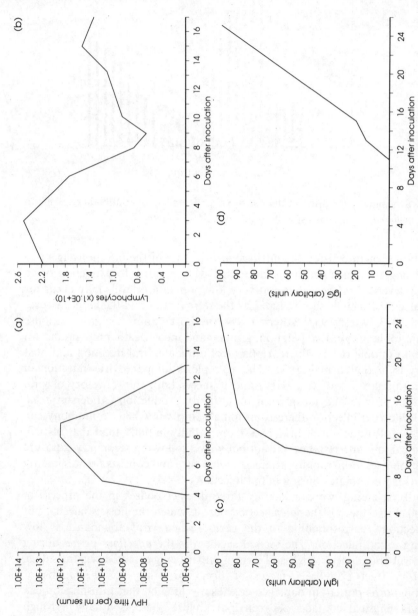

Fig. 3.2. Changes through time in virus titres, antibody specific to viral antigens, and total lymphocyte counts in patients following first exposure to human parvovirus infection (data from Anderson *et al.* 1985). Graphs (a) to (d) record respective changes in viraemia, total lymphocyte counts, and IgG and IgM antibodies.

Table 3.1 Incubation, latent and infectious periods (in days) for a variety of viral and bacterial infections. Data from Fenner and White (1970), Christie (1974), and Benenson (1975)

Infectious disease	Incubation period	Latent period	Infectious period
Measles	8–13	6–9	6–7
Mumps	12–26	12–18	4–8
Whooping cough (pertussis)	6–10	21–23	7–10
Rubella	14–21	7–14	11–12
Diphtheria	2–5	14–21	2–5
Chicken pox	13–17	8–12	10–11
Hepatitis B	30–80	13–17	19–22
Poliomyelitis	7–12	1–3	14–20
Influenza	1–3	1–3	2–3
Smallpox	10–15	8–11	2–3
Scarlet fever	2–3	1–2	14–21

(see Fig. 2.2). Table 3.1 lists the latent, incubation, and infectious periods of a variety of common viral infections of humans. The third segment is host recovery during which viral abundance decays to zero or very low levels and antibody titres (antibodies specific to viral antigens) rise to high levels. Recovered hosts are almost invariably fully immune to further infection in the case of viral parasites. Furthermore, the duration of human immunity against many viral infections appears to be lifelong. Whether such immunity is maintained via constant exposure to infection (where infections subsequent to the initial one do not result in overt symptoms of disease but simply act to bolster acquired immunity), via long-lived clones of lymphocytes (memory T and B cells) that are able to recognize specific viral antigens and maintain antibody production in the absence of repeated exposure, or via the persistence of the virus at low levels of abundance within the host such that antibodies to viral antigens are constantly produced, remains unclear at present. The most popular hypothesis is that based on the presence of so-called long-lived memory cells (Roitt *et al.* 1985). However, some recent theoretical work questions this belief, suggesting that immunological memory may be a dynamic state arising either from regulatory networks within the immune system, or from the continual persistence of the infectious agent within the host (Hoffman 1975; Anderson and May 1988*b*).

Immunological memory is clearly an important topic in any consideration of the interaction between host and parasite, both at the individual and at the population levels. For example, the degree of specific population immunity, often referred to as *herd immunity*, is a major determinant of the transmission dynamics of most microparasitic organisms. A detailed understanding of the basis of immunological memory is not central to the discussions and analyses presented in later chapters. However, we make a small diversion at this point to illustrate some of the interesting conceptual insights that can be generated by simple analyses of the dynamic interaction between a population of microparasites within a host and the immune system of the host. We address this issue by reference to the growth of a virus population within an individual host and the response of a population of immune 'effector' cells to changes in viral abundance. For the purposes of illustration, we define the population of effector cells as those entities within the host's immune system (such as T and B lymphocytes which specifically recognize viral antigens) which act to restrict viral population growth. This is clearly a gross oversimplification of the many cell types and chemical factors involved in an immune response and their action in producing the specific antibodies that help to kill the virus. We consider two different approaches to the description of the interaction: namely, one based on an *antigen-driven* view of the immune system and the other based on the *network regulation* of interactions between different cell types within the immune system and the replicating antigen (the virus).

3.1.1.1 *Antigen-driven systems*   The respective densities of the virus and the effector cells within an individual are defined as $V(t)$ and $E(t)$ at time t. We assume that effector cells are recruited at a constant rate Λ (which mimics, for example, the production of primordial lymphocytes in the bone marrow of vertebrates) and die at a per capita rate μ, where $1/\mu$ denotes life expectancy of the effector cells. Effector cells are assumed to proliferate at a net rate dependent on their contact with the virus, εVE where ε denotes the coefficient of proliferation. Our assumption concerning effector cell proliferation is based on the theory of lymphocyte clonal selection (Burnett 1957). The specificity of the adaptive immune system is based on the specificity of the antibodies and lymphocytes. It is believed that each lymphocyte is only capable of recognizing one particular antigen. Since the immune system as a whole can specifically recognize many thousands of antigens this means that the lymphocytes recognizing any particular viral antigen are a very small proportion of the total. An adequate response to viral infection is achieved via clonal selection and expansion. A viral antigen binds to the small number of cells that initially recognize it and induces them to proliferate so that they now constitute sufficient cells to mount (via antibody production by the B cells) an effective immune response. That is, an antigen selects the specific clones of antigen-bonding cells and causes their proliferation. This process occurs both for the B lymphocytes, which proliferate and mature into antibody-producing cells, and for the T lymphocytes, which are involved in the recognition and destruction of virally infected cells. Broadly speaking, the immune system regards all molecules not belonging to the individual as 'non-self' and reacts against them. It recognizes many of the individual's own molecules as 'self' but does not react against them. Clearly the body must both 'tolerate' its own tissues and react effectively against all infectious agents if disease is to be avoided.

The viral population is assumed to have per capita birth and death rates b and d respectively; we define the natural intrinsic growth rate of the virus, r, as $r = b - d$. Effector cells are assumed to kill viruses at a net rate σVE where σ is a coefficient denoting the degree of contact between effector cell and virus and the efficacy of the killing process. These assumptions lead to the following differential equations to describe changes in $V(t)$ and $E(t)$ with respect to time:

$$dE/dt = \Lambda - \mu E + \varepsilon VE, \tag{3.1}$$

$$dV/dt = rV - \sigma VE. \tag{3.2}$$

In the absence of the virus ($V = 0$), the effector cell population settles to a stable equilibrium $\hat{E}$ where

$$\hat{E} = \Lambda/\mu. \tag{3.3}$$

When the host is infected by the virus, the effector cell population is stimulated to proliferate. The viral population will not increase in size above the magnitude of the initial infecting inoculum (V_0) unless

$$r > \hat{E}\sigma. \tag{3.4}$$

In other words, its intrinsic growth rate r must be greater than the product of the equilibrium effector cell density in the naive host ($\hat{E}$) times the coefficient representing the efficacy of virus killing by effector cells. If eqn (3.4) is satisfied, the system will settle to an equilibrium with the virus persisting, where

$$E^* = r/\sigma \tag{3.5}$$

and

$$V^* = \mu(r - \hat{E}\sigma)/\varepsilon r. \tag{3.6}$$

This equilibrium is locally stable but the system has a strong propensity to exhibit oscillatory behaviour (the system is weakly stable). The model predicts large-amplitude oscillations in viral and effector cell abundances (Fig. 3.3). The period, T, between peak viraemias (for $r \gg \mu$, Λ, or σ) is approximately given by

$$T \simeq 2\pi(r\mu - \Lambda\sigma)^{-1/2}. \tag{3.7}$$

The derivation of T follows similar lines to those outlined in a later chapter for the interepidemic period of viral epidemics in populations of hosts (the details are given in Appendix C). Note that provided eqn (3.4) is satisfied (i.e. the viral population is able to initially grow in size), the period between peak viraemias gets longer as the life expectancy of the effector cells increases. For example, if $1/\mu$ is of the order of a few years then T may be longer than human life expectancy.

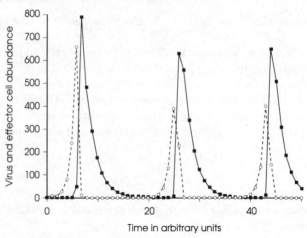

Fig. 3.3. Temporal changes in virus and effector cell abundance as predicted by the model defined in eqns (3.1) and (3.2). Following infection of the host at time $t = 0$, viral abundance ($\times 10$) grows exponentially until the effector cell population (stimulated to proliferate by the presence of the virus) is of sufficient size to cause a decline in the size of the virus population (parameter values $V_0 = 1$, $E_0 = 2$, $\Lambda = 1$, $\mu = 0.5$, $\varepsilon = 0.01$, $\sigma = 0.01$). Recurrent outbreaks or epidemics of viraemia are triggered by the decay in effector cell abundance (due to the cells' short life expectancy) once the stimulus of proliferation (the virus) is at low abundance. If the life expectancy of the effector cells is long ($1/\mu$ large) then the interval between peak viraemias may be longer than the life expectancy of the host.

Bearing in mind the caution that the model is a very crude caricature of the true complexities of the interaction of the immune system with a replicating antigen, two broad conclusions may be drawn. First, provided effector cell life expectancy is not too short in relation to host life expectancy, the immunological memory created by their proliferation is sufficient to suppress viral abundance to very low levels following the initial 'epidemic' within the host. In crude terms the latent period of infection can be viewed as the earlier stages of viral population growth (the lag phase before a viraemia becomes detectable is determined by r), while the infectious period can be viewed as the period which coincides with the phase of high viral abundance in the first 'epidemic' inside the host (the duration and magnitude of the 'epidemic' is determined by r, ε, and σ). Following the suppression of viral population abundance to a very low level, immunological memory is created by the high abundance of long-lived, or relatively long-lived, effector cells. The second point concerns the prediction that the effector cells, even at high abundance, are unable completely to eliminate the virus from the host. This provides some support for the view that immunological memory may, in part, be a consequence of viral persistence (very low levels of viral abundance are probably undetectable by current methods).

However, it may be that viral abundance drops to such a low level following the initial population explosion that chance effects (i.e. demographic stochasticity) inevitably lead to parasite extinction.

3.1.1.2 *Network-regulated systems* Once an immune response is initiated by viral infection, the components of that response, such as the B and T cells, are capable of immense replication. Experiments involving the transfer of stimulated lymphocytes into irradiated recipient hosts (i.e. the immunological system of the recipient is effectively inactivated) demonstrate that, if given the opportunity, a clone of B cells will continue to expand indefinitely (Bach *et al.* 1979). It is thus evident that some form of feedback mechanism must act to regulate the immune system. In the previous section, the feedback control was the density of the replicating antigen (= virus) itself. An alternative hypothesis, advanced by Jerne (1974), is that regulation is achieved even in the absence of foreign antigens by interactions between cell and antibody types within the host. In its simplest form, such regulation is envisaged as a symmetric network in which cell type 1 acts as antigen to cell type 2, and vice versa. Thus 1 mounts an immune response to 2 and suppresses its abundance and 2 mounts an immune response to 1 which concomitantly limits 1's abundance. A useful conceptual analogy is to envisage 1 and 2 operating in a two-way predator–prey interaction in which 1 is both predator and prey to 2, and vice versa. In its original form, Jerne's so-called network regulation theory was asymmetrical in form, such that cell type 1 acted as antigen to 2, 2 acted as antigen to 3, 3 acted as antigen to 4, and so on (Jerne 1974). More recently, the idea of symmetric interactions has gained credence (see Hoffman 1975; Urbain 1986). The reality may well be complex networks, in which all manner of loops and reciprocities are found.

A central observation in support of the network theory of regulation is that an antibody's variable and hypervariable regions may act as antigenic determinants. Thus it is possible to demonstrate the presence of antibodies (called anti-idiotypic antibodies) which specifically bind with other antibodies produced by the host. The experimental induction of anti-idiotypic antibodies shows that lymphocytes exist which are capable of recognizing and responding to the combining sites of antibodies and receptors on other lymphocytes (Eichmann 1978). The possibility is thus presented for regulatory (= predator–prey) interactions between the cells and antibodies of the immune system via their antigen combining sites. The network hypothesis is still the subject of much controversy, but evidence is mounting that idiotypic–anti-idiotypic interactions can modulate the immune response. The question of central importance, however, concerns the relative roles of network regulation versus foreign antigen regulation in the *resting state* (the virgin or unstimulated state denoted by $\hat{E} = \Lambda/\mu$ in the antigen-driven model, see eqn (3.3)) and the active *immune state* (arising from exposure to and recovery from infection). One view is that foreign antigen is of prime importance in regulating the active immune state, but that idiotypic regulation is more important in determining activity in the virgin or resting state.

Theory based on simple mathematical models cannot resolve this controversy, but it can help to clarify what forms of dynamical behaviour can arise in a network-regulated system. The issue is a complex one, but the principal properties of network regulation are well illustrated by the following model. We define two types of effector cells (i.e. lymphocytes) whose abundances are denoted by $E_1(t)$ and $E_2(t)$ at time t. New cells of type i are recruited from the bone marrow at a constant rate Λ_i and they die at a per capita rate μ_i. We assume that cell type 1 is triggered to proliferate by contact with cell type 2, and vice versa. In other words, both cell types act as antigenic stimulants to each other in a symmetric manner. We further assume that the respective proliferation responses saturate to a maximum net rate which is dependent on the product of their respective densities. These assumptions, in the absence of foreign antigens, lead to the following pair of predator–prey-like interaction equations,

$$dE_1/dt = \Lambda_1 - \mu_1 E_1 + a_1 E_1 E_2/(1 + b_1 E_1 E_2), \tag{3.8}$$

$$dE_2/dt = \Lambda_2 - \mu_2 E_2 + a_2 E_1 E_2/(1 + b_2 E_1 E_2). \tag{3.9}$$

The terms a_i and b_i are arbitrary constants that determine the degrees of proliferation arising from the cell–cell interaction and the levels at which the net rates of proliferation saturate. This is a very simple mimic of the basic concepts of network regulation, but the model nevertheless has a number of properties that provide a caricature of some important dynamical features of the immune system. These properties are best understood by reference to the phase plane of E_1 and E_2 defined by eqns (3.8) and (3.9) when $dE_1/dt = dE_2/dt = 0$. Isoclines of E_1 and E_2 are depicted in Fig. 3.4. For certain sets of

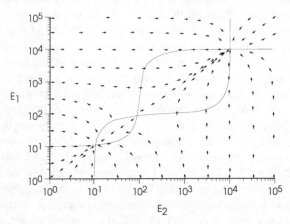

Fig. 3.4. Phase plane of E_1 and E_2 (effector cell types 1 and 2) defined by eqns (3.8) and (3.9) when $dE_1/dt = dE_2/dt = 0$ (the full lines on the graph). The plane records three positive equilibrium states; the lower and upper states (with respect to the vertical axis) are stable and they are separated by an unstable state. The arrows record directions of flow or movement in the phase plane (see text for further details).

parameter values three positive equilibrium states exist; two of these are stable and they are separated by an unstable state. The lower one defines the virgin or resting state of the immune system where $E_i^* \simeq \Lambda_i/\mu_i$. The upper stable state is the active immune state at which the abundances of the two types of effector cells are elevated to high levels. As indicated by the arrows in Fig. 3.4, showing the 'flow lines' along which trajectories move, there are now two distinct domains in this 'phase space'. Broadly speaking, initial points in the region to the lower left of Fig. 3.4 are 'attracted' to the virgin state, whereas initial points to the upper right are attracted to the immune state. Disturbance from the virgin state that, as indicated by the arrows in Fig. 3.4, are attracted back to it represent 'low-zone tolerance'.

How can the system be switched from the virgin to the immune state? Suppose the host is infected by a viral pathogen which possesses an antigen which is identical to that expressed by cell type 1. Once the virus has undergone a phase of replication the net outcome will be to substantially shift the density of cell type 1, and hence antigen type 1, upwards (along the horizontal axis in Fig. 3.4) so that the system leaves the 'attractive zone' of the virgin state, and moves towards the immune state. Once there the host is actively immune. This state is stable and hence the rapid elimination of the virus will leave the system with elevated levels of effector cell abundance. In other words immunological memory is in essence a dynamic state created by network regulation via cell–cell interactions.

In the paradigm presented by this model, the state of active immunity and the existence of immunological memory are independent of the expected lifespans of the effector cells (i.e. $1/\mu_i$ may be large or small). The system is driven to an active immune state by the presence of the replicating antigen, but once the state is attained the system remains in it; maintenance of the immune state does not depend on the continued presence of the infectious agent.

The very simple model captured in eqns (3.8) and (3.9) therefore has the following properties: a resting and an active immune state; low-zone tolerance (where changes in antigen density over a defined range do not elicit an immune response); and immunological memory. It is very remarkable that such a simple representation of the concept of network regulation can reflect such a wide range of properties. The lessons to be learned from this example are twofold. First, it generates an alternative hypothesis to explain the existence of immunological memory. Second, it argues that the interpretation of observed immunological responses to infectious agents can be greatly facilitated by investigations of the population dynamics of cell–cell and cell–antigen interactions within an individual host. Research of this nature is in its infancy at present but it holds great promise for helping to unravel, and perhaps to simplify, the ever more complex hypotheses that are proposed to explain observed immunological phenomena.

3.1.2 *Bacteria*

Human defences against pathogenic bacteria consist of a variety of specific and non-specific mechanisms. When bacteria gain access to host tissues, the effectiveness of an immune response depends to a large degree on the ability to damage the components of the bacterial cell wall. Antibody is often produced which is specific to receptors on the bacterial cell wall, or to toxins produced by the bacteria. Surface receptors or the transport of molecules across the bacterial cell wall can be blocked by antibody binding. Ultimately, almost all bacteria are killed by phagocytic cells (polymorphs and macrophages). The pathogenicity of some non-invasive infections of epithelial surfaces (e.g. *Coryne-bacterium diphtheria* and *Vibrio cholerae*) depends on toxin production, and neutralizing antibody is thought to be sufficient for immunity, though antibody blocking adhesion to the epithelium is also important. The pathogenicity of invasive organisms does not tend to rely on a single toxin, so that immunity requires killing of the organism itself. Antibody and phagocytic cells are the main effector mechanisms. Certain species which are resistant to phagocytic cells (*Myco-bacterium tuberculosis*) or are obligate intracellular parasites (*Mycobacterium leprae*) are killed by other mechanisms that are poorly understood at present.

Bacteria are clearly more complex antigenically than viruses and it is often the case that acquired immunity following infection is neither so complete nor of such long duration as that for most viral infections.

3.1.3 *Protozoa*

Protozoa invariably stimulate more than one immunological defence mechanism (i.e. antibody and cell mediated immunity). Their large size relative to viruses and bacteria entails the existence of more antigens, both in number and kind. Protozoan infections tend to be more persistent (than the transient viral diseases) and chronic in character. This implies the long-term presence of circulating antigens, persistent antigenic stimulation, and the formation of immune complexes. Levels of immunoglobulins are typically raised in malaria (IgG and IgM), visceral leishmaniasis (IgG), and trypanosomiasis (IgM). Many protozoan species have evolved mechanisms to help evade the host's immuno-logical defences. Antibody seems to be the most important part of the immune response against those parasites that live in the bloodstream, such as the malarial parasites and the African trypanosomes. Cell mediated immunity is active against those like *Leishmania* that live in the tissues. Antibody can damage parasites directly, enhance their clearance by phagocytosis, activate complement, or block their entry into host cells. Transfer of γ-globulin from immune adults to a child infected with *Plasmodium falciparum*, for example, causes a sharp drop in parasitaemia. Once inside the cell, the parasite is safe from antibody, but oxygen metabolites and other cytotoxic factors are thought, for example, to play a role in killing the intracellular stages of malaria.

Certain protozoan species persist within their hosts via successive waves of parasitaemias (e.g. the malarial and trypanosome parasites) induced by im-munologically distinct populations of parasites. Protection is not afforded by antibody against preceding waves. Evasion of the host's defences is therefore achieved by antigenic variation. In the case of the African trypanosomes each variant (arising during asexual replication) possesses an antigenically distinct glycoprotein which forms its surface coat (Vickerman 1978; Cross 1979). Some malarial parasites also show antigenic variation but not, it seems, of antigens of the sporozoites or merozoites (Brown 1983). Other species are protected from the host's defences by their occupancy of refugia, such as host cells, where they avoid the effects of antibody (e.g. *Leishmania* spp.).

The consequence of the evolution of well tuned immune evasion mechanisms implies that protozoan infections are often able to persist within the human host for considerable periods of time. Acquired immunity is therefore rarely fully protective against reinfection and its efficacy appears to depend on the duration and intensity of past exposure to infection. In many instances the mechanisms that facilitate parasite persistence and repeated host infection are poorly understood at present. Genetic variability within protozoan parasite populations (many antigenically distinct variants) and its maintenance by sexual reproduction is probably of great significance to the maintenance of transmission within human communities (Walliker *et al.* 1987).

3.2 Epidemiological data

Epidemiological research on microparasitic infections is largely based on two distinct measures of parasite abundance within communities of people. The first of these is the *incidence* of infection or of disease (infection is not always synonymous with disease and in some circumstances inapparent infection may arise that produces no overt symptoms). Incidence is defined as the *rate* of appearance of new cases (of infection or disease) per unit of time. The second measure is the *prevalence* of infection or disease. This is a 'standing crop' statistic (i.e. not a rate) and it records the proportion of people infected (or with symptoms of disease) at one point in time, or over a short sampling interval. The measurement of incidence or prevalence is often based on the stratification of the population under study with respect to a variety of factors such as age, sex, social status, etc. Stratification by age is of particular importance since age reflects time; changes in prevalence with host age therefore represents a further measure of the *rate* at which individuals acquire infection. Surveys of incidence or prevalence may be carried out longitudinally (i.e. through time) or horizontally (at one point in time or over a short interval of time). If sampling is based on the stratification of the population into a series of classes, the sample design is referred to as a stratified longitudinal survey or a stratified horizontal survey.

A further epidemiological statistic of great value in the study of transmission is the proportion of individuals within a population who possess antibodies specific to a particular microparasite's antigens. The presence of such antibodies can be detected via various serological techniques which are based on immunological assay. Measures may be qualitative (i.e. presence or absence) or quantitative (i.e. antibody titres). The detection of antibodies implies that the individual is either currently infected or, more commonly, has experienced the infection at some time in earlier life. Their absence, however, does not necessarily imply that the individual has never experienced the infection. Duration of measurable levels of antibody production following recovery is clearly of central importance. Surveys of the proportion seropositive may again be horizontal or longitudinal in nature and they may be stratified according to age, sex, etc.

In this section we briefly review the kinds of data that are available (or can be collected) to test theoretical predictions, to estimate the rate-determining parameters of transmission, and to guide model formulation.

3.2.1 *Longitudinal and horizontal changes in incidence*

In many developed countries, public health authorities have well-developed systems for the collection of data on the incidences of various microparasitic infections. Many viral, bacterial, and protozoan diseases, for example, are classified as notifiable in the sense that a general practitioner must inform some central authority of the occurrence of cases of these infections within patients in his or her practice. A list of the notifiable infections in the United States (as at 1984) is recorded in Table 3.2. The details of such notifiable infections vary somewhat between different countries.

Cases are normally tabulated by age, sex, and geographical locality either weekly, monthly, or annually. In certain countries these records extend back to the early part of the current century. Some examples of changes in disease incidence within England and Wales over long periods of time are recorded in Fig. 3.5. These infectious disease notifications constitute some of the best records of long-term fluctuations in population abundance that are available for any animal or plant species. In some instances even longer-term records can be acquired via reference to causes of human mortality. For example, the London Mortality bills of the seventeenth century record deaths per week stratified by cause, such as various infectious diseases like smallpox and bubonic plague (Fig. 3.6). Clearly such records contain many inaccuracies since the identification of cause of death was in early times subject to much error. However, they do provide qualitative indices of longitudinal trends in incidence for the more easily identified infections such as smallpox and plague (Fig. 3.7).

What can be learned from these notification records? First, they enable one to pose a simple statistical question, namely, are observed changes in disease incidence more regular through time than would be expected on the basis of chance fluctuations alone? In other words, long runs of changes in incidence facilitate the measurement of the mean and variance of the interepidemic period (the time interval between major peaks in disease incidence). As we shall see

Table 3.2 Notifiable infections in the United States (1984)

Acquired Immunodeficiency Syndrome (AIDS)
Amoebiasis
Anthrax
Aseptic meningitis
Botulism
Brucellosis
Chancroid
Cholera
Diphtheria
Encephalitis, primary
Encephalitis, post infectious
Gonorrhoea
Granuloma inguinale
Hepatitis, serum
Hepatitis, infectious
Hepatitis, unspecified
Leprosy
Leptospirosis
Lymphogranuloma venereum
Malaria
Measles
Meningococcal infections
Mumps
Pertussis
Plague
Poliomyelitis
Psittacosis
Rabies, animal
Rabies, human
Rheumatic fever, acute
Rubella
Rubella Congenital Syndrome
Salmonellosis
Shigellosis
Smallpox
Streptococcal sore throat and scarlet fever
Syphilis
Tetanus
Trichinosis
Tularemia
Typhoid fever
Typhus fever, flea borne
Varicella
Yellow fever

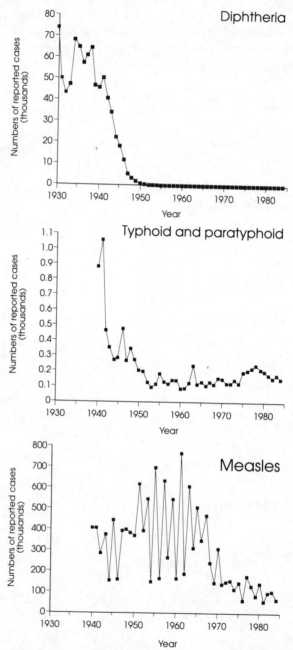

Fig. 3.5. Longitudinal records of the incidence (defined as reported cases of infection per annum) of various infectious diseases (diphtheria, polio, typhoid and paratyphoid, scarlet fever, measles, and whooping cough (pertussis)) in England and Wales over the

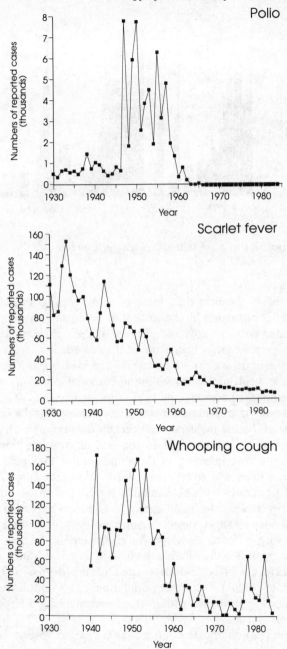

period 1930 to 1985 (from the Registrar-General's weekly infectious disease returns for England and Wales).

44   *Microparasites*

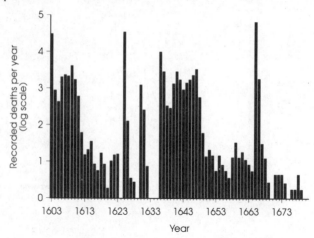

Fig. 3.6. Reported deaths from bubonic plague in London over the interval 1603 to 1679 (Brayley 1722).

later, simple theory predicts that, for certain microparasitic infections, these intervals are determined, not by chance, but by processes intrinsic to the biology of the interaction between host and parasite at the individual and population levels (see Chapter 6). On a finer scale, if the records are based on weekly or monthly compilations, we can also examine the evidence for seasonal periodicities in disease incidence. Many viral and bacterial infections of humans, for example, show marked seasonal changes in incidence (Fig. 3.8).

The second use is in providing a means of examining the relationship between the magnitude of disease incidence and certain demographic characteristics of a human community. For example, in the case of viral infections that induce lifelong immunity to reinfection in those individuals that recover, we might expect incidence to be related to the net birth rate of the community (the rate at which new susceptibles arise). Similarly, for infections that are transmitted by contact between hosts, we might expect incidence to be related to population density. Such ideas can be tested against records of disease incidence in communities with differing demographic characteristics (i.e. in developed or developing countries with differing birth and survival rates). Longitudinal changes in incidence may also be related to the degree of isolation of a community from contact with other populations. This notion can be tested by examining trends in incidence within island communities and populations on large continents.

Thirdly, stratification of case notifications enables an assessment to be made of how incidence changes not just in time but with age or sex within a community. For most common viral and bacterial infections, incidence changes substantially with host age owing to a variety of factors, not least of which is the duration of time over which an individual is exposed to infections within a

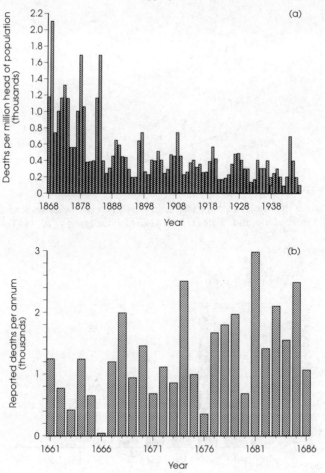

Fig. 3.7. (a) Recorded deaths from smallpox in Calcutta, India over the years 1868 to 1947. Data from Annual Reports of the Public Health Commissioners with the Government of India (1930 to 1946/47) Calcutta, Government of India Central Publications Branch. (b) Reported deaths from smallpox in London over the interval 1661 to 1686 (data from Brayley 1722).

population (Fig. 3.9). Incidence may also vary due to environmental, behavioural, or sociological factors such as family size (Fig. 3.10). Age-related changes are of particular importance since, as mentioned earlier, the dimensions of age and time are in some ways equivalent. Horizontal age-related changes in incidence therefore represent rates of acquisition of infection. Longitudinal cohort studies of changes in incidence provide similar information.

Finally, the pattern of a single epidemic recorded by notification is of central importance in determining the relationship between the net rate of transmission

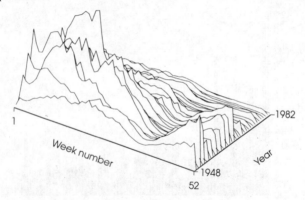

Fig. 3.8. Surface showing seasonal patterns in the incidence of measles (based on weekly case reports) in England and Wales, 1948–82 (from Anderson *et al.* 1984).

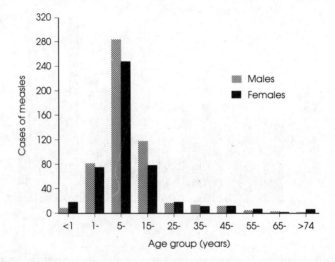

Fig. 3.9. The age- and sex-stratified incidence of measles (weekly reports) in England and Wales prior to the introduction of mass vaccination in 1967.

of infection and the density of susceptible individuals within a population. The epidemic curve has been the subject of much study both in the epidemiological and biomathematical literatures (Fig. 3.11). Its geometry provides many clues concerning the dynamics of parasite transmission (see Bailey 1975; Fine 1979). The determinants of the shape of the curve will be discussed in detail in later chapters.

In the interpretation of epidemiological trends it is clearly important to take account of the accuracy of the data base. Longitudinal trends in incidence based on case notification are clearly subject to much error. It is often the case, for example, that notification efficiency (i.e. accuracy) is better during periods of

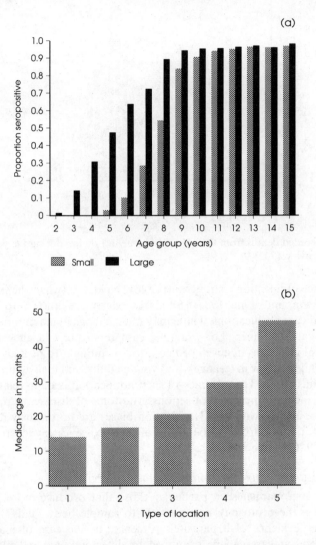

Fig. 3.10. (a) The proportion of an age group with antibodies specific to measles virus antigens in children from small and large families in the United States in 1957 prior to the introduction of mass vaccination (data from Black 1959). Family size clearly has an important influence on immunity to measles at different ages. (b) Median age of measles infection by urban–rural classification in West and Central Africa (data from Walsh 1983). The type-of-location numbers, 1–5, represent respectively dense urban, urban, dense rural, rural, and isolated rural.

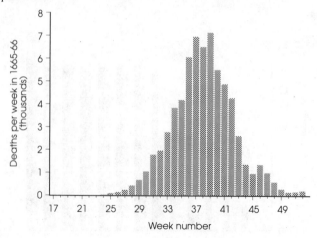

Fig. 3.11. Recorded deaths from the bubonic plague in London during the year 1665–6 (data from Brayley 1722).

high incidence of infection than periods of low incidence (when the infection is rare) (Clarkson and Fine 1985). Similarly biases are known to occur in age-stratified case notifications. These may often change in magnitude with age in a complicated manner. For example, case reporting efficiency for many common viral infections in developed countries is thought to be high in infants and young children, low in teenagers and young adults, and high again in elderly people (Collins 1929). The accuracy of such notification is often related to the manner in which the incidence of serious symptoms of disease, as opposed to just infection, change with age. Notification biases are notoriously difficult to quantify but it is important to be aware of their existence (Sydenstricker and Hedrich 1929; Crombie 1983).

3.2.2 *Longitudinal and horizontal changes in prevalence*

For certain microparasites, in particular those that produce more persistent infections (e.g. the protozoa), it is possible to sample body fluids, tissues, or secretions for evidence of a parasite's presence. In the case of malaria, for example, blood smears can be examined to detect infected red blood cells. Presence or absence can be recorded and, if desired, a more quantitative measure of parasite abundance (such as the number of infected red blood cells per unit volume of blood) may in some instances be obtained (Fig. 3.12).

Recent advances at the molecular and biochemical levels of biological study have produced new techniques for the detection of the presence (or absence) of the very small microparasites such as viruses and bacteria (e.g. DNA probes). In the case of hepatitis B viral infection, for example, it is now possible to identify those individuals who harbour persistent infections (called carriers) via tests to detect the presence or absence of viral antigens (Fig. 3.13).

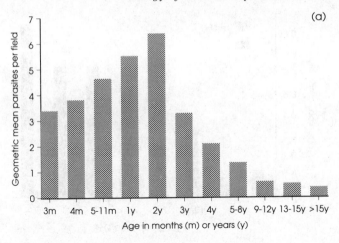

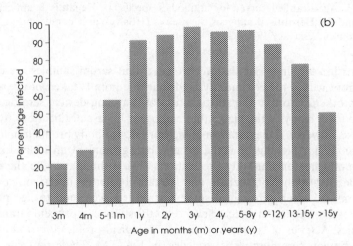

Fig. 3.12. Intensity and prevalence of malaria among Nigerians in various age groups (data from Putnam 1931). (a) The intensity of infection by reference to the geometric mean number of parasites per thick blood film among persons carrying parasites in fewer than 25 microscope fields. (b) The percentage of persons carrying parasites in fewer than 25 microscope fields.

Changes in parasite prevalence with respect to host age (either horizontally or longitudinally) provide valuable information on the rate at which individuals acquire infection (i.e. the 'force' of transmission or infection).

3.2.3 *Serological surveys*

For many common viral and bacterial infections that induce lifelong immunity in those that recover, serological surveys for the presence or absence of antibodies specific to parasite antigens provide very precise information on

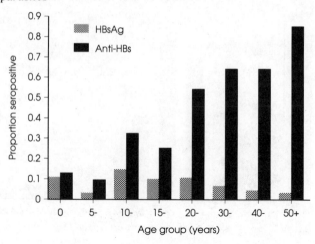

Fig. 3.13. Age-stratified survey for antibodies specific to Hepatitis B antigens (Anti-HBs), and for Hepatitis B antigens themselves (HBsAg), in a population in Thailand (data from Sobeslavsky 1980).

transmission within a population. Provided that serum samples are collected at random within the community, and that due note is taken of age, sex, and various other factors in the stratification of sampling design, serological data are free from many of the biases that can occur in case notifications. Problems can arise, however, if the duration of measurable antibody production following infection is not lifelong or if the genetic background of an individual has a strong influence on antibody production. This is thought to be the case, for example, for many protozoan and certain bacterial infections. For viral infections, however, serological surveys stratified according to age provide a wealth of information of direct relevance to the study of a parasite's transmission dynamics. A series of typical horizontal serological profiles for viral infections within human communities is recorded in Fig. 3.14. These patterns reveal a number of important points. First, the proportion that is seropositive decays rapidly with age following birth within a community with endemic infection. This initial phase of decay is a consequence of the loss of maternally derived protection in those children born to mothers who had experienced the infection. Maternal antibodies (IgG) are acquired during a child's development in the uterus of the mother. Such maternally derived antibodies (IgG) have a half-life of approximately 3–6 months, irrespective of the type of viral infection that has induced their production (Fig. 3.15). The proportion seropositive for such antibodies decays to zero over a period of approximately one year in the absence of infection.

Second, in communities in which the viral infection is endemic, following the decay in maternally derived protection, the proportion seropositive rises steadily with age (as a consequence of the acquisition of infection) often

Table 3.3 Average age at infection (in years) for different diseases in different localities (Anderson and May 1985*c*)

Infectious disease	Average age, *A*	Geographical location and time period
Measles	5–6	USA, 1955–8
	4–5	England and Wales, 1948–68
	2–3	Morocco, 1962
	2–3	Ghana, 1960–8
	2–3	Pondicherry, India, 1978
	1–2	Senegal, 1964
	1–2	Bangkok, Thailand, 1967
Rubella	9–10	Sweden, 1965
	9–10	USA, 1966–8
	9–10	Manchester, England, 1970–82
	6–7	Poland, 1970–7
	2–3	Gambia, 1976
Chicken pox	6–8	USA, 1921–8
Poliovirus	12–17	USA, 1955
Pertussis	4–5	England and Wales, 1948–68
	4–5	USA, 1920–60
Mumps	6–7	England and Wales, 1975–77
	6–7	Netherlands, 1977–9

attaining a plateau close to 100 per cent in elderly people. The rate of rise in seropositivity with age is a direct measure of the age-specific rates or forces of infection pertaining in that community (in the absence of vaccination). The force of infection is defined as the per capita rate at which susceptibles acquire infection (i.e. convert from seronegativity to seropositivity) and it often varies according to an individual's age. Statistical methods, involving maximum likelihood techniques, are available to estimate the age-specific forces of infection from age-stratified serological data (Griffiths 1974; Grenfell and Anderson 1985). The paper by Grenfell and Anderson contains a discussion of the assumptions on which such methods are based and the biases in estimation that can arise from the use of case notification and serological data.

A very useful summary statistic can be derived from age-stratified serological data, namely, the average age, *A*, at which an individual typically acquires a specific infection in a given community. Statistical methods for its calculation from serology surveys are again described in Grenfell and Anderson (1985). The magnitude of *A*, which inversely measures the net force of infection within a community, varies greatly for different infections and for the same infection between different communities. In illustration of this point, Table 3.3 records a wide range of values of *A* for a great variety of different microparasites in various geographical localities.

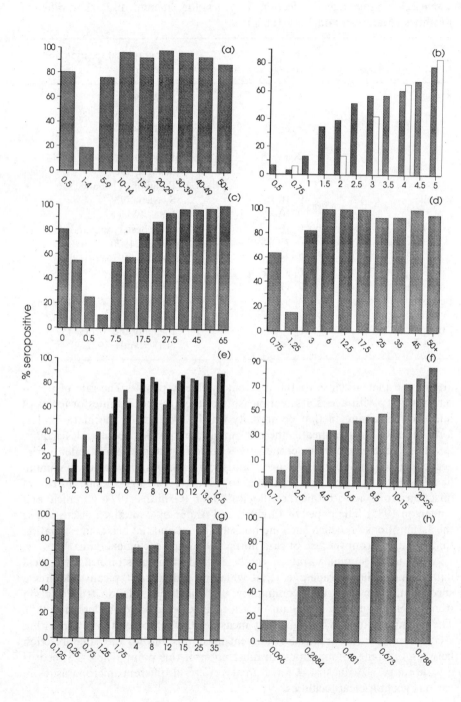

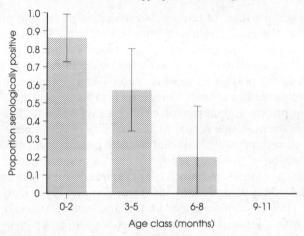

Fig. 3.15. The decay in maternally-derived antibody to antigens of the rubella virus (+95 per cent confidence limits) over the period from birth to 11 months of age (data from Nokes *et al.* 1986).

Third, in the absence or presence of mass vaccination the area under the curve denoting changes in the proportion seropositive with age is a direct measure of the degree of herd immunity to an infection prevailing in the population. Conversely the area above the seropositive curve reflects the degree of susceptibility in the community. The monitoring of changes in herd immunity under the impact of a mass vaccination programme is an important guide to the success of the control programme. Unfortunately, far too little attention has been paid to this area of epidemiological study in past immunization programmes. We wish to stress the point that the collection of serological data, finely stratified according to age, is of vital importance in any quantitative assessment of disease transmission and the impact of mass vaccination. Ideally, serological surveys should be carried out before as well as during the course of an immunization programme.

Fig. 3.14. Age-stratified (horizontal) serological profiles of the percentage of people in different age groups with antibodies to the antigens of various infectious disease agents in developed and developing countries (data sources given in Anderson and May (1985*c*)): (a) measles in the United States in 1955–8; (b) measles in India (left-hand histograms) and Nigeria (right-hand histograms); (c) rubella in England and Wales in the 1960s and 1970s; (d) rubella in The Gambia in the late 1970s; (e) mumps in England and Wales (left-hand histogram) and The Netherlands (right-hand histogram); (f) polio in the United States in 1955; (g) Hepatitis B (HBV) in Senegal; and (h) malaria (*Plasmodium falciparum*) in Nigeria. The vertical axis denotes the cumulative percentage of people who have experienced infection. Note that in (a)–(h) the scales of the *x* axes are not always identical and in certain cases record unequal age-class divisions.

Before leaving the topic of serology we wish to mention two problems that can complicate the interpretation of observed patterns. The first of these has been alluded to earlier, namely, genetically based variability in the intensity and the duration of antibody production following infection. It is sometimes the case that the proportion seropositive never attains 100 per cent in the older age classes, but saturates to some lower level (e.g. 90–95 per cent). The reasons are unclear at present and may involve either a substantial decline in exposure to infection in the older age groups or the inability to detect measurable levels of antibody in certain individuals due to their genetic background. Research on the production of antibody following immunization against various viral infections such as measles and rubella, for example, has revealed an association between HLA antigens and antibody titres (Nokes 1987; Dorf 1981). The second, but related, problem concerns the duration of antibody production following infection. Quantitative studies of antibody titres in patients of different ages reveal that the mean titre of antibody specific to a particular virus tends to decay in old individuals who experienced infection early in life (Fig. 3.16). This implies that there is often a greater chance of falsely identifying an individual as seronegative, when in fact he or she has experienced infection, in elderly individuals than in younger people. Such a bias can of course influence the accuracy of estimates of age-specific rates of infection (Nokes *et al.* 1986). Similar problems arise in individuals vaccinated against viral infections at a young age. This is especially true if immunization is administered in early life when maternal antibodies are still present. In these circumstances, vaccination may fail to adequately protect an individual against infection (Albrecht *et al.* 1977).

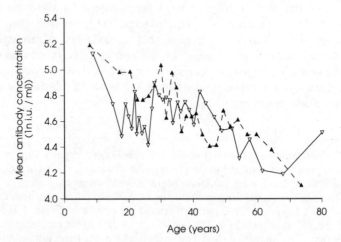

Fig. 3.16. The decay in mean antibody concentration to rubella virus antigens with the age and sex of the individual from whom serum has been collected: ▲ = males, ▽ = females (data from Nokes *et al.* 1986).

3.2.4 *Incubation, latent, and infectious periods*

In Section 3.1.1 we discussed the typical course of a transient microparasitic infection within an individual patient. We defined a series of quantities that described the durations of various stages of the infection such as the latent, incubation, and infectious periods. The latent period is the time from initial infection to the point at which the individual becomes infectious to others, the incubation period denotes the time from initial infection to the point where symptoms of disease typically appear (or are diagnosed), and the infectious period is, as its name implies, the period of time during which an infected individual is infectious to others. In practice these periods vary for any particular infection among individuals within a population. However, for many common viral and bacterial infections the degree of variability appears to be small relative to the average length of the period. It is therefore not unreasonable to define average values for a given infectious agent. These quantities are, as we shall see in later chapters, of central importance as determinants of the transmission dynamics of microparasitic organisms. Of particular significance are the generation time of the disease agent, defined as the sum of the average latent and infectious periods, and the latent period itself, which introduces a form of time-delay into the dynamics of parasite transmission. It is well understood in population biology that time delays of significant magnitudes relative to the generation time of an organism can induce oscillatory fluctuations in population abundance (May 1974).

The statistical estimation of latent, incubation, and infectious periods is fraught with many problems, not least of which are those relating to the collection of adequate samples of data. It is usually very difficult, for example, to assess the duration of infectiousness in the case of micro-organisms via the detection of viral particles or bacteria in host secretions or excretions. Many of the documented records of these epidemiological parameters are therefore rather anecdotal in nature and arise from relatively few observations. Inferences are often based on rather heterogeneous collections of observations. The data are best for the incubation period, and the papers and bibliographies of Sartwell (1950, 1966) provide extensive information on a wide variety of infections. Sartwell found that lognormal distributions gave good descriptions of the variation in incubation periods for a considerable number of childhood infections (Fig. 3.17).

With respect to latent and infectious periods, an extensive review of models and estimation procedures is provided by Bailey (1975). The ideal types of data are those concerning the transmission of an infection within a household from person to person following the introduction of a single infective. Such case-to-case studies, however, are rarely attempted. Three exceptions are the work on measles transmission in 264 households by Hope-Simpson, the work on smallpox by Abakaliki, and the research on Hepatitis A by Petersen (all discussed in Bailey (1975)). One of the data sets, namely that on measles, is

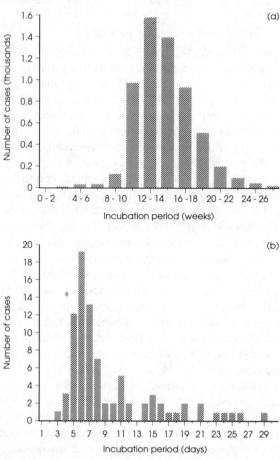

Fig. 3.17. The distribution of the incubation period in days (defined as the interval from infection to the appearance of symptoms of disease) for Hepatitis B (data from Sartwell 1950) and for typhoid (data from Miner 1923) in graphs (a) and (b) respectively.

presented in Table 3.4. This information, collected in the Cirencester area of England during the years 1946–52 (before immunization), records the distribution of the observed time interval between two cases of measles in 219 families with two children under the age of 15 years. The bulk of these observations represent case-to-case transmission within a family. However, in a small number of families, where the observed interval is only a few days, it may be assumed that these cases are double primaries; both children having been simultaneously infected from some outside source. Early work on the estimation of latent periods was based on chain binomial models where it is assumed there is a constant incubation period which is terminated by a very short interval of infectiousness. This assumption is based on the belief that once symptoms

Table 3.4 Observed time intervals between two cases of measles in families of two children. Data from Cirencester, England, 1946–52 (Hope-Simpson 1952)

Time interval between the two cases (days)	Total number of observations	Presumed double primaries	Presumed case-to-case transmission
0	5	5	
1	13	13	
2	5	5	
3	4	4	
4	3	2	1
5	2		2
6	4		4
7	11		11
8	5		5
9	25		25
10	37		37
11	38		38
12	26		26
13	12		12
14	15		15
15	6		6
16	3		3
17	1		1
18	3		3
19			
20			
21	1		1

appear, the case is promptly removed from circulation (Abbey 1952; Greenwood 1949; Bailey 1956). Recently, more sophisticated models have been developed based on a continuous time framework, which assume that the latent and infectious periods are variable, with say a lognormal or Weibüll distribution (see Bailey 1975; Becker 1976, 1977; Gough 1977; Anderson *et al.* 1987*b*). We refer the reader to Bailey (1975) for methods of parameter estimation and the details of model formulation.

In rare instances, very good data are available from studies of infection in volunteers who have been infected at a known point in time. The work of Anderson *et al.* (1985), for example, on human parvovirus infection provides good data on the latent and infectious period (determined by viral excretion). A summary of the available data is presented in Table 3.1. Some of these estimates are based on detailed statistical analyses of transmission within households, some are based on volunteer infection studies, while the remainder are more speculative in character.

3.3 A simple model and its biological basis

For a quantitative discussion of infection processes at the population level, we begin by apportioning the total host population into three classes:

$$X(a, t) = \text{number susceptible, of age } a, \text{ at time } t;$$

$$Y(a, t) = \text{number infected, of age } a, \text{ at time } t;$$

$$Z(a, t) = \text{number immune, of age } a, \text{ at time } t.$$

The total number of hosts of age a, at time t, is of course the sum of these three:

$$N(a, t) = X(a, t) + Y(a, t) + Z(a, t). \tag{3.10}$$

A basic set of partial differential equations describing the dynamical behaviour of this system is:

$$\partial X/\partial t + \partial X/\partial a = -(\lambda(t) + \mu(a))X(a, t), \tag{3.11}$$

$$\partial Y/\partial t + \partial Y/\partial a = \lambda X - (\alpha(a) + \mu(a) + v(a))Y(a, t), \tag{3.12}$$

$$\partial Z/\partial t + \partial Z/\partial a = vY - \mu(a)Z(a, t). \tag{3.13}$$

These equations differ slightly from the conventional set (Bailey 1975; Dietz 1975, 1976; Hoppenstaedt 1976; Waltman 1974) in that disease-induced mortality is explicitly included. The demographic and epidemiological parameters in these equations, which are discussed further below, are:

$\mu(a) = $ age-specific host death rate, per capita,

$v(a) = $ per capita recovery rate (which may be age-specific),

$\alpha(a) = $ per capita disease-induced death rate (possibly age-specific),

$\lambda(t) = $ 'force of infection' at time t (discussed below).

An intuitive interpretation of this system of equations is straightforward. The number of susceptibles at a given point in time may change with age ($\partial X/\partial a$), and likewise the number at a given age may change over time ($\partial X/\partial t$), as susceptibles are lost by 'natural' deaths (that is, deaths not associated with this infection) at a rate μ, or as they are transferred to the infected class at a rate λ. Infected individuals either die (naturally at the rate μ or from infection at the rate α) or recover into the immune class (at the rate v).

To complete a description of this system, sets of initial or boundary conditions are needed. Usually these conditions are provided by specifying X, Y, Z for age zero at all times, and for time zero at all ages. That is, one condition is typically provided by assuming that all hosts are born susceptible, so that at $a = 0$ we have $Y(0, t) = Z(0, t) = 0$ for all t, while $X(0, t) = B(t)$ where B is the net birth rate of the population at time t. The second condition is usually that at $t = 0$ expressions for $X(a, 0), Y(a, 0), Z(a, 0)$ are given, for all a.

3.4 Some complications

We now proceed to catalogue the biological factors that are—and are not—incorporated in this basic model. Many of the features omitted from the basic model will be added on, and their consequences discussed in detail, later. We believe, however, that it is a good idea to list these things at the outset.

3.4.1 *Latent and other classes*

Other classes of hosts can obviously be added within the compartmental framework of these models. The most usual such additional class is for hosts who are infected but not yet infectious, or 'latent'. This complicates the analysis, and in most situations does not add qualitatively new features to the dynamics, so we omit the latent class from the basic model.

If the number of hosts in the latent class, $H(a, t)$, is acknowledged, eqns (3.11) and (3.13) of the basic model remain unchanged, but eqn (3.12) is replaced by two equations:

$$\partial H/\partial t + \partial H/\partial a = \lambda X - (\sigma + \mu(a))H(a, t), \tag{3.14}$$

$$\partial Y/\partial t + \partial Y/\partial a = \sigma H - (\alpha + \mu + v)Y(a, t). \tag{3.15}$$

Here σ is the rate at which hosts move out of the latent class into the infectious class; the average duration of the latent period is $1/\sigma$. Latent periods for some common infections are listed in Table 3.1.

3.4.2 *Maternal antibodies*

Maternal antibodies may protect newly born infants for the first 3–9 months of life. This fact is important in the design of some immunization programmes, because a lasting response is not evoked by immunization during this protected period; as a result, immunization cannot usefully be implemented as a routine part of postnatal care, which otherwise would be administratively convenient. It also means that the useful immunization 'window' between decline in maternal antibodies and the early acquisition of infections in many developing countries is narrow.

Thus, for detailed analysis of some immunization programmes it is desirable to add an initial class of protected or immune hosts, into which class all infants are born. Hosts typically pass out of this class into the susceptible class in the first 3–9 months of life. Incorporation of such a class, and tests of the ensuing models against serological data for measles, is deferred to the next chapter.

3.4.3 *Vertical transmission*

For some infections, there can be a degree of 'vertical transmission', whereby the infection is passed directly to the new-born offspring of an infected parent (usually an infected mother, but also possibly an infected father). This phenomenon has been discussed by Fine (1975), Anderson and May (1979*b*, 1981) and others. Vertical transmission lowers the threshold host density required for the infection to maintain itself, and may play a part in the population biology of some microparasites of humans.

Vertical transmission can be included in the system of eqns (3.11)–(3.13) by modifying the boundary condition at $a = 0$, so that some fraction of births are into the infected class: $X(0, t) = B_1(t)$, $Y(0, t) = B_2(t)$, $Z(0, t) = 0$. These births, $B_2(t)$, in turn would represent some fraction of the births from infected people, and thus would depend in a complicated way on the number infected up to 9 months ago (with the details dependent on whether vertical infection takes place at conception, during gestation, or during passage down the birth canal).

3.4.4 *Males and females treated separately*

There are many situations where male and female host populations need to be treated separately, with distinct equations for X_i, Y_i, Z_i ($i = 1, 2$) for males and females. Such two-sex models are often required for the accurate discussion of sexually transmitted diseases, or when infections affect the two sexes differently, or when vertical transmission takes place from infected mothers (but not infected fathers) as in rubella. Sometimes the complications of a two-sex model can be avoided by assuming a 1:1 sex ratio at all ages, but sometimes the complications are unavoidable.

3.4.5 *Recovery*

The recovery rate, $v(a)$, is usually treated as an age-independent constant, in which case the average duration of infectiousness is $D = 1/v$. While this assumption is mathematically convenient, it is rarely realistic. More commonly, recovery may be after some defined period of time, D, has elapsed. These two extremes are illustrated in Fig. 3.18(a) and (b): Fig. 3.18(a) corresponds to a constant recovery rate, v, and the probability for a given host to remain in the infected class declines exponentially with the passage of time, t; Fig. 3.18(b) corresponds to a defined interval of illness, and a host remains infected for a time D and then recovers. More generally, most infections have aetiology intermediate between these two extremes (but closer to Fig. 3.18(b)), and a truly accurate model would employ some empirically determined distribution of recovery times. One such set of data is illustrated in Fig. 3.17. Some characteristic recovery times are listed in Table 3.1.

As discussed by Hoppenstaedt (1974) and others, a more accurate model such as this would have the simple vY term of eqns (3.12) and (3.13) replaced by an integral, leading to integro-differential equations. Hoppenstaedt (1974), Grossman (1980) and others have shown that—with exceptions in a few situations—there is not much difference between results obtained using what we henceforth call 'Type A recovery' (constant rate; Fig. 3.18(a)) and those with 'Type B recovery' (defined interval; Fig. 3.18(b)). In most of what follows, we use Type A recovery with an age-independent v.

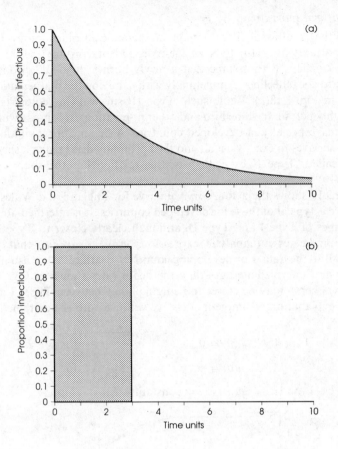

Fig. 3.18. Schematic representation of (a) Type A recovery from the infectious state and (b) Type B recovery from the infectious state. See text for details.

3.4.6 *Loss of immunity*

Equations (3.11)–(3.13) assume that immunity, once acquired, is lifelong. As discussed earlier, this is not the case for all microparasites.

Loss of immunity can be included in the basic model, to a good approximation, by terms describing the rate of transition from the immune to the susceptible class. Specifically, we add a term γZ to the right-hand side of eqn (3.11) describing changes in X, and we subtract a corresponding term γZ from the right-hand side of eqn (3.13) for Z. The parameter γ represents the rate of loss of immunity: if $\gamma = 0$, immunity is lifelong; if $\gamma \to \infty$, there is no immune response; and in general the average duration of immunity is $1/\gamma$.

3.4.7 *Natural mortality*

Most of the traditional literature on mathematical epidemiology takes the natural mortality rate, $\mu(a)$, to be an age-independent constant (see, for example, Bailey 1975). This is to assume that a newly born individual's probability of surviving to age a declines exponentially with a, having the mathematical shape depicted in Fig. 3.18(a). While such 'Type II' survival (in ecologists' jargon) may roughly pertain to some bird and other populations, it is grossly unrealistic for humans, especially in developed countries. A better approximation is that everyone survives to exactly age L, and then promptly dies (giving a survivorship relation called 'Type I' by ecologists; this relation has the shape shown in Fig. 3.18(b)).

Figure 3.19 shows the actual survival curve for England and Wales in 1977. This curve is typical of those for developed countries. It is intermediate between the extremes of Type I and Type II, although clearly closer to Type I. Figure 3.19 also indicates an analytic expression, $\mu(a) = c\exp(da)$, that gives an excellent fit to the data. For developing countries, death rates are usually higher at young and intermediate ages than the death rates shown in Fig. 3.19, and the survival curve may be closer to being half-way between Types I and II.

In our explanation of simple models, we will use both the extreme forms, as follows:

Type I: $\mu(a) = 0,$ for $a < L$ (3.16)

$\mu(a) = \infty,$ for $a > L$

Type II: $\mu(a) = \mu = \text{constant}(1/L).$ (3.17)

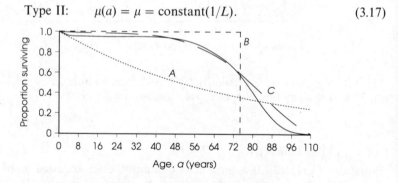

Fig. 3.19. Examples of Type I (short-dashed curve B) and Type II (dotted curve A) survivorship (or mortality) functions. The graph records the proportion of a cohort surviving to age a. The full curve records the age-dependent survivorship of females and males (combined) in England and Wales in 1977 (data from the Registrar-General's Statistical Review for 1977). The age-specific mortality, $\mu(a)$, is the logarithmic derivative of this curve with respect to age a. Average life expectancy from birth is 75 years. The Type I and Type II survivorship curves are set to give identical life expectancy. Curve C (long dashes) is a Gompertz function that assumes that the death rate, $\mu(a)$, rises exponentially with age. (From Anderson and May 1983*a*.).

In detailed calculations, we often use actual survival data or the analytic approximation indicated in Fig. 3.19.

3.4.8 *Disease-induced mortality*

The disease-induced mortality rate, $\alpha(a)$, has been omitted from most studies, and when it is included it is usually treated as a constant, $\alpha(a) = \alpha$ (Anderson and May 1979b). In reality, the mortality associated with malaria, smallpox, measles, infant diarrhoeas, and many other infections are typically greater among infants, especially in developing countries where such mortality is appreciable. We put $\alpha = 0$ in Chapters 4–12, and return to these questions in Chapter 13.

3.4.9 *Transmission*

The 'force of infection', λ, is the per capita rate of acquisition of infection. That is, $\lambda(t)\Delta t$ represents the probability that a given susceptible host will become infected in the small time interval Δt.

Sometimes, λ can be deduced directly or indirectly from epidemiological data. In other contexts, we may wish to close the system of equations by relating λ to the number of infected individuals. In this case, the usual assumption (e.g. Bailey 1975; Dietz 1975, 1976; Hoppenstaedt 1976; Waltman 1974) is that λ is linearly proportional to the total number of infectious individuals:

$$\lambda = \beta \int_0^\infty Y(a, t)\, \mathrm{d}a. \tag{3.18}$$

Here β is a transmission parameter, which combines a multitude of epidemiological, environmental, and social factors that affect transmission rates.

For an endemic infection, measurement of λ is, in principle, easy. In contrast, direct measurement of β is essentially impossible for most infections. But if we wish to predict the changes wrought by public health programmes, we need to know β. Such programmes change levels of susceptibility and infection, and thus change λ; β, on the other hand, is a constant characterizing the infection, and it is not changed by programmes of immunization or chemotherapy (although it can be altered by changes in personal or public hygiene, such as greater cleanliness or sanitation). Thus the procedure for attempting to make predictions about programmes of control or eradication, on the basis of eqns (3.11)–(3.13) and (3.18), is: (1) determine λ in the pre-control population; (2) thence determine the underlying parameter β (or some equivalent combination of parameters); (3) now calculate the new values of X, Y, Z, and λ for the new situation (which may, for instance, correspond to vaccinating a proportion p of all children essentially at birth). The main point here is that λ changes as epidemiological circumstances change, and so determining the value of λ is of predictive use only in so far as it leads to an assessment of the basic parameter β (which itself usually cannot be measured directly).

The conventional assumptions embodied in eqn (3.18) imply that λ does not vary with age. As reviewed in Chapters 8 and 9, this is rarely the case; λ is usually larger in the school ages, around 5 to 15 years, than at earlier or later ages. More generally, eqn (3.18) takes the form:

$$\lambda(a, t) = \int_0^\infty \beta(a, a') Y(a', t) \, da'. \tag{3.19}$$

Here $\beta(a, a')$ represents the probability that an infective of age a' will have contact with, and successfully infect, a susceptible of age a.

In these more general circumstances, which are discussed in detail in Chapter 9, the scheme outlined above for making predictions remains valid in its essentials (although the technical aspects of the calculations can become tricky). One problem is already clear. We need to infer $\beta(a, a')$ from the pre-intervention values of $\lambda(a)$. But if $\beta(a, a')$ is a two-dimensional matrix of quantities, depending on the ages of infecter and infectee, while $\lambda(a)$ is a one-dimensional vector depending only on a, we cannot infer β from the one-dimensional shadow it casts as λ. This problem is pursued in Chapter 9.

3.4.10 *Seasonality*

Many microparasites exhibit marked seasonality in transmission. Such seasonal patterns can derive from the effects of temperature or humidity on the survival of transmission stages of the viral, bacterial, or other parasite, or from the effects of weather either on the population biology of an intermediate vector or on the social habits of the human hosts. Temporal patterns in human activity, most notably in the bringing of children together at the start of the school year, can also produce annual cycles in transmission efficiency.

Whatever the cause, such seasonal variations in the effective magnitude of the transmission parameter β have been documented for measles, pertussis, chicken pox, and other microparasites. Some of these data are surveyed in Chapter 6, where some of the epidemiological consequences are also explored.

3.4.11 *Nutritional state*

We have implicitly regarded recovery rates, disease-induced death rates, rates of loss of immunity (v, α, γ, respectively), and other such parameters simply as biological entities that depend on the nature of the interaction between the infectious agent and the individual host. But such interactions in general depend on the nutritional state of the host. A poorly nourished individual will be usually more prone to acquire infection, slower to shake it off (slower to mount an effective immune response), and more likely to die of a severe infection, than a well-fed host. It is the combination of malnutrition and measles that makes measles a leading child-killer in many developing countries, while it is a relatively insignificant infection in those developed countries where it is still found to a significant degree.

We return to these complications in Chapter 13. But for most purposes we take no account of the important influence that nutrition can exert on the parameters v, α (and γ if immunity is not lifelong). Even in Chapter 13, the approach is to include observed values of the disease-induced mortality, α, rather than to let α be dependent on nutrition in some explicit way.

3.4.12 *Homogeneous mixing*

Probably the most significant and the most questionable assumption involved in eqns (3.11)–(3.13) and (3.18), and their friends and relatives, is that of homogeneous mixing. All the local details—school groupings, family size, geographical location, social habits—are averaged out, and epidemiological and demographic processes are treated as occurring at rates that depend only on the average number or density of susceptibles, infectives, and immunes. In particular, if λ is given by eqn (3.18), new infections appear at a rate that depends only on the product of the total numbers of susceptibles and of infectives, $\beta X Y$; infection is described as if by binary collisions in an ideal gas. The underlying philosophy is well expressed by Bartlett (1960): 'even if a multiplicity of detailed causes is operating to produce the observed broad classes of events, it is often an economy of thought . . . to ignore these and appeal merely to the operations of chance and the laws of averages'.

In this sense, the assumption of homogeneous mixing is a sensible starting point for theoretical studies. Tests against data, however, lead us to the conclusion that inhomogeneities associated with age-specific differences in contact rates, geographical location (cities versus villages), social and cultural factors (family size; number of sexual partners), and genetic heterogeneity within the host population (leading, for example, to 'carriers' versus normal infectives) all can be important in particular applications. These complications are discussed in Chapters 8–12.

3.5 Summary

We began by discussing the processes governing immunity in individuals. From this, we turned to herd immunity, and surveyed the sorts of epidemiological data that are sometimes available, emphasizing those kinds of information that help us understand infection processes at the population level. A basic model, comprising a homogeneously mixed population of susceptibles, infectives, and immunes, was then described. Various realistic refinements to this basic model were then outlined one by one; most of these refinements will be pursued in later chapters.

4

The basic model: statics

In this chapter, we restrict attention to the steady state of the basic model defined in Chapter 3. That is, we assume there is no time dependence in the variables X, Y, Z of eqns (3.11)–(3.13), so that they depend only on host ages, a: $X(a)$, $Y(a)$, $Z(a)$.

Such analysis of the statics of host–microparasite interactions is accompanied by two assumptions that are so routinely made that they usually pass unremarked in the literature (for example, Bailey 1975). The first assumption is that births and deaths are exactly balanced, to give a constant host population of magnitude N. The second assumption is to ignore mortality associated with the infection; that is, to assume $\alpha = 0$ in eqn (3.12). With $\alpha = 0$, the first assumption corresponds to the net birth rate, B, being given by

$$B = \int \mu(a)N(a)\,\mathrm{d}a. \tag{4.1}$$

Here $N(a)$ is given by eqn (3.10), $N(a) = X(a) + Y(a) + Z(a)$, the time dependence having dropped out. For a constant (Type II) mortality, eqn (4.1) reduces to $B = \mu N$, with $N = \int N(a)\,\mathrm{d}a$. For Type I mortality (defined by eqn (3.16)) the calculation is a bit more subtle (by virtue of the abrupt discontinuity at $a = L$), but it gives the commonsense result $B = N/L$. As μ may be related to life expectancy L by $\mu = 1/L$ for Type II survival, both results boil down to

$$B = N/L. \tag{4.2}$$

Under these assumptions, the static versions of eqns (3.11)–(3.13) reduce to the system of ordinary differential equations (Bailey 1975; Dietz 1975, 1976):

$$\mathrm{d}X/\mathrm{d}a = -(\lambda + \mu(a))X(a), \tag{4.3}$$

$$\mathrm{d}Y/\mathrm{d}a = \lambda X - (v + \mu(a))Y(a), \tag{4.4}$$

$$\mathrm{d}Z/\mathrm{d}a = vY - \mu(a)Z(a). \tag{4.5}$$

Adding these three equations, we get a differential equation for the number of hosts of age a:

$$\mathrm{d}N/\mathrm{d}a = -\mu(a)N(a). \tag{4.6}$$

The boundary conditions, as discussed earlier, are $X(0) = N(0)$ and $Y(0) = Z(0) = 0$, where $N(0) = B$ is the net birth rate, or number of hosts of age zero.

Integration of these linear equations is straightforward. Equation (4.6) gives simply

$$N(a) = N(0)\ell(a). \tag{4.7}$$

Here $\ell(a)$ is defined for notational convenience as

$$\ell(a) = \exp\left(-\int_0^a \mu(s)\,ds\right). \tag{4.8}$$

That is, $\ell(a)$ gives the probability of surviving to age a; it is the ecologists' and demographers' 'survivorship function'.

The age-specific number of susceptibles then follows from eqn (4.3), and is

$$X(a) = N(0)\ell(a)\,e^{-\lambda a}. \tag{4.9}$$

The corresponding *fraction* of hosts of age a who are susceptible is

$$x(a) \equiv X(a)/N(a) = e^{-\lambda a}. \tag{4.10}$$

Here we adopt a convention, followed henceforth throughout the book, of writing proportions or fractions (of susceptibles, infectives, etc.) in lower case letters, while writing total numbers or densities in upper case letters. (The expressions of eqns (4.9) and (4.10) can clearly be generalized to the case when the force of infection depends on age, $\lambda(a)$.)

The numbers of infected and of immune individuals are also easily found:

$$Y(a) = \lambda N(0)\ell(a)(e^{-va} - e^{-\lambda a})/(\lambda - v), \tag{4.11}$$

$$Z(a) = N(0)\ell(a)[1 - (\lambda\,e^{-va} - v\,e^{-\lambda a})/(\lambda - v)]. \tag{4.12}$$

(The generalization to an age-dependent $\lambda(a)$ is no longer trivial, which is why such complications are deferred to Chapter 9.)

These age-dependent patterns of susceptibility, infection, and immunity are illustrated in Fig. 4.1, with the parameters λ and v chosen to be representative of rubella (notice that the age-specific mortality, $\mu(a)$, has no effect on the proportions $x(a)$, $y(a)$, $z(a)$). Figure 4.2 shows corresponding data for rubella in southeast England in the early 1980s, before any significant vaccination of the male segment of the population.

4.1 Basic reproductive rate, R_0

In Chapter 2, we gave a general argument relating R_0 for a microparasite in a homogeneously mixed host population to the overall fraction who are susceptible at equilibrium, x^*:

$$R_0 = 1/x^*. \tag{4.13}$$

It should be stressed that this result, eqn (4.13), depends on assuming what might be called 'weak homogeneous mixing'; it assumes only that the rate at

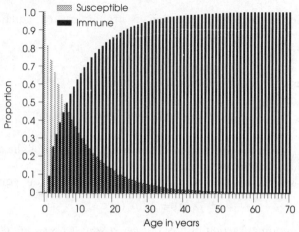

Fig. 4.1. Changes in the proportion of susceptibles, $x(a)$, and immunes, $z(a)$, as predicted by eqns (4.9) and (4.12) (the numbers $X(a)$ and $Z(a)$ divided by $N(0)$). Parameter values: $\lambda = 0.1$ year; $v = 31.74$ year; $\ell(a) = 1$, $0 \leqslant a < 70$, $\ell(a) = 0$ for $a > 70$.

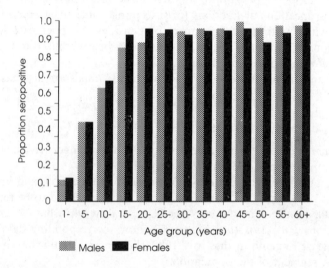

Fig. 4.2. Serological profile for rubella antibodies in a sample of sera collected in southeast England over the period 1980–4, which is stratified by sex and age (from Nokes *et al.* 1986).

which new infections appear is directly proportional to the total number of susceptibles, $\bar{X}$ (here and elsewhere the bar on $\bar{X}$ denotes the total number, integrated over all ages: $\bar{X}(t) = \int X(a, t) \, da$). In contrast, 'strong homogeneous mixing' makes the greater demand that infection rates depend both on the total number of susceptibles and on the total number of infectives, $\beta \bar{X} \bar{Y}$. It seems to us more plausible that the net rate of acquisition of new infections is proportional to $\bar{X}$ than to $\bar{Y}$; doubling the number of susceptibles in a school is arguably more likely to double the incidence of infection than is doubling the number of infectious individuals.

Be this as it may, we proceed to give simple expressions for, and numerical estimates of, R_0 based on eqn (4.13).

For the kinds of age-specific information about serology or case notifications that is described at the start of Chapter 3, we can calculate x^*:

$$x^* = (\bar{X}/\bar{N})_{\text{equilibrium}}. \tag{4.14}$$

Here $\bar{X}$ and $\bar{N}$ are the total numbers of susceptibles and of hosts, respectively, integrated over all ages:

$$\bar{N} = \int_0^\infty N(a)\, da, \tag{4.15}$$

$$\bar{X} = \int_0^\infty X(a)\, da. \tag{4.16}$$

The outcomes of such calculations for a variety of microparasitic infections are given in Table 4.1.

It is also interesting to note the analytic relations between R_0 (which characterizes the infection in a fundamental way, but which usually cannot be measured directly) and λ (which is essentially a derived quantity, depending on the number infectious, but which can be measured directly), for various assumptions about the mortality rate $\mu(a)$.

For Type I mortality, we have from eqn (4.8) that

$$\ell(a) = 1 \qquad \text{for } a < L, \tag{4.17a}$$

$$\ell(a) = 0 \qquad \text{for } a > L. \tag{4.17b}$$

It follows trivially from eqn (4.7) that $N(a) = N(0)$ up to $a = L$, and zero thereafter, whence

$$\bar{N} = N(0)L. \tag{4.18}$$

Substituting the appropriate form of eqn (4.9) for $X(a)$ into eqn (4.16) likewise gives

$$\bar{X} = N(0)(1 - e^{-\lambda L})/\lambda. \tag{4.19}$$

Thus for Type I mortality, which is a good approximation to reality in developed countries, R_0 is given by

$$R_0 = \frac{\lambda L}{1 - e^{-\lambda L}}. \tag{4.20}$$

Table 4.1 Estimated values of the basic reproductive rate, R_0, for various infections (data from Anderson (1982*b*), Anderson and May (1982*d*, 1985*c*, 1988), Anderson *et al.* (1988), Nokes and Anderson (1988)).

Infection	Geographical location	Time period	R_0
Measles	Cirencester, England	1947–50	13–14
	England and Wales	1950–68	16–18
	Kansas, USA	1918–21	5–6
	Ontario, Canada	1912–13	11–12
	Willesden, England	1912–13	11–12
	Ghana	1960–8	14–15
	Eastern Nigeria	1960–8	16–17
Pertussis	England and Wales	1944–78	16–18
	Maryland, USA	1943	16–17
	Ontario, Canada	1912–13	10–11
Chicken pox	Maryland, USA	1913–17	7–8
	New Jersey, USA	1912–21	7–8
	Baltimore, USA	1943	10–11
	England and Wales	1944–68	10–12
Diphtheria	New York, USA	1918–19	4–5
	Maryland, USA	1908–17	4–5
Scarlet fever	Maryland, USA	1908–17	7–8
	New York, USA	1918–19	5–6
	Pennsylvania, USA	1910–16	6–7
Mumps	Baltimore, USA	1943	7–8
	England and Wales	1960–80	11–14
	Netherlands	1970–80	11–14
Rubella	England and Wales	1960–70	6–7
	West Germany	1970–7	6–7
	Czechoslovakia	1970–7	8–9
	Poland	1970–7	11–12
	Gambia	1976	15–16
Poliomyelitis	USA	1955	5–6
	Netherlands	1960	6–7
Human Immunodeficiency Virus (Type I)	England and Wales (male homosexuals)	1981–5	2–5
	Nairobi, Kenya (female prostitutes)	1981–5	11–12
	Kampala, Uganda (heterosexuals)	1985–7	10–11

Usually we have $\lambda L \gg 1$ (before the advent of immunization), so that to an excellent approximation

$$R_0 \simeq \lambda L. \tag{4.21}$$

For Type II mortality, eqn (4.8) gives the survivorship function to be

$$\ell(a) = \exp(-\mu a). \tag{4.22}$$

The consequent expression for R_0 is even simpler than eqn (4.20). Equations (4.7) and (4.15) give

$$\bar{N} = N(0)/\mu, \tag{4.23}$$

and eqns (4.9) and (4.16) give

$$\bar{X} = N(0)/(\lambda + \mu). \tag{4.24}$$

Thence

$$R_0 = 1 + (\lambda/\mu). \tag{4.25}$$

Recalling the earlier identification $\mu = 1/L$, we can rewrite eqn (4.25) as

$$R_0 = 1 + \lambda L. \tag{4.26}$$

Thus an estimate of R_0 based on Type II survivorship is typically greater, by unity, than that based on Type I survivorship (eqn (4.21)). The slightly smaller, Type I, estimate is likely to be more reliable, especially in developed countries.

All this assumes a stationary population, with births exactly balancing deaths. If the host population is experiencing net population growth, things are complicated (as discussed in Chapter 13). But a good approximation can be obtained by observing that the life expectancy parameter, L, enters the above expression as the ratio $\bar{N}/N(0) = L$. In the more general case of a growing population, $N(0)$ represents the net number of births, $N(0) = B$, and L should be replaced by the reciprocal of the per capita birth rate, $G = \bar{N}/B$ (we are running out of letters of the alphabet!):

$$R_0 \simeq \lambda G \quad \text{for Type I,} \tag{4.26a}$$

$$R_0 \simeq 1 + \lambda G \quad \text{for Type II.} \tag{4.26b}$$

The difference between L and G can be significant, especially in some developing countries. For example, in a country like India life expectancy L is around 40 years, while births are around 40 per 1000 per annum which corresponds to $G \sim 25$ years. Use of L rather than G would give rough estimates of R_0 that were too high by almost a factor of two.

4.2 Average age at infection

It is intuitively plausible that the average age at which individuals acquire infection, A, is the reciprocal of the force of infection λ.

More rigorously, suppose we have serological studies of the host population, which determine empirically the number of hosts of age a who are susceptible, $X(a)$. Of these susceptibles, the number acquiring infection between age a and da (that is, 'at age a') is $\lambda X(a)\,da$, whence A is the first moment of the $\lambda X(a)$ distribution:

$$A \equiv \int_0^\infty a\lambda X(a)\,da\left(\int_0^\infty \lambda X(a)\,da\right)^{-1}. \tag{4.27}$$

For the relatively realistic Type I survival, substitution of eqns (4.9) and (4.17) into eqn (4.27) gives

$$A = \frac{1}{\lambda}\left(\frac{1 - (1 + \lambda L)\exp(-\lambda L)}{1 - \exp(-\lambda L)}\right). \tag{4.28}$$

Figure 4.3 illustrates this relation between A and λ. For λL significantly in excess of unity, eqn (4.28) gives

$$A \simeq 1/\lambda. \tag{4.29}$$

The correction terms are of relative order $\exp(-L/A)$, which will typically be less than 1 per cent for L in the range 50–75 years and A around 3–15 years

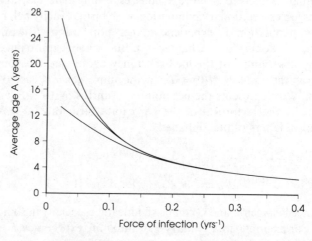

Fig. 4.3. The relationship between the average age at infection, A, and the force of infection, λ, as defined by eqn (4.28). The top line is for $L = 70$, the middle line $L = 50$, and the bottom line $L = 30$ years.

(before immunization). For Type II survival, eqns (4.9) and (4.22) together with eqn (4.27) give the simpler result

$$A = 1/(\lambda + \mu). \tag{4.30}$$

Again, eqn (4.29) will be a good approximation, although now the correction terms are of relative order A/L rather than $\exp(-L/A)$.

The definition of A given by eqn (4.27), which is based on the age distribution of acquisition of infection in the actual population, corresponds to what would normally be meant by 'average age at infection'. But public health information is commonly compiled to give the *proportions* susceptible in each age class, $x(a)$. By averaging the incidence of infection over the age-specific fractions susceptible, we define $\hat{A}$ as the first moment of the $\lambda x(a)$ distribution:

$$\hat{A} \equiv \int_0^\infty a\lambda x(a)\, da \left(\int_0^\infty \lambda x(a)\, da \right)^{-1}. \tag{4.31}$$

For Type I survival, A and $\hat{A}$ are identical, because all hosts survive to age L. For developed countries, this will be close to reality. For the opposite extreme of Type II survival, eqn (4.31) in conjunction with eqn (4.10) gives

$$\hat{A} = 1/\lambda. \tag{4.32}$$

That is, the approximate result of eqn (4.29) is exact in this case.

Anticipating Chapters 8 and 9, we observe that λ is rarely seen to be an age-independent constant, but rather is $\lambda(a)$. We can, however, still integrate eqn (4.3) for $X(a)$, to replace eqn (4.10) for $x(a)$ by

$$x(a) = \exp\left(-\int_0^a \lambda(s)\, ds \right). \tag{4.33}$$

By substituting this into the numerator in eqn (4.31) for $\hat{A}$, performing a partial integration, and ignoring boundary effects associated with the upper age limit (that is, taking the ∞ sign literally in eqn (4.31)), we arrive at

$$\hat{A} \simeq \int_0^\infty x(a)\, da \left(\int_0^\infty \lambda(a)x(a)\, da \right)^{-1}. \tag{4.34}$$

That is, in this more general case,

$$\hat{A} \simeq 1/\langle\lambda\rangle. \tag{4.35}$$

Here $\langle\lambda\rangle$ is defined as the mean value of $\lambda(a)$, averaged over the $x(a)$ distribution.

Table 3.3 lists the average age at infection for a variety of microparasites, at different times and places. The available data are such that some of these average ages are A (defined by eqn (4.27)), but most are $\hat{A}$ (defined by eqn (4.31)).

The average age at infection, A (or $\hat{A}$), is of intrinsic interest. Beyond this, rough knowledge of A and L can be used to estimate λ, and thence R_0. This is useful, both because A is a more intuitively evident quantity than λ, and because (partly for this reason) information about A is often available when it is not for λ, as such. For Type I survival, the appropriate relations, eqns (4.21) and (4.29), combine to give

$$R_0 \simeq L/A. \tag{4.36}$$

The correction terms, as above, are of relative order $\exp(-L/A)$. For Type II survival, the exact expressions, eqns (4.25) and (4.30), give eqn (4.6) as an exact relationship. For any general mortality function, $\mu(a)$, λ may be computed as a function of A from eqns (4.9) and (4.27), and thus R_0 computed for given A from eqn (4.13); eqn (4.36) will remain a good approximation in the general case. For host populations undergoing population growth, $R_0 \simeq G/A$ will, as before, be a better estimate than will eqn (4.36).

We conclude this discussion of R_0 and A by giving a simple, intuitive derivation of the approximate relation $R_0 \simeq L/A$. This pictorial method will be used repeatedly in what follows, to give intuitive insight into the more formal results. In Fig. 4.4, we first assume Type I survival: all hosts survive to exactly age L, and then die. Next we replace the continuously rising curve of age-specific seropositivity (fraction recovered and immune) of Figs. 4.1 and 4.2 by the crude assumption that all hosts remain susceptible up to age A, at which age they all acquire infection. The assumption of 'weak homogeneous mixing' gave us eqn (4.13), $R_0 = 1/x^*$, as discussed earlier. But in Fig. 4.4 the fraction susceptible is obviously A/L, whence $R_0 = L/A$.

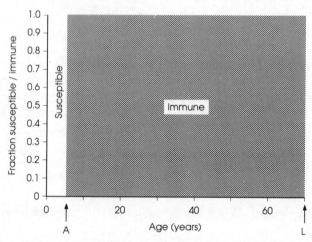

Fig. 4.4. As discussed in the text, this figure illustrates an intuitive way of estimating the fraction susceptible (and thence R_0) from knowledge of the average age at infection, A, and the life expectancy, L. It is assumed that everyone is susceptible (the unshaded area) up to age A, with everyone immune and surviving to age L thereafter (the shaded area). The fraction susceptible is clearly estimated as $x \simeq A/L$, whence $R \sim L/A$.

4.3 Transmission parameter, β

More formally, the force of infection, λ, is to be related to the underlying parameter, β, that captures the aetiology of the infection process. This relation is given, in the simplest case, by eqn (3.18):

$$\lambda = \beta \int_0^\infty Y(a)\, da \equiv \beta \bar{Y}. \tag{4.37}$$

From the explicit expression for $Y(a)$ given in eqn (4.11), we can calculate the total number of infectives, $\bar{Y}$, once the survival function, $\ell(a)$, is specified.

For Type II survival, $\ell(a) = \exp(-\mu a)$, and integration of eqn (4.11) over all ages gives

$$\bar{Y} = \frac{\mu \lambda \bar{N}}{(v + \mu)(\lambda + \mu)}. \tag{4.38}$$

Here we have used eqn (4.23) to write $N(0) = \mu \bar{N}$, where $\bar{N}$ is the total host population density. Equations (4.37) and (4.38) thus enable us to express λ as

$$\lambda = \mu \left(\frac{\beta \bar{N}}{(v + \mu)} - 1 \right). \tag{4.39}$$

Comparing this with eqn (4.25) for R_0 under Type II survival, we have an explicit relation between R_0 and β:

$$R_0 = \beta \bar{N}/(v + \mu). \tag{4.40}$$

Alternatively we could argue that the criterion for the infection to persist is that $\lambda > 0$, whence the first term inside the large brackets in eqn (4.39) can be identified with R_0. This approach is revisited in Chapter 6, when we look at the dynamics of infection.

For Type I survival, integration of eqn (4.11) gives

$$\bar{Y} = (\bar{N}/vL)[1 - (v\,e^{-\lambda L} - \lambda\,e^{-vL})/(v - \lambda)]. \tag{4.41}$$

As L is measured in decades, while $1/v$ (the duration of infection) is days or weeks, $\exp(-vL)$ is utterly negligible, except for a few long-lasting infections. To a less excellent, but still good, approximation we can neglect λ in comparison with v (because $A = 1/\lambda$ is typically a few years, at least). Then eqn (4.37) applied to eqn (4.41) gives λ in terms of β:

$$\frac{\lambda L}{1 - \exp(-\lambda L)} \simeq \beta \bar{N}/v. \tag{4.42}$$

Comparing this with eqn (4.20) for R_0 under Type I survival, we have an identification of R_0 in terms of β:

$$R_0 \simeq \beta \bar{N}/v. \tag{4.43}$$

The correction terms are of relative order λ/v or R_0/vL.

4.4 Latent periods and maternal antibodies

The above analysis can be extended, in a routine way, to include the effects both of a latent period (during which individuals are infected but not yet infectious) and of maternal antibodies (which protect new-borns, typically for 3–9 months). Although their inclusion is straightforward from a mathematical point of view, addition of these features makes for cluttered equations and tends to render the results less transparent. That is why we restricted the bulk of the presentation to the basic model (with only susceptible, infected-and-infective, and immune individuals). We now, however, indicate the essential consequences of including latent periods and maternal antibodies, placing most of the detailed results in Appendix A.

In the previous chapter we indicated explicitly (eqns (3.14) and (3.15)) how a class of latent hosts, $H(a, t)$, can be included. We also explained, in more general terms, how protection by maternal antibodies may be included in the model by assuming that hosts are born into an immune class, $I(a, t)$, from which they pass to the susceptible class at a rate d; $M = 1/d$ is then the average duration of such protection. In the equilibrium state, the numbers of protected, susceptible, latent, infectious, and immune individuals depend only on age a: $I(a)$, $X(a)$, $H(a)$, $Y(a)$, $Z(a)$, respectively. The appropriately extended version of eqns (4.3)–(4.5) is:

$$dI/da = -(d + \mu(a))I, \tag{4.44}$$

$$dX/da = dI - (\lambda + \mu(a))X, \tag{4.45}$$

$$dH/da = \lambda X - (\sigma + \mu(a))H, \tag{4.46}$$

$$dY/da = \sigma H - (v + \mu(a))Y, \tag{4.47}$$

$$dZ/da = vY - \mu(a)Z. \tag{4.48}$$

The equation for $N(a)$ is as before, eqn (4.6), and it still has the solution (4.7). These linear, first-order differential equations are easily solved, subject to the boundary condition $I(0) = N(0)$, $X(0) = H(0) = Y(0) = Z(0) = 0$ (which says all births are into the protected class, which is a reasonable approximation if essentially all adults have experienced infection). The solutions are listed in Appendix A. In particular, the number protected by maternal antibodies, as a function of age, is

$$I(a) = N(0)\ell(a)\,e^{-da}. \tag{4.49}$$

Here $\ell(a)$ is the survivorship function of eqn (4.8). The number of susceptibles (which is zero at age zero) is now

$$X(a) = N(0)\ell(a)d[e^{-\lambda a} - e^{-da}]/(d - \lambda). \tag{4.50}$$

Notice that the age-specific fraction who are susceptible attains its maximum value at an age a_m given by:

$$a_m = \frac{\ln (d/\lambda)}{d - \lambda}. \tag{4.51}$$

When the latent and infectious periods are short compared with other time-scales, as they usually are, this age a_m also represents the dip in the age-specific serological profiles. We see that if the average age at infection, A, is significantly larger than the duration of maternal protection, M (λ significantly smaller than d), the dip in the age–serology profile lies noticeably above M (specifically, $a_m \simeq M \ln (A/M)$). For instance, for measles in developed countries, where $A \simeq 5$ years and $M \simeq 0.5$ year, eqn (4.51) suggests a dip at around age 1.3 years.

4.4.1 *Maternal antibodies*

The assumption that—at the population level—protection by maternal antibodies decays exponentially at a roughly constant rate is reasonable. Figure 4.5 shows the decline, over the first year of life, in the number of infants serologically positive for rubella for serum samples collected in England. The data are well fitted by an exponential decay curve, eqn (4.49), with an average duration of protection $M = 1/d = 3$ months.

Figure 4.6 shows that this simple model is capable of giving quite a good description of actual data. The data are for the proportion serologically positive to rubella virus (that is, $(I(a) + Z(a))/N(a)$), as a function of age, in two Gambian villages. The theoretical curve is for the model defined by eqns

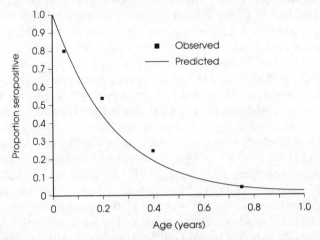

Fig. 4.5. The prevalence (proportion) of rubella IgG antibody in different age groups of infants from the Manchester area of England in 1977. The predicted curve assumes an expected duration of stay in the maternally-protected class of 3 months (from Anderson and May 1983*a*).

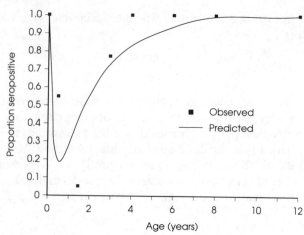

Fig. 4.6. Changes in the proportion of children with antibody to rubella virus with age in two Gambian villages (data from Clark *et al.* 1980). Solid squares, observed rates; full curve, predictions of the simple model defined in eqns (4.44)–(4.48) in the main text. ($A = 2.5$ years, $d = 0.25$ years, and $L = 50$ years) (from Anderson and May 1983*a*).

(4.44)–(4.48), with the Gambian parameter values $A \simeq 2.5$ years, $L \simeq 50$ years, and with d, σ, v having the values for the rubella virus ($d = 4\ \text{yr}^{-1}$, and σ and v from Table 3.1).

Figure 4.6 also points vividly to a problem confronting programmes of immunization in countries like The Gambia, where infection rates are high (that is, where the average age at infection, A, is low). The problem is that the age 'window' for effective immunization is narrow: immunization at too young an age will fail to evoke a lasting response, by virtue of the effects of maternal antibodies; immunization at too old an age is likely to find the child has already experienced infection. For rubella in The Gambia, for example, this age window (as shown in Fig. 4.6) is around one, or at most two, years wide.

Once the average age at infection becomes large relative to the duration of protection by maternal antibodies (A significantly in excess of M), the inclusion of such initial protection becomes a relatively unimportant refinement. This is seen in Fig. 4.7, which shows age-specific data for the proportion of young people (around Manchester in 1977) with antibodies specific to rubella virus. The accompanying theoretical curve in Fig. 4.7 takes no explicit account of those with maternal antibodies, but instead assumes that all 'susceptibles' remain uninfectible up to the age of one year; the ensuing curve is a reasonable fit to the data, for most practical purposes. The basic difference between the Gambian rubella data in Fig. 4.6 and the Manchester rubella data in Fig. 4.7 is that in the former case $A \simeq 2.5$ years (with a correspondingly narrow age window for effective vaccination), while in the latter case $A \simeq 9$ years (resulting in a wide age window).

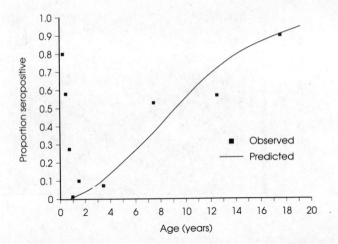

Fig. 4.7. Prevalence of antibodies to the rubella virus in infants, children, and young adults from the Manchester area of England in 1977. The solid squares are observed values and the full curve is the fit of the model with an age-dependent force of infection, $\lambda(a)$, which rises linearly over the age range 1–20 years (see Anderson and May 1983a).

In Appendix A, we use eqn (4.50) for the age-specific susceptibility to calculate the average age at infection, A, from eqn (4.27). The resulting formula is

$$A \simeq (1/d) + (1/\lambda). \tag{4.52}$$

The corrections to this formula are of relative order $\exp(-\lambda L)$ and $\exp(-dL)$ for Type I survival, and of relative order μ/λ and μ/d for the less realistic Type II survival; under Type II survival the formula is an exact result for $\hat{A}$, the average over the $\lambda x(a)$ distribution defined by eqn (4.31). That is, λ and A are related by

$$\lambda = 1/(A - M). \tag{4.53}$$

This result is in accord with common sense, representing a simple correction to allow for the fact that infants are not susceptible for an initial period of duration roughly M (whence A effectively becomes $A - M$).

Using eqn (4.52), rather than the earlier eqns (4.29) or (4.30), to substitute for λ in the appropriate equation for R_0, we obtain the result

$$R_0 \simeq (L - M)/(A - M). \tag{4.54}$$

This result is derived in Appendix A, where the simple approximation of eqn (4.54) is shown to differ negligibly from the exact expressions for either Type I or Type II survival. Equation (4.54) is to be compared with the earlier result $R_0 \simeq L/A$, obtained in the limit $M = 0$. From the viewpoint of the microparasite, the effect of protection of new-borns by maternal antibodies is to remove entirely individuals of age less than M from the host population; hence eqn (4.54).

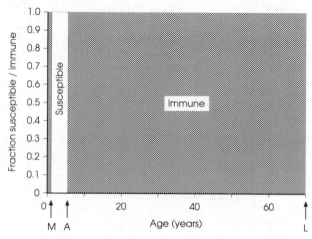

Fig. 4.8. This figure is similar to Fig. 4.4, except that the effects of maternal antibodies are caricatured by assuming that no one is a candidate for infection until age M is attained. The argument of Fig. 4.4 now gives $x^* \simeq (A - M)/(L - M)$, as discussed in the text.

Figure 4.8 extends the intuitive argument presented earlier in Fig. 4.4, including now a period of protection by natural antibodies that is of duration exactly M for everybody (in place of the less individually predictable reality shown by the data in Fig. 4.5). As everyone is always immune up to age M, the total population of hosts is effectively proportional to $L - M$ (rather than to L), and the number susceptible is similarly proportional to $A - M$ (rather than to A). Thus $x^* = (A - M)/(L - M)$, whence eqn (4.54) follows from the basic eqn (4.13) for R_0.

4.4.2 *Latent periods*

All the calculations relating R_0 and A to λ in the equilibrium state depend on various integrals involving $X(a)$. But the parameters characterizing the latent or pre-infective period do not enter into $X(a)$—see eqn (4.50)—so that all the above results hold true whether or not a latent period is acknowledged.

The latent period does affect the dynamics of the system, as will be seen in Chapter 6.

Even for the statics, it must be remembered that λ ultimately depends on the number of infectious individuals, and this number is affected by the presence of a latent class. Thus the latent period (of average duration $1/\sigma$) does affect the relation between λ and β, and thus can affect expressions like eqn (4.40) or (4.43) relating R_0 and β. As shown in Appendix A, for Type I survival the expression $R_0 \simeq \beta \bar{N}/v$ is unaffected (up to correction terms of order $\exp(-\lambda L)$,

$\exp(-\sigma L)$, $\exp(-dL)$, and $\exp(-vL)$). For Type II survival, eqn (4.40) is modified to

$$R_0 = \left(\frac{d}{d + \mu}\right)\left(\frac{\sigma}{\sigma + \mu}\right)\left(\frac{\beta \bar{N}}{v + \mu}\right). \tag{4.55}$$

Other things being equal, the existence of a latent period or protection by maternal antibodies, in a population with roughly Type II survival, tends to diminish R_0 (and thus to raise threshold host densities). These effects will be very slight, unless the duration of latency or protection is relatively long (such that $1/\sigma L$ or $1/dL$ is not negligible compared with unity).

4.5 Stochastic aspects of persistence of infection within a population

Having $R_0 > 1$, or host population densities above the threshold density corresponding to this criterion, does not guarantee that the parasite will be able to persist within the population in the long term. As briefly mentioned in Chapter 2, such persistence is dependent on the magnitude of stochastic fluctuations around the endemic equilibrium state.

Moreover, as will be discussed in more detail in Chapter 6, the equilibrium association between host and microparasite is not necessarily constant, but can often be a 'stable limit cycle' of some kind, in which numbers of susceptibles and infecteds wax and wane in well-determined periodic oscillations. Such phenomena commonly arise (in theory and in practice) in predator–prey associations, and they are likely to appear in microparasite–host interactions when transmission efficiency is high (large β), when the infection is short-lived, so that hosts rapidly recover to join an immune class or else rapidly die (v or α large), or when transmission involves long-lived infective stages (see Anderson and May 1979b, 1981, 1986). Many microparasitic infections of invertebrates and non-human vertebrates, as well as humans, possess these characteristics, and thus tend to induce oscillations (which can have large magnitudes) in the incidence of infection, and even in host abundance. What happens essentially is that, following a phase of relatively high susceptibility, infection spreads rapidly and causes the number of susceptibles to decline to low levels such that the reproductive rate of the infection is below unity; the next mini-epidemic of infection must await the replenishment of the susceptible population by births or by loss of immunity.

During the troughs in such cycles, the incidence of infection may fall to low levels and extinction can occur by stochastic effects. The probability of such extinction depends on the size of the host population and on the rate of replenishment of susceptibles.

A concrete illustration of these ideas is given by measles in human communities of differing sizes (Bartlett 1960a; Black 1966). From Bartlett's studies of cities in North America and Black's studies of island communities, before widespread

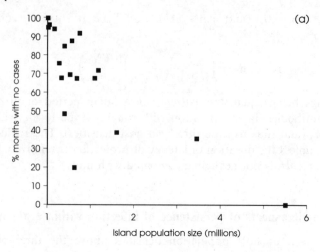

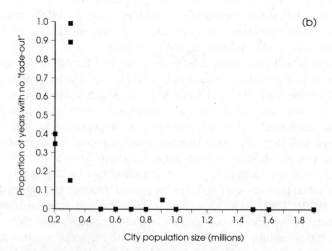

Fig. 4.9. The persistence of measles in island communities (a) and cities in the USA (b) of various population sizes. (a) records the percentage of months in which no cases of measles were reported in 19 island communities (data from Black 1966). (b) records the proportion of years in which no cases of measles were reported in one or more months for various cities in the USA for the period 1921–40.

vaccination, it appears that the measles virus is unable to remain endemic in communities of less than a quarter to a half a million people; see Fig. 4.9.

The critical community size for persistence depends not simply on total numbers, but also on demographic characteristics such as the net birth rate (which determines the rate of replenishment of susceptibles). A further twist in the problem of long-term persistence of infection in the absence of repeated re-introduction can be seen in the data for measles incidence in a large island

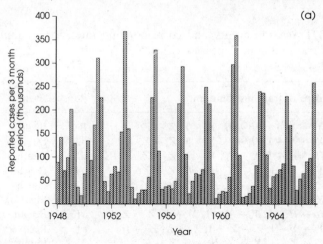

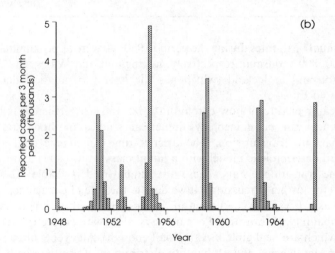

Fig. 4.10. Recurrent epidemics of measles as observed (cases per three-month period) (a) in England and Wales over the interval 1948–66 and (b) in Iceland over the same period (data from the Registrar-General's Statistical Review for England and Wales, and from Cliff *et al.* 1981).

(such as Britain) and in a smaller island (such as Iceland). As shown in Fig. 4.10(a), the measles virus persists endemically in England and Wales, showing recurrent two-year cycles in incidence (before mass vaccination, which began in 1968). In Iceland, however, the virus cannot persist endemically and the relatively infrequent epidemics are triggered by introductions by travellers (Fig. 4.10(b)); these miniature epidemics occur at roughly four-year intervals, presumably dependent on the net birth rate in the community, and between epidemics the virus often vanishes from the island (Cliff *et al.* 1981). The population sizes

Table 4.2 Transition events, and corresponding rates, for a simple stochastic model of transmission of measles virus ($N = X + H + Y + Z$) (Anderson and May 1986)

Label	Type of transmission event	Rate	Event
1	$X \to X + 1, H \to H, Y \to Y, Z \to Z$	B	Birth
2	$X \to X - 1, H \to H, Y \to Y, Z \to Z$	μX	Death
3	$H \to H - 1, X \to X, Y \to Y, Z \to Z$	μH	Death
4	$Y \to Y - 1, X \to X, H \to H, Z \to Z$	μY	Death
5	$Z \to Z - 1, X \to X, H \to H, Y \to Y$	μZ	Death
6	$X \to X - 1, H \to H + 1, Y \to Y, Z \to Z$	$\beta X Y$	Infection
7	$H \to H - 1, Y \to Y + 1, X \to X, Z \to Z$	σH	Becoming infectious
8	$Y \to Y - 1, Z \to Z + 1, X \to X, H \to H$	$v Y$	Recovery
9	$Y \to Y + 1, X \to X, H \to H, Z \to Z$	Λ	Immigration of infectives

and annual birth rates during the period 1960–70 were approximately 49 million and 700–800 thousand, respectively, in England and Wales, and 200 000 and 4–5 thousand in Iceland (which has the lowest population density of any country in Europe).

A clearer picture of how community size and net birth rate influence virus persistence can be gained by numerical studies of stochastic models of microparasite transmission. The discrete-time, stochastic equivalent of our standard deterministic model with a latent class (eqns (3.11) and (3.13)–(3.15)) has nine transition events. These are summarized in Table 4.2 (see Bartlett (1960a) for further discussion). If we denote the rate of occurrence of transition event i as r_i ($i = 1, 2, \ldots, 9$), then in the small interval of time from t to $t + \Delta t$ the probability of transition i occurring is $r_i \Delta t$ (with correction terms of order $(\Delta t)^2$, which are negligible if Δt is small enough). All events are assumed to be independent, whence the probability distribution of the time between any two successive events, $f(t)$, is

$$f(t) = r\,e^{-rt}. \tag{4.56}$$

Here $r \equiv \sum_i r_i$. The probability that the next event is of type i, p_i, is $p_i = r_i/r$. This comparatively simple stochastic model is difficult to study analytically, and is best investigated using standard Monte Carlo methods (Tocher 1963; Anderson and May 1986).

Figure 4.11 presents two examples of stochastic studies of temporal changes in measles incidence, for communities of 250 000 and 100 000 individuals. The other demographic and epidemiological parameters in Table 4.2 are assigned values roughly corresponding to measles in Iceland: $1/\mu = 70$ years; $1/\sigma = 7$ days; $1/v = 7$ days; $\Lambda = 7 \text{ yr}^{-1}$; $\beta = 0.008 \text{ yr}^{-1}$ (corresponding, via eqn (4.43) and the threshold condition $R_0 = 1$, to a threshold population of 6500 for persistence of the population in the deterministic case); and $B = \mu N$ (giving birth rates of 3570 and 1430 per year for the larger and smaller communities, respectively).

In the smaller community, Fig. 4.11(b), stochastic extinction occurs and the

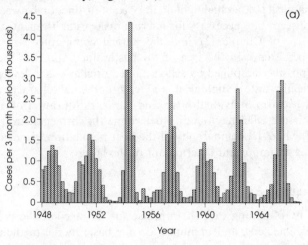

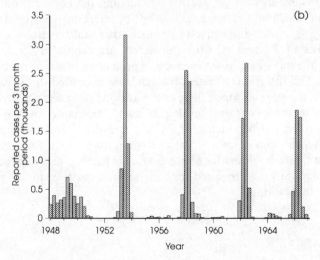

Fig. 4.11. Temporal realizations of a stochastic model of the transmission of measles (see text and Anderson and May (1986) for further details). The graphs record predicted cases of measles for a three-month period for two realizations. In (a) the community size is set at 230 000 people, while in (b) it is set at 100 000 people. Parameter values: latent and infectious periods, 7 days each; life expectancy 70 years; rate of immigration of infectives 7 per year; annual birth rate 3571 for the large community and 1428 for the smaller community; $N = 15\,000$ for (a) and 6500 for (b).

recurrent epidemics are triggered by the immigration of infectives. Notice that the interval between epidemics is around 4 years in the smaller community, and is roughly 2–3 years in the larger community within which the virus can maintain itself; this period falls to around 2 years in communities of half a million.

Such numerical studies highlight an important distinction between the critical density of susceptibles necessary for microparasite establishment (the threshold density of N_T of Chapter 2), and the critical community size required for long-term persistence in the face of stochastic fluctuations in the number of infectives (possibly amplified by self-sustained oscillations in levels of infection in the endemic state). Biological and environmental characteristics of the interaction between individual hosts and parasites (duration of infectiousness and transmission efficiency) tend to determine the former quantity (the N_T of Chapter 2), while the demography of the host population (particularly the net birth rate) is an important determinant of the latter.

4.6 Summary

We began by obtaining explicit formulae for the age-specific proportions of susceptibles, infecteds, and immunes for our basic model in the steady state. These results are used to get expressions relating the basic reproductive rate, the force of infection, the average host age at infection, and the transmission parameter (R_0, λ, A, β respectively) to each other and to serological or other data. Values of R_0 and A, thus calculated, are tabulated for a variety of infections. We show next how the effects of protection of newborns by maternal antibodies, and the effects of latent periods, may be added to the basic model; we focus on the ways in which these complications can affect the earlier results, and we test these ideas against serological data. The chapter ends by discussing stochastic aspects of persistence of a microparasite within a host population, using numerical simulations to draw an important distinction between the deterministic threshold density of hosts, N_T, for parasite establishment and the critical community size required for long-term persistence in the presence of stochastic fluctuations.

5

Static aspects of eradication and control

Implementation of a vaccination or other immunization programme has two main effects. The first and most obvious is the *direct* effect whereby a fraction of the host population is removed directly into the immune class by successful immunization. Such direct protection will, by itself, clearly result in fewer infections. The second and less obvious effect is *indirect*: a smaller number of infections implies a weaker force of infection, λ. Unimmunized individuals are indirectly protected, to a degree, by the diminution in the number of their fellows who are candidates for spreading infection. In essence, mass immunization has the indirect effect of creating a smaller population of hosts; in this sense, it decreases the microparasites' basic reproductive rate.

One important consequence of these indirect effects is that it is not necessary to immunize everyone in order to eradicate an infection. Once the vaccination coverage has reached some critical level, the microparasite will be unable to maintain its reproductive rate above unity. As it will never be possible to immunize every last individual, such indirect effects of 'herd immunity' are crucial in eradication programmes.

5.1 Overall criterion for eradication

The above considerations lead directly to a criterion for the overall fraction of the population that must be protected to achieve eradication, assuming 'weak homogeneous mixing'.

If a proportion p is successfully immunized, the proportion remaining susceptible is at most $x^* = 1 - p$ (it may be less by virtue of immunity acquired following natural infection). The effective reproductive rate of the microparasite is therefore

$$R \leqslant R_0(1 - p). \tag{5.1}$$

If the right-hand side of eqn (5.1) is less than unity, then $R < 1$, and the infection will not be able to maintain itself. Thus the critical proportion of the population to be immunized, for eradication to be attained, is

$$p_c = 1 - (1/R_0). \tag{5.2}$$

Figure 5.1 illustrates the dependence of this critical level, p_c, on R_0. Equivalently, Fig. 5.1 shows how p_c varies with A, using the relation $R_0 \simeq L/A$ to re-express eqn (5.2) as

$$p_c \simeq 1 - (A/L). \tag{5.3}$$

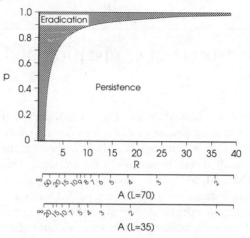

Fig. 5.1. The dependence of the critical level of vaccination coverage required to halt transmission, p_c, on the basic reproductive rate R_0, or, equivalently, on the average age at infection, A (see eqns (5.2) and (5.3)).

Table 5.1 Approximate estimates of the vaccination coverage (the degree of herd immunity) required to eradicate a variety of viral, bacterial, and protozoan infections in developed and developing countries (eqn (5.2) in the main text)

Infectious disease	Critical proportions (p_c) of the population to be immunized for eradication
Malaria (*P. falciparum* in a hyperendemic region)	99%
Measles	90–95%
Whooping cough (pertussis)	90–95%
Fifths disease (human parvovirus infection)	90–95%
Chicken pox	85–90%
Mumps	85–90%
Rubella	82–87%
Poliomyelitis	82–87%
Diphtheria	82–87%
Scarlet fever	82–87%
Smallpox	70–80%

Table 5.1 uses the previously derived estimates of R_0 for various infections (see Table 4.1) to give a rough assessment—using eqn (5.2)—of the overall level of coverage required for eradication.

Although the values of p_c given in Table 5.1 are only rough estimates, based on the assumption of homogeneous mixing, they point to some interesting trends.

Smallpox appears to have one of the smallest values of R_0 of these tabulated diseases, suggesting that a vaccination coverage of around 70–80 per cent in the neighbourhood of known cases is sufficient for eventual eradication. This fact, in conjunction with the apparency of the disease and the availability of an effective vaccine, may help explain the success of the global eradication programme.

Arita *et al.* (1986) have given a careful analysis of epidemiological data recorded for the smallpox eradication programme in African and Asian countries. They conclude that the persistence of smallpox after mass immunization, as revealed by a continuing incidence of cases, depended on population density as well as on the coverage level. These findings are summarized in Table 5.2, which condenses the data reviewed by Arita *et al.* (1986). The information in Table 5.2 helps explain why coverage levels of around 80 per cent succeeded in essentially eradicating smallpox in Africa, but not in Asia: for the three largest countries of the Indian subcontinent, the lowest population density of susceptibles remained around 17 per km^2 (in Pakistan, 1973), which was higher than the highest value observed in Africa (13 per km^2 in Nigeria, which significantly is the most densely populated country in western Africa, in 1969). In essence, the data in Table 5.2 testify to the dependence of R_0, and thus the immunization coverage needed for eradication, on population density.

Arita *et al.* (1986) note further that such association between population

Table 5.2 Estimates of population densities, densities of susceptibles, and reported cases of smallpox in countries in Africa and the Indian subcontinent, around 1968–73 (condensed from Arita *et al.* 1986)

Country	Population[a] (thousands)	Area ($km^2 \times 10^{-3}$)	Population density (km^{-2})	Vaccination coverage[b] (per cent)	Density of susceptibles[b] (km^{-2})	Reported cases of smallpox per km^2 ($\times 10^5$) 1973		
Bangladesh	72 000	143	502	80	100	22 875		
India	574 000	3280	175	80	35	2686		
Pakistan	67 000	304	83	80	17	3045		
						1967	1969	1970
Nigeria	53 730	924	58	77	13.4	514	22	7
Sierra Leone	2510	72	35	84	5.6	2357	111	0
Ghana	8440	239	35	93	2.5	48	0	0
Togo	1900	56	34	88	4.1	593	148	0
Benin	2650	113	23	80	4.7	721	51	0
Guinea	3840	246	16	90	1.6	622	7	0
Liberia	1490	111	13	83	2.3	5	0	0
Mali	4930	1240	4.0	95	0.2	24	0.1	0
Niger	3910	1267	3.1	79	0.6	94	2	0
Chad	3570	1284	2.8	78	0.6	7	0	0

[a] Population in 1973 for Asian countries, in 1969 for African.
[b] Vaccination coverage and density of susceptibles in 1973 for Asian countries, and around 1969 for African.

density and reduction in smallpox incidence for a specified coverage holds at the local level. For instance, a survey in Bolivia in 1958 demonstrated that, given the same vaccination coverage, there was a higher density of pockmarks in densely than in sparsely populated regions. Arita *et al.* stress, however, that their analysis shows this association between population density and continuing transmission also obtains at the regional and country-wide level.

As is often emphasized, the eventual global eradication of smallpox rested on the strategy of surveillance and containment by intensive vaccination in a 'ring' surrounding identified cases. Commenting that 'no adequate analysis appears to have been made as to why mass vaccination appeared to have been effective in some countries but not in others', Arita *et al.* (1986) make the case that the success of surveillance–containment rested on earlier achievements of high levels of herd immunity by mass vaccination, even though the actual such levels varied with population density. The smallpox story is more complicated, and tells us more about population-level aspects of epidemiology, than the conventional wisdom admits. Too many of the putative facts known to public health planners rest on enthusiastic retelling of plausible tales, rather than on controlled experiments or careful analysis of data. The study of Arita *et al.* is exemplary.

Even though the aetiology of measles is similar to smallpox, with the infection always apparent and running a relatively short course, the tentative estimate that R_0 is probably around 15 (corresponding to a critical coverage, p_c, around 90–95 per cent or more) for measles in developing countries is likely to make its global eradication much more difficult than was the case for smallpox.

The relatively small R_0 value, of around 6, for poliomyelitis was probably a contributing factor to the success of the immunization programmes that have essentially eradicated this infection from most developed countries. In contrast, immunization against pertussis (whooping cough) presents many problems, including questions about the efficacy of the vaccine, the need for several shots, and worries about possible neurological side-effects (albeit only in something like 1 in 300 000 instances); the relatively high value of R_0 for pertussis, which necessitates coverage of 90–95 per cent or more for eradication, is nevertheless a substantial additional problem.

The very high values of R_0 for malaria suggest that its eradication is likely to be very difficult, whatever the control method. In particular, a campaign against *P. falciparum* in certain regions of Nigeria based wholly on use of an effective vaccine would seem to require 99 per cent of the population to be protected for eradication to be achieved (see Molineaux and Gramiccia 1980).

5.2 Immunization programmes and new equilibria

To get a more explicit idea of how the indirect effects of herd immunity work, we show how the force of infection changes as a result of an immunization programme that falls short of eradicating infection.

For simplicity, we first suppose that a fraction p of each age-cohort of hosts is successfully immunized, effectively at birth. If we work with the simple susceptible-infected-recovered, or SIR, model of Chapter 4, this immunization scheme amounts to assuming a fraction $1 - p$ of hosts are born susceptible, while the remaining fraction p of new-borns move directly into the immune class: $X(0) = (1 - p)N(0)$ and $Z(0) = pN(0)$. Once this system has settled to its new equilibrium state, we denote the new (and smaller) force of infection by λ'. The new expression for the age-specific susceptibility, $X'(a)$, is a simple modification of eqn (4.9):

$$X'(a) = (1 - p)N(0)\ell(a) \exp(-\lambda' a). \tag{5.4}$$

Here the age-specific survivorship, $\ell(a)$, is as defined earlier by eqn (4.8). The total number of hosts of age a is $N(a) = N(0)\ell(a)$, as before.

So long as the infection continues to persist at some new equilibrium state following the implementation of the immunization programme, eqn (4.14) relating R_0 to the equilibrium values of $\bar{X}$ and $\bar{N}$ continues to hold. For relatively realistic Type I mortality, $\ell(a)$ is given by eqn (4.17) and we find

$$R_0 = \frac{\lambda' L}{(1 - p)[1 - \exp(-\lambda' L)]}. \tag{5.5}$$

For Type II mortality, the corresponding expression is

$$R_0 = \frac{\lambda' + \mu}{(1 - p)\mu}. \tag{5.6}$$

Unless social or environmental changes have accompanied the immunization programme in such a way as to change the basic biology of infection, these values of R_0 are as they were before any immunization. Thus for any specified death rate—be it the idealized Type I or Type II, or actual mortality data—the force of infection, λ', at equilibrium under a given immunization programme is found by first estimating R_0 from pre-immunization data, and then using the appropriate equation (eqn (5.5), eqn (5.6), or some generalization) to get λ' in terms of p and R_0.

For Type II survival, λ' decreases linearly as p increases:

$$\lambda' = \mu R_0(p_c - p), \tag{5.7}$$

with p_c given by eqn (5.2). The formula (5.5) for λ' cannot be inverted analytically, but the dependence of λ' on p is shown for a representative value of R_0 in Fig. 5.2. In both eqn (5.7) and Fig. 5.2, it is clear that $\lambda' \to 0$ as $p \to p_c$, as by definition it must.

More generally, if less transparently, we next consider the case where a fraction p of each age cohort are immunized at age b. Running through the

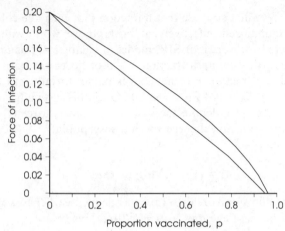

Fig. 5.2. The pattern of decline in the force of infection, λ', as the proportion vaccinated in the population, p, rises (see eqn (5.7)). The rate or force of infection declines to zero as $p \to p_c$ (see text). Two cases are recorded: in the top line the average age at vaccination, b, was set at 2 years while in the bottom line it was set at 0 years (immediately after birth). The value of R_0 was fixed at 15.

above arguments, but with this additional complication, we arrive at the expressions

$$R_0 = \frac{\lambda' L}{[1 - p\exp(-\lambda' b) - (1 - p)\exp(-\lambda' L)]} \qquad (5.8)$$

and

$$R_0 = \frac{1 + (\lambda'/\mu)}{\{1 - p\exp[-(\lambda' + \mu)b]\}} \qquad (5.9)$$

for Type I and Type II survival, respectively. These equations are derived in Appendix B. Equations (5.8) and (5.9) clearly reduce to eqns (5.5) and (5.6), respectively, in the limit $b \to 0$. The dependence of λ' on p given by eqn (5.8) with $b = 0.027L$ (corresponding to $b \simeq 2$ years in a developed country) is illustrated in Fig. 5.2, together with the result for $b = 0$.

Other kinds of immunization programmes, such as vaccination at some constant rate or according to some prescribed schedule of ages, can be similarly assessed. Some details of these more general calculations are set out in Appendix B.

5.3 Immunization programmes and average age at infection

The above expressions for age-specific susceptibility, eqn (5.4) for immunization essentially at birth, $b = 0$, or in Appendix B for $b \neq 0$, may be substituted into eqn (4.27) to find the new average age at infection, A', in the post-immunization population.

For Type I survival and immunization at birth, $b = 0$, we get

$$A' = \frac{1}{\lambda'}\left(\frac{1 - (1 + \lambda'L)\exp(-\lambda'L)}{1 - \exp(-\lambda'L)}\right). \tag{5.10}$$

From eqn (5.5), λ' can be found from R_0 and p, and thence A' can be calculated as a function of p for given R_0. Notice that in the eradication limit we have $\lambda' \to 0$, whence from eqn (5.10) $A' \to \frac{1}{2}L$. This is intuitively understandable: when the infection is on the brink of extinction, there is essentially no dependence of susceptibility on age among those remaining unimmunized, and infection is equally likely at any age; thus for a flat, Type I survival function A' is the average host age, $\frac{1}{2}L$. For small values of p, A' can be seen to behave as $A' = A/(1 - p)$. The more general expression for A' when immunization is at some finite age, $b \neq 0$, can be routinely calculated. Figure 5.3 illustrates the dependence of A' on p for the same values of R_0 and b used in Fig. 5.2.

For Type II survival and $b = 0$, we obtain the very simple result $A' = 1/(\lambda' + \mu)$. Combining this with eqn (5.6) relating λ' to R_0, and eqn (4.36) relating R_0 to the pre-immunization value of A, we get

$$A' = A/(1 - p). \tag{5.11}$$

In the limit $p \to p_c$ (corresponding to $\lambda' \to 0$), eqn (5.11) reduces to $A' \to L$.

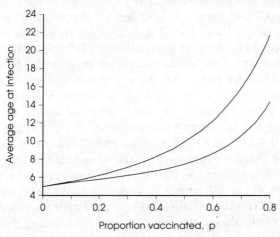

Fig. 5.3. The dependence of the average age at infection in a vaccinated population, A', on the proportion vaccinated in the community, p, for two different values of b, the average age at which children are vaccinated (see eqn (5.10)). The top line is for $b = 0$ and the bottom for $b = 2$; in both cases R_0 was 15 and L (human life expectancy) was set at 75 years. Note that the increase in A' as p rises is less severe when the average age at vaccination is set at 2 years as opposed to immediately after birth.

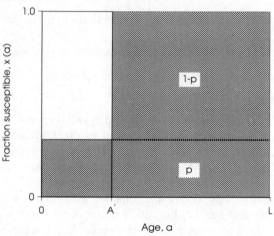

Fig. 5.4. This figure extends the intuitive arguments presented in Figs. 4.4 and 4.8, to show how the average age at infection is affected by immunizing a fraction of all new-borns. Again, the unshaded area represents those remaining susceptible (namely, the unimmunized fraction, $1 - p$, who are below the age of infection, A'). The fraction susceptible is now $x^* = (1 - p)(A'/L)$. If no other epidemiologically relevant changes accompany the immunization programme and if $p < p_c$, then we still have $x^* = 1/R_0 = A/L$, hence the results for A' that are discussed in the text.

This limiting result has the same intuitive explanation as the earlier $A' \to \frac{1}{2}L$ for Type I survival, with the technical difference that the average host age is $\frac{1}{2}L$ for Type I survival to age L, and is L for Type II survival with $\mu \equiv 1/L$.

We end this section by deriving the relation (5.11) between the average ages at infection before and after an immunization programme, by an intuitive argument along the lines of Fig. 4.4. As in Fig. 4.4, in Fig. 5.4 we make the crude assumption that all those who are not immunized effectively at age zero acquire infection at exactly age A'. The susceptibles are thus represented by the unhatched rectangle in the upper left-hand corner of Fig. 5.4, and they clearly constitute a fraction $(1 - p)A'/L$ of the total population. But if R_0 itself is not altered by social changes accompanying the immunization programme, this fraction susceptible is the same as for the pre-immunization state, which (from Fig. 4.4 or eqn (4.36)) is A/L. Hence $A' = A/(1 - p)$. As we noted above, this result is exact for Type II mortality, and is a good approximation for Type I if p is relatively small, always assuming homogeneous mixing. We will return to test this eqn (5.11) for A' against data in Chapter 8.

5.4 Programme-specific criteria for eradication

In the previous section, we obtained expressions for the equilibrium value of the force of infection, λ', under a programme that immunized a proportion p of each age cohort at age b. The critical level of coverage, p_c, that just produces eradication can be found from these expressions by taking the limit $\lambda' \to 0$.

Specifically, for the relatively realistic Type I survival, $\lambda' \to 0$ in eqn (5.8) gives the critical proportion to be immunized, p_c, as

$$p_c = \frac{1 - (1/R_0)}{1 - (b/L)}. \tag{5.12}$$

Using the excellent approximation $R_0 \simeq L/A$ (eqn (4.36) for Type I survival), we can rewrite eqn (5.12) as

$$p_c = \frac{L - A}{L - b}. \tag{5.13}$$

The corresponding expressions for Type II survival follow from $\lambda' \to 0$ in eqn (5.9), and are

$$p_c = [1 - (1/R_0)] \, e^{b/L}, \tag{5.14}$$

or equivalently

$$p_c = [1 - (A/L)] \, e^{b/L}. \tag{5.15}$$

As b/L is usually quite small, $\exp(b/L) \simeq 1/[1 - (b/L)]$, and the expressions (5.12) and (5.14) are effectively identical, as are eqns (5.13) and (5.15). Moreover, the assumptions of Type I and Type II mortality are extremes which bracket reality—see Fig. 3.19—so eqns (5.12) and (5.13) are likely to be robust results for this kind of immunization schedule. In Appendix B, we derive the analogous results for a programme that immunizes a proportion p of the population at a constant rate c (corresponding to an average age at immunization of V years), rather than at a defined age. The results are again identical with those above, up to correction terms of relative magnitude $(b/L)^2$ or, equivalently, $(V/L)^2$.

In short, these results are encouragingly insensitive to the details of the age-specific immunization schedules and survival probabilities. The reader may care to derive eqn (5.12) by the rough pictorial reasoning illustrated in Figs. 4.4 and 5.4, to check that these ideas have been grasped.

Equation (5.12), or (5.13), makes plain the unsurprising fact that eradication is easier if people are immunized at the earliest feasible age, b (allowing for the complications of maternal antibodies, which for pedagogical reasons have not been included in the illustrative analysis above). Eradication is simply impossible once $b > A$. Again, this is reasonable; to eliminate infection one must on average immunize people before they catch the infection. In the limit $b \to 0$ we of course obtain the earlier result $p_c = 1 - (1/R_0)$, eqn (5.2).

In Appendix B, we set out more general calculations for a situation in which a proportion p of hosts are immunized according to some arbitrary age-specific schedule, $c(a)$, while the remaining proportion, $1 - p$, escape immunization. In this more general (and correspondingly more realistic) framework we also allow for a crude kind of age dependence in the force of infection, by assuming the transmission parameter is some fixed function of age, $\beta(a)$; that is, we put $\lambda(a) = \beta(a)\bar{Y}$ in eqn (4.37). As briefly indicated in Chapter 3, the actual causes of age-specific variation in $\lambda(a)$ are likely to be more complicated than this, and we explore more realistic models in Chapter 9.

In these more elaborate models, the basic procedure for calculating the force of infection at equilibrium under a prescribed immunization schedule, and thence for estimating p_c (via $\lambda' \to 0$), follows the lines laid down in the relatively transparent calculations above. First, the age-specific force of infection, $\lambda(a)$, in the pre-immunization community is deduced from observed serological profiles or other information about susceptibility as a function of age. Second, the age-specific number of infectives, $Y(a)$, and thence the total number, $\bar{Y}$, are calculated in terms of this $\lambda(a)$. Third, the transmission parameter, $\beta(a)$, which describes the unchanging biological processes that govern transmission rates, is deduced (under the assumptions of this model) from $\beta(a) = \bar{Y}/\lambda(a)$. With $\beta(a)$ thus evaluated, we have a closed set of four equations for the four variables $X'(a)$, $Y'(a)$, $Z'(a)$, $\lambda'(a)$ under any defined immunization strategy; the fourth step is to solve these equations for $\lambda'(a)$ (adding equations for latent or maternal-antibody-protected individuals is simple in principle, although it complicates the computations). The fifth and final step is to find the critical coverage, p_c, for which $\lambda' \to 0$ and infection is extinguished.

This procedure is expounded more explicitly in Appendix B. Figure 5.5, however, gives a sense of the similarities and differences between such a relatively realistic calculation and the simpler, but more understandable, situations analysed above. Figures 5.5(a) and 5.5(b) are based on case notifications of measles and pertussis, respectively, in England and Wales in the years indicated; the figures give the force of infection in the period before or just after vaccination against these infections were introduced. These data indicate that $\lambda(a)$ does depend on age a, at least for the first few years. Figure 5.5(c) correspondingly shows the actual age-specific survivorship function, $\ell(a)$, for England and Wales (which is intermediate between Types I and II, though much closer to Type I). The actual age-specific schedules of vaccination against measles and pertussis is shown in Figs. 5.5(d) and 5.5(e), respectively.

If we now turn the handle on the machinery described above (estimating $\beta(a)$ from the information in Figs. 5.5(a)–(c)), and also make the dubious assumption that vaccines are 100 per cent effective, we find that the coverage—the overall proportion vaccinated—required to eradicate measles from England and Wales is around 96 per cent if the age-specific schedule of vaccinations has the shape of Fig. 5.5(d). For pertussis, with a vaccination schedule having the age-dependent form of Fig. 5.5(e), the critical coverage also turns out to be 96 per cent. These percentages could be reduced to the low nineties by concentrating vaccination on one-year-olds, but they would remain well above the levels actually attained under voluntary vaccination in Britain. Calculations that take more accurate account of the way transmission rates vary with the ages of infector and infectee will be pursued in Chapter 9, but we think Fig. 5.5 helps to motivate our discussion of relatively simple models (even though it is no longer 'state of the art').

5.5 Stochastic effects in the eradication of endemic infections

As we mentioned in Chapter 2, and in more detail in Chapter 4, the requirement that the reproductive rate exceed unity is a necessary, but not a sufficient, condition for a microparasite to maintain itself endemically in a host population. Even if the average number of infectious individuals is not oscillating in some systematic way (see Chapter 4), it is necessary for this average number at any one time to be sufficiently large that stochastic fluctuations (associated with the demography of small numbers) have a low probability of interrupting the chain and extinguishing infection.

Such possibility of 'endemic fade-out' has been discussed, in the context of mass immunization, by Katzmann and Dietz (1985). The rough requirement is that the average number of people carrying the infection (latent plus infectious) be of the order of 20–100. Since in simple models the number of such individuals in the steady state before any immunization is $N[1 - (1/R_0)](D + D')/L$, with $D + D'$ the average duration of infectious plus latent periods (see Chapter 6), the criterion for eradication by endemic fade-out is very roughly that $1 - p$ times the above expression should be brought below 20–100. On essentially this basis Katzmann and Dietz (1985) obtain the estimates of critical coverage, p_c, as a function of population density, N, that are summarized for measles in Table 5.3. Notice, incidentally, that the presence of a latent class

Table 5.3 Minimum proportion p_c to be vaccinated against measles in a population of size N ($R_0 = 15$, $D = 1$ week, $L = 70$ years) (from Katzmann and Dietz 1985)

N	p_c
5×10^6	0.75
6×10^6	0.83
7×10^6	0.86
8×10^6	0.88
9×10^6	0.89
10×10^6	0.90
25×10^6	0.92
50×10^6	0.93
75×10^6	0.93

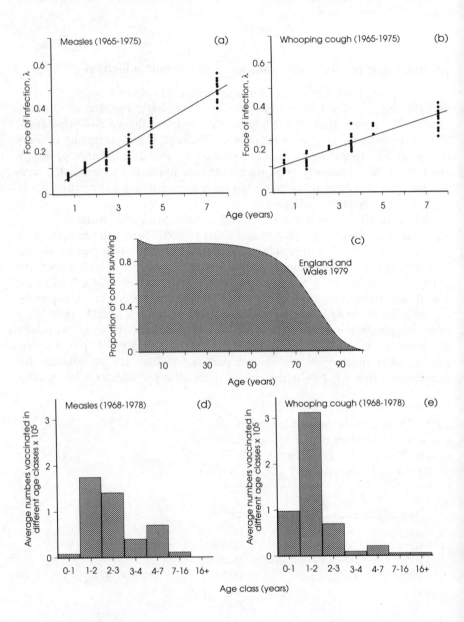

Measles (1965-1975)   (a)

Force of infection, λ

Age (years)

Whooping cough (1965-1975)   (b)

Force of infection, λ

Age (years)

Proportion of cohort surviving

England and Wales 1979

Age (years)   (c)

Measles (1968-1978)   (d)

Average numbers vaccinated in different age classes x 10⁵

0-1 1-2 2-3 3-4 4-7 7-16 16+

Whooping cough (1968-1978)   (e)

Average numbers vaccinated in different age classes x 10⁵

0-1 1-2 2-3 3-4 4-7 7-16 16+

Age class (years)

(infected but not yet infectious) helps to make stochastic fluctuation to extinction less likely, and in this sense acts to facilitate the persistence of a microparasite.

We will return to this topic, and present some Monte Carlo studies of this aspect of eradication, in the next two chapters.

5.6 The effects of immunization when the risk of serious illness depends on the age at infection

As a result of the direct and indirect effects of immunization, fewer people will experience infection. But the weaker force of infection in the community after immunization (produced by the indirect effects of the programme) means the smaller number who do acquire infection will on average do so at an older age.

If deaths or serious complications are more likely at older ages, it is thus possible that some immunization programmes could actually increase the incidence of serious cases. The likelihood of such a perverse outcome is not easily guessed, but rather requires a close analysis of the detailed interplay among several factors: the way serious illness depends on age, and the way age-specific incidence of infection is altered by the immunization programme (which in turn depends on the details of the programme and on the basic biology of the transmission process, captured by R_0).

It is often suggested that the history of poliomyelitis in developed countries represents a 'natural experiment' of this general kind. The argument was that, in earlier times, most people contracted this infection in the first few years of life, when it is less likely to have serious consequences. Increasingly high standards of cleanliness in Western societies in the middle decades of this century led to lower values of R_0, and thence to a diminished force of infection and a rise in the average age at which infection was acquired (albeit by fewer

---

Fig. 5.5. (a) The 'force', or instantaneous rate, of infection, λ, is shown as a function of age for measles in England and Wales between 1965 and 1975. The rate λ is estimated from data presented in the *Registrar General's Statistical Reviews*, by methods described by Griffiths (1974); λ is defined per annum per susceptible. The dots represent yearly estimates of the age-dependent rates, while the full line is the best linear fit. The relation between λ and age, a, up to the age of 10 years, is indeed described well by the linear expression $\lambda(a) = \alpha + ba$, where α and b are constants: $\alpha = 0.030$ and $b = 0.07$ (and $r^2 = 0.99$). (b) The conditions are as for (a), except that the data are for whooping cough (pertussis). The linear relation between λ and a here has coefficients $\alpha = 0.109$ and $b = 0.033$ (and $r^2 = 0.95$). (c) The age-dependent survival curve for the population of England and Wales in 1979. The age-specific mortality rate, $\mu(a)$, is the logarithmic derivative of this curve with respect to a. (d) The average number of individuals, in various age classes, who are vaccinated against measles is shown. These average values are for the span 1968 to 1978, and are calculated from data supplied by the Department of Health and Social Security, United Kingdom. (e) As for (d), except that the data are for whooping cough from 1965 to 1978 (from Anderson and May 1982*d*).

people, in total). Since paralysis and other complications are apparently more likely for infections in teenage or older individuals, poliomyelitis paradoxically became more troublesome as its transmissibility declined. Or so the story commonly goes. More recently, of course, in a notable triumph, the advent of safe, effective, and cheap vaccines has effectively eradicated poliomyelitis in North American and many European countries.

Rubella (German measles) is a particularly striking example of an infection whose seriousness depends on the age at infection. Usually a mild infection, rubella can cause the damaging congenital rubella syndrome (CRS) in the offspring of women who experience the infection in the first trimester of pregnancy. Encephalitic complications associated with measles infections are rare, but the probability of their occurring appears to increase as the age at infection increases. Conversely, in those developing countries where many children are poorly nourished, and where immunocompetence rises relatively slowly in the first few years of life, the risk of dying from measles is often higher for very young children than for those over 2 years or so; in these circumstances, disproportionate gains may be realized from programmes that raise average ages at infection without achieving eradication.

Motivated by these thoughts, we now present a formal framework for discussing such complications. The framework is then applied to an empirically oriented discussion of CRS, measles encephalitis, paralytic poliomyelitis, and orchitis arising from infection by the mumps virus.

5.6.1 *Age and risk of serious infection*

To get an intuitive feeling for the above-mentioned effects, we define $w^*(a_1, a_2)$ to be the number of cases arising in the age range a_1 to a_2 at equilibrium after the immunization programme is established, divided by the corresponding number of cases in this age range before any immunization. A programme that raises this ratio above unity is a candidate for concern. For the homogeneously mixed models discussed so far, new infections in the age class a appear at the rate $\lambda' X'(a, \lambda')$ at equilibrium in the post-immunization population, so that

$$w^*(a_1, a_2) = \int_{a_1}^{a_2} \lambda' X'(a, \lambda') \, da \left(\int_{a_1}^{a_2} \lambda X(a, \lambda) \, da \right)^{-1}. \qquad (5.16)$$

Thus defined, $w^*(a_1, a_2)$ can be calculated for any specific set of assumptions about the vaccination programme; λ' is given by the earlier results in this chapter.

In particular, for Type I survival, a policy that successfully immunizes a proportion p of all children at some age b (with $b < a_1$) leads to the result

$$w^*(a_1, a_2) = (1 - p) \frac{[\exp(-\lambda' a_1) - \exp(-\lambda' a_2)]}{[\exp(-\lambda a_1) - \exp(-\lambda a_2)]}. \qquad (5.17)$$

Here λ' is given implicitly as a function of R_0 (as is λ) by eqn (5.8) above. A

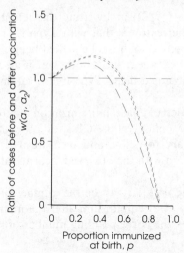

Fig. 5.6. The ratio $w(a_1, a_2)$ of cases after vaccination of a proportion, p, of children at birth, divided by those before vaccination, in the age range $a_1 = 16$ years to $a_2 = 40$ years. Long-dashed curve, prediction of eqn (5.17) in which survival is assumed to be type A of Fig. 3.19. Short-dashed curves, predictions of eqn (5.17) in which survival is assumed to be either type B or type C. The predictions are virtually identical (from Anderson and May 1983a).

similar expression can easily be obtained for Type II survival.

In eqn (5.17), the factor $1 - p$ comes from the direct herd effects of immunization, and acts to decrease w^* as p increases. In contrast, as p increases, indirect effects act to decrease λ', as illustrated earlier in Fig. 5.2. As a result, the factor inside the square brackets in the numerator in eqn (5.17) becomes increasingly larger than the corresponding factor inside square brackets in the denominator as p increases. Whether the net outcome of these countervailing effects causes w^* to increase or to decrease with increasing p depends on a_1, a_2, and R_0.

Figure 5.6 illustrates eqn (5.17), and similar results with other assumptions about the survival curve, in the case where immunization is essentially at birth. The ratio w^* is plotted against p for the parameter values $a_1 = 16$ and $a_2 = 40$ years, $L = 75$ years, and $R_0 = 8$; this roughly corresponds to the situation of interest for rubella in developed countries (where A was around 9 years before vaccination was begun). Several interesting points emerge from Fig. 5.6. First, as originally observed by Knox (1980), in this circumstance the equilibrium ratio w^* rises above unity for low to moderate levels of vaccination coverage, p. Second, calculations based on the assumption of an age-independent, Type II, mortality rate (as conventional in much of the literature on mathematical epidemiology, and as used in studies of rubella by Dietz (1981) and Hethcote (1983)) give results somewhat different from those obtained by using Type I survival (as did Knox (1980)) or by using the actual death rates in England and Wales in 1977; the reason is that with Type II survival a significant (and unrealistically high) number of hosts have died before becoming candidates for infection in the 16–40 year age range. Third, there is an encouraging concordance between the results obtained using Type I survival and those based on actual survivorship data.

To assess the impact of mass immunization on the incidence of measles encephalitis, paralytic poliomyelitis, CRS, or other serious complications of infection, it is necessary to define and measure a risk function whose value varies with age in accord with the observed facts about such complications. We call this risk function $r(a)$.

We may now define $\rho^*(a_1, a_2)$ to be the number of cases of serious disease in the age range a_1 to a_2 at equilibrium after the immunization programme is established, divided by the corresponding number of such serious cases before immunization:

$$\rho^*(a_1, a_2) = \int_{a_1}^{a_2} r(a)\lambda'X'(a, \lambda')\,\mathrm{d}a\left(\int_{a_1}^{a_2} r(a)\lambda X(a, \lambda)\,\mathrm{d}a\right)^{-1}. \quad (5.18)$$

We will usually be interested in the ratio of the total number of serious cases after versus before immunization: this ratio is formally $\rho^*(0, \infty)$. Clearly, all such calculations follow the lines laid down above for ratios of age-specific infections, $w^*(a_1, a_2)$. We now proceed to an explicit discussion of these ideas in relation to rubella, measles, and poliomyelitis.

5.6.2 Rubella

Rubella is worldwide in distribution, except in remote and isolated communities. Transmission is direct, by droplet spread or direct contact, and virus may be recovered from the nasopharyngeal secretions, blood, urine, and faeces of infected people. The incubation time (time from infection to appearance of symptoms) is about 14–21 days, and the infectious period is about 7 days before the onset of symptoms (rash) until at least 4 days after such onset. In other words, the latent period is 7–14 days and the infectious period is 11–14 days.

Symptoms of rubella are few in children, and as many as 20–50 per cent of the cases may occur without an evident rash. It is the hazard of significant congenital defects in offspring of women who acquire rubella during pregnancy that motivate efforts to control the disease by immunization. This association between congenital abnormalities and maternal rubella during pregnancy was first made in Australia in 1941 (Gregg 1941). Congenital rubella syndrome (CRS) occurs among 80 per cent of infants born to women who contract apparent or inapparent rubella during the first trimester of pregnancy, with the probability decreasing thereafter (Benenson 1975; South and Sever 1985). The syndrome includes cataracts, mental retardation, deafness, and cardiac defects (see Hanshaw and Dudgeon (1978) for a thorough review).

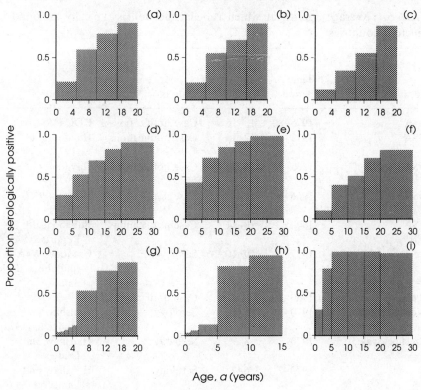

Fig. 5.7. Age–prevalence curves (based on horizontal studies) of the proportions of different age classes who have experienced an attack of rubella. (a)–(c) Data from Illinois, Massachusetts, and New York City, USA for three different periods: (a) 1966–8; (b) 1969–71; and (c) 1972–4. Immunization was initiated in 1969 (Hayden *et al.* (1977); based on case notification records). (d) Data from West Germany 1970–7 (Hanshaw and Dudgeon (1978); based on serology). (e) Data from Poland 1970–7 (Hanshaw and Dudgeon (1978); based on serology). (f) Data from United Kingdom 1970–2. (g) Data from Baltimore 1943 (based on case notifications). (h) Data from Scotland (based on case notifications). (i) Data from The Gambia 1966–76 (Clarke *et al.* (1980); based on serology). In all graphs, immunity resulting from maternal antibodies is not recorded.

The epidemiology of rubella, as revealed by cross-sectional serological surveys (stratified by age) or by case-notification records, varies from place to place, depending on such things as community size, net birth rate, and social and environmental conditions. Figure 5.7 illustrates this, recording nine examples of the prevalence of those who have had rubella, in various age classes in different communities throughout the world. As documented in Table 5.4, the average age at infection, *A*, varies from 2–3 years in The Gambia in 1976 to 13–16 years in the USA during 1978–80 (following the beginning of systematic vaccination). Notice that CRS is not a cause for concern in The Gambia, since virtually

Table 5.4 Average age, A, at which rubella infection is typically acquired in different countries

Location	Time period	Average age, A (years)	Data base	Data source
USA	1978–80	13–16	Case notifications	CDC (1981a)
USA	1972–4	12–14	Case notifications	Haydon et al. (1977)
USA	1969–71	10–11	Case notifications	Haydon et al. (1977)
USA	1966–8	9–10	Case notifications	Haydon et al. (1977)
USA	1943	10–11	Case notifications	Public Health Reports USA
England and Wales	1977	9–10	Serology	Cradock–Watson (unpublished data)
Scotland	1950–60	6–7	Case notifications	
West Germany	1970–7	11–12	Serology	Hanshaw and Dudgeon (1978)
Czechoslovakia	1970–7	8–9	Serology	Hanshaw and Dudgeon (1978)
Poland	1970–7	6–7	Serology	Hanshaw and Dudgeon (1978)
The Gambia	1976	2–3	Serology	Clark et al. (1980)

100 per cent of people over the age of 5 years have experienced infection (Clark *et al.* 1980). In contrast, in the UK prior to the introduction of immunization in 1970, roughly 10–15 per cent of 20-year-old women were susceptible to infection (Urquhard 1980; Clark *et al.* 1980; Nokes *et al.* 1986).

As discussed earlier (see Fig. 4.5) protection against rubella by maternal antibodies characteristically lasts about 3–6 months, but with considerable individual variation (Nokes *et al.* 1986). Such protection is not a key ingredient for models of rubella in developed countries (see Fig. 4.7 and the accompanying discussion), but it would be important for the kind of situation found in The Gambia (see Fig. 4.6). In what follows, we take rough account of protection by maternal antibodies simply by assuming that all infants enter the susceptible class at the age of 1 year.

The force of infection is taken to rise linearly with age in the pre-vaccination community, from age 1 to age 20 years (specifically, $\lambda(a) = c_1 + c_2 a$, with $c_1 = 0.032$ and $c_2 = 0.0118$; for $a > 20$, $\lambda = \lambda(20)$). This is done to provide a better fit to the serological data in the UK and the USA. Such age dependence is derived from an underlying $\beta(a)$, as discussed earlier. This leads to an average

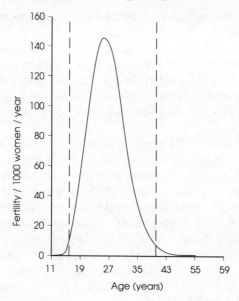

Fig. 5.8. The age-specific fertility of women, $m(a)$, in England and Wales in 1980. The fertility rate is defined per 1000 women per year. A precise empirical fit to the data in the age range 16–40 years of age (encompasses 99 per cent of all recorded births) is obtained by the polynomial $m(a) = c_1 + c_2 a + c_3 a^2 + c_4 a^3 + c_5 a^4 + c_6 a^5 + c_7 a^6$ with coefficients $c_1 = 5256.0$, $c_2 = -1058.0$, $c_3 = 78.47$, $c_4 = -2.59$, $c_5 = 0.0342$, $c_6 = -0.0$, $c_7 = -0.2523 \times 10^{-5}$ ($r^2 = 0.997$). The data are from the *Registrar General's Statistical Review* for 1980.

age at infection, before vaccination, of $A = 9.2$ years (Anderson and May 1983a). Our value is somewhat less than the value assumed by Knox (1980), and following him by Dietz (1981) and Hethcote (1983). Knox's value is based on the single, qualitative observation that around 70 per cent of 14-year-olds are immune; although seminal in its ideas, Knox's paper—and subsequently Dietz's formal elaboration of it—is also notable for this being the only datum to intrude into it.

We take the annual number of cases of CRS in infants born to mothers of different ages to be proportional to the age-specific fertility rates. For most developed countries today, the pattern of age-specific fertility is similar to that for England and Wales in 1980, which is shown in Fig. 5.8. Peak fertility occurs around 25 years of age, and 99 per cent of all births take place in the maternal age range 16–40 years. As ρ^* involves the ratio between cases after and before vaccination, we can simply define the risk function, $r(a)$, for CRS to be the age-specific fertility rate.

Finally, in the absence of clear evidence to the contrary, we assume that successful immunization induces permanent immunity to infection (Preblud *et al.* 1980).

With these important factual preliminaries disposed of, we now turn to use eqn (5.18) to evaluate $\rho^*(16, 40)$, which is an excellent approximation to the ratio between the total incidence of CRS after and before implementation of a defined vaccination programme. The quantities $v(a)$ and $\lambda(a)$ are obtained from data in the manner just described, and $\lambda'(a)$ is computed by the methods explained above.

We consider first the USA immunization policy, which aims (successfully it would seem) to eradicate rubella by vaccinating essentially all girls and boys before they enter pre-school kindergarten or elementary school (but after the age of 15 months, to guard against maternal-antibody protection). Idealizing this to be a policy of vaccinating a proportion p of each age cohort at exactly 1 year of age ($b = 1$), but otherwise retaining the realistic elements just described, we obtain the full curves in Figs. 5.9(a) and 5.9(b) for the equilibrium ratio ρ^* as a function of the proportion vaccinated, p. The different curves are, as indicated, for different assumptions about the average age at infection, A, before any vaccination; the curve labelled $A = 9$ corresponds to the actual situation in the USA and the UK.

Notice that ρ^* drops to zero as p approaches the critical level of coverage, which by virtue of the indirect effects of herd immunity is always below 100 per cent (this particular feature is presented wrongly in Knox's (1980) paper, which has $\rho^* \to 0$ only as $p \to 1$). Notice also that coverage levels of less than 50 per cent would perversely lead to an increase in the incidence of CRS in the USA and UK (the $A = 9$ curve).

In the UK, where vaccination of children has never been required for entrance to school or kindergarten (as it is now in all 50 states of the USA), p for rubella vaccination has been around 60 per cent, rising to 80–90 per cent in recent years. Consequently, the immunization strategy in the UK has been to vaccinate a proportion p of girls, and only girls, in the age range 10–15 years, thus taking advantage of the immunity acquired by natural infection in the first 10–15 years of life. Such a policy may be idealized as vaccinating a fraction $p/2$ of the population at age 12 years (assuming a 1:1 sex ratio at this age). The formula (5.17) still has the full factor $1 - p$ appearing on the right-hand side, because all cases of CRS come from the unvaccinated females. The dashed curves in Figs. 5.9(a) and 5.9(b) show the value of the ratio ρ^* as a function of p, the proportion of 12-year-old girls vaccinated; as A varies from 3 to 18 years, the differences among the curves for the UK policy are less than the thickness of the dashed line.

This ρ^*–p relation for the UK policy may be easily understood. The policy of vaccinating at most half the population at age 12 has little impact on the force of infection ($\lambda' \simeq \lambda$), and so it cannot eradicate rubella even at high levels of coverage. But it does protect females directly, without the offsetting indirect effects that characterize the 'everybody-at-age-one' policy at modest values of p.

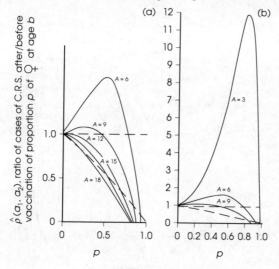

Fig. 5.9. (a) Rubella. The equilibrium ratio $\hat{\rho}(a_1, a_2)$ of rubella cases in pregnant women in the age range 16–40 years after vaccination of a proportion p at age b, divided by the cases before vaccination. The age-specific fertility function, $m(a)$, employed to calculate $\hat{\rho}(a_1, a_2)$ is as defined in Fig. (5.8), and we assume a type B survival function with a life expectancy of 75 years. Full curves show changes in the ratio for various values of p under the US policy where boys and girls are vaccinated at age 1 year ($b = 1.0$), for various values of the average age at infection, A, prior to vaccination, ranging from 6 to 18 years. The broken line intersecting the horizontal axis at $p = 1.0$ is the ratio for the UK policy where girls and only girls are vaccinated at age 12 years ($b = 12$). For A values between 6 and 18, the value of the ratio $\hat{\rho}(a_1, a_2)$ is virtually identical for the UK policy for all values of p. The horizontal broken line denotes the ratio value of unity. (b) Rubella. Identical to (a) but including changes in $\hat{\rho}(a_1, a_2)$ for an average age at infection, A, of 3 years (to mirror events in the Gambian community discussed in the main text) (from Anderson and May 1983a).

This tendency for vaccination of girls, and girls only, after the average age at infection to have little impact on the overall level of herd immunity is illustrated in Fig. 5.10. Here the pattern of herd immunity from 1969 to 1985 in South Yorkshire in the United Kingdom is reflected in a longitudinal (through time) and horizontal (across age classes) study of seropositivity for antibodies to the rubella virus. Note that vaccination of teenage girls against rubella was started in 1970 (see Nokes *et al.* 1987).

Figure 5.11 summarizes much of this work, by showing the value of p at which 'UK' and 'USA' policies are equally effective (in the sense of leading to the same incidence of CRS), for various values of A. The cross-over point is at around 85 per cent coverage: below this level (as in the UK), the UK policy affords better protection against CRS; above this level (as in the USA) the USA policy is better. Intuitive arguments can suggest these general trends, but they cannot produce quantitative estimates such as the 85 per cent cross-over level.

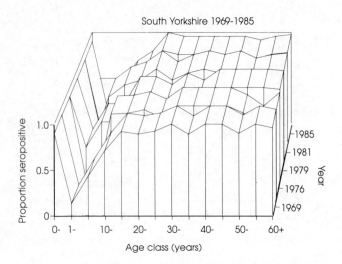

Fig. 5.10. Cross-sectional serological profiles of rubella antibodies in South Yorkshire, 1969–85. Little change can be seen in the age–serological profiles when observed longitudinally, from pre-vaccination 1969 through a number of post-vaccination years. (Note that sample sets for each of the years are independent.) From Nokes (1987).

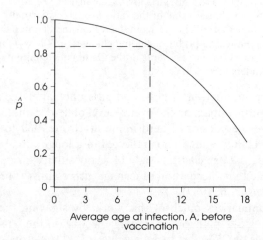

Fig. 5.11. Rubella. The critical level of immunization, $\hat{p}$, above which the US policy has a greater impact on the incidence of CRS than UK policy, for various values of the average age at infection, A, prior to vaccination. Broken line shows the current situation in the UK and US where $A = 9$ years.

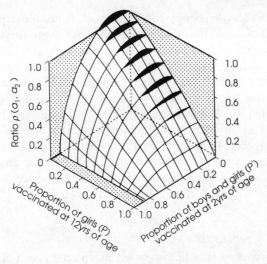

Fig. 5.12. The ratio $\rho(a_1, a_2)$ of the predicted number of CRS cases arising from pregnancies in the age range 16–40 years after vaccination, divided by the number in the same age range before control, plotted as a function of the proportion (p_a) of boys and girls vaccinated at 2 years of age and the proportion (p_g) of girls vaccinated at 12 years of age. The average age at infection before immunization was assumed to be 9 years and the methods used in the calculation of $\rho(a_1, a_2)$ are detailed in Anderson and May (1983a). In the shaded regions a two-stage policy is predicted to increase the number of CRS cases over the number of cases arising under the current policy.

With coverage approaching 80 per cent of 12-year-old girls in recent years in the UK, there is thought of combining continued such coverage with vaccination of as many 1- to 2-year-old boys and girls as possible. Figure 5.12 endeavours to show the consequent two-dimensional surface of ρ^* values as a function both of the proportion p_g of 12-year-old girls and of the proportion p_a of all 2-year-olds so vaccinated. It will be seen that such an extended vaccination policy is unlikely to increase CRS in the UK (provided the current 80 per cent coverage of 12-year-old girls is maintained), but neither is it likely to do much good unless high coverage is achieved among 2-year-olds.

As part of the global initiative toward immunization against childhood infections, it is sometimes suggested that measles vaccine might be better administered as MMR (measles, mumps, rubella). After all, the argument runs, why not have the extra protection? Figure 5.9(b) shows why it would be foolish to immunize young children against rubella in a country like The Gambia where current values of A are around 3 years; 80 per cent coverage of 1- to 2-year-olds against rubella could increase the (admittedly small) incidence of CRS in The Gambia by a factor 10 or more.

The above calculations, and their biological background, are presented much more fully in Anderson and May (1983a).

We are all familiar with some of the differences between group interests and individual interests with respect to vaccination. Thus most people have an intuitive appreciation that the best vaccination programme, from an individual's point of view, is one where almost everyone else is vaccinated while they are not, so that they are indirectly protected without incurring any of the risks or inconveniences associated with direct protection. The situation for CRS, however, can stand this thinking on its head: at, say, 30 per cent coverage, it is best for an individual female to be protected by vaccination; but, on average, each individual case of CRS thus prevented produces more than one case of CRS in the unprotected female population. That is, if better than 30–50 per cent coverage of young children is not possible, it is in the group's interest to have no vaccination, but in an individual's interest to be vaccinated (and better still, of course, to adopt a UK or other policy).

5.6.3 *Measles encephalitis*

The epidemiology of measles has attracted much attention, partly because the characteristic symptoms of this acute and highly communicable viral infection facilitate accurate diagnosis. Transmission is by droplet spread on direct contact, and the latent and infectious periods are around 6–9 and 6–7 days, respectively.

Death from measles in developed countries, resulting from respiratory or neurological complications, has been low over the past 30 years (1 in 3000–5000 notified cases), but the morbidity is often high. The severity of measles is greatly affected by the child's nutritional state, and very high case fatality rates (up to 20–30 per cent) are recorded in developing countries where malnutrition is rife. Measles is also thought to be a common cause of blindness in communities with vitamin A deficiencies, and to increase susceptibility to secondary infections as a result of its severe impact on the immune system of the patient.

In developed countries, measles encephalitis occurs in approximately 1 of every 2000 reported cases (CDC, 1981b). Survivors often have permanent brain damage and mental retardation. The risk of measles encephalitis is known to increase with age: Fig. 5.13(a) shows data for the incidence of measles encephalitis per case of measles, as a function of age, in the USA in 1973–5; Fig. 5.13(b) shows similar data from the UK in 1980 (Anderson and May 1983a). In both cases, the risk factor rises roughly linearly with age, although somewhat more steeply in the UK. Unfortunately, both figures are based on relatively few cases of measles encephalitis (a total of 151 for Fig. 5.13(a) and 58 for Fig. 5.13(b)); the UK data in the 1–15 year age range are consistent with the slope of the USA risk factor, with the overall slope being set higher by the single outlying point at age 43. In what follows, we take the risk factor $r(a)$ of eqn (5.18) to be given as a function of age by the straight-line relation shown in Fig. 5.13(a).

The average age at infection, A, varies from place to place, depending on differing social and environmental circumstances. From the studies summarized

Table 5.5 Average age, A, at which measles infection is typically acquired in different countries

Location	Time period	Average age A (years)	Type of data	Reference
England and Wales	1944–65	4.5–5.5	Case notifications	*Registrar General's Statistics*
Various localities in North America	1912–28	4.0–6.0	Case notifications	Collins (1929)
Zambia, Rhodesia and South Africa (urban centres)	1960–8	3.0–4.0	Serology	Davis (1982)
Nepal (Terai)	1977	3.0–4.0	Serology	Davis (1982)
Ghana	1960–8	2.0–3.0	Case notifications	Morley (1969)
Eastern Nigeria	1960–8	2.0–3.0	Case notifications	Morley (1969)
India (Pondicherry area)	1978	2.0–3.0	Serology	Davis (1982)
Morocco	1960	2.0–3.0	Serology	Davis (1982)

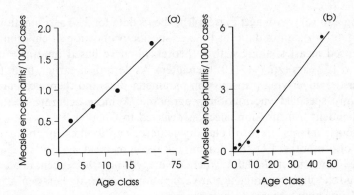

Fig. 5.13. Measles. (a) The age dependency in the ratio of measles encephalitis cases to 1000 measles cases in the US between 1973 and 1975 (CDC 1981*a*). Dots show observed values; the line is the best-fit linear model of the form $m(a) = c_1 + c_2 a$, where $c_1 = 0.23$, $c_2 = 0.0717$ ($r^2 = 0.95$). (b) Identical to (a) but recording the case ratio for England and Wales in 1980 ($c_1 = -0.308$, $c_2 = 0.127$, $r^2 = 0.99$ (see text).

in Table 5.5, we see that A is around 2–3 years of age in communities in Africa and India, and around 4–6 years of age in developed countries before the advent of vaccination. In particular, A was around 5 years of age in urban communities in the USA and UK before vaccination. A value $A \simeq 5$ gives a force of infection $\lambda \simeq 0.2 \text{ yr}^{-1}$. As shown in Fig. 5.14, the UK data are somewhat better fit by

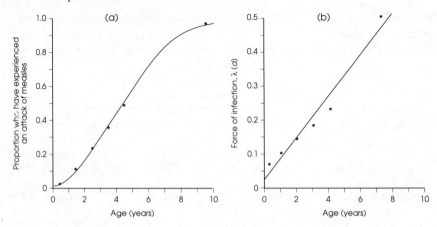

Fig. 5.14. Measles. (a) Proportion of children who had experienced an attack of measles at various ages in England and Wales in 1958 (based on case notification records). Dots, observed values; full curve, predictions of a simple catalytic model with age-dependent rates of infection (see text). (b) The age dependency in the rate or force of infection $\lambda(a)$. Dots, calculated values; full curve, best-fit linear model of the form $\lambda(a) = m + va$, where $m = 0.0178$ and $v = 0.063$ ($r^2 = 0.96$).

allowing λ to vary with age: Fig. 5.14(b) shows data for $\lambda(a)$ as a function of age, and Fig. 5.14(a) shows data for the age-specific proportion of children to have experienced measles, along with a theoretical curve based on $\lambda(a) = c_1 + c_2 a$ for up to 10 years ($\lambda(a) = \lambda(10)$ thereafter). As described earlier, from this $\lambda(a)$ we infer the underlying transmission parameter $\beta(a)$, and thence calculate $\lambda'(a)$ under any specified vaccination programme. A more accurate treatment of age-dependent transmission effects is deferred to Chapter 9.

Newborn infants are protected by maternal antibodies for, on average, a period of 6 months. For this reason, the recommended age for vaccination is around 15 months; in the USA, where coverage is now 96 per cent of all children entering school, the average age at vaccination is currently between 1.5 and 2.5 years. Protection appears to be lifelong.

Given these data and assumptions, we can calculate the ratio, ρ^*, of cases of measles encephalitis at equilibrium after, versus before, implementing a defined programme of vaccination against measles.

Figure 5.15 shows ρ^* as a function of p, the proportion of children vaccinated at age 2 years ($b = 2$), for three values of the average age at infection before vaccination ($A = 5$ corresponds to the $\lambda(a)$ of Fig. 5.14(b), while $A = 4$ and 6 correspond to appropriately higher and lower values, respectively, of the constant c_1). For measles encephalitis, there are none of the perverse effects noted for CRS. Vaccination against measles always reduces the overall incidence of measles encephalitis, although for coverage levels below about 80 per cent the reduction is significantly less than would be guessed by assuming it

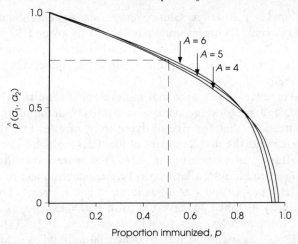

Fig. 5.15. Measles. The equilibrium ratio $\hat{\rho}(a_1, a_2)$ of measles encephalitis cases in the age range 0–75 years after vaccination of a proportion p at age b, divided by the cases before vaccination (see text). The age-dependent risk function $m(a)$ employed to calculate $\hat{\rho}(a_1, a_2)$ is as defined in Fig. (5.14(a)) and we assume a type II survival function with a life expectancy of 75 years. Three curves are recorded for three different values of the average age A at infection prior to control ($A = 4$, 5, and 6). Broken line shows the current situation in the UK, with a p value of approximately 0.5. The age at vaccination, b, was set at 2.0 years ($a_1 = 0$, $a_2 = 75.0$).

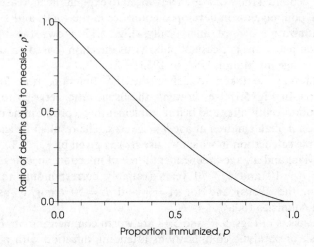

Fig. 5.16. The ratio, ρ^*, of measles deaths at equilibrium after, versus before, establishment of a programme that vaccinates a proportion p of all children at age 1.5 years (see text) (parameter values, $\lambda = 0.4 \, \mathrm{yr}^{-1}$, $L = 45$ years, $\alpha = 1.5$ years, and maternally derived protection set at 0.5 year).

proportional to $1 - p$; at 80 per cent coverage, measles encephalitis is reduced by about 50 per cent. If current uptake in the UK is around 50 per cent at an average age of 2.2 years, this should reduce the incidence of measles encephalitis by about 20 per cent. This work is presented in much greater detail in Anderson and May (1983*a*).

Before leaving measles, we note that in developing countries the problem is measles itself, and measles encephalitis is relatively unimportant. Moreover, there are indications that the risk of dying from measles infection decreases with age throughout the first few years of life. Lacking good data, we present a purely illustrative calculation in Fig. 5.16. This figure shows the ratio, ρ^*, of measles deaths at equilibrium after, versus before, establishment of a programme that vaccinates a proportion p of all children at age 1.5 years. The risk factor, $r(a)$, is arbitrarily assumed to have the form $r(a) = \exp(-r/\alpha)$, with $\alpha = 1.5$ years. Apart from measles, survivorship is assumed to be Type I with life expectancy $L = 45$ years; protection by maternal antibodies is allowed for by assuming susceptibles first appear at age 6 months; the pre-vaccination value of A is 3 years, giving an age-dependent force of infection $\lambda = 0.40\ \mathrm{yr}^{-1}$.

Only the qualitative trends in Fig. 5.16 are to be taken seriously. These trends are, however, interesting; they illustrate that disproportionate gains may accrue to intermediate levels of coverage, because of the way in which the risk factor declines with age.

5.6.4 *Paralytic poliomyelitis*

We earlier recounted the story often advanced to explain the increased incidence of paralytic poliomyelitis in developed countries in the 1940s and 1950s, before mass immunization. More analytically, Fig. 5.17 shows the incidence of paralytic complications per case of polio virus infection (based on serology), as a function of age, in Miami, USA in 1953.

The data may be taken to define the risk function, $r(a)$, for paralytic poliomyelitis. In Fig. 5.18 we show ρ^*, the usual ratio between total cases of paralytic poliomyelitis after and before implementing a programme of immunizing a fraction p of all children at age $b = 2$ years. The results in Fig. 5.18 derive from a simple calculation in which we use $r(a)$ as given by Fig. 5.17, along with Type I survival and an age-independent force of infection: specifically we show results for $A = 10$ and $L = 70$ years (roughly corresponding to developed countries in the 1950s) and for $A = 3$ and $L = 50$ (roughly as for some developing countries today).

Several aspects of Figs. 5.17 and 5.18 are worth commenting on. First, notice that the risk of paralytic complications attending infection with poliomyelitis does indeed increase with age into the teen years, but in a gradual and decelerating way. As the curves in Fig. 5.18 show, upward changes in the average age at infection (produced either by better hygiene or by mass immunization) do not—with the risk function of Fig. 5.17—lead to a perverse increase in the

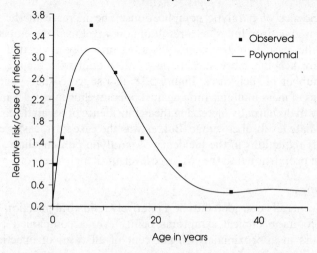

Fig. 5.17. The relative risk (or incidence) of paralytic poliomyelitis per case of infection of polio virus (type II) as a function of age, based on serological data and paralytic complication data collected in Miami, USA in 1953 (from Paul 1953 and Nathanson and Martin 1979).

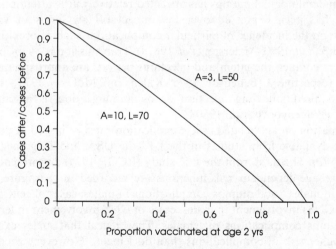

Fig. 5.18. Ratio of cases of paralytic poliomyelitis after, divided by cases before, implementing a programme of immunizing various fractions of children at age 2 years, for two sets of parameter values which mirror respectively a developed country ($A = 10$, $L = 70$ years) and a developing country ($A = 3$, $L = 50$ years). In both examples the calculations were based on the risk function portrayed in Fig. 5.17, type I survival, on cases over the age range of 0 to L years ($L = 50$ or 70 years) and an age-independent force of infection.

overall incidence of paralytic complications. The increase in the number of people encased in 'iron lungs' as a result of poliomyelitis in developed countries in the middle decades of this century is most probably associated with better medical care keeping more such patients alive than with an increase in the intrinsic number of such cases. Figure 5.18 also suggests that—unlike CRS—programmes of mass immunization against poliomyelitis in developing countries are unlikely to do harm by increasing the net incidence of paralytic complications at intermediate levels of coverage. But, as was the case for measles encephalitis in Fig. 5.15, reductions in the incidence of paralytic poliomyelitis are likely to be less than proportional to the coverage level, until high levels of p are attained.

5.6.5 *Mumps*

Mumps is generally considered to be a relatively mild viral infection of children, the most common clinical symptoms being fever accompanied by parotitis which occurs in approximately 60 per cent of all cases of infection. Several complications are associated with mumps virus infection, of which meningo-encephalitis and orchitis are the most common (CDC 1984). The former occurs in approximately 10 per cent of all diagnosed clinical cases, and the latter occurs in about 27 per cent of clinical cases in post-pubertal males (Beard *et al.* 1977; CDC 1984). Case complication rates appear to depend on both age and sex (RCGP 1974; Beard *et al.* 1977).

The epidemiology of mumps has attracted relatively little attention, although concern has been expressed over the impact of low levels of vaccination coverage on the incidence of particular complications such as orchitis in males (Galbraith *et al.* 1980; Anderson *et al.* 1987a). Transmission is by droplet spread and direct contact; the latent and infectious periods are approximately 13 and 6 days, respectively (Benenson 1975; Kalen and McLeod 1977). Immunity, either acquired following infection or by immunization, is assumed to be life-long (Wagenvoort *et al.* 1980).

Information on age-related case complication rates is limited at present, but data are available from studies in the UK, the USA, and Belgium (Anderson *et al.* 1987a). The data from the UK study (RCGP 1974) are presented in Fig. 5.19. Five age-dependent risk functions are recorded in the figure, denoting orchitis in males, total mumps complications in males, cases of central nervous system (CNS) involvement in males, cases of CNS involvement in females, and total mumps complications in females. They reveal that males experience a much higher risk of complications than do females. However, when the data are partitioned to reveal complications owing to meningitis and encephalitis in both sexes (these are considered together since the diagnosis depends on clinical judgement and is often arbitrary (CDC 1984, RCGP 1974)), and orchitis in males, it becomes apparent that the risk of CNS involvement is similar for males and females. Much of the total risk experienced by males is due to orchitis in post-pubertal males (Anderson *et al.* 1987a).

The average age at infection, A, varies among countries but was between 6

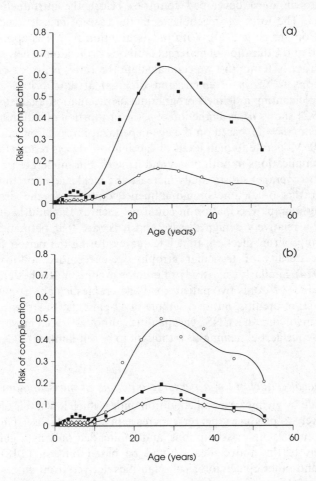

Fig. 5.19. The age- and sex-dependent risk of serious complications arising from infection by the mumps virus. The points represent the proportion of cases of mumps, admitted to hospitals in England and Wales in 1958–9, that presented with complications (data from RCGP (1974)), adjusted to mirror the proportion of the total number of cases of mumps in each age class (see text for further details). The recorded risk values denote relative as opposed to absolute changes with respect to age. Full curves, best-fit polynomials of the form $m(a) = b_0 + b_1 a + b_2 a^2 + b_3 a^3 + b_4 a \cdots b_n a^n$. (a) solid squares, males, and open circles, females, denote the total relative risk of complications. (b) Complications divided into the risk of meningitis and/or encephalitis in males (solid squares) and females (open diamonds), and the risk of orchitis in males (open circles). Parameter values as defined in Anderson *et al.* (1987a).

and 7 years in most developed countries before the introduction of mass vaccination. The force of infection, as in the case of measles and rubella, is dependent on age (Fig. 5.20). With the assumption that A is approximately 7 years and that the duration of maternal antibody protection in new-born infants is of the order of 6 months, we can calculate the ratio, ρ^*, of cases of mumps complications (CNS involvement and orchitis) at equilibrium after, versus before, implementing a defined programme of vaccination against mumps.

Figure 5.21 shows ρ^* as a function of p, the proportion of children vaccinated at age 2 years ($b = 2$), based on the age-dependent forces of infection recorded in Fig. 5.20. Moderate to high levels of vaccination always reduce the incidence of CNS complications in both males and females, but moderate levels (around 60 per cent coverage) substantially increase the incidence of orchitis in males.

Whether this prediction should influence opinion on the desirability of introducing mumps vaccination in countries such as England is questionable. Mumps is a relatively benign disease and it is rare that permanent sequelae follow mumps virus infection. In a UK survey during the period 1958–69, no permanent sterility or testicular atrophy were recorded following orchitis (RCGP 1974). Similarly, in a study of mumps orchitis in Rochester, USA, over the period 1935–74, only two patients had bilateral testicular atrophy, following the diagnosis of orchitis, out of a sample of 47 patients (Beard *et al.* 1977). Of the cases involving the CNS, encephalitis, although rare, may give rise to persistent sequelae, but meningitis is thought to be self-limiting (RCGP 1974).

5.6.6 *General criterion for a perverse outcome of mass immunization*

We conclude by giving a general condition under which low levels of immunization are likely to produce a perverse increase in serious disease. This condition is derived under simple assumptions, and is intended only as a guide. Serious applications of the above ideas should be based on eqn (5.18), with risk functions and other epidemiological quantities derived from data.

The essential question is whether ρ^* increases, rather than decreases, at low levels of coverage. That is, we need to know whether the slope of ρ^* against p is positive (perverse) or negative in the limit p tends to zero. From eqn (5.18), and noting that $\lambda' \to \lambda$ as $p \to 0$, we can write:

$$(d\rho^*/dp)_{p=0} = -1 + e^{-\lambda b} \int_{a_1}^{a_2} r(a)(\lambda a - 1)\, e^{-\lambda a}\, da \left(\int_{a_1}^{a_2} r(a)\, e^{-\lambda a}\, da \right)^{-1}.$$

$$(5.19)$$

Here we have assumed Type I survival and an age-independent force of infection. It is further assumed that immunization takes place at age b, so that $d\lambda'/dp \to -\lambda \exp(-b\lambda)$ in the limit $p \to 0$ (see eqn (5.8)). The '−1' term on the right-hand side of eqn (5.19) comes from the direct effects of immunization, which of course always tend to reduce the incidence of serious infection.

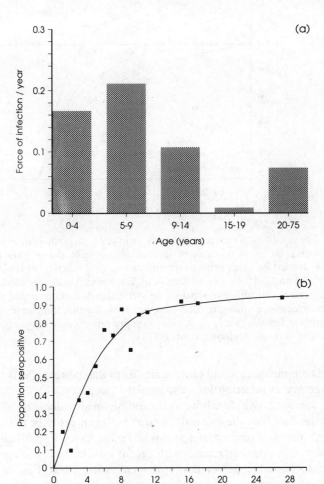

Fig. 5.20. Age-related changes in the per capita force of infection (the rate at which susceptibles acquire infection per unit of time) derived from serological data collected in London and the Home Counties in 1977–8 (data from Mortimer 1978). (a) The average values of $\lambda(a)$ (defined per year) for various age classes estimated by the maximum likelihood technique described in Grenfell and Anderson (1985). (b) Age-related changes in the proportion seropositive for antibodies to the mumps virus: solid squares, observed values; full curve, values predicted on the basis of the average forces of infection recorded in (a).

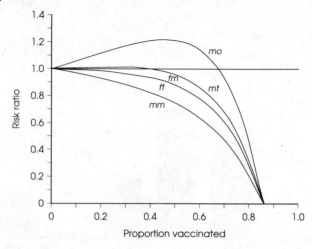

Fig. 5.21. The equilibrium or steady state risk ratio $\rho^*(a_1, a_2)$ (where $a_1 = 0$ and $a_2 = 75$ years), denoting the ratio of cases of serious disease after the introduction of mass vaccination divided by cases prior to immunization, as a function of the proportion of 2-year-old boys and girls immunized each year. The five curves denote model predictions of the equilibrium ratio for five separate age-related risk functions: mo, male orchitis; mt, total complications, males; ft, total complications, females; mm, meningitis in males; fm, meningitis in females (see text). A value of unity reflects no change after the start of mass vaccination (from Anderson *et al.* 1987*a*).

The more complicated second term comes from the indirect effects (which raise the average age at infection for unimmunized people).

For a specified risk function, $r(a)$, and defined values of b and λ (or, equivalently, $A \simeq 1/\lambda$), the integrals in eqn (5.19) can easily be evaluated to see whether ρ^* increases or decreases at low coverage levels. In particular, suppose the risk of serious disease increases with age (at least in the age-range of interest) according to a simple power law, $r(a) = ca^v$, with $v > 0$. For immunization essentially at age zero ($b \simeq 0$), and considering all ages ($a_1 \to 0$, $a_2 \to \infty$), we then have:

$$(d\rho^*/dp)_{p=0} = v - 1. \tag{5.20}$$

The indirect effects (represented by v) will prevail over the direct benefits (represented by -1), to give a perverse outcome at low coverage levels, if $v > 1$; that is, if the risk function increases faster than linearly with age over the age interval of interest to us. More generally, if the age at immunization, b, is not close to zero, eqn (5.20) is replaced by

$$(d\rho^*/dp)_{p=0} = v \, e^{-\lambda b} - 1. \tag{5.21}$$

Risk functions somewhat steeper than linear will not necessarily lead to perverse outcomes, provided the age at vaccination is appreciable ($b > A \ln v$).

Alternatively, for the artificially simple case where the risk of serious disease is essentially zero below age α and roughly constant above it ($r(a) = 0$ for $a < \alpha$, $r(a) = C$ for $a > \alpha$), which crudely corresponds to CRS, eqn (5.19) gives

$$(d\rho^*/dp)_{p=0} = \lambda\alpha - 1. \tag{5.22}$$

Remembering $\lambda \simeq 1/A$, we see that low levels of immunization will tend to produce a perverse result if $\alpha > A$, i.e. if the age at which serious complications become likely exceeds the average age at infection before immunization. This is virtually always the case for rubella and CRS. More generally, if immunization is at age b rather than close to birth, eqn (5.22) is modified to

$$(d\rho^*/dp)_{p=0} = \lambda\alpha\, e^{-\lambda b} - 1. \tag{5.23}$$

A perverse outcome can be avoided by postponing immunization to around age b, provided $b > A \ln(\alpha/A)$.

These deliberately oversimplified results do indeed give some insight into the results for rubella, measles, mumps, and poliomyelitis, above. For detailed applications, however, we need more precise computations, of the kind indicated for these infections.

5.7 Summary

We began by distinguishing between the direct and indirect effects that immunization has on population-level immunity. A criterion for the overall fraction of the population that must be protected by immunization, in order to achieve eradication, is given; estimates of this critical level of coverage are given for various infections, with particular emphasis on the global eradication of smallpox. We also discuss the way in which the force of infection, and the average age at infection, are affected by specific immunization programmes that fall short of eradication. Eradication criteria are discussed for specific programmes, such as immunization of a proportion p of each age cohort according to some defined age-schedule. Stochastic effects of 'endemic fade-out' are mentioned, in relation to eradication criteria.

The second, and larger, part of the chapter deals with the effects that herd immunization may have on the incidence of serious disease, particularly in those cases (such as CRS) where the risk of serious complications rises with the age at which infection is experienced. A general approach to these issues is developed, and applied in some detail to congenital rubella syndrome, measles encephalitis, paralytic poliomyelitis, and mumps orchitis.

6

The basic model: dynamics

6.1 Introduction

At the beginning of Chapter 3, we wrote down a set of partial differential equations describing the way in which the numbers of susceptibles, infectives, and immunes change with time, t, and age, a, under specified circumstances. The subsequent Chapters 4 and 5 have focused on the equilibrium or static properties of these equations and various elaborations on them.

We now turn to consider the dynamics of the basic model defined by eqns (3.11)–(3.13). It is easier to begin by integrating over all ages, and examining the way in which the total numbers of susceptible, infectious, and immune hosts ($X(t)$, $Y(t)$, $Z(t)$, respectively) change over time in response to various disturbances. In such studies, it is usual to assume Type II survival, with a constant mortality rate μ, whence (integrated over all ages) eqns (3.11)–(3.13) become

$$dX/dt = \mu N - (\lambda(t) + \mu)X(t), \tag{6.1}$$

$$dY/dt = \lambda X - (v + \mu)Y(t), \tag{6.2}$$

$$dZ/dt = vY - \mu Z(t). \tag{6.3}$$

Here we have assumed that all births are into the susceptible class, and that births exactly balance deaths (so that the total population $N = X + Y + Z$ is constant). In this chapter we drop the 'bars' that heretofore have sat on top of variables like X to denote total numbers (summed over all ages) as distinct from numbers in a particular age class; we have decided to set convenience and uncluttered type-setting above consistency (Emerson would have found us pleasingly free of hobgoblins, while some readers may have other views). Although rarely discussed in the literature on mathematical epidemiology, other assumptions about the mortality rate, $\mu(a)$, lead to a system of equations similar to eqns (6.1)–(6.3), although usually with minor complications that require some hand-waving before approximate results can be obtained analytically: see the explicit discussion in Appendix C.

Under the simple assumption of an age-independent transmission parameter that was discussed earlier, eqn (3.18), this set of equations is closed by the relation

$$\lambda(t) = \beta Y(t). \tag{6.4}$$

As $Z(t) = N - X(t) - Y(t)$ for all t, and $\lambda(t)$ and $Y(t)$ differ only by a proportionality constant, the dynamical behaviour of this system is described simply by a pair of non-linear, first-order differential equations for $x(t)$ and $\lambda(t)$ (or, equivalently, $X(t)$ and $Y(t)$):

$$dx/dt = \mu - (\mu + \lambda(t))x(t),\qquad(6.5)$$

$$d\lambda/dt = (v + \mu)\lambda(t)(R_0 x(t) - 1).\qquad(6.6)$$

Here $x(t)$ is defined as the *proportion* of the population remaining susceptible at time t,

$$x(t) \equiv X(t)/N.\qquad(6.7)$$

R_0 appears here as the parameter combination

$$R_0 \equiv \beta N/(v + \mu).\qquad(6.8)$$

This is, of course, the basic reproductive rate of the microparasite, as fully discussed earlier.

We have laboured over the derivation of eqns (6.5) and (6.6), because they serve to illustrate some basic ideas about the changes that immunization programmes and other perturbations can bring about, and also because they serve as a point of departure for more complicated and realistic models (whose dynamics are less transparent).

Equations (6.5) and (6.6), or similar systems, are conventionally studied in either one of two limits. The mathematical theory of *epidemics* is essentially concerned with the introduction of a 'seed' of infection into a largely susceptible population. Things happen on a fast time-scale following such an introduction, and the analysis tends to deal with such questions as the total fraction of hosts who have experienced infection before the epidemic dies out. Such an epidemic is commonly treated as a discrete event, happening on a time-scale much faster than that governing the recruitment of new susceptibles ($\mu = 1/L$); these studies usually employ a simpler version of eqns (6.5) and (6.6) in which $\mu = 0$. Conversely, studies of *endemic* infections—such as those in Chapters 4 and 5—in effect deal with the properties of eqns (6.5) and (6.6) at or near equilibrium.

Figure 6.1 is unusual in showing a numerical solution of eqns (6.5) and (6.6), over a span of time long enough to enable us to see both epidemic and endemic phases of the dynamics. In order to do this with a linear time-scale, we have for pedagogical purposes invented an infection with modest R_0 and long duration of infectiousness ($R_0 = 5$, $v = 10 \text{ yr}^{-1}$) in a population with a high birth and death rate ($\mu = 0.014 \text{ yr}^{-1}$); if we used the actual R_0 and v values for measles, for example, the initial epidemic phase would be lost in the thickness of the y-axis.

The initial precipitous drop in density of susceptibles, x, and the rise and fall of the force of infection, λ (and in the number infected, $Y = \lambda/\beta$), corresponds to the classical epidemic. The predatory microparasite finds a superabundance of susceptible 'prey'; infection levels grow rapidly as the microparasite initially

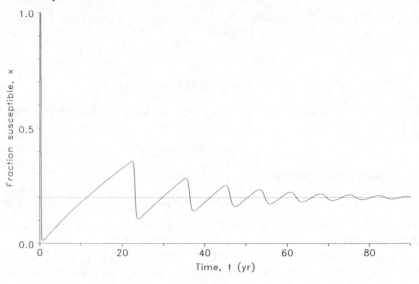

Fig. 6.1. This figure illustrates the relation between 'epidemic' and 'endemic' phases of an infection within a host population, as described by the simple dynamical eqns (6.5) and (6.6); the figure shows the fraction susceptible, $x(t)$, as a fraction of time, t. The relevant epidemiological and demographic parameters are chosen to be $v = 10 \, \text{yr}^{-1}$ (duration of infectiousness, $D = 1/v$, is around one month, with no latent period), Type II survival with $\mu = 1/70 \, \text{yr}^{-1}$ (life expectancy, L, of 70 years), and $R_0 = 5$ (so that the average age at infection once the infection is endemic is $A \simeq L/R_0 \simeq 14$ years). The infection is introduced here at $t = 0$ with an initial 'seed' corresponding to $\lambda(0) = 10^{-4} \, \text{yr}^{-1}$, and an epidemic spreads on the fast, $1/v$ (one month) time-scale until nearly everyone has been infected. There is then a comparatively long phase, of duration very roughly $2A \sim 28$ yr, until the pool of susceptibles has been replenished by births to the point where a second epidemic can spread, again on the fast, $1/v$, time-scale; the second epidemic is less severe than the first, because the bulk of the population is immune, following the earlier epidemic. Successive epidemics are less and less severe, and the pattern of oscillation becomes more sinusoidal, with a period, T, that is the geometric mean of the fast and slow time-scales of the early episodes: $T = 2\pi(AD)^{1/2}$. In this simple model, the oscillations eventually damp out, and $x(t)$ settles to its endemic value of $1/R_0$ (indicated by the broken line). For details, see the text and Appendix C.

realizes its basic reproductive rate, R_0; and eventually the exponentiating microparasite numbers overexploit their susceptible prey, whose numbers fall well below the long-term equilibrium level ($x^* = 1/R_0$, as shown by the horizontal broken line in Fig. 6.1).

Some details of this epidemic phase will be pursued further in the next section, but for the moment we note that the initial, roughly exponential, rise in $\lambda(t)$ and $Y(t)$ is at the rate

$$\Lambda = v(R_0 - 1). \tag{6.9}$$

For largish R_0, the epidemic has a characteristic duration time of order $1/v$, and the peak value of λ is roughly vR_0. These results can be justified intuitively (at least for large R_0): initially each infective produces R_0 offspring in a time equal to the duration of infectiousness, $D = 1/v$, and then recovers, whence the initial doubling rate is of order $(R_0 - 1)/D$; essentially everyone acquires infection at this fast rate (faster than v), and then infection is lost relatively slowly over a time of typical length $D(= 1/v)$ which thus sets the time-scale for the epidemic; and at the peak of the epidemic virtually everyone is infected, whence $\lambda \sim \beta N = vR_0$.

The boom and bust of the initial epidemic in Fig. 6.1 is followed by an episode in which the pool of susceptibles is restocked by births. As can be seen in Fig. 6.1, during this episode $x \simeq \mu t$. Eventually, after a time that is approximately $t \sim 2/\mu R_0$ (when $x \simeq 2/R_0$; see Appendix C), a new, but less severe, epidemic is triggered. The comparative absence of boom-and-bustiness in this second epidemic is because now there are initially fewer susceptibles than there were at the start of the first epidemic, and so the overshoot is less dramatic.

After this second epidemic has waned, susceptibles again build up, and the process repeats itself. The excursions above and below the long-term equilibrium state become progressively less noticeable.

In the long run, this simple system settles to an equilibrium state. The equlibrium values of x and y can be found easily by putting $dx/dt = 0$ and $d\lambda/dt = 0$ in eqns (6.5) and (6.6), respectively, to get:

$$x^* = 1/R_0, \tag{6.10}$$

$$\lambda^* = \mu(R_0 - 1). \tag{6.11}$$

These, of course, are results we obtained and discussed earlier. The corresponding equilibrium formula for $y^* = (Y/N)^*$ and $z^* = (Z/N)^*$ are:

$$y^* = \left(\frac{\mu}{\mu + v}\right)\left(1 - \frac{1}{R_0}\right) \tag{6.12}$$

$$z^* = \left(\frac{v}{\mu + v}\right)\left(1 - \frac{1}{R_0}\right). \tag{6.13}$$

Notice that as the epidemic phase gives way to the endemic phase in Fig. 6.1, the rapid fall and slow rise in susceptibility that characterizes the epidemic phase is replaced by a pattern of roughly sinusoidal (though slowly damped) oscillations about the endemic state. As shown in Appendix C, these relatively small-amplitude oscillations have a period T given by:

$$T \simeq 2\pi[L(D + D')/(R_0 - 1)]^{1/2}. \tag{6.14}$$

Here, as before, $D = 1/v$ is the duration of infectiousness and $D' = 1/\sigma$ is the duration of the latent period, so that $D + D'$ is the total duration of infection. We choose to include the latent period explicitly in the analysis leading to eqn

(6.14) (which in this sense is a new result), even though we omitted it in eqns (6.1)–(6.4) and Fig. 6.1, in order to undertake a more accurate comparison with data below. As always, $L = 1/\mu$. Using the approximate relation $A = 1/\lambda$ in conjunction with eqn (6.11), we can rewrite this period T in terms of the average age at infection and the duration of infection:

$$T \simeq 2\pi[A(D + D')]^{1/2}. \tag{6.15}$$

One qualitative feature of Fig. 6.1, which derives from the non-linear nature of the underlying eqns (6.5) and (6.6), is worth emphasizing. In the epidemic phase, far from the steady state, there is effectively a decoupling of time-scales for spread of infection and replenishment of susceptibles: the actual epidemic takes place on a characteristic time-scale D, and restocking of the pool of susceptibles takes place on the slower time-scale $A(\sim 1/\mu R_0)$. In the endemic phase, the damped oscillations about the equilibrium state have a period that is essentially the geometric mean of A and D.

6.2 Dynamics of epidemics

Mathematical aspects of both deterministic and stochastic models for epidemics are reviewed thoroughly and lucidly by Bailey (1975). Since we are mainly interested in dynamic properties of programmes of immunization or other intervention against endemic infections, we do not dwell on this material. We will, however, mention a few results that will be useful later (in Chapter 11).

Consider first the beginning stages of the epidemic, following the introduction of a very small number of infectives, $Y(0)$, into an otherwise wholly susceptible population. In these early stages, we can put $x \simeq 1$ in eqn (6.6) to get

$$d\lambda/dt \simeq v(R_0 - 1)\lambda. \tag{6.16}$$

Here we have replaced the factor $v + \mu$ with v, because usually $v \gg \mu$. Equation (6.16) describes exponential growth in λ,

$$\lambda(t) = \lambda(0) \exp(\Lambda t). \tag{6.17}$$

The initial value $\lambda(0) = \beta Y(0)$, and the growth rate $\Lambda = v(R_0 - 1)$, are as defined in eqn (6.9) or, in a more general context earlier, eqn (2.3).

For the simple epidemic described by eqns (6.5) and (6.6) with $\mu = 0$, a direct relation between the fractions susceptible and infected at time t, $x(t)$ and $y(t)$, can be obtained by dividing eqn (6.5) into eqn (6.6) and remembering that $\lambda = \beta N y = v R_0 y$:

$$dy/dx = -1 + 1/(R_0 x). \tag{6.18}$$

Integrating this equation (subject to the initial conditions that $y(0) = Y(0)/N \simeq 0$ and $x(0) \simeq 1$) gives

$$y(t) = 1 - x(t) + (\ln x(t))/R_0. \tag{6.19}$$

The peak value of y may now be found easily: y is stationary—poised between increasing and decreasing—when $dy/dt = 0$; from eqn (6.6), this happens when $x = 1/R_0$. Putting this value of x into eqn (6.19) gives

$$y_{max} = 1 - (1 + \ln R_0)/R_0. \qquad (6.20)$$

Equation (6.20) supports our earlier assertion that essentially everyone is infected at the height of the epidemic, provided R_0 is not too close to unity.

In such a 'closed' epidemic, where there is no recruitment of new susceptibles ($\mu = 0$ in eqns (6.5) and (6.6)), the infection eventually dies out, leaving a fraction $1 - I$ of the population remaining susceptible. The magnitude of the fraction who experience infection, I, can also be read off from eqn (6.19), in the limit $t \to \infty$. In this limit, $y \to 0$ and $x \to 1 - I$, whence I is seen to depend only on R_0 via the expression

$$I = 1 - \exp(-R_0 I). \qquad (6.21)$$

Some generalizations of this relation, to allow for disease-induced deaths and/or recovery followed by re-infection, are given elsewhere (May and Anderson 1983a; May 1990).

The above expressions for the peak fraction infected, y_{max}, and the fraction ever infected, I, are plotted as functions of R_0 in Fig. 6.2.

The discussion in this section has been given primarily to serve as a background, against which in Chapter 11 we will present new work on epidemics of sexually transmitted diseases (such as AIDS) in heterogeneously mixed populations.

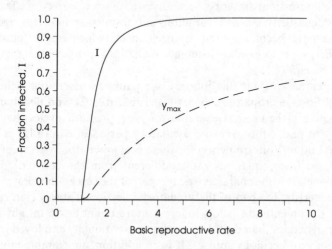

Fig. 6.2. The peak fraction infected, y_{max}, and the fraction ever infected, I, plotted as functions of R_0 (see text and eqns (6.20) and (6.21)).

6.3 Dynamical behaviour in the endemic state

As we have just mentioned, the basic model predicts that disturbances about the endemic equilibrium state will tend to show weakly damped oscillations, whose period is to a good approximation given by eqn (6.14) or eqn (6.15). More explicitly, the oscillations are damped by the factor $\exp(-t/T_D)$, where the characteristic damping time is approximately $T_D \simeq 2A$. This damping time is longer than the oscillatory period, by a factor of the order $[(D + D')/A]^{1/2}$. Although the duration of infection is typically a lot less than the average age at infection (usually a factor of 10^2 to 10^3), by the time the square root is taken the damping is significant, usually producing noticeable effects over the span of a few cycles (as can be seen in Fig. 6.1).

The fact that simple models give only damped oscillations was discouraging to Soper (1929), who first studied such models with a view to explaining the rather regular two-year cycles in the annual incidence of measles. Other such non-seasonal cycles are seen in the annual incidence of various endemic infections of childhood. The inter-epidemic periods for a collection of such endemic infections, at different places and times, are summarized in Table 6.1, and a careful analysis of some of the underlying data is given below.

Table 6.1 also shows the inter-epidemic periods that may be calculated (to varying degrees of accuracy, depending on available information about $D + D'$ and A) from the simple formula (6.15). The facts and the simple theoretical estimates are in good agreement. In the next two sections, we first present time-series analyses of data for measles, pertussis, and mumps; these analyses verify the occurrence of such non-seasonal cycles, thus substantiating earlier and more impressionistic work. Secondly, we survey a variety of effects—demographic stochasticity, seasonal variations in transmission, time lags, age structure, etc.—that have been proposed as mechanisms which might 'pump' such a system, driving it to exhibit sustained oscillations at its characteristic periods, as given by eqn (6.15).

Before embarking on this journey, we pause to assert our belief that the sustained host–microparasite cycles listed in Table 6.1 and documented more fully below are the clearest examples of prey–predator cycles that ecologists are likely to find. Moreover, the oscillatory period of eqn (6.15) is essentially the basic Lotka–Volterra period for these prey–predator systems, even though it is derived from equations rather different from the conventional Lotka–Volterra ones: A is the characteristic lifespan of the susceptible prey, and $D + D'$ the characteristic lifespan of the predatory infection. Table 6.1, in conjunction with the documentation below, offers a more quantitative insight into prey–predator dynamics than do the examples conventionally employed in introductory biology and ecology courses. It is, in addition, an example more likely to engage the attention of pre-medical students!

Table 6.1 Inter-epidemic period, T, of some common infections (from Anderson and May 1985c) and theoretical predictions of the period (eqn (6.15))

Infection	Inter-epidemic period, T, (years) (observed)	Geographical location and time period	Average age at infection, A	Latent plus infectious period, $D + D'$, (days)	Inter-epidemic period, T, (years) (calculated)
Measles	2	England and Wales, 1948-68	4-5	12	2
	2	Aberdeen, Scotland, 1883-1902	4-5		2
	2	Baltimore, USA, 1900-27	4-5		2
	2	Paris, France, 1880-1910	4-5		2
	1	Yaounde, Cameroun, 1968-75	2		1-2
	1	Ilesha, Nigeria, 1958-61	2		1-2
Rubella	3.5	Manchester, UK, 1916-83	11	18	4-5
	3.5	Glasgow, Scotland, 1929-64	11		4-5
Parvovirus (HPV)	3-5	England and Wales, 1960-80	?	?	
Mumps	3	England and Wales, 1948-82	6-7		3
	2-4	Baltimore, USA, 1928-73	8-9	16-26	3-4
Poliomyelitis	3-5	England and Wales, 1948-65	11-12	15-23	4-5
Echovirus (type II)	5	England and Wales, 1965-82	?	?	–
Smallpox	5	India, 1868-1948	12	10-14	4-5
Chickenpox	2-4	New York City, USA, 1928-72	6-8	18-23	3-4
	2-4	Glasgow, Scotland, 1929-72	6-8		3-4
Coxsackie virus (type B2)	2-3	England and Wales, 1967-82	?	?	
Scarlet fever	3-6	England and Wales, 1897-1978	10-14	15-20	4-5
Diphtheria	4-6	England and Wales, 1897-1979	11	16-20	4-5
Pertussis	3-4	England and Wales, 1948-85	4-5	27	3-4
Mycoplasma pneumoniae	4	England and Wales, 1970-82	?	?	

6.4 Periodicities in the incidence of endemic infections: data

This section summarizes a paper by Anderson *et al.* (1984), which uses two complementary techniques—autocorrelation and spectral analysis—to look carefully at secular trends in the incidence of infection. The methods are applied to three childhood diseases: pertussis and mumps (using disease-incidence data from England and Wales), and measles (using data from England and Wales, Scotland, North America, and France).

Autocorrelation analysis is based on the construction of a series of sample autocorrelation coefficients, r_k ($k = 0, 1, \ldots, N - 1$, where N is the length of the time-series), which measure the correlation between observations at different distances k (and thence times) apart, within the series. That is, r_k (with $-1 < r_k < 1$) measures the correlation between the original data and the same series with a displacement, or lag, of k steps. Autocorrelations are usually interpreted via a correlogram, which is a plot of r_k against the lag, k. Confidence limits for a correlogram based on randomly distributed data, and tests for the significance of departures from randomness, can be constructed to help interpret the results. For a fuller discussion, see Anderson *et al.* (1984).

The correlogram is a natural tool for analysing periodicities in time. By contrast, spectral analysis is less intuitive, in that it examines the contributions to the observed time-series of oscillations at different frequencies. Spectral analysis is based on the idea of a theoretical 'power spectrum', which partitions the total variance (or power) of the series among sinusoidal components (up to a maximum frequency of one cycle every two measurements). A number of earlier authors have used a harmonic (Fourier) analysis to calculate the contribution of various frequency components to observed patterns of disease incidence; for a process with a continuous frequency spectrum, however, such harmonic analysis does not produce a consistent estimate of the theoretical spectrum (Jenkins and Watts 1968). We therefore calculate the spectral estimate as the Fourier transform of the autocovariance function, using a 'Tukey spectral window' as a noise filter (for details see Anderson *et al.* (1984)). To strike a balance between variance and discrimination, we present the results for a range of 'windows', which essentially represent increasing degrees of spectral smoothing. As before, a much fuller discussion is given in Anderson *et al.* (1984).

Figures 6.3–6.13 are selected from the larger set in Anderson *et al.* (1984). We now proceed to look seriatim at measles, pertussis, and mumps—all before widespread vaccination.

6.4.1 *Measles*

Figure 6.3 shows longitudinal records of measles incidence for the period 1948–68 (before vaccination), from weekly case-notification data (see Anderson *et al.* (1984) for background to this and other data).

The correlogram derived from the data of Fig. 6.3 is given in Fig. 6.4. This

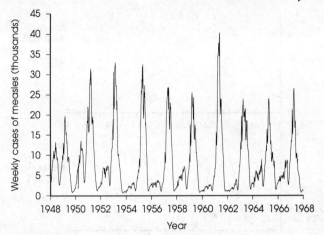

Fig. 6.3. Weekly case notifications of measles in England and Wales for the period 1948 to 1968 prior to the introduction of mass vaccination.

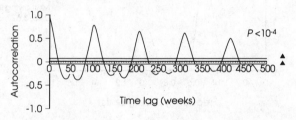

Fig. 6.4. Correlogram of weekly measles reports for England and Wales, 1948–68. Here, and in subsequent correlograms, the solid triangles indicate the 95 per cent confidence limits for the zero correlogram from a completely random series, and p is the probability that such data could generate the observed correlogram (see Appendix in Anderson *et al.* (1984)).

correlogram is based on serial correlation coefficients calculated from logarithmically transformed data, which has the effect of making the oscillations in Fig. 6.4 somewhat more symmetrical than an arithmetic plot. The correlogram has a smooth two-peak oscillating curve, with a major period of 2 years and a minor period of 1 year (the seasonal component). Note the smoothness of the correlogram, which indicates great regularity in both seasonal and two-year cycles. Note also the dominance of the amplitude of the longer-term cycle over the seasonal component.

Figure 6.5 shows the corresponding spectral density for Fig. 6.3, with a Tukey window chosen to give a relatively narrow bandwidth (see Anderson *et al.* 1984). This spectrum has a sharp peak at a frequency of 0.5 yr^{-1}, corresponding to a two-year cycle, and a smaller but nevertheless pronounced peak at a frequency of 1 yr^{-1}, corresponding to the annual cycle.

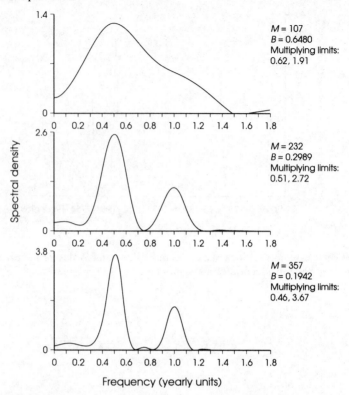

Fig. 6.5. Spectral density for the data presented in Fig. 6.3. Data were mean-corrected before the spectra were constructed. Here, and in subsequent spectra, the results are presented at a range of window cut-off points (*M*), and therefore bandwidths (*B*, cycles per year); multiplicative 95 per cent confidence limits for the spectra are also given (called multiplying limits).

Similar analyses of measles data from Aberdeen (1883–1902) and Baltimore (1910–27), along with measles mortality data from Paris (1880–1910) and London (1910–39), are discussed in Anderson *et al.* (1984). From this work, we select two further figures. Figure 6.6 shows the spectral density of monthly case notifications of measles in Baltimore (1900–27); the seasonal and two-year frequencies again are conspicuous, but here the annual component is more pronounced than the two-year oscillation. Figure 6.7 is a correlogram from the yearly totals of deaths from measles in London (1910–39). Again the two-year cycle stands out strongly. It is noteworthy that the period of this non-seasonal cycle in England remained at 2 years from 1910 (London only) to 1968 (England and Wales).

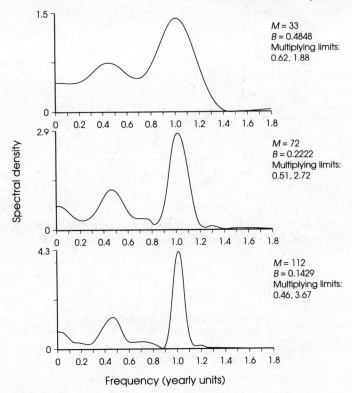

Fig. 6.6. Spectral density of monthly case notifications of measles in Baltimore from 1900–27 (from Anderson *et al.* 1984).

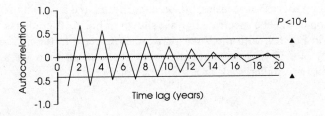

Fig. 6.7. Correlogram from the yearly total deaths from measles in London from 1910–39 (from Anderson *et al.* 1984).

6.4.2 *Pertussis (whooping cough)*

Figure 6.8 shows the weekly case notifications of pertussis in England and Wales for the time-period 1948–82. Vaccination was introduced in 1956.

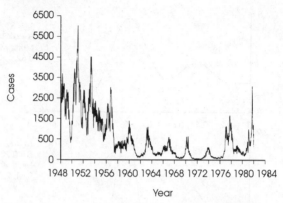

Fig. 6.8. Weekly case notifications of pertussis (whooping cough) in England and Wales for the time period 1948–82. Mass vaccination was introduced in 1956.

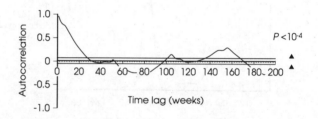

Fig. 6.9. Correlogram for the pre-vaccination pertussis data recorded in Fig. 6.8 (1948–56) (from Anderson *et al.* 1984).

The correlogram for the pre-vaccination data in Fig. 6.9 is less smooth than the clear-cut patterns for measles, but seasonal cycles and a dominant three-year peak are apparent. The spectral analysis, shown in Fig. 6.10, confirms the trends evidenced in Fig. 6.9, with the three-year cycle (reflected in the marked peak at a frequency of 0.33 yr^{-1}) significantly more pronounced than the annual one (reflected in the smaller peak at a frequency of 1 yr^{-1}).

6.4.3 *Mumps*

The mumps data for England and Wales (1962–81) are in the form of yearly case records, and thus do not allow us to investigate seasonal trends. These annual totals (from reports by general practitioners) are shown in Fig. 6.11.

The spectral density corresponding to the data in Fig. 6.11 is displayed in Fig. 6.12 (with annual data, the maximum frequency is one cycle every 2 years, and so the frequency spectrum terminates at 0.5 yr^{-1}). The spectral density in Fig. 6.12 shows a significant cycle, with an average period of 3 years (corresponding to a frequency of 0.33 yr^{-1}).

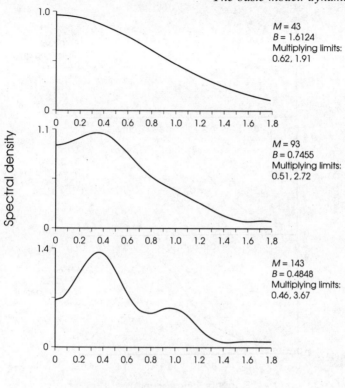

M = 43
B = 1.6124
Multiplying limits:
0.62, 1.91

M = 93
B = 0.7455
Multiplying limits:
0.51, 2.72

M = 143
B = 0.4848
Multiplying limits:
0.46, 3.67

Frequency (yearly units)

Fig. 6.10. Spectra for the pre-vaccination pertussis data from England and Wales (1948–56) (from Anderson *et al.* 1984).

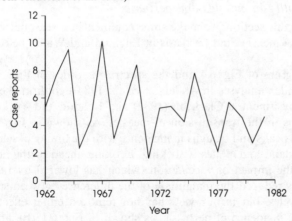

Fig. 6.11. Annual general practitioner reports of mumps (consultation rates per 1000 population) in England and Wales, 1962–81.

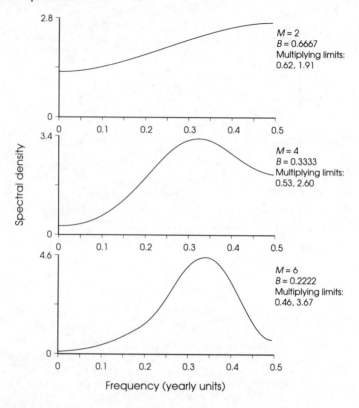

Fig. 6.12. Spectra for the England and Wales mumps data (from Anderson *et al.* 1984).

6.4.4 *Seasonality in measles and pertussis*

Before leaving this section, we make some comments on seasonal variations in the incidence of measles and pertussis in England and Wales, before and after vaccination.

The correlogram of Fig. 6.4 and the spectral densities of Figs. 6.5 and 6.6 (and other similar analyses in Anderson *et al.* (1984)) confirm the interesting observations by Fine and Clarkson (1982) and London and Yorke (1973) on annual patterns in the transmission of measles. As shown in Fig. 6.13(a), the associations of peaks and troughs in incidence with the timing of school holiday periods in England and Wales is striking. Looking ahead to the next chapter, we note that the impact of vaccination (which has lowered overall incidence since 1968) has reduced the magnitude of the difference between seasonal and longer-term cycles, but in our view has not removed either effect. Observed patterns in the incidence of pertussis, as shown in Fig. 6.13(b), are, however, very different from measles; the relatively high levels of vaccine uptake in the late 1950s and early 1970s totally removed the seasonal trend. We find this

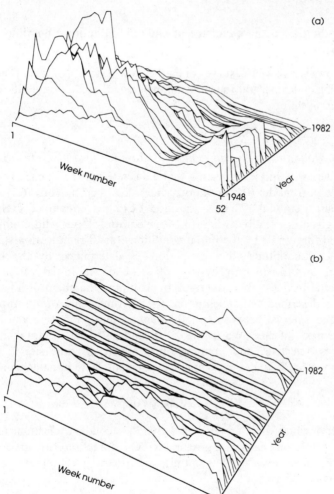

Fig. 6.13. Surfaces showing seasonal patterns in measles and pertussis incidence, based on weekly case reports in England and Wales, 1948–82: (a) measles, (b) pertussis. 1 = first week in January.

observation somewhat puzzling. It could be that the aggregation and dispersal of schoolchildren is not the main cause of seasonality in pertussis, and that climatic factors are important. But it remains unclear to us why these differences should exist between seasonal patterns of incidence of measles and pertussis.

6.5 Periodicities in the incidence of endemic infections: possible mechanisms

What follows is a very brief survey of mathematical studies of various non-linear mechanisms that can lead to sustained non-seasonal oscillations in the incidence of endemic infection.

6.5.1 *A pedagogic preliminary: neutral stability in a discrete-time model*

Some readers will find it interesting that a discrete-time analogue of the simple epidemiological model (in continuous time) described by eqns (6.1)–(6.4) has purely neutral stability. That is, the model exhibits undamped cycles whose period is given essentially by eqn (6.14) or eqn (6.15), but whose amplitude is determined forever (!) by the initial conditions (as distinct from a stable limit cycle, whose amplitude—like its period—is determined by the biological parameters, and to which the system will settle for any initial state).

The model in question is obtained by assuming the chain of infection and ·recovery is described as happening in discrete time steps, of duration D: D is the (average) interval between an individual acquiring infection and passing it on to the next infectee. We define X_t, Y_t and Z_t to be the total number of susceptibles, infecteds, and immunes, respectively, at time step t; the total population, $N = X_t + Y_t + Z_t$, is assumed constant. With homogeneous mixing, we have

$$Y_{t+D} = (R_0 X_t/N) Y_t. \tag{6.22}$$

Each case, of which there are Y_t, would give R_0 secondary infections if all hosts were susceptible, and each case gives $R_0(X_t/N)$ if a fraction X_t/N are susceptible and no infections 'overlap'. Susceptibles are lost·by infection, eqn (6.22), and gained by new births:

$$X_{t+D} = X_t - Y_{t+D} + B. \tag{6.23}$$

Here B represents net births in the interval D. If births equal deaths, and occur at the per capita annual rate μ, then $B = \mu DN$. (Equations (6.22) and (6.23) essentially say $\Delta Y = Y(R_0 X/N - 1)$ and $\Delta X = B - R_0 XY/N$, where ΔX means 'change in X over the time interval D'; if instead we pass to the continuous limit, and take ΔX to mean $D\, dX/dt$, and similarly for ΔY, we recover the previous eqns (6.5) and (6.6) in continuous time.)

A routine linearized stability analysis now shows the system of eqns (6.22) and (6.23) possesses neutral stability, oscillating like a frictionless pendulum, with periods given approximately by eqn (6.15). This result is established in Appendix C.

This model is of pedagogical interest only. Its dynamical behaviour is structurally unstable. The slightest modification, for instance allowing for the possibility that some infections 'overlap' (see eqn (6.24) below), tips the dynamics off the razor's edge of neutral stability.

6.5.2 *Demographic stochasticity*

Soper's (1929) model and the generalizations of it discussed above (Bailey 1975; our Appendix C) are deterministic, with birth, death, and infection all occurring at fixed rates. Although it may be mathematically inconvenient, humans in fact come quantized in integer units, so that ultimately it does not make sense to talk of a fraction of a birth or infection. Accounting for this fact introduces stochastic elements into the description of epidemiological processes, along the lines discussed and illustrated (see, for example, Fig. 4.11) at the end of Chapter 4.

A variety of studies have shown that such 'demographic stochasticity' (as distinct from 'environmental stochasticity', whose effects do not become smaller as population sizes increase; see May (1974)) can tip the kind of models discussed above from neutral stability or damped oscillations into *sustained* oscillations in the incidence of infection. These results are for populations large enough to avoid stochastic extinction of infection, and the indefinitely maintained cycles have a period given approximately by eqn (6.14) or eqn (6.15); see, in particular, Bailey (1975, Section 7.61). For smaller populations, as we saw earlier, there is stochastic 'fade-out', and repeated epidemics depend on introductions from outside the population; the inter-epidemic period now tends to scale as A, which measures the time taken for susceptibles to be replenished by birth processes. In a rough sense, the stochastic fade-out situation corresponds to the far-left (epidemic) phase in Fig. 6.1 (whence the inter-epidemic interval $\sim A$), while the stochastically driven sustained oscillations correspond to the far-right (endemic) phase in Fig. 6.1 (whence the inter-epidemic period T of eqn (6.15)).

A seminal study of this kind is by Bartlett (1957, 1960a). He began with a discrete model similar to eqns (6.22) and (6.23) above, modified by replacing the infection probability, $R_0 Y_t / N$, in eqn (6.22) by the expression

$$1 - (1 - R_0/N)^{Y_t}. \tag{6.24}$$

The expression (6.24) gives a more accurate account of the binomial infection process, and reduces to the previous expression when $R_0 Y_t / N$ is very small. By itself, this modification serves to carry the neutrally stable model discussed above into (weakly) damped oscillations. Bartlett, however, showed that further incorporation of a term representing the variability introduced by demographic stochasticity had the effect of producing sustained oscillations (unless the population is too small to perpetuate the infection, which then exhibits 'fade-out'). Bartlett's work has been extended in a variety of elegant mathematical studies, many of which are surveyed by Bailey (1975).

Extensive numerical studies, originally by Bartlett (1956, 1960b) and more recently by ourselves and others, have likewise shown that demographic stochasticity tends—in populations large enough to avoid fade-out—to produce sustained, if slightly irregular, oscillations with period T close to that given by eqn (6.14) or eqn (6.15). The basic procedure for generating such simulations, and some specific examples, are set out at the end of Chapter 4.

6.5.3 *Seasonal variation in transmissibility*

As mentioned in Chapter 3, a variety of biological effects (virus survival in droplets dependent on temperature and humidity, and the like) and social effects (particularly the aggregation of schoolchildren in obedience to the patterns of the school year) can produce marked seasonal variations in the transmission rate, and thus in the incidence of infection. Such annual variations are a pronounced feature of the data analysed in the previous section.

Beginning with Yorke and London (1973) and London and Yorke (1973), several studies have shown that such seasonality is capable of 'pumping' the system to produce longer-term oscillations, with peaks separated by integer numbers of years, close to the basic period T of eqn (6.15). The mechanism is most transparent when the basic period T is around 2 years, when it is readily excited as a sub-harmonic of the annual cycle (Dietz 1975; Grossman 1980; Schwartz and Smith 1984; Aron and Schwartz 1984; Schwartz 1985).

6.5.4 *Age structure in transmision rates*

In Chapter 8 we review the evidence for age dependence in the transmission parameter β. If the transmission rates do indeed vary significantly according to the ages of infectee and infector, $\beta(a, a')$, the analysis of the dynamical properties of epidemiological models becomes considerably more complicated than for the basic models studied above.

Our own numerical studies, of the kind reported in Chapter 9, suggest that such age structure in the underlying transmission rates can result in the system's basic propensity to oscillate being very weakly damped. But damped it still is. If the numerical studies are not run for a long enough time (or if they are run with too coarse a time step in the finite-difference approximation to continuous time), the cycle may appear undamped.

Other authors have conjectured that such age-structured transmission rates might, by themselves, produce sustained oscillations (e.g. Dietz, private communication). To the contrary, Greenhalgh has recently made a linearized stability analysis of the age-structured systems described in Chapter 9, and finds essentially no unstable regions of parameter space (the exceptions arise in very special circumstances, and probably have more to do with actual discontinuities in rate processes—such as arise in Type I survival—than with age-structured transmission as such) (Greenhalgh 1987).

In short, the question of whether sustained cycles can be driven by age structure in transmission processes seems to us an interesting and still-open one. Whether or not such effects can, by themselves, 'pump' oscillations at the basic period T of eqn (6.15), they can certainly greatly reduce the damping found in the simpler Soper equations. Our guess is that these effects do not, by themselves, drive the observed cycles, but that they make it significantly easier for seasonality or stochasticity to do so.

6.5.5 *Time lags*

Time delays in epidemiological processes, or defined intervals in the duration of latency or infectiousness (in contrast with constant rates; see Fig. 3.17), also in some extreme circumstances appear to be capable of 'pumping' the system at around the period T discussed above. These effects, which have been studied by Hethcote and Tudor (1980), Hethcote *et al.* (1981), Grossman (1980), Gripenberg (1980), Busenberg and Cooke (1978), Stech and Williams (1981), Green (1978), Smith (1978), and others can be complicated, and there seems room for additional formal work here. We doubt, however, that these often quite delicate effects are commonly responsible for the inter-epidemic cycles that are so widely observed.

6.5.6 *Functional dependence of incidence of infection on X and Y*

In the standard models, the incidence rate is bilinear, being proportional to the total number or density of susceptibles, X, and infectives, Y. More generally, it seems reasonable to assume the rate at which new cases appear is proportional to the number of susceptibles, X, and to the fraction of their contacts who are infectious, Y/N, even though the transmission coefficient may have some complicated dependence on total population density N (rather than being βN, as assumed above): in this case, the incidence rate is still $\beta(N)XY$.

Lui *et al.* (1987) have analysed what happens when this linear dependence of incidence on X and Y is replaced by some more general functional relationship. They show that the outcome can result in a wide variety of dynamical behaviour, including many creatures from the zoological gardens of dynamical systems theory (Hopf bifurcations, saddle-node bifurcations, homoclinic loop bifurcations), depending on the functional dependence of incidence rates on X and Y.

Lui *et al.* (1987) begin with a comprehensive review of previous studies of this general kind, which we will not recapitulate. They go on to deal mainly with the case where the incidence rate is equal to $\beta X^q Y^p$, where p and q are positive constants. The array of dynamical behaviour mentioned above can then ensue, depending on the values of p and q. Of particular interest is the case, which can arise for $p > 1$, when there are two alternative equilibrium states: one corresponds to extinction of the infection, and the other to stable cycles; whether the infection will die out or remain endemic in autonomously-driven cycles depends on the initial densities of susceptibles and infectives.

The essential conclusion of Lui *et al.* is that periodic solutions may occur naturally if 'an effective cooperativity exists among infectives; that is, if the dependence of the incidence rate on the number of infectives is faster than linear' ($p > 1$). They go on to suggest some ways in which such non-linearity could arise. First, it could be, for viruses that live outside the host for only a short time, that significant incidence levels arise only when virus concentration in the environment exceeds a threshold level; when Y is small, the threshold is never exceeded, whereas increasing values of Y raises the concentration above threshold. Such a mechanism in effect gives $p > 1$. A similar situation would arise if individuals could harbour low-level infections that did not make them infectious, but did increase their susceptibility; the incidence rate would then again rise faster than linearly with Y. Second, for some vector-borne diseases, the vector may have to attack on average p individuals before acquiring a level of infective stages sufficient to render its next attack effective in transmittng the infection. In this event, the incidence rate will be proportional to Y^p, with $p > 1$ (provided the attacks are independently random).

In summary, changes from a linear dependence of incidence rates on X and Y can result in qualitative changes in dynamical behaviour. This important point has been made independently by Mollison (private communication). Whether such departures from bilinearity are plausible depends on the infection in question. Lui *et al.* (1987) make a case for the relevance of their results, especially to some vector-borne infections, but we doubt if the mechanisms they have elucidated are the reason for the observed cycles in measles and other such directly transmitted viral infections.

6.5.7 *More general considerations*

Recent years have seen increasing understanding of the way in which simple systems of difference equations (for discrete time) or differential equations (for continuous time) can exhibit an astonishing array of dynamical behaviour, ranging from the familiar stable points, through stable cycles, to cascading bifurcations of period-doublings, into apparently 'chaotic' regimes where the trajectories can be effectively indistinguishable for the sample function of a random process (Lorenz 1963; May 1976, 1987; Holden 1986; Sugihara and May 1990; for a more general review, see Gleick 1987). As a result of this work, phenomenological techniques have been developed for analysing apparently complicated, irregularly periodic, dynamical behaviour (in turbulent fluids, electrical circuits, and so on) to see if it can be generated by some relatively low-dimensional relationship or 'map'. Such studies do not aim to tease out the basic mechanisms, but rather to see if simple heuristic relations can describe the observed phenomenon.

Schaffer and Kot (1986) and Olsen (1987) have applied these heuristic

methods to the time-series data for measles and other infections. They find that
the observed oscillations can indeed be well described by a one-dimensional
map. Although not focused on underlying mechanisms in the first instance, such
work holds promise both of enabling predictions to be made, and of pointing
the way to a more basic understanding (by explaining the heuristically derived
'map'). For a recent and general review, see Sugihara *et al.* (1990).

6.6 Summary

We begin by drawing a rough distinction between epidemic and endemic phases
of infection within a population (see Fig. 6.1). After some brief remarks on
dynamical properties of epidemics, we focus attention on the non-seasonal
cycles in incidence that are observed for many infections. Techniques of
autocorrelation and spectral analysis are applied to data for measles, pertussis,
and mumps, to show that well-determined cycles do indeed account for most
of the variablity in these data. The basic model for endemic infections exhibits
damped oscillations, with a period $T \simeq 2\pi[(D + D')A]^{1/2}$; $D + D'$ is the duration
of the latent plus infectious intervals, and A the average age at infection. The
period T, thus estimated, is in good agreement with the observed inter-epidemic
periods for a variety of infections (see Table 6.1). A variety of mechanisms that
may be capable of 'pumping' this propensity to oscillate, thus sustaining cycles
with roughly the period T, are reviewed. Some will find the agreement between
the observed period and the above rough estimates pleasing (and a good
illustration of basic prey–predator principles); others may believe we understand
little until we comprehend the exact mechanism driving the cycles.

7

Dynamic aspects of eradication and control

We have just seen that host–microparasite associations have a strong propensity to oscillate, so that even the endemic equilibrium state is often one of self-sustained cycles. The initiation of a programme of immunization, by its nature, constitutes a perturbation to such a host–microparasite system, and consequently is likely to evoke oscillations even if they are absent in the pre-immunization state. In other words, it is not to be expected that the incidence of infection will change smoothly and monotonically from its pre-immunization equilibrium value to some new and lower value (or to zero if eradication is achieved) under immunization, but instead we should often expect to see oscillations—sometimes quite pronounced—superimposed on the trends. If the equilibrium states before and after immunizations are not too different, the oscillations thus evoked should have periods given roughly by eqn (6.15), $T \simeq 2\pi[(D + D')A]^{1/2}$. But for stronger perturbations, non-linear effects and changes in the average age at infection will typically cause the period to be longer than given by this linearized estimate.

There have been few such studies of the epidemiological dynamics of immunization programmes; most work has been confined to the kind of static analyses outlined in Chapter 5. The work of Knox (1980) and of Cvjetanovic *et al.* (1978, 1982) are important exceptions, which will be discussed further at the end of this chapter. The oscillatory effects foreshadowed in the previous paragraph are often not intuitively obvious to the clinical practitioner. Yet, as we shall see, some of these short-term dynamical phenomena have practical implications.

We now proceed to study an artificially simple example which illuminates some of the basic ideas. We then discuss more realistic models (mainly for congenital rubella syndrome (CRS) in this chapter, and more generally in Chapter 9).

7.1 An illustrative example

We consider the dynamical behaviour, following implementation of an immunization programme, of the simple system of eqns (6.1)–(6.4) studied in the previous chapter. More specifically, we focus on eqns (6.5) and (6.6) for the fraction susceptible, $x(t)$, and the force of infection, $\lambda(t)$, at time t. At time $t = 0$ we introduce a programme which immunizes a proportion p of each age cohort, essentially at birth. The resulting equations (repeating eqn (6.6) for convenience) are, for $t > 0$:

$$dx/dt = \mu(1 - p) - (\mu + \lambda(t))x(t), \tag{7.1}$$

$$d\lambda/dt = v\lambda(t)(R_0 x(t) - 1). \tag{7.2}$$

Immunization has the effect of removing a proportion p of all births directly to the immune class, so that susceptibles are now gained at the rate $\mu(1 - p)$. Apart from this, all the assumptions are as for eqns (6.5) and (6.6). Equations (7.1) and (7.2) have the initial conditions $x(0) = 1/R_0$, $\lambda(0) = \mu(R_0 - 1)$, which comes from eqns (6.10) and (6.11) for the pre-immunization equilibrium.

Equations (7.1) and (7.2) can, of course, easily be integrated numerically. It is, however, instructive to look at some analytic results and at a linearized approximation of the dynamics.

Notice first that eqns (7.1) and (7.2) give the asymptotic ($t \to \infty$) values of $\lambda(\infty)$ and $x(\infty)$ that were found in Chapter 5. By putting the left-hand side of eqn (7.2) equal to zero, $d\lambda/dt = 0$, we get $x(\infty) = 1/R_0$. The fact that the fraction susceptible is the same after the immunization programme has come to equilibrium as it was before immunization (unless, of course, coverage was high enough to achieve eradiction) is implicit in our original derivation of the relation $R_0 x^* = 1$ (in Chapter 2), which made no reference to whether susceptibility was lost naturally by infection or artificially by immunization. The asymptotic value of $\lambda(\infty)$ is found by putting $dx/dt = 0$ in eqn (7.1), and is $\lambda(\infty) = \mu[R_0(1 - p) - 1]$; this is the result found earlier (eqn (5.6)).

Equation (7.2) can be integrated directly, to get

$$\lambda(t) = \lambda(0) \exp\left(v \int_0^t (R_0 x(s) - 1) \, ds\right). \tag{7.3}$$

Notice that the kernel of the integral in eqn (7.3) vanishes both at $t = 0$ and at $t \to \infty$ because $R_0 x \to 1$ at these times. But $\lambda(\infty)$ is less than $\lambda(0)$. Therefore $R_0 x(t)$ must, on average, dip below unity at times intermediate between $t = 0$ and $t \to \infty$.

A linearized analysis of eqns (7.1) and (7.2) is outlined in Appendix C. Under the usual approximation that $v \gg \mu R_0$ (that is, $A \gg D$), and assuming p is small, we get:

$$x(t) = (1/R_0)[1 - p(2\alpha/\omega) \, e^{-\alpha t} \sin(\omega t)], \tag{7.4}$$

$$\lambda(t) = \mu[R_0 - 1 - pR_0(1 - e^{-\alpha t} \cos(\omega t))]. \tag{7.5}$$

Here terms of relative order p^2 have been discarded. The quantities ω and α are the oscillatory frequency and damping rate, respectively, for perturbations to this basic system, as discussed in Chapter 6: $\omega = 2\pi/T$ (with the inter-epidemic period T given by eqn (6.14)) and $\alpha = 1/2A$ (with the average age at infection $A = 1/\mu R_0$).

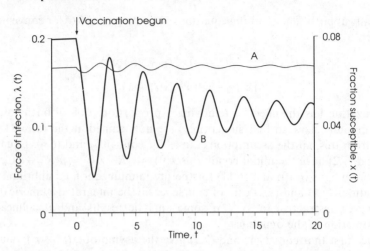

Fig. 7.1. This figure shows the changes in the fraction of the host population who are susceptible, $x(t)$ (the thin curve A), and in the force of infection, $\lambda(t)$ (the thick curve B), following the introduction of a programme in which 40 per cent of each cohort are successfully immunized at birth, beginning in year 0. Specifically, the figure illustrates the dynamical behaviour of the linearized version of eqns (7.1) and (7.2) that is discussed in Appendix C, with the demographic and epidemiological parameters having the values $\lambda_0 = 0.2 \text{ yr}^{-1}$, $\mu = 1/70 \text{ yr}^{-1}$ (whence $R_0 = 15$), and $v = 25 \text{ yr}^{-1}$; it follows that the damping rate, α, and oscillatory frequency, ω, in eqns (7.4) and (7.5) have the values $\alpha = 0.11 \text{ yr}^{-1}$ and $\omega = 2.23 \text{ yr}^{-1}$. The numerical values are fairly representative of many childhood infections. The incidence of infection at time t is proportional to $\lambda(t) x(t)$, and therefore exhibits roughly the same dynamical behaviour as $\lambda(t)$.

This linearized approximation, eqns (7.4) and (7.5), is illustrated in Fig. 7.1 for $p = 0.4$ and for epidemiological parameters specified in the caption, which amount to $\alpha = 0.11 \text{ yr}^{-1}$ and $\omega = 2.23 \text{ yr}^{-1}$. Notice that the perturbations to the fraction susceptible, $x(t)$, are very small even for this relatively large value of p. This is because the disturbance term scales relatively as $p\alpha/\omega$ in eqn (7.4), and α/ω is of the order of $(D/A)^{1/2}$ which typically is small (and is ~ 5 per cent in this example). The amplitude of the oscillations in the force of infection, $\lambda(t)$, as it moves from $\lambda(0)$ to $\lambda(\infty)$ are of significant magnitude, initially scaling simply with p relative to $\lambda(0)$ itself. All this shows plainly in Fig. 7.1.

7.2 Dynamics of age-specific susceptibility, and other quantities, following immunization

More generally, we may wish to know how age-specific levels of infection, susceptibility, and so on, change over time following the introduction of some defined policy of immunization. Such understanding of the dynamics of age-specific incidence of infection is particularly important for those diseases, such as CRS, where age at infection is important.

Our studies of the dynamical behaviour of infection, in the years after immunization is begun, are based on the set of partial differential equations discussed in Chapter 3. These equations, which we repeat here for convenience, describe how quantities like susceptibility change with time, t, and age, a:

$$\partial X/\partial t + \partial X/\partial a = -(\lambda(t) + c(a) + \mu(a))X(a, t), \tag{7.6}$$

$$\partial H/\partial t + \partial H/\partial a = \lambda X - (\sigma + \mu(a))H(a, t), \tag{7.7}$$

$$\partial Y/\partial t + \partial Y/\partial a = \sigma H - (v + \mu(a))Y(a, t), \tag{7.8}$$

$$\partial Z/\partial t + \partial Z/\partial a = vY + cX - \mu(a)Z(a, t). \tag{7.9}$$

The one new thing in these equations is the presence of the age-specific immunization rate, $c(a)$, which describes the transfer of susceptibles, X, directly into the immune class, Z, by successful immunization. We have assumed here that the age-specific immunization schedule does not vary over time (so that c is $c(a)$, with no dependence on t); this is, at best, only approximately true for real programmes. Equations (7.6)–(7.9) embody all the other assumptions made in Chapters 4–6 about the flows from susceptibility, through latent and infectious intervals, to the immune state. In particular, we have neglected disease-induced deaths ($\alpha = 0$), and assume (via the boundary conditions) that births exactly balance deaths, so that the total population, $N = X + H + Y + Z$, remains constant. The possibility of protection by maternal antibodies is not included in eqns (7.6)–(7.9); it could be incorporated either by adding on explicit equations (as discussed in Chapter 3), or more roughly by modifying the boundary conditions (in the next paragraph) to have everyone effectively 'born' into the susceptible class of age M instead of age zero.

Two sets of boundary or initial conditions are required in order to specify the solutions of eqns (7.6)–(7.9). One of these is usually that all births are into the susceptible class, at all times: $X(0, t) = N(0)$, $H(0, t) = Y(0, t) = Z(0, t) = 0$, for all t. The other condition here is that at $t = 0$, just before immunization is initiated, $X(a, 0)$, $H(a, 0)$, $Y(a, 0)$, and $Z(a, 0)$ all have the pre-immunization equilibrium distributions obtained Chapter 4.

The system of eqns (7.6)–(7.9), along with boundary conditions, does not by itself give a complete description of the time- and age-dependent changes that follow initiation of an immunization programme. We must also specify an explicit relation governing the subsequent changes in the force of infection over time, $\lambda(t)$. To this end, we make the previously discussed assumption of homogeneous mixing, namely (see eqn (3.18))

$$\lambda(t) = \beta \bar{Y}(t). \tag{7.10}$$

Here the transmission parameter, β, is a constant, and $\bar{Y}$ is the total number of infectives ($\bar{Y}(t) = \int Y(a, t)\,da$). Note that we have resumed the convention of denoting totals—integrated over all ages—by placing a 'bar' over the variable in question. As we shall see in the next chapter, the assumption that λ is independent of age (which is explicit in homogeneous mixing) is often violated in practice; we retain the simple assumption in this chapter, and move to more realistic and detailed studies in Chapter 9.

The system of eqns (7.6)–(7.9), with $\lambda(t)$ related to $\bar{Y}(t)$ by eqn (7.10), can be solved numerically for any given immunization schedule (specified by $c(a)$). As we emphasize at the end of the chapter, the numerical methods must be chosen with care; several different time-scales are important in eqns (7.6)–(7.9), and numerical approximation of the continuous derivatives by an inappropriately coarse finite time-step, for example, can generate spurious results.

7.3 Some analytic results

We can do a bit better than simply integrate eqns (7.6)–(7.9) numerically. As shown below and in Appendix C, an explicit formula for $X(a, t)$ can be obtained in terms of $\lambda(t)$. The partial differential equations for $X(a, t)$, $H(a, t)$, and $Y(a, t)$ can be integrated over all ages, and eqn (7.10) can be used to express $\lambda(t)$ in terms of $\bar{Y}(t)$; this leads to a set of three ordinary, first-order differential equations for $\bar{X}(t)$, $\bar{H}(t)$, and $\lambda(t)$. These three equations can be integrated numerically, to give a computation of $\lambda(t)$, and thence $X(a, t)$, that is much simpler and more efficient than integration of the full set of partial differential equations. For many applications, such as calculation of the overall risk ratio $\rho(a_1, a_2)$ of Chapter 5 as a function of time, the quantities $\lambda(t)$ and $X(a, t)$ are all we need.

Equation (7.6) can be integrated using the method of characteristics (Hoppensteadt 1974; Anderson and May 1983a), which is essentially a mathematical consequence of the biological fact that as time t passes each individual's age advances from a to $a + t$. Equivalently, Laplace transform techniques or Green's functions can be used. In any event, the solution is

$$X(a, t) = N(0) \exp(-\Psi(a, t)). \tag{7.11}$$

Here Ψ is defined as

$$\Psi(a, t) = \int_0^a \mu(s)\,\mathrm{d}s + \int_{a-t}^a c(s)\,\mathrm{d}s + \int_{t-a}^t \lambda(s)\,\mathrm{d}s. \tag{7.12}$$

In the integrations in eqn (7.12), it is to be understood that $c(s) = 0$ for $s < 0$, and that $\lambda(s) = \lambda_0$ (the force of infection in the initial, pre-immunization population) for $s < 0$. In the frequently met special case where a proportion p of hosts are successfully immunized at age b, eqns (7.11) and (7.12) take the explicit form given in Appendix C.

These formulae give $X(a, t)$ in terms of known quantities and the time-dependent force of infection, $\lambda(t)$. We can no longer use the equilibrium conditions $R_0 x^* = 1$ to determine λ, as was done in Chapter 5, but instead we relate $\lambda(t)$ to $\bar{Y}(t)$ via eqn (7.10). As explained in general terms above, three ordinary differential equations for $\bar{X}(t)$, $\bar{H}(t)$, and $\lambda(t)$ can be obtained by integrating eqns (7.6)–(7.8) over all ages. These three equations are given explicitly in Appendix C, for Type I and for Type II survival, under the above-mentioned programme of immunizing a proportion p of hosts at age b.

These three analytically expressed equations, along with the explicit result for $X(a, t)$, are all given in Appendix C, and are the basis for the results in the next section. But these results could equally well have been obtained (albeit a bit more expensively) by integrating eqns (7.6)–(7.11) directly. If the rate of immunization is itself changing over time, $c(a, t)$, we have no alternative but to proceed by direct integration of the partial differential equations.

7.4 An example: dynamics of CRS following immunization

We estimate the change in the number of cases of CRS, as a function of the time elapsed since starting a programme of immunizing either a proportion p of all girls at age $b = 12$ years (assumed equal to vaccinating $p/2$ of all 12-year-olds for calculating changes in $\lambda(t)$) or a proportion p of all children at age $b = 1$ year. We call the former the 'UK programme' and the latter the 'USA programme'. In either event, we use the methods described above to calculate $X(a, t)$ and $\lambda(t)$ for a programme initiated at time $t = 0$, and assume the age-specific risk function for CRS, $r(a)$, is proportional to the age-specific fertility. Then the ratio of the number of cases of CRS at time t to that before immunization is:

$$\rho(a_1, a_2; t) = \int_{a_1}^{a_2} r(a)\lambda'(t)X'(a, t)\, da \left(\int_{a_1}^{a_2} r(a)\lambda_0 X(a, 0) da \right)^{-1}. \quad (7.13)$$

As before, the primes indicate post-immunization variables; λ_0 is the (constant) force of infection before any immunization.

The outcome of this procedure is depicted in Fig. 7.2, which shows the relative incidence of CRS at time t after a 'UK' vaccination programme is started (proportion p of girls successfully immunized at age 12). In the trajectories illustrated for various values of p in Fig. 7.2, there is initially a pronounced oscillation, with a period of around 4–5 years. This period is in accord with the estimate of the basic inter-epidemic period for rubella in Table 6.1. As time goes on, these oscillations tend to damp out, and the system settles to the post-immunization equilibrium state discussed in Chapter 5 (remember that there are no seasonal or other effects acting to 'pump' the oscillations in these basic models).

Figure 7.3 shows data for the annual number of reported cases of CRS in

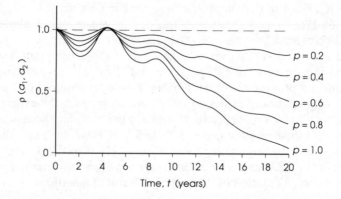

Fig. 7.2. Rubella. Temporal trends, under the past United Kingdom policy (up to October 1988) of vaccinating girls, and girls only, at around 12 years of age, of the ratio $\rho(a_1, a_2; t)$ are shown over a period of 20 years for five different levels of vaccination coverage ($p = 0.2, 0.4, 0.6, 0.8$, and 1.0). For details of the parameter values employed in the numerical simulations see Anderson and May (1983a). The calculations were made to mirror the situation in the United Kingdom from the initiation in 1970 of a programme to vaccinate teenage girls. The level of vaccination coverage attained in recent years is around 90 per cent.

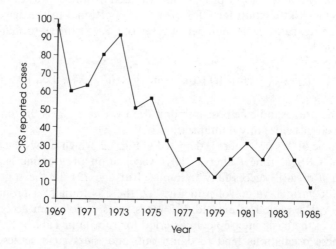

Fig. 7.3. The annual number of reported cases of congenital rubella syndrome in the years 1970–85 in England, Scotland, and Wales. For a given year the total number of cases is based on diagnoses up to 4 years after the birth of the child (the figures for 1981 onwards are therefore incomplete).

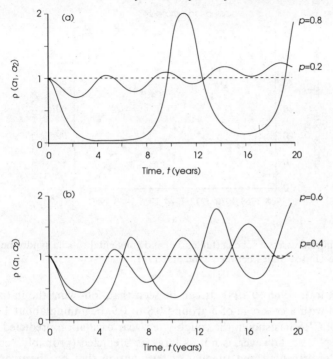

Fig. 7.4. Rubella. Temporal trends in the ratio $\rho(a_1, a_2; t)$ under the United States vaccination policy, with vaccination of boys and girls at the age of 1 year ($b = 1.0$). Graphs (a) and (b) show temporal changes under four different levels of vaccine coverage ($p = 0.2, 0.4, 0.6$, and 0.8). Other parameter values are the same as employed in Fig. 7.4 and as reported in Anderson and May (1983a).

England and Wales, from 1969 to 1985. The reality is less tidy than the theory, partly because the pre-vaccination state already shows oscillations (as discussed earlier) and the vaccination programme was gradually implemented starting around a 'trough'. Even so, there is indication of the existence of the predicted oscillation in incidence of CRS (with a 4–5 year period). This is a consequential feature of the dynamics of the vaccination programme that could not easily be guessed on purely intuitive grounds.

Similarly, though more dramatically, Fig. 7.4 shows the relative number of cases of CRS, $\rho(a_1, a_2; t)$, as a function of time, t, after the institution of a 'USA' vaccination programme (proportion p of all children successfully immunized at age 1 year) (Anderson and May 1983a). The results are displayed in two figures, to avoid confusing the curves for various p values. For small p there are weakly damped oscillations with the by-now familiar period of around 4–5 years; at large p the non-linear effects become pronounced, both lengthening the period (essentially by the factor $1/(1 - p)^{1/2}$) and modifying the amplitude.

Figure 7.5 shows data for the total number of cases of rubella and of CRS

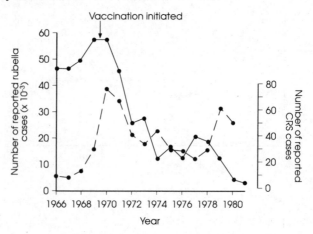

Fig. 7.5. Reported cases of rubella (full curve) and congenital rubella syndrome (broken curve) in the United States between 1966 and 1981.

in the USA from 1966 to 1981. It can be seen that, following the initiation of vaccination with a coverage of p around 0.8 to 0.9, beginning about 1969, the incidence of CRS has shown the roughly ten-year oscillation predicted by Fig. 7.4; the amplitude, however, is not as large as predicted (probably because of the policy of screening and pregnancy termination that has been operating along with vaccination).

The agreement between theory and data in Figs. 7.2–7.5 is qualitative rather than quantitative, but is nevertheless encouraging in view of the simplicity of the mathematical model. More realistic studies of this problem are pursued in Chapter 9, after the evidence for age dependence in transmission rates has been reviewed and after such age dependence has been incorporated in the models.

7.5 Two cautionary tales

Most previous studies have focused on comparisons between the equilibrium states before and after mass immunization. Two pioneering exceptions are the studies of rubella by Knox (1980) and of measles by Cvjetanovic *et al.* (1982), both of which present computer studies of the impact of immunization on the population dynamics of infection. We believe that both these studies offer important and new insights, but that some of their major conclusions may be seriously in error in ways that are illuminating.

Knox's (1980) study of the dynamics of rubella following the introduction of mass vaccination employs a set of difference equations, which describe changes in the number of cases of CRS under different regimes. In particular, Knox uses the apparently harmless approximation of changing the magnitude of the force of infection in 1-year time steps (the changes depend on the total number of cases in the previous year). But many of the essential dynamical processes in this system are, in fact, keyed to the time-scale T described by eqn (6.15); the inter-epidemic period is one natural time-scale for the system of equations in question. Up-dating λ annually corresponds, in effect, to assuming that $D + D' = 1$ year in eqn (6.15), when actually for rubella $D + D' \simeq 2\text{-}3$ weeks ($D + D'$ is the average value of the latent plus infectious periods). Because the natural time-scale T depends on $(D + D')^{1/2}$, Knox's procedure—which does not at first glance seem unreasonable—has the effect that the epidemiological changes generated by his computer models all take place on time-scales that are about four to five times too long (the ratio of the square roots of 1 year and 2–3 weeks). This mistake is repeated in Dietz's (1981) mathematical elaborations of Knox's work. If their simulations of rubella vaccination programmes are repeated with λ up-dated every 3 months, we obtain virtually the same graphical results except the time axes are halved; if λ is up-dated every 4 years, the time axes are doubled. All this can be read as a cautionary tale: the time steps used in approximating the partial differential equations (7.6)–(7.9) must be chosen carefully.

Cvjetanovic *et al.* (1982) also used a set of difference equations to examine the impact of various levels of vaccination coverage on the dynamics of measles within large populations. Making extensive use of public health data for measles in Britain, Germany, and elsewhere, they concluded that immunization of 60–70 per cent of successive cohorts of infants could eventually (in 10–20 years) eradicate measles. This is a surprising conclusion, being much lower than other estimates that use essentially the same data to estimate the age at infection, A, and other such parameters (Anderson and May 1982*d*, 1983*a*; see also Chapter 9). Cvjetanovic *et al.* use a reasonably appropriate time-step (up-dating all relevant variables every 10 days, which is a bit coarse), but they do not describe how the force of infection is modified in response to changes in the number of infectious individuals and other such factors. It appears to us that in some parts of the computation they hold λ fixed, at age-specific values deduced from data from a community in which a roughly 60 per cent level of immunization had been sustained for some time. Under this assumption of fixed λ, any increase in the proportion immunized, no matter how small, will lead to eventual eradication: at the initial equilibrium, the effective reproductive rate is unity, $R = 1$, and now vaccination removes susceptibles without any compensating decrease in λ being allowed, whence R falls below unity and the infection dies out. This interpretation explains why Cvjetanovic *et al.* obtain an eradication criterion (60–70 per cent coverage) just in excess of the level (60 per cent) corresponding to the empirical λ values they employ.

The work of Cvjetanovic *et al.* is exemplary in the way the model is solidly based on data. Assessment of the dynamical consequences of an immunization programme, however, ineluctably needs more than existing data; it also needs some concrete assumption about how the force of infection will change in response to other epidemiological changes.

We have told these two stories in order to make a constructive point. Most people recognize that mathematical models are not much use if they are not grounded on a real understanding of the epidemiological data and the public health problems. But a similar shoe fits the other foot: the complexities of herd immunity are such that years of practical experience and loads of data will not guarantee a sensible answer if the basic dynamics of the system are not understood. It is clearly insufficient for the mathematician to have a quick chat with a medical friend, or to expect elegance to be a guide. But it is similarly insufficient for the medical practitioner or public health worker to write a computer program that appears realistic because it is complicated, and then expect sensible answers automatically to emerge.

7.6 Summary

When a programme of immunizing a proportion of each yearly cohort of children is begun, it will often take 20 years or more before most of the children and adolescents have been given the option of immunization. In this and other situations, the degree of artificially induced herd immunity within the total population will tend to change gradually over a period of years, as will the force of infection. The total density of susceptibles is likely to remain roughly constant over this period (see Fig. 7.1), but the proportion immune will change in character from being largely naturally acquired to being acquired by immunization. Moreover, many microparasitic infections of childhood have a marked propensity to oscillations in incidence, and strong perturbations (such as extensive immunization) can induce complex dynamical behaviour that is not easy to predict by intuition alone; immunization may at first produce a marked reduction in the incidence of disease, but in the longer run the community may experience oscillations between low and high incidence (with many years between peaks) before infection settles to a new equilibrium level or is eradicated.

This chapter begins by illustrating these ideas with a simple example. We then explain how more realistic calculations may be carried out. As an example, we show how the incidence of CRS may be expected to change over time, under various immunization schedules; the theoretical work is compared with data from the USA and UK. We end with two cautionary tales, which testify to the need to understand the mathematics as well as the biological and medical details.

8

Beyond the basic model: empirical evidence for inhomogeneous mixing

The assumption of homogeneous mixing leads to predictions about the way in which the fraction susceptible, the average age at infection, and the inter-epidemic period change under mass immunization. It also necessarily implies that the force of infection is not dependent on age. In this chapter, these implications of homogeneous mixing are tested against available facts.

8.1 Fraction susceptible, following immunization

In Chapter 2, the argument that led to the relation (2.1) between R_0 and the equilibrium fraction who are susceptible, $R_0 x^* = 1$, was entirely independent of how susceptibility was lost. That is, under the assumption of weak homo-geneous mixing (incidence of infection linearly proportional to X), the fraction remaining susceptible at equilibrium under an immunization programme that does not achieve eradication is the same as the pre-immunization fraction. We noted this earlier, for example in Fig. 7.1.

Fine and Clarkson (1982a) have tested this idea for measles. Analysing information that is available for age-specific incidence and immunity levels for measles in England and Wales since 1950, they find the 'total number of individuals susceptible to measles has remained relatively constant', at around 4 to 4.5 million. This corresponds to about 9 per cent of the population being susceptible, implying R_0 is around 11, which roughly accords with other independent estimates (Table 4.1). As Fine and Clarkson emphasize, there are biases and deficiencies in the data, having to do mainly with the notification of cases. Their methods of correcting for such biases depend to a degree on the assumption of homogeneous mixing. Thus their test of this assumption is not altogether free of some circularity. Fine and Clarkson's work is nevertheless important, pointing the way to empirical tests of the homogeneous mixing assumption.

8.2 Average age at infection, following immunization

In Chapter 5, we saw that the average age at infection, A, rises under a programme of mass immunization. In particular, Fig. 5.3 illustrates how A increases with the proportion p who are immunized (at birth or at age b = 0.05L years), assuming relatively realistic Type I survival. More generally, we saw that at low levels of coverage A will tend to increase as $A' = A/[1 - p \exp(-b/A')]$; here A and A' are the average ages at infection, at equilibrium, before and after mass immunization at age b, respectively.

Fine and Clarkson (1982a) also studied the change in A for measles in England and Wales. Roughly 50 per cent of each cohort has been vaccinated at around age 2.2 years, since about 1969 (Anderson and May 1983a). The analysis in Appendix B (eqns (4.27), (B.6), (5.8)) or interpolation in Fig. 5.3 therefore suggests that A should have increased from its pre-vaccination value of around 5 years to about 8.1 years. Fine and Clarkson document an upward shift in A, but they emphasize that this increase is much less than the simple estimate would suggest.

A more detailed analysis of changes in the mean age of attack by measles in England and Wales, 1948–82, is presented in Fig. 8.1 (Grenfell and Anderson 1985). Although the overall average age at infection has risen only from 5.0 years in the pre-vaccination epoch (1948–68) to 5.3 years post-vaccination (1969–82), these gross averages conceal much of the structure evident in Fig. 8.1. The average age at infection rose from around 4.8 years in 1948 to 5.1 years in 1960, then fell to 4.6 years in 1968 before rising to a plateau around 5.5 years in the 1980s. This shift remains too small to be accounted for by the homogeneous mixing model. The comparatively low value of A in the late 1940s is probably a consequence of the post-war 'baby-boom', although a change in notification practices may also be involved. The reduction of A during the 1960s is thought to be produced by a combination of increased birth rates, further changes in recording practice, and changes in social habits whereby more

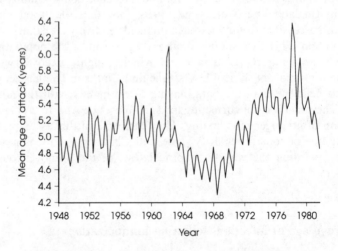

Fig. 8.1. Estimated mean age at attack, by quarter, for measles in England and Wales in the period 1948–82; based on quarterly measles notifications (from Grenfell and Anderson 1985).

children attend pre-school kindergartens (Griffiths 1974; Fine and Clarkson 1982*b*; Anderson and May 1982*d*). The increase in *A* since 1968 reflects the impact of mass vaccination. Figure 8.1 also indicates a marked annual periodicity in the value of *A*; the longer two-year cycles have virtually no effect on *A*, being averaged out by the process determining *A*.

8.3 Interepidemic period, following immunization

After a system has settled to a new equilibrium state under mass immunization (insufficient for eradication), the basic model suggests that the period of the non-seasonal oscillations should lengthen. The new period should be approximately $T' = 2\pi[(D + D')A']^{1/2}$, where A' is the new average age at infection.

Anderson *et al.* (1984) have analysed the data for measles and pertussis in this light, using the techniques described in Chapter 6.

Figure 8.2(a) shows the correlogram of weekly reports of measles in England and Wales, 1968–82. Fig. 8.2(b) shows a corresponding spectral density (with, as before, a Tukey window chosen to give a relatively narrow bandwidth, for high discrimination). Two substantial changes are evident in comparison with the pre-vaccination data in Figs. 6.4 and 6.5. First, as the spectral density makes particularly clear, the period of the longer-term cycles has shifted up from 2 years (frequency peak at $0.5 \, \text{yr}^{-1}$ in Fig. 6.5) towards 2–3 years (frequency peak at $0.4 \, \text{yr}^{-1}$ in Fig. 8.2). The theoretical expectation, from the basic model, is for the period to lengthen by a factor of about 1.3, which is slightly more than actually observed. Second, the inter-epidemic peak is no longer significantly more pronounced than the seasonal one, in contrast with the case before immunization (Fig. 6.5).

Vaccination against pertussis in England and Wales reached high levels in 1957. Uptake declined, however, between 1975 and 1976 following the widely publicized concern over the safety of the vaccine (HMSO 1981; Anderson and May 1982*b*). Low levels of vaccine acceptance persisted from that time to 1982. The vaccination era in England and Wales has therefore been divided into two periods: 1957–76 and 1977–82. During the former period, 70–80 per cent of each yearly cohort of children were vaccinated between the ages of 1 and 3 years; during the latter period, coverage fell to 40 per cent or less.

The correlogram and spectral densities for weekly case notifications for pertussis in the former epoch (1957–76) are shown in Figs. 8.3 and 8.4, respectively. These are to be compared with the pre-vaccination results of Figs. 6.9 and 6.10. Again, two points are striking. First, the period of the inter-epidemic cycles has lengthened, from around 3 years before vaccination to 3–4 years (the frequency peak is at $0.33 \, \text{yr}^{-1}$ in Fig. 6.10, and is shifted to about $0.27 \, \text{yr}^{-1}$ in Fig. 8.4). This increase in the period is as expected, but the magnitude of the shift is significantly less than the basic model with homogeneous mixing would suggest (the prediction is a period of around 5 years, or a frequency peak around $0.21 \, \text{yr}^{-1}$). Second, the seasonal peaks in incidence

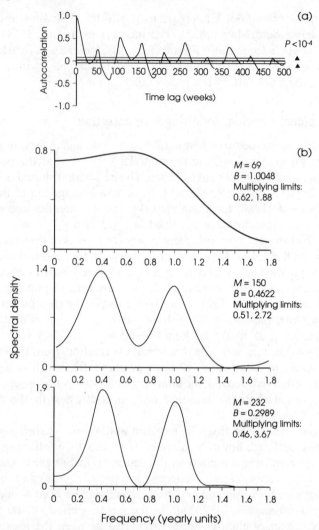

Fig. 8.2. (a) Correlogram of weekly measles reports for England and Wales, 1968–82. (b) Spectral density (spectra) for the same series. Data used trend-corrections before spectral analysis (from Anderson *et al.* 1984) (*M* denotes window cut-off point and *B* denotes cycles per year).

of pertussis seen in the pre-vaccination era (Figs. 6.9 and 6.10) are completely absent in the post-vaccination Figs. 8.3 and 8.4.

The 1977–82 section of relatively low vaccination is too short a span of time for the detection of changes in the longer-term cycles. We nevertheless show the spectral density in Fig. 8.5, to illustrate the continued suppression of the

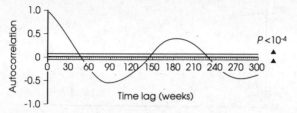

Fig. 8.3. Correlogram of weekly pertussis case reports for England and Wales, 1957–76 (from Anderson *et al.* 1984).

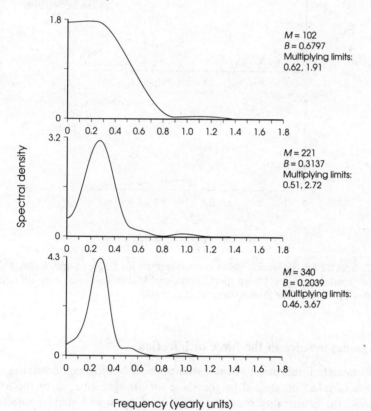

Fig. 8.4. Spectra for the weekly pertussis case reports for England and Wales, 1957–76 (from Anderson *et al.* 1984) (*M* denotes window cut-off point and *B* denotes cycles per year).

seasonal cycles. The puzzling difference whereby vaccination against measles makes the seasonal cycles relatively more pronounced, while for pertussis it virtually eliminates the seasonal cycles, is discussed earlier (Fig. 6.13 and p. 136).

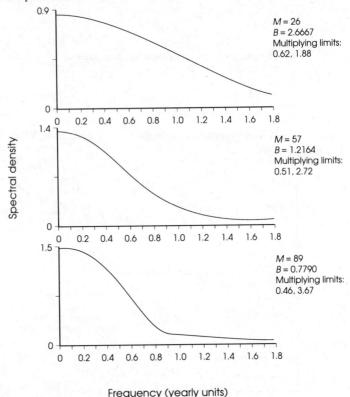

Fig. 8.5. Spectra for the weekly pertussis case reports for England and Wales, 1977–82. Data use trend-corrections before spectral analysis; *M* denotes window cut-off point and *B* denotes cycles per year (See Anderson *et al.* 1984).

8.4 Age-dependence in the force of infection

One immediate implication of the assumption of homogeneous mixing is that the force of infection should be the same for all ages. Studies of the force of infection—the probability that a susceptible of age a will acquire infection at that age—thus provide a direct test of the assumption.

Empirical evidence of age-related changes in λ have been documented for childhood infections by Collins (1929), Griffiths (1974), and Anderson and May (1982*d*); a critical evaluation of this earlier work is given in Grenfell and Anderson (1985). Grenfell and Anderson (1985) have presented a maximum-likelihood method that gives an operational way of assessing changes in λ with a, from serological data or from records of case notification.

Figure 8.6(b) shows the data for the cumulative proportion infected with measles, as a function of age, for England and Wales; the data are averages

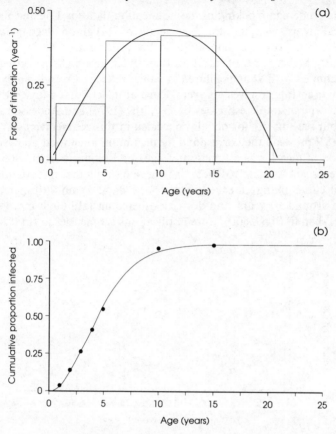

Fig. 8.6. Analysis of measles notifications for England and Wales, 1948–68. (a) The best fit polynomial (full curve) to the observed forces of infection $\lambda(a)$; the histograms represent average values in the age ranges 0.5–5 years, 5–10 years, etc). The average values are derived from the best fit polynomial (full curve) to the observed point values of $\lambda(a)$ (full circles) as recorded in (b) (see Grenfell and Anderson 1985).

over the pre-vaccination period from 1948 to 1968. The quadratic curve shown in Fig. 8.6(a) is the maximum-likelihood fit for $\lambda(a)$ in the age range 0–25 years (for details of the procedure, see Grenfell and Anderson (1985)). This functional form for $\lambda(a)$ generates the curve in Fig. 8.6(b), which captures the age-specific trends in case notifications well. Figure 8.6(a) also shows the values assigned to $\lambda(a)$ if it is constrained to have a series of constant values in five-year age blocks (except for the first block, which runs from 0.5 to 5 years, allowing for maternal antibodies by assigning $\lambda = 0$ for the first 6 months of life). Figure 8.6(a) shows a rise of λ up to around 10 years of age, followed by a decline at older ages. The Fine and Clarkson (1982*b*) analyses of a more finely age-stratified data set from London reveal a decline in $\lambda(a)$ after about 7–8 years of age; the crude age-blocking of the notification data for England and Wales does not allow us to explore the finer details of $\lambda(a)$ among teenage and adult age classes. It is probable that adults in the rough range 20–35 years of age have slightly higher rates of infection than older groups as a consequence of frequent contact with young children in family settings. Overall, analysis of the measles data in Fig.8.6 gives an average age at infection at 5.0 years, in broad agreement with a simple estimates by Griffiths (1974) and Anderson and May (1982*a*); but see Fig. 8.1 for details concealed in this coarse average.

Figure 8.7 presents the corresponding maximum-likelihood analysis of case notification of measles as a function of age, for Baltimore from 1906 to 1915. The patterns are similar to those in Fig. 8.6, with the smooth maximum-likelihood curve giving an excellent fit to the data. Again $\lambda(a)$ increases with age up to around 10 years, and decreases thereafter (although more slowly in Fig. 8.7(a) than in Fig. 8.6(a)). Case notifications for measles in rural Maryland

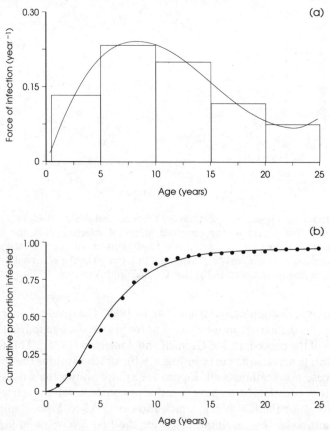

Fig. 8.7. Analysis of measles notifications for Baltimore, USA from 1906 to 1915. Parts (a) and (b) are as defined in the legend to Fig. 8.6 (see Grenfell and Anderson 1985).

(1908–17), Aberdeen (1883–1902), and England and Wales after vaccination (1969–82), along with serological data for small and large families in New Haven, show similar trends, albeit with a tendency for $\lambda(a)$ to increase more slowly with age in low-density rural communities than in large urban ones ($A = 6.7$ years in Baltimore versus $A = 9.3$ years in Maryland as a whole, at the turn of the century).

Table 8.1 (from Anderson and May (1985a) where the sources are cited) summarizes crude analyses of age-stratified data for incidence of measles infection, giving values of $\lambda(a)$ in five-year age blocks for a variety of places and times.

More generally, Fig. 8.8 shows the age-specific force of infection for pertussis in England and Wales, from case reports in 1956 (before widespread vaccination) and in 1980 (after more than 20 years of vaccination at varying coverage). Figure 8.9 illustrates $\lambda(a)$ for scarlet fever in England and Wales in 1977, again from age-stratified case reports. Lastly, Fig. 8.10 gives a melange of λ values for measles, mumps, chicken pox, and rubella, as deduced from case records in Baltimore in 1963.

The most striking feature of the information presented above is the consistency in the patterns of change in $\lambda(a)$ with age, for measles and other infections. The force of infection rises to a peak roughly around 5–15 years of age, and declines thereafter. This pattern holds for measles in different geographical locations and at different times, and broadly similar patterns hold for pertussis, mumps, chicken pox, rubella, and scarlet fever. These trends probably reflect age-related changes in the degree of mixing and contact, within and among age classes. School attendance is undoubtedly an important component in generating such changes.

Such social and behavioural factors should not, however, be accepted uncritically as the sole determinants of the observed changes in $\lambda(a)$ with age. The patterns could equally well derive largely from a consistent bias in case reporting with age; it is widely believed, for example, that the probability of a case of measles being reported is higher for young children than for adolescents or adults (Fine and Clarkson 1982b). Another problem is that the above analyses assume a roughly flat age distribution in the host population, from birth to an age around the average life expectancy. This is a reasonable assumption for many developed countries in the past decade or so, but can be less good for earlier periods; some of the data from case notifications may be somewhat biased by uneven age distributions.

In addition to these essentially technical problems, there is the interesting biological possibility that the host population may have genetic or behavioural heterogeneities that render some people intrinsically more liable to infection than others. If this were the case, a majority of more 'infectable' individuals could on average suffer illness at earlier ages, while less infectable individuals experienced illness at lower per capita rates (corresponding to older average ages); this effect, by itself, could generate most of the patterns documented above.

Table 8.1 Measles; age-dependent forces of infection (λ_i yr^{-1})

Geographic location and data	Age classes, λ_i						Type	Source of data Reference
	0–5	5–10	10–15	15–20	20–75	λ		
Aberdeen, Scotland, 1883–1902	0.172	0.400	0.149	0.121	0.105	0.133	Case notifications	Wilson (1904)
Willesden, London, England, 1913	0.089	0.340	0.143				Case notifications	Butler (1913)
Maryland, USA, 1808–17	0.078	0.250	0.195	0.131	0.030	0.065	Case notifications	Fales (1928)
Massachusetts, USA, 1930–40	0.074	0.370	0.150	0.150	0.0914	0.117	Case notifications	Wilson and Worcester (1941)
Shetlands, UK, 1977–8	0.049	0.100	0.109	0.045	0.057		Case notifications	Macgregor et al. (1981)
Baltimore, USA, 1963	0.200	0.582	0.379					*Baltimore Public Health Reports*
London, Ontario, Canada, 1912–13	0.088	0.240	0.220				Case notifications	Henderson (1916)
Baltimore, USA, 1900–31	0.124	0.320	0.176				Case notifications	Hedrich (1933)
Providence, RI, USA, 1917–24	0.190	0.440	0.114				Case notifications	Chaplin (1925)
England and Wales, 1966	0.184	0.579	0.202	0.100			Case notifications	*Registrar General Annual Reports*
England and Wales, 1980	0.148	0.348	0.268	0.101			Case notifications	*Registrar General Annual Reports*
Denmark, 1971–2	0.171	0.278	0.155				Case notifications	Horwitz et al. (1974)
New Haven, Conn. USA, 1955–8	0.100	0.240	0.362	0.086			Serlogy	Black (1959)
Average values	0.121	0.345	0.201	0.114	0.068			

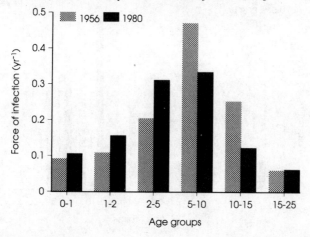

Fig. 8.8. Age-specific forces of infecion (yr^{-1}) for pertussis in England and Wales, derived from case reports during 1956 and 1980 (from Anderson and May 1985*c*).

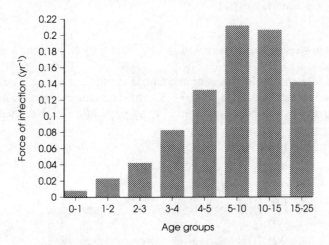

Fig. 8.9. Similar to Fig. 8.8 but representing scarlet fever in England and Wales during 1977 (from Anderson and May 1985*c*).

Motivated by this range of possibilities, we turn to survey two kinds of data that could help resolve the ambiguities.

8.4.1 *Epidemics in 'virgin' populations*

Outbreaks of infection in populations that have not experienced the disease agent before (or at least not for several decades) can provide valuable information about age-specific attack rates. We are aware of three such sets of

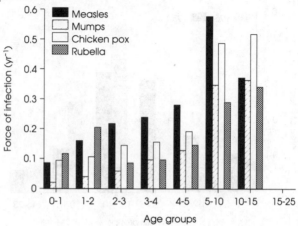

Fig. 8.10. A comparison of the age-specific forces of infection for measles, mumps, chicken pox, and rubella in Baltimore, USA during 1963, derived from case notifications (see Anderson and May 1985*c*).

data, which we summarize here and review more fully elsewhere (Anderson and May 1985*a*).

Figure 8.11 shows the forces of infection as a function of age for an outbreak of measles in the Shetlands in 1977–8. Although some exposure to infection had occurred in the past, and some of the population had been immunized,

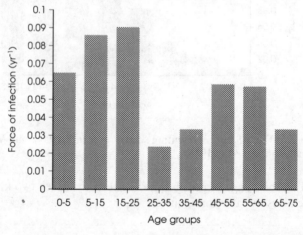

Fig. 8.11. Epidemics in 'virgin' populations. An epidemic of measles in the Shetlands, UK during the period 1977–8 (data source Macgregor *et al.* 1981) resulted in widespread infection across a broad band of age classes. The figure records estimates of the age-specific forces of infection acting during the epidemic (see Anderson and May 1985*c*).

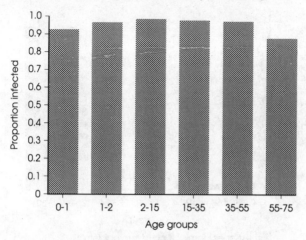

Fig. 8.12. Epidemics in 'virgin' populations. The estimated age-specific forces of infection based on proportions in each age class who experienced an attack of measles (Christensen *et al.* 1953) during an epidemic in southern Greenland during 1951 (see Anderson and May 1985*c*).

this population had an unusually high proportion of susceptibles before the epidemic. As can be seen from Fig. 8.11, λ does vary with age, but much less markedly than is the case for endemic measles. In particular, λ remains high (relative to its value in the 5–15 age group) in the adult age classes; λ actually reaches its peak value in the 15–25 age range, although this value is only marginally greater than for the 5–15 age range.

Figure 8.12 shows the proportion in each age class who experienced measles in a population in Greenland in 1951. This population was essentially 100 per cent susceptible before the epidemic. The attack rate is uniformly high, with just a hint of lower λ in the very young (0–1 age group) and the old (55–75 age group).

The third example is for a rubella outbreak on St Paul's Island in Alaska in 1963; a previous epidemic had occurred 20 years earlier, but the population was largely susceptible. Unlike the first two examples, which were based on case notifications, the Alaskan data give the proportion seropositive for rubella antibodies, both before and after the epidemic. These data are shown in Fig. 8.13. As with the measles outbreak in Greenland, the attack rate in Fig. 8.13 is uniformly high across all age groups.

These three examples suggest that age-related changes in the force of infection are weak or absent in previously unexposed populations. Most importantly, they reveal a much less marked decline in λ for adults relative to children than do the studies in Figs. 8.6–8.10 and Table 8.1. It is tempting to read this as support for the notion that the apparent changes in $\lambda(a)$ with age in endemic situations are produced by genetic or behavioural heterogeneities, as suggested above. It should be remembered, however, that social and environmental factors within these

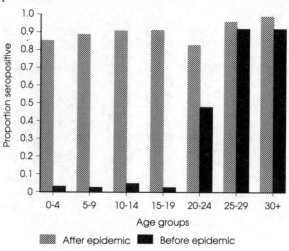

Fig. 8.13. Epidemics in virgin populations. Proportions serologically positive for rubella antibodies prior and post an epidemic of rubella in Alaska, USA during 1963 (see Broady *et al.* 1965).

isolated communities may affect the observations. For one thing, the climate in the Shetlands, Greenland, and Alaska is such that people are likely to spend more time in close contact within buildings than they would in England and Wales (to take a generous view of the latter climates). For another thing, small island communities typically have larger family sizes and fewer rooms per person than do more affluent mainland communities. Such factors may conspire to keep λ at a relatively high level among adults.

8.4.2 *Serological evidence for heterogeneity in susceptibility and resistance to infection*

Genetically based or other variablity in the level and duration of antibody production following infection would seriously complicate the interpretation of age–serological profiles (Aaby *et al.* 1981). Associations between HLA type and antibody titres following vaccination against rubella and measles provide evidence for the existence of such complications (Spencer *et al.* 1977; Kato *et al.* 1982). Little is understood, at present, about the importance of such factors in the design of vaccination programmes.

Figure 8.14(a) presents the proportion seropositive, by age, from a serological study of measles in 302 individuals in New Haven, in the pre-vaccination era (Black 1959). The figure shows clearly the decay in maternal antibodies in early life, followed by a rapid rise in positive scores to attain a plateau at around 96 per cent in the early adult age groups; thereafter the proportion positive falls to around 86 per cent in the 50+ age classes.

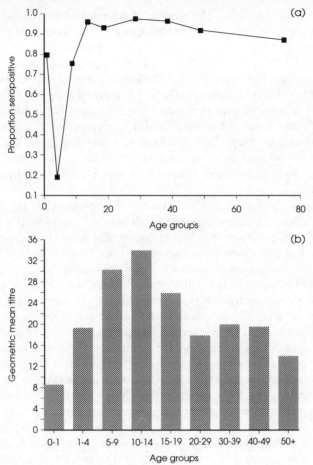

Fig. 8.14. Cross-sectional survey for the prevalence of measles antibodies in the population of New Haven, Connecticut, USA during 1957 (data source Black (1959)) (sample size = 302). (a) Proportion serologically positive by age; (b) geometric mean neutralizing antibody titres by age.

The geometric mean values of the neutralizing antibody titres, as shown in Fig. 8.14(b), rise during childhood to reach a peak in the 5–10 year age group, and then exhibit a significant decrease in later years. Black (1959) notes that a significant correlation was found between the presence of measles antibodies and a recorded history of infection, but that this association did not hold invariably: this confirms worries about the reliability of case-notification data.

The most intriguing question raised by these serological results, however, concerns the 4–5 per cent of individuals in the 15–30 year class who seem never to have experienced infection. The presence of these individuals is largely responsible for the low estimates of λ among older age groups. There are several possible explanations for these older individuals showing up as negative in serological tests. Black (1959) concluded that the individuals probably had experienced measles, but that their antibody titres had since decayed to undetectable levels. Alternatively, it could be that the serological tests gave false negatives, particularly when antibody titres were low. The possibility remains, however, that a small percentage of the population simply are not susceptible to apparent infection by measles, either for behavioural reasons (people who escape infection by living very isolated lives) or for genetic reasons (which could involve the level of antibody production following exposure, and the capacity to infect others).

The general patterns found in Black's work—particularly the few per cent who appear never to have experienced infection—are also found in more recent serological studies (for review, see Anderson and May (1985a) and Nokes *et al.* (1986)). The interpretation of these results is, however, made difficult by the impact of vaccination on the prevailing rates of infection.

If Fig. 8.14 is taken at face value, the calculated values of λ show the same variation with age (rising to a peak around age 5–15 years and then falling to low values in later life) that was noted earlier (see Table 8.1). We believe, however, there is need for further serological investigation of possible genetic variability in responses to infection. It is not inconceivable that community-level diagnostic programmes may, in the future, be aimed at the identification of relatively immunodeficient individuals, allowing vaccination to be targeted (at least for some viral and bacterial infections) to those children who are genetically predisposed to infection and severe morbidity.

Against this background, we go on in Chapter 9 to explore models in which the basic transmission rates (and consequently the force of infection) depend explicitly on age. We observed above that genetic heterogeneity with respect to infection could be partly responsible for the apparent dependence of λ on age; this and other kinds of heterogeneity are explored in Chapters 10–12.

8.5 Summary

We review some ways in which the basic model's assumption of homogeneous mixing can be tested against various kinds of data. Under an immunization programme that stops short of eradication, the fraction susceptible appears to remain roughly constant (consistent with homogeneous mixing), but the average age at infection and the period of the non-seasonal cycles in incidence usually increase less markedly than would be predicted. The most direct evidence against the homogeneous mixing assumption comes from studies showing that the force of infection, $\lambda(a)$, tends to increase with age up to about 5–15 years, and then to decrease in later years. This evidence is reviewed; potential biases and confounding effects are noted, and possibly supported by evidence from epidemics in 'virgin' populations and from serological studies.

Age-related transmission rates

9.1 Introduction

In this chapter, we generalize the basic model of Chapters 3–7, to include the effects of age-dependent variation in the force of infection (which ultimately derives from age dependence in the underlying transmission coefficients). We are particularly interested in how these realistic refinements, with parameter values based on the data surveyed in the preceding chapter, affect quantitative predictions about immunization programmes.

A qualitative feeling for the effects of variation of λ with age may be obtained as follows. Under the assumption of homogeneous mixing, λ is an age-independent constant, and the critical level of immunization coverage required for eradication is equal to the equilibrium fraction who are immune in the pre-immunization population; $p_c = 1 - x_0^*$ (eqns (2.1) and (5.2), where we have written the original population seropositive as x_0^*). This is no longer true if λ varies with age: if λ is high in the younger age classes, then p_c is *less* than would be estimated from $1 - x_0^*$; if λ is relatively higher in older age groups, then p_c is *greater* than estimated by $1 - x_0^*$. This observation, first made by Schenzle (1984), can be explained intuitively in the following way. As we discussed earlier, the indirect effect of immunization is to raise the average age at infection. But if the infection is intrinsically less transmissible among older age groups, it will be easier to eradicate than it would be if transmission were equally effective at all ages. Conversely, if infection is more efficiently transmitted at older ages, the indirect effects of immunization push transmission on average into an age range where eradication is relatively more difficult.

All this has clear implications for the design of immunization programmes. The critical levels of coverage estimated from the basic model (with homogeneous mixing) in Table 5.1 will be too pessimistic if $\lambda(a)$ decreases with age, and too optimistic if $\lambda(a)$ increases with age. Unfortunately, as we have just seen in Chapter 8 in some detail, $\lambda(a)$ in reality tends initially to increase with age, to peak in the 5–15 age range, and then to decrease at older ages. Depending on the relative magnitudes of these countervailing tendencies, the estimates of p_c in Table 5.1 could be too high or too low.

The rough pictorial arguments employed earlier in Figs. 4.4, 4.8, and 5.4 may again be helpful here. Figure 9.1 is a schematic representation of a hypothetical population in which infection cannot be acquired below age a_1 or above age a_2 (that is, $\lambda(a) = 0$ for $a < a_1$ or $a > a_2$). In the infectable age band $a_1 < a < a_2$, there is homogeneous mixing and $\lambda(a)$ is constant. This is clearly an artificially extreme case of the force of infection being lower at younger and at older ages!

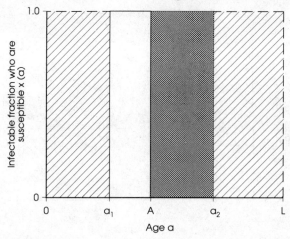

Fig. 9.1. Using the approach previously seen in Figs. 4.4, 4.8, and 5.4, this figure gives intuitive insight into the relation between the basic reproductive rate, R_0, of an infectious agent and the average age at infection, A, in the extreme case where transmission—far from being by homogeneous mixing among all ages—occurs only between ages a_1 and a_2. In this crude picture, the relevant fraction who are susceptible is $(A - a_1)/(a_2 - a_1)$, whence $R_0 = (a_2 - a_1)/(A - a_1)$; for further discussion see the text.

We further assume that individuals all remain susceptible up to the average age at infection, A, whereupon all are infected. Within the infectable age range, we may apply the same reasoning as was used in Figs. 4.4, 4.8, and 5.4, to deduce that the susceptible fraction of the at-risk population is $(A - a_1)/(a_2 - a_1)$. But this is the fraction by which the basic reproductive rate must be discounted to get an equilibrium rate of unity, whence (for hosts in the infectable range)

$$R_0 = (a_2 - a_1)/(A - a_1). \tag{9.1}$$

If we blithely assumed homogeneous mixing for the entire population, we would make the incorrect assessment $\tilde{R}_0 = L/A$. We see that true values of R_0 will be lower than our earlier estimates, $R_0 < \tilde{R}_0$, if

$$A > a_1/[1 - (a_2 - a_1)/L]. \tag{9.2}$$

In this event, eradication will be easier than estimated from $\tilde{R}_0$. Conversely, if A is less than the right-hand side of eqn (9.2), R_0 will be higher than crudely estimated under homogeneous mixing assumptions, and eradication will be correspondingly harder. Equation (9.2) shows that in the limit $a_1 \to 0$ (λ decreases with age), the critical coverage for eradication is always less than the rough (homogeneous mixing) estimate $1 - x_0^*$, while in the limit $a_2 \to L$ (λ increases with age) it is always greater. More generally, the answer depends on the details of A in relation to a_1, a_2, and L.

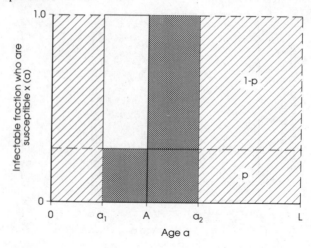

Fig. 9.2. This figure bears the same relation to Fig. 9.1 as Fig. 5.4 does to Fig. 4.4; it gives an intuitive impression of how the average age at infection, A', changes under an immunization programme in which the proportion immunized, p, is insufficient for eradication. The fraction susceptible is now roughly $(A' - a_1)(1 - p)/(a_2 - a_1)$, which remains equal to $1/R_0$. The resulting rough relations between A' and R_0 or A are as discussed in the text.

Figure 9.2 extends Fig. 9.1 to the case where a proportion p of the population have been immunized, which has the effect, *inter alia*, of increasing the average age at infection to $A'(p)$. By applying the earlier arguments to the at-risk population between the ages of a_1 and a_2, we see that A' and A are roughly related by

$$R_0 = \frac{a_2 - a_1}{(1 - p)(A' - a_1)}. \tag{9.3}$$

That is

$$A' = (A - pa_1)/(1 - p). \tag{9.4}$$

Depending on the relative magnitudes of A and a_1, $A'(p)$ can increase quite slowly with small-to-intermediate values of p, in contrast to the roughly $1/(1 - p)$ increase under the homogeneous mixing assumption. This can explain the observations about changes in A following vaccination which were discussed in Chapter 8.

Figures 9.1 and 9.2 are, of course, purely for exposition. They are far too extreme to be taken seriously.

In the next section, we outline the procedure for generalizing the basic model to include age dependence in the force of infection. These methods are then used to analyse static and dynamic aspects of mass vaccination against measles and rubella, with emphasis on the implications for programmes of control or

:radication. The chapter ends with a mathematical *jeu d'esprit*, in which we lraw some interesting conclusions from a simple model in which $\lambda(a)$ has two :omponents: a constant background component (as for homogeneous mixing) ind a component focused on contacts within the individual's own age cohort.

).2 Epidemiological models with age-dependent transmission rates

\s we explained when first defining $\lambda(a)$, eqn (3.19), the force of infection may n general be written (May 1986; May and Anderson 1984; Schenzle 1984; \nderson and May 1985a)

$$\lambda(a, t) = \int \beta(a, a') Y(a', t) \, da'. \qquad (9.5)$$

Γhe transmission rate, $\beta(a, a')$, describes the probability that an infective of age ι' will infect a susceptible of age a, per unit time. Under the 'mass action' ιssumption embodied in eqn (9.5), we obtain $\lambda(a)$—the net probability that a :usceptible individual of age a will acquire infection, per unit time—by ntegrating the transmission rate times the number of infectives of age a' over ιll ages a'.

The assumption of homogeneous mixing amounts to taking β to be constant, ndependent of a and a'. Another assumption making for simple calculations is that β depends only on a and not on a', so that $\lambda(a, t) = \beta(a) \bar{Y}(t)$. Although we did, in effect, use this assumption to carry out some relatively accurate calculations in Chapters 4 and 5 (see, for example, Figs. 5.5 and 5.13), it is hard to justify the assumption that transmission efficiency depends only on the age of the infectee and not at all on the age of the infector. The assumption that $\beta(a, a')$ separates into a symmetrical product, $\beta(a, a') = b(a)b(a')$, allows some elegant mathematics to be done, but has the drawback of explicitly denying the possibility of correlations in the ages of infector and infectee; such correlations are surely important. A common assumption—which we will make in essentially all of what follows—is that β is symmetrical, $\beta(a, a') = \beta(a', a)$. While there are obvious symmetries in the contact process, this particular assumption means that the process of development of a full-blown infection, following exposure, is independent of age (or is precisely mirrored by age dependence in production of infective stages by infectives). We suspect, although we cannot be sure, that age-related changes in contact probabilities are more important than age-related changes in inherent susceptibility or infectiousness.

In practice, the host population is usually divided into n discrete age classes (0–5, 5–10, etc.), which may be labelled by an index i ($i = 1, 2, \ldots, n$). The transmission rates are then defined by the elements of an $n \times n$ matrix, β_{ij}, where β_{ij} represents the probability that an infective in age class j will infect a susceptible in age class i, per unit time. For brevity, we refer to this 'who acquires infection from whom' matrix as the WAIFW matrix.

Once $\beta(a, a')$ or β_{ij} has been specified, the calculation of all epidemiological quantities of interest proceeds essentially as before. Starting with the usual set of partial differential equations that describe changes with time, t, and age, a, along with appropriate boundary conditions, we integrate numerically to find $X(a, t)$, $Y(a, t)$, $Z(a, t)$ (and also $H(a, t)$ and $I(a, t)$ if latent and maternal-antibody-protected categories are included). At each time-step, the force of infection, $\lambda(a)$, is updated by using eqn (9.5). This procedure can be time-consuming (and expensive in computer time), but it is straightforward.

There remains one problem in this otherwise routine procedure. Very rarely, if ever, do we have enough information to determine the WAIFW matrix, β_{ij}. In the case of homogeneous mixing, we can determine the (constant) value of λ in particular situations, and can thus infer the (constant) value of β. But in the present more general circumstances, we are likely to have n pieces of information—the n values of λ_i found from serological studies or age-stratified case records for each of the n age classes labelled by i—which is obviously insufficient to determine the n^2 elements of the matrix β_{ij} (except when $n = 1$). In effect, we observe a one-dimensional shadow (the $\lambda(a)$) cast by a two-dimensional object (the $\beta(a, a')$); in principle we could conceivably assess the distribution of ages of infectives who infected a particular age class of susceptibles, but in practice this is usually impossible.

A solution to this problem is implicit in Schenzle's pioneering work, and explicit in our own subsequent studies: the WAIFW matrix β_{ij} is constrained in such a way that it has only n distinct elements. The usual symmetry assumption, mentioned above, reduces the number of distinct elements to $n(n + 1)/2$. More severe restrictions are, however, needed to reduce the number down to n, once n gets up to around 3 to 6 or more.

Four possible structures for the WAIFW matrix, thus constrained, are set out below, for an epidemiological situation in which five age classes are distinguished. We shall use these 5×5 matrices in our later study of measles in England and Wales, where the five age categories are: 0–5 years, 5–10 years, 10–15 years, 15–20 years, and 20–75 years (Type I survival); these categories are labelled 1, 2, 3, 4, 5, respectively. The matrix called WAIFW 1, for example, embodies the prevailing opinion that the main route of transmission for many directly transmitted viral and bacterial infections is within the school playground or classroom: there is a unique coefficient (β_2) to describe the (presumed high) transmission among susceptibles and infectives in age class 2 (5–10 years), and two other coefficients (β_1 and β_3) for other contacts among children under 15 years of age; adolescents and adults are described as likely to acquire infection from a wider range of age groups. The matrix WAIFW 2 is a minor variation on WAIFW 1. The third form, WAIFW 3, simply corresponds to the situation discussed earlier, where transmission rates depend only on the age of the susceptible, $\beta(a, a') = \beta(a)$; this structure is included in order to compare its predictions with those of more plausible structures. Lastly, WAIFW 4 corresponds to the transmission process for those in the first four age classes (below

20 years) being primarily from contacts within their own age class, against a general background common to all individuals (the β_5 rate).

WAIFW 1

β_1	β_1	β_3	β_4	β_5
β_1	β_2	β_3	β_4	β_5
β_3	β_3	β_3	β_4	β_5
β_4	β_4	β_4	β_4	β_5
β_5	β_5	β_5	β_5	β_5

WAIFW 2

β_1	β_1	β_1	β_4	β_5
β_1	β_2	β_3	β_4	β_5
β_1	β_3	β_3	β_4	β_5
β_4	β_4	β_4	β_4	β_5
β_5	β_5	β_5	β_5	β_5

WAIFW 3

β_1	β_1	β_1	β_1	β_1
β_2	β_2	β_2	β_2	β_2
β_3	β_3	β_3	β_3	β_3
β_4	β_4	β_4	β_4	β_4
β_5	β_5	β_5	β_5	β_5

WAIFW 4

β_1	β_5	β_5	β_5	β_5
β_5	β_2	β_5	β_5	β_5
β_5	β_5	β_3	β_5	β_5
β_5	β_5	β_5	β_4	β_5
β_5	β_5	β_5	β_5	β_5

To study the impact of a specified immunization programme, we proceed as follows. *Step 1:* from serological studies or case records, determine the values of the forces of infection, λ_i, in the various age classes, before any immunization. *Step 2:* assign a structure to the WAIFW matrix, β_{ij}, and calculate the n distinct coefficients from the statics of infection before immunization. *Step 3:* solution of the partial differential equations, to unfold the dynamical trajectories after implementing a given immunization policy, now proceeds along the lines spelled out above; at each time-step, $\lambda(a)$ is updated, using eqn (9.5) or its discrete analogue with the unchanging values of the age-specific transmission rates as evaluated in Step 2. Notice, incidentally, that one or more of the matrix elements β_{ij} deduced in Step 2 may be negative; this indicates that a matrix structure inappropriate to the observed age dependence in λ has been chosen.

The next section makes these ideas more concrete, by running through the above recipe for the simple case where the WAIFW matrix is 2×2, distinguishing only two age classes. Appendix D gives details, and some analytic short-cuts, for the general cases of continuously varying ages, $\beta(a, a')$, and of n discrete age classes, β_{ij}.

9.3 A model with two age categories

Consider, as a special case of the more general treatment presented in Appendix D, a population divided into two age classes: class 1 and class 2, containing individuals in the age ranges 0 to a_1 years and a_1 to L years, respectively (where L is the life expectancy under Type I survival). At equilibrium, the number of susceptibles of age a is

$$X(a) = N(0) \exp(-\lambda_1 a) \qquad \text{if } a_1 > a, \qquad (9.6a)$$

$$X(a) = N(0) \exp[-\lambda_1 a_1 - \lambda_2(a - a_1)] \qquad \text{if } L > a > a_1. \qquad (9.6b)$$

Here, as always, $N(0)$ is the annual input of susceptibles by births, and λ_1 and λ_2 are the age-specific forces of infection for the age classes 1 and 2, respectively.

The age-specific forces of infection, λ_i ($i = 1, 2$), are related to the coefficients β_{ij} of the 2×2 WAIFW matrix by eqn (9.5):

$$\lambda_1 = \int \beta(1, a') Y(a') \, da' = \beta_{11} \bar{Y}_1 + \beta_{12} \bar{Y}_2, \qquad (9.7a)$$

$$\lambda_2 = \int \beta(2, a') Y(a') \, da' = \beta_{21} \bar{Y}_1 + \beta_{22} \bar{Y}_2. \qquad (9.7b)$$

Here $\bar{Y}_1$ and $\bar{Y}_2$ are the total number of infectious people in age classes 1 and 2, respectively. We could substitute from eqns (9.6) for $X(a)$ into the equilibrium equations describing the age dependence of $H(a)$ and $Y(a)$, and so obtain $Y(a)$ and thence $\bar{Y}_i$ to substitute in eqns (9.7). Alternatively, for most viral and bacterial infections of childhood where latent and infectious periods are very short compared with the average age at which infection is acquired ($\sigma \gg \lambda_i$, $v \gg \lambda_i$), we can use the approximation (see Appendix D)

$$\bar{Y}_i \simeq \lambda_i \bar{X}_i / v. \qquad (9.8)$$

The total number of susceptibles in age class i is easily calculated from eqns (9.6). Thus if λ_1 and λ_2 are estimated from data, we can calculate $\bar{Y}_1$ and $\bar{Y}_2$ (either directly or via the approximation of eqn (9.8)), and thence determine all the coefficients in eqns (9.7). Equations (9.7), however, then represent *two* equations in *four* unknowns ($\beta_{11}, \beta_{12}, \beta_{21}, \beta_{22}$). By imposing some structure on the matrix (for instance, $\beta_{11} \equiv \beta_1$ and $\beta_{12} \equiv \beta_{21} \equiv \beta_{22} \equiv \beta_2$), as discussed above, eqn (9.8) can be reduced to two equations in two unknowns, and the basic transmission rates thus determined. If either β_1 or β_2 is found to be negative, an inappropriate matrix structure has been chosen. This fulfils steps 1 and 2 of the programme outlined above.

Some other quantities of epidemiological interest are as follows. The total proportion of the population who are susceptible, in the equilibrium state, is

$$x = (\bar{X}_1 + \bar{X}_2)/\bar{N}. \qquad (9.9)$$

Here $\bar{N} = LN(0)$ is the total population size. The average age at infection, A, can be calculated from eqn (4.27) with eqns (9.6) for $X(a)$. The resulting expression is given in Appendix D. The concept of a basic reproductive rate needs some modification when the rate of transmission is different for different age classes. It is then necessary to define an age-specific basic reproductive rate, $R_{0,i}$, which is the average number of secondary cases (in all age classes) generated by one primary case in the ith age class, when the population is essentially wholly susceptible. With this definition,

$$R_{0,i} = (1/v) \int N(a)\beta(i, a) \, da. \tag{9.10}$$

Here $N(a)$ is the number of hosts in age class a. For our two-age-class model with Type I survival, eqn (9.10) reduces to

$$R_{0,1} = [\beta_{11}a_1 + \beta_{12}(L - a_1)]\bar{N}/vL, \tag{9.11a}$$

$$R_{0,2} = [\beta_{21}a_1 + \beta_{22}(L - a_1)]\bar{N}/vL. \tag{9.11b}$$

As pointed out by Dietz (1982b; Dietz and Schenzle 1985), the simple expression for R_0 with age-dependent $\lambda(a)$ given in our early studies of these complications is wrong (Anderson and May, 1982a).

With the transmission coefficients determined by the above procedure, the dynamics and eventual steady state of the system, following any specified disturbance (such as introduction of a vaccination scheme), may be determined by integrating the relevant equations. Of particular interest is the eradication criterion that replaces the simple $p_c = 1 - (1/R_0)$ of the homogeneously mixed models. We sketch how this criterion is found.

Suppose a fraction p of each cohort is immunized, essentially at birth. At equilibrium (if it exists) under this programme, the number of susceptibles at age a will be given by eqn (9.6) with two changes: the effective birth rate into the susceptible category is reduced to $(1 - p)N(0)$, and the force of infection is λ' (reduced below the original λ by the indirect effects of immunization). When the infection is teetering on the brink of eradication, $\lambda'_1 \to 0$ and $\lambda'_2 \to 0$. It follows that, in this limit, $\bar{X}_1 \to (1 - p)N(0)a_1$ and $\bar{X}_2 \to (1 - p)N(0)(L - a_1)$. Putting these expressions for $\bar{X}_i$ into eqn (9.8) for $\bar{Y}_i$, and then substituting into eqns (9.7) which relate λ'_i to β_{ij}, we have, in the limit $\lambda'_i \to 0$:

$$\lambda'_1 = \tilde{\beta}_{11}(1 - p)a_1\lambda'_1 + \tilde{\beta}_{12}(1 - p)(L - a_1)\lambda'_2, \tag{9.12a}$$

$$\lambda'_2 = \tilde{\beta}_{21}(1 - p)a_1\lambda'_1 + \tilde{\beta}_{22}(1 - p)(L - a_1)\lambda'_2. \tag{9.12b}$$

Here we have written $\tilde{\beta}_{ij} = \beta_{ij}N(0)/v$, to avoid unnecessary clutter. Equations (9.12a) and (9.12b) are homogeneous linear equations in λ'_1 and λ'_2, and they are consistent only if the determinant of the matrix formed from their coefficients vanishes:

$$\det \begin{vmatrix} \tilde{\beta}_{11}a_1(1 - p) - 1 & \tilde{\beta}_{12}(L - a_1)(1 - p) \\ \tilde{\beta}_{21}a_1(1 - p) & \tilde{\beta}_{22}(L - a_1)(1 - p) - 1 \end{vmatrix} = 0. \tag{9.13}$$

This amounts to a quadratic equation for p; the largest root in the range 0–1 represents the critical coverage, p_c, that we sought. More generally, and in more elevated language, we can show that $p_c = 1 - 1/\rho$, where ρ is the dominant eigenvalue of the $n \times n$ matrix whose elements are $\tilde{\beta}_{ij}\Delta a_j$ (where Δa_j is the width of the jth age class).

9.4 An example: measles in England and Wales, 1966–82

These methods are now applied to study the population biology of measles in England and Wales, from the days before vaccination (1966) to the early 1980s, as a concrete example (Anderson and May 1985*a*). For assessing $\lambda(a)$ and $\beta(a, a')$, the population is partitioned into five age categories: 0–5, 5–10, 10–15, 15–20, and 20–75 years. Some values of λ in these categories, as inferred from various data, were given and discussed in Table 8.1.

9.4.1 *Determining the transmission rates*

We present results for each of four choices for the structure of the 5×5 WAIFW matrix, β_{ij}, in order to get an idea of how sensitive the answers are to this somewhat arbitrarily imposed structure. These four matrices, labelled WAIFW 1–4, are depicted and discussed in Section 9.2. Mainly, however, we will work with WAIFW 1. As listed in Table 9.1, three different sets of λ_i values are used to calculate the five independent elements of the WAIFW matrix: those derived from case notifications in England and Wales in 1966, those derived from the serological data collected by Black (1959) in New Haven in 1955–8, and the mean age-specific values obtained by averaging over all the data recorded in Table 8.1. As Table 8.1 makes plain, estimates of λ are not often available for the adult age groups (20–75 years), and are frequently missing for the 15–20 year age group. Unfortunately, such absence of data compounds the problems of bias and ambiguity of biological interpretation that—as discussed in

Table 9.1 Estimates of age-specific forces of infection from various sources, and consequent predictions about vaccination coverage to achieve eradication (from Anderson and May 1985*a*)

Data source (for references see Anderson and May (1985*a*))	Age groups					Average age at infection, A (year)	Proportion immune before immunization, $1 - x^*$	Critical vaccination coverage for eradication, ρ_c
	0–5	5–10	10–15	15–20	20–75			
	Forces of infection, λ_i (yr^{-1})							
	λ_1	λ_2	λ_3	λ_4	λ_5			
Case reports, England and Wales, 1966	0.184	0.579	0.202	0.100	0.100	4.3	0.94	0.89
Serological studies, USA, 1955–8	0.100	0.240	0.362	0.086	0.086	6.6	0.91	0.86
Average values of studies summarized by Anderson and May (1985*a*)	0.121	0.345	0.201	0.144	0.068	5.9	0.92	0.83

Table 9.2 Parameter values used in the various models for static and dynamic aspects of measles in England and Wales (see Anderson and May 1985*a*)

Parameter	Symbol	Value
Life expectancy	L	75 years
Duration of infectiousness	$1/v$	7 days
Duration of latency	$1/\sigma$	7 days
Duration of protection by maternal antibodies	$1/d$	3 months
Total population size	N	49 600 000

Chapter 8—already affect estimates of the apparently lower values at λ_i at older ages. In Table 9.1, we simply assume $\lambda_5 = \lambda_4$ for the England/Wales and New Haven data. As for the different WAIFW structures, these different sets of λ_i values are explored to see how sensitive to details the answers are; in subsequent calculations, we mainly use the λ_i values for England and Wales in 1966.

For the other relevant epidemiological and demographic parameters in the models, we assign average values appropriate for measles in Britain; these are set out in Table 9.2.

9.4.2 *Long-term steady state under vaccination*

Having deduced the WAIFW matrix elements under a particular set of assumptions, we can estimate (as shown generally in Appendix D) the critical proportion, p_c, of each age cohort that must be vaccinated at around one year of age, eventually to eradicate measles.

The results of one such equilibrium calculation are set out in Table 9.1, which gives p_c for each of the three sets of λ_i values (assuming the transmission matrix has structure WAIFW 1). The net effect of the lower infection rates among young children and adults is to reduce the critical level of coverage somewhat below the predictions based on homogeneous mixing (which are $\tilde{p}_c = 1 - x^* \simeq 1 - L/A$). Using the data for England and Wales, for example, the basic model suggests that 94 per cent need be immunized close to birth, while the model with age-dependent forces of infection predicts a critical level of 89 per cent. A similar 5 per cent difference is found for the calculations based on serological data. A larger 9 per cent discrepancy arises between p_c from the age-structured calculation and $\tilde{p}_c$ from the basic model when λ_i values are obtained by averaging over all entries in Table 8.1; the discrepancy comes primarily from the unusually low value of λ_5 (20–75 age class), which itself is determined as an average over four rather dodgy sets of data (see Table 8.1).

In view of our earlier worries that estimates of the force of infection in the 20–75 age class, λ_5, are less reliable than those in other age classes, Table 9.3 examines the sensitivity of the predictions to changes in λ_5. As the value of λ_5 is reduced from slightly below λ_3 down to essentially zero (from 0.15 to

Table 9.3 Predictions of the model, under various assumptions about the force of infection in the age group 20–75 years, λ_5; the values of λ_i for the younger age groups are set equal to those from case reports in England and Wales in 1966 (first row in Table 9.1). As discussed in the text, these results illustrate how sensitive the predictions can be to the value of λ_5

λ_1	λ_2	λ_3	λ_4	λ_5	Average age at infection, A (years)	Proportion immune before immunization $1 - x^*$	Critical vaccination coverage for eradication, p_c
0.184	0.579	0.202	0.100	0.150	4.25	0.94	0.92
0.184	0.579	0.202	0.100	0.100	4.27	0.94	0.89
0.184	0.579	0.202	0.100	0.080	4.28	0.94	0.87
0.184	0.579	0.202	0.100	0.050	4.29	0.94	0.85
0.184	0.579	0.202	0.100	0.010	4.22	0.94	0.84
0.184	0.579	0.202	0.100	0.001	4.15	0.94	0.84

Age-specific forces of infection (yr^{-1})

Table 9.4 The effect of the form of the WAIFW matrix (from p. 177) upon predictions about eradication criteria, and other such epidemiological indicators

WAIFW matrix	Average age at infection, A (years)	Average age at infection, at the point of eradication, A_c (years)	Critical vaccination coverage for eradication, p_c
1	4.3	33.1	0.89
2	4.3	33.0	0.89
3	4.3	28.2	0.91
4	4.3	17.8	0.97

$0.001 \, \text{yr}^{-1}$), the differences between the basic model, $\tilde{p}_c$, and the more accurate age-structured model, p_c, increase from about 2 per cent to about 10 per cent. If the value of λ_5 is really very low, we would predict that an 85 per cent level of successful immunization would eradicate measles. We believe, however, that a λ_5 value of around $0.1 \, \text{yr}^{-1}$ is more realistic, leading to a critical coverage of 89 per cent or more.

Table 9.4 presents results obtained by varying the structure of the transmission matrix, from WAIFW 1 to WAIFW 4 (see Section 9.2); in all cases the λ_i were determined from the first row (England and Wales 1966) in Table 9.1. There is no significant difference between the predictions from the structures 1 and 2, which we believe represent the most reasonable approximations to current ideas about age-specific contact rates. The structure WAIFW 3 was included for comparison, and also because it corresponds to the crude way in which age-dependent effects were introduced into some of our earlier calculations (Chapter 5); this less-reasonable structure gives results only 2 per cent different from the others for p_c. The structure WAIFW 4 assumes that transmission has essentially two components, one concentrated within age classes and the other deriving from homogeneous mixing among all age classes. In comparison with the other WAIFW matrices, WAIFW 4 requires very significantly higher levels of coverage, around 97 per cent, for eradication. This is essentially because, with WAIFW 4 and any of the λ_i values in Table 9.1, most individuals in the age class 2 (5–10 years) experience infection, leaving relatively few susceptibles in the later years; for λ_3 to be as large as observed, this WAIFW 4 structure thus implies that β_3 (transmission within the 10–15 year class) must be very high (higher than β_2). This, in turn, means that as an immunization programme pushes the average age at infection higher, transmission is perversely enhanced (by the higher β_3 in the 10–15 year range), and eradication is therefore harder. Hence the conclusion that, for WAIFW 4 and the λ_i values in Table 9.4, 97 per cent coverage is needed for eradication (with the average age of infection near eradication being just past the 15-year-old boundary). An analytic model for within-cohort transmission is discussed at the end of this chapter, and it provides further insight into the interesting—and probably relevant—complications that such age-focussed transmission may produce. For the time being, however, we note that caution can be needed in interpreting results based on the assumption that much of the transmission is confined within age classes.

9.4.3 *Short-term dynamics*

This subsection sketches the results of numerical studies of the dynamical behaviour of the full set of partial differential equations for numbers protected by maternal antibodies, susceptible, latent, infectious, and recovered-and-immune at age a and time t ($I(a, t)$, $X(a, t)$, $H(a, t)$, $Y(a, t)$, and $Z(a, t)$, respectively), with age-dependent transmission rates, eqn (9.5). These equations are set out in Appendix D, and a much more complete discussion of the analysis is in Anderson and May (1985a).

Figure 9.3 shows the oscillations in the incidence of measles that are produced by the model described above, with the WAIFW 1 matrix and λ_i values from England and Wales in 1966 (row 1, Table 9.1). The simulation was started by reducing the fraction susceptible in each age class below the equilibrium value by 20 per cent. These oscillations have a much longer damping time than was found for the basic model in Chapter 6. Indeed, if the simulations are not run for long enough (a century or more!), the oscillations may appear to be self-sustaining limit cycles. This, we believe, is the basis for the claims mentioned in Section 6.5.4 (derived apparently from numerical studies) that age structure in transmission rates can produce limit cycles. Greenhalgh's (1987) analytic

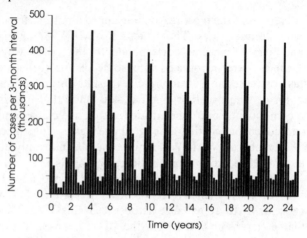

Fig. 9.3. Predicted changes in the reported number of cases of measles (in three-monthly intervals) over a time span of 25 years, following a perturbation of the system from its equilibrium state. In this computation, the transmission matrix has the form WAIFW 1 and the forces of infection, λ_i, are given by the top row in Table 9.1. The total population size was held constant at 5×10^7, maternally derived antibodies were assumed to provide protection for an average period of 3 months, and the incubation and infectious periods were set at 7 days each. After Anderson and May (1984), where fuller details are given.

studies show that this is not so. But age-structure effects certainly do enhance the system's propensity to oscillate, probably making it easier for other mechanisms (such as demographic stochasticity or seasonality) to sustain the oscillations indefinitely.

The periods of the cycles in Fig. 9.3 are almost exactly 2 years. This is shorter than the estimate based on homogeneous mixing (Table 6.1), and fits the observed facts better. The average age at infection, A, calculated from Fig. 9.3 and others like it, also accords with the observed values, varying between 4.3 and 4.7 years depending on whether the estimate is made in a 'peak' or 'trough' year (compared with the 1966 data in Fig. 8.1).

Using the same age-structured model as for Fig. 9.3, in Fig. 9.4 we display predicted trends under the impact of vaccination. The first ten years are before vaccination, and are identical with the first ten years in Fig. 9.3. Vaccination is begun in year 10, and for the next 15 years the age-specific vaccination rates were set at the values actually recorded for England over the period 1968–82 (see Anderson and May 1985a). For the last five years, the vaccination levels were set equal to the 1982 figures. The observed data, plotted as case notifications per three-month interval, are shown in Fig. 9.5.

In two respects, Fig. 9.4 provides a much better fit to the facts about measles vaccination in England and Wales than did the basic model discussed in Chapters 6 and 8. First, the age-dependent model predicts a marked reduction

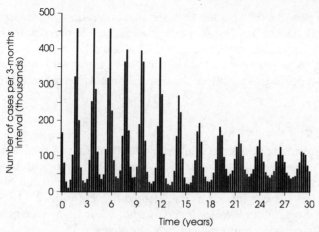

Fig. 9.4. As for Fig. 9.3, except that an immunization programme is begun in year 10. The rates of immunization for each age class in each year are extracted from recorded levels of coverage in England and Wales, 1968–82. Of each yearly cohort, approximately 50–55 per cent were immunized by their sixth year of life (after Anderson and May 1984).

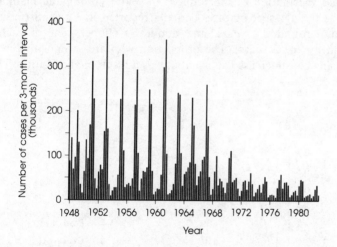

Fig. 9.5. Longitudinal trends in measles incidence, following the introduction of immunization in 1968. The figure shows the number of reported cases of measles, per three months, in England and Wales from 1948 to 1982. (After Anderson and May 1984).

in the amplitude of the 'epidemics', and a slight increase in the inter-epidemic period from around 2 to around 2.5 years. This matches with the facts; see Figs. 8.2 and 8.3. Second, the increase in A is from an average of 4.5 years to around 5.6 years, which is much closer to reality than the value of $A \sim 9$ years suggested by the basic model; in fact A was 4.4 years in 1968 and between 5.2 and 5.5

years in the period 1980–2, after 15 years of vaccination. On the negative side, the predicted decline in overall average incidence of measles in Fig. 9.4 is somewhat less than observed, in Fig. 9.5. This could be owing to a fault in the model (such as the omission of seasonality in transmission), or it could arise from under-reporting of cases (see the discussion in Anderson and May 1985*a*).

9.4.4 *Impact of vaccination*

Figure 9.6 presents a detailed test of the model's accuracy in predicting changes in the number seropositive as a function of age. The serological data are from various places in England over the period 1979–83 (Anderson and May 1985*a*). The theoretical curve is for our age-structured model (using WAIFW 1 and λ_i values from England and Wales in 1966), after 12 years of vaccination at the rates actually pertaining in England over those years. The agreement between theory and data is heart-warming.

Figure 9.7 shows the predictions of the same age-structured model as was used in Fig. 9.6 for the impact of vaccination on age–serological profiles for measles antibodies in England and Wales. In the calculations leading to this figure, mass vaccination was introduced in year 1 (1968), and maintained for 16 years at the age-specific rates actually reported in England (mean age at vaccination around 2.2 years, and about 50–60 per cent of each cohort immunized by age 5 years). The proportion who are seropositive in the 1–6 year age range has increased substantially as a result of vaccination. The figure

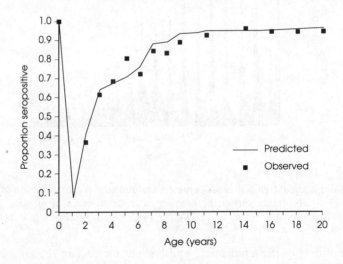

Fig. 9.6. Predicted and observed serological profiles for measles antibody after 12 years of mass immunization. The levels of immunization coverage were taken to be as reported in England for the years 1968–79. The observed data are as compiled in Anderson and May (1985*a*).

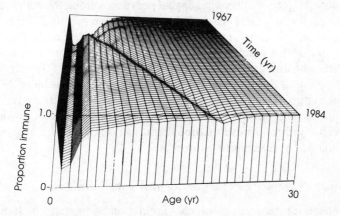

Fig. 9.7. This figure shows the predictions made by our model for the impact of mass immunization upon age–serological profiles for measles antibodies (i.e. the proportion in each age class who are immune as a result of maternally derived protection (among infants), recovery from natural infection, or vaccination), in England and Wales. Mass immunization was begun in 1968, and maintained here up to 1984 at the age-specific rates actually recorded in England and Wales (mean age at vaccination is 2.2 years and around 50–55 per cent of each cohort are immunized by age 5); the 1967, pre-vaccination profile was used to estimate the magnitude of the elements of the age-specific transmission matrix. The x axis measures age, in one-year steps. Notice how mass immunization (in the age range 1–3 years) acts to decrease the proportion seropositive in the older age classes (by reducing the overall force of infection within the community below the pre-immunization level). The valley of seronegativity running diagonally across the surface corresponds to the ageing of the last cohorts of young children to be excluded from mass immunization. For further details see Anderson and May (1985*a, c*).

also shows, however, that those who were not immunized are exposed to a reduced force of infection, and hence have a greater chance of remaining seronegative during their teenage and adult years than was the case before mass immunization. The valley of seronegativity running diagonally across the surface corresponds to the last cohorts of young children who escaped immunization. All this bears out in detail the points made earlier, in Chapter 5.

All the work in this section is presented more fully elsewhere (Anderson and May 1985*a*). We conclude that the age-structured models are capable of providing a good fit to the facts about serological profiles and temporal trends under vaccination for measles in a developed country. The predictions as to critical levels of coverage for eradication are relatively insensitive to the choice of the WAIFW matrix among reasonable alternatives, but they do depend significantly on the estimate of λ in older age classes before immunization.

Past estimates of p_c, based on models with homogeneous mixing and assuming vaccination at around one year of age, were around 94–96 per cent (Anderson and May 1982*a*). The more accurate estimates presented above suggest a lower figure of approximately 89 per cent. Among the many remaining factors which further complicate such estimates, we mention three. First, in Britain vaccination against measles is typically in the second or third year of life; if continued, this practice would raise p_c. Second, current vaccines are not perfectly efficient, and probably protect roughly 95 per cent of those immunized; this factor, by itself, would require 94 per cent coverage to achieve 89 per cent protection. Third, and cutting against the other two, stochastic fade-out becomes increasingly likely as incidence falls under vaccination, which could possibly result in local or even national eradication of measles at levels below those estimated by deterministic thresholds.

9.5 Another example: vaccination against rubella in Britain

The counter-intuitive way in which vaccination of young children against rubella can, at moderate levels of coverage (less than ~50 per cent), lead to an increase in the incidence of CRS was discussed in Chapter 5. The consequent differences in vaccination policies between the USA (where vaccination is essentially compulsory, and where high coverage of 2- to 3-year-olds has been achieved) and the UK (where vaccination is voluntary) were also discussed in Chapters 5 and 7 (see Figs. 5.9–5.11 and 7.2–7.5).

In the UK, the policy has been to vaccinate girls, and only girls, between the ages of 10 and 15 years. By the mid-1980s, the average age at vaccination was 12 years, and roughly 85 per cent of each cohort was vaccinated by age 15 years. This strategy has been supplemented by selective post-partum vaccination of women found to be susceptible to rubella, and by encouraging women in the child-bearing years to be screened for rubella antibodies and vaccinated if seronegative. As emphasized earlier, although the UK policy may result in lower incidence of CRS than the USA policy at all but very high coverage levels, it can never eradicate rubella. The currently high levels of vaccine uptake among girls in the UK has therefore prompted discussion of alternative policies that might further reduce the incidence of CRS.

One such suggestion is a two-stage policy in which continued vaccination of 12-year-old girls is combined with vaccination of 2-year-old girls and boys, in the form of a combined measles-mumps-rubella, MMR, vaccine (and thus presumably at levels of coverage similar to measles vaccination in the UK, which in the mid-1980s was around 50–60 percent). Such a programme of immunization of pre-school children with MMR, rather than simply measles, vaccine was begun in the UK in late 1988. An alternative two-stage policy combines vaccination of 12-year-old girls with vaccination of susceptible women at an average age of around 25 years. These two policies could be combined in a three-stage scheme. Table 9.5 summarizes these options, labelling them for ease in subsequent reference.

We now show how our age-structured models can be applied to give a comparative analysis of these options (Anderson and Grenfell 1986).

Table 9.5 Some policies for vaccination against rubella

Type of policy	Description
Single-stage (policy 1)	A UK policy in which girls, and girls only, are vaccinated between the ages of 10–15 years.
Two-stage—Type A (policy 2)	A combined UK and USA policy in which girls and boys are vaccinated at 2 years of age, and girls at between 10–15 years of age
Two-stage—Type B (policy 3)	A UK policy plus the vaccination of susceptible women at around the age of 25 years.
Three-stage (policy 4)	A combined UK and USA policy plus vaccination of susceptible women of age 25 years.

9.5.1 *Estimating the model's parameters*

Because infection in the child-bearing years is so important, we employ one more age class than in the measles models by subdividing the 20–75 year class into 20–30 years (Class 5) and 30–75 years (Class 6).

We mainly use a 'who acquires infection from whom' matrix whose structure is a direct extension of WAIFW 1 (Section 9.2), obtained by adding a row (β_6) at the foot and a column (β_6) to the right; we call this 6×6 matrix WAIFW A. Likewise, we generalize WAIFW 4 by having five diagonal elements (β_1–β_5) against a background of β_6s; we call this WAIFW B. To explore the sensitivity of the predictions to the shape chosen for the transmission matrix, we also consider WAIFW C, which is the same as WAIFW B except that $\beta_{51} = \beta_{52} = \beta_{15} = \beta_{25} = \beta_5$ (which says that adults in the 20–30 year age group have essentially as much contact with 0- to 10-year-olds as within their own age group). These matrix structures are summarized in Table. 9.6.

Table 9.6 The principal features of virus transmission captured by the different WAIFW matrices

Configuration	Transmission characteristic
WAIFW A	High levels of mixing within age classes are a unique feature of the child age groups.
WAIFW B	Mixing within age classes is greater than mixing between age classes in child, teenage and adult classes.
WAIFW C	Adults in the principal-parent age class (20–30 years) have a high degree of contact with the infant and child age groups.

Table 9.7 Age-specific forces of infection for rubella in England

| Data source | Forces of infection (λ_i (yr^{-1})) by age class in years | | | | | |
	0–4	5–9	10–14	15–19	20–29	30+
Serological studies in southeast England, 1980–1 (from Nokes *et al.* 1985)	0.081	0.115	0.115	0.083	0.067	0.067
Case notifications (data summarized in Anderson and Grenfell (1986))	0.089	0.134	0.151	0.148	0.126	0.126

The age-specific forces of infection, λ_i, from which the coefficients of the underlying transmission matrix are calculated, are based on two sources of data. They are summarized in Table 9.7. One set of values comes from a serological survey of over 3000 people with a range of ages, and the other comes from age-stratified case records. Both sets of data are for males only, in the hope that their age–serological profiles are essentially as they were before vaccination of 12-year-old girls; the age-structured models suggest this assumption is reasonably accurate.

The average duration of protection by maternal antibodies is taken to be 3 months, and the duration of latent and infectious periods 10.5 days and 11.5 days, respectively. We use Type I survival, with $L = 75$ years; births and deaths are assumed to balance. As before, the age-specific risk function for CRS, $r(a)$, is taken to be proportional to the age-specific fertility rates in the UK.

9.5.2 *Impact of vaccination on rubella and CRS*

With the pre-vaccination state defined by the above choice of parameters, the impact of vaccination can be studied by numerical integration of our age-structured model. Figures 9.8(a) and 9.8(b) compare the observed age-specific serological profiles for rubella antibodies in females and males, respectively, in England and Wales in 1984 with the predictions of the model after 15 years of vaccination. These theoretical predictions are generated using the form WAIFW A for the matrix of transition rates and the serological data for λ_i (first row in Table 9.7); the age-specific vaccination rates are set equal to those actually recorded for girls between the ages of 10 and 15 years in the UK over the period 1970–84. The agreement between theory and data in Fig. 9.8 lends some credibility to the projections into the future now to be presented.

Once the age-specific susceptibilities and forces of infection have been computed at any given time after the implementation of a given vaccination policy, the ratio between the number of cases of CRS at that time and the number before vaccination, $\rho(a_1, a_2; t)$, can be calculated from eqn (5.18).

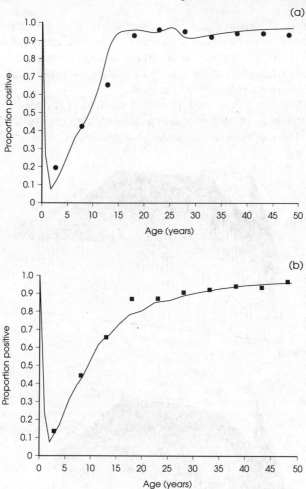

Fig. 9.8. A comparison of the observed and predicted horizontal serological profiles for rubella, stratified by age, in (a) the female and (b) the male population of the UK in 1980–1. The observed data are from Nokes *et al.* (1986). As discussed more fully by Anderson and Grenfell (1986), the predictions are based on time-dependent solutions of the model described in the text. The intrinsic forces of infection were estimated from serological data for males before the advent of immunization, and age-specific immunization rates were set at the levels reported in England and Wales over the period 1970–84.

The long-term equilibrium prediction for this ratio, ρ^*, was shown earlier in Fig. 5.11 for the two-stage 'UK plus USA' programme defined as policy 2 in Table 9.5 (this figure anticipated the present discussion, in that it is calculated from an age-structured model using serological data for λ_i and WAIFW A). Figure 5.11 depicts the two-dimensional surface of values of ρ^*, as a function of the coverage of girls at age 12 years and of the coverage of boys and girls at age 2 years. This surface gives a measure of the achievements of a particular programme. It will be seen that, at 80–90 per cent coverage of 12-year-old girls, little is gained (though nothing is lost) by adding vaccination at age 2 years, until the coverage exceeeds 50–60 per cent.

Figures 9.9(a) and 9.9(b) show predicted serological surfaces, for the female and male segments of the population respectively, over the 20-year span 1984–2003. The calculations show the changes in age–serological profiles to

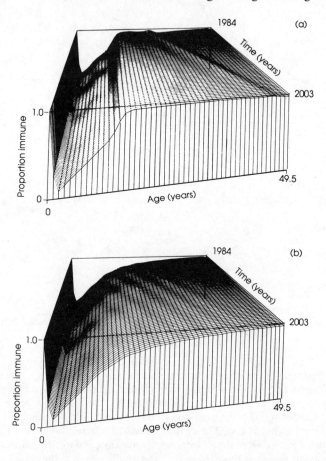

Fig. 9.9. As discussed in the text, these figures show the age-specific serological profiles for rubella for (a) females and (b) males, over the time span 1984–2003, under a continuation of the one-stage UK policy (policy 1 of Table 9.5). These calculations are based on models with age-dependent forces of infection. The parameters are estimated from serological data, assuming the WAIFW matrix A of Table 9.6; vaccination levels in each year are set equal to the actual rates in the UK in 1984. After Anderson and Grenfell (1986).

be expected if the one-stage UK vaccination policy (policy 1 of Table 9.5) were continued, maintaining the age-specific levels of vaccination at 1984 levels (roughly 85 per cent). Again, these estimates employ the serological data for λ_i and the structure WAIFW A for β_{ij}. The ripple running diagonally across the surface in Fig. 9.9(a) corresponds to the initiation of vaccination back in 1970.

Figures 9.10(a) and 9.10(b) are similar to Figs. 9.9(a) and 9.9(b), except now a combined UK and USA vaccination programme (policy 2 of Table 9.5) is instigated in 1985, with 60 per cent coverage of boys and girls at age 2 years and the 1984 levels of vaccination of girls between 10 and 15 years of age.

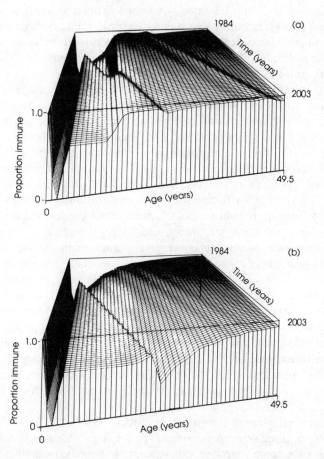

Fig. 9.10. As for Fig. 9.9, except now the predicted serological surfaces for rubella for (a) females and (b) males in 1984–2003 are for a two-stage UK–USA immunization policy (policy 2 of Table 9.5) begun in 1985, with 60 per cent coverage of boys and girls at 2 years of age and the 1984 levels of immunization of girls between 10 and 15 years of age. The features of this figure are discussed in the text; for further details see Anderson and Grenfell (1986).

Comparison of Figs. 9.10(a) and 9.10(b) with Figs. 9.9(a) and 9.9(b) shows a marked increase in immunity among pre-teen children, as obviously expected. But policy 2 increases the proportion of females remaining seronegative in the late teenage and adult years (Fig. 9.10(a)) in comparison with policy 1 (Fig. 9.9(a)). On the one hand, policy 2 does reduce the incidence of CRS (as shown in Fig. 5.11 and in Fig. 9.12 below), yet on the other hand it reduces the level of herd immunity among women in the child-bearing years. This paradox arises because the incidence of rubella is greatly reduced by the vaccination of children at a young age, which has a direct impact on the incidence of CRS; but this reduced incidence of rubella results in fewer people acquiring immunity by natural infection, and—as illustrated—ends up leaving more females susceptible at older ages. This fact points to a danger latent in the two-stage policy: once begun, strenuous efforts must be made to maintain high levels of vaccination among 2-year-olds, lest the increased susceptibility of women in the age-range 16–40 years result in serious outbreaks of CRS.

The best example of immunization increasing the average age at infection and inducing ripples in the age-stratified serological profile is provided by the history of rubella immunization in Finland. The programme adopted in this country was as follows. From 1975 to 1982 immunization was targeted at girls and girls only (to prevent congenital rubella syndrome (CRS) in babies born to mothers who contract rubella during the first trimester of pregnancy) in the age range of 12–18 years. Vaccination took place after the average age at infection (7–9 years prior to the start of immunization) and hence had little impact on the overall transmission of the virus. In November 1982 an additional programme of vaccination was introduced (using the triple measles, mumps, and rubella vaccine, MMR) to cover young children in the age ranges 1–6 years. This new programme had an immediate effect on the net rate of transmission and it acted to shift the age distribution of cases upwards, increasing the average age of infection from 1983 onwards (Fig. 9.11(a)). In addition the major perturbation introduced by this sudden reduction in transmission induced a ripple in the age-stratified serological profile such that a cohort of susceptible children, just older than the age range covered by the vaccination introduced in 1982, is clearly discernible in the serological profiles for 1984 onwards (Fig. 9.11(b)). The data displayed in Fig. 9.11 are described in an excellent publication by Ukkonen and von Bronsdorff (1988).

The dangers inherent in the two-stage UK + USA policy 2 can be reduced by adopting a three-stage programme (policy 4 of Table 9.5), which adds vaccination of women who are still susceptible to rubella in their twenties. Figure 9.12 is similar to Figs. 9.9(a) and 9.10(a), except that policy 4 is initiated in 1985, with 50 per cent of still-susceptible women vaccinated at age 25 years. Close comparison of Figs. 9.12 and 9.10(a) shows the three-stage policy substantially reduces the band of susceptibility among women of child-bearing ages.

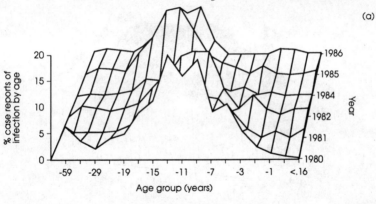

(a)

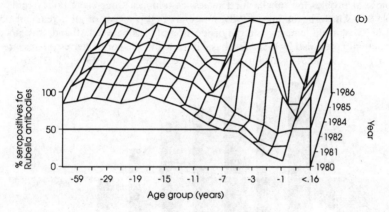

(b)

Fig. 9.11. (a) Occurrence of virologically proven rubella infection in different age groups, males and females combined, in Finland from 1980 to 1986 (from Ukkonen and von Bronsdorff (1988)). See text for details. (b) Occurrence of rubella IgG antibodies (evidence of past infection) in different age groups, males and females combined, in Finland from 1980 to 1986 (Ukkonen and von Bronsdorff (1988)). See text for details.

9.5.3 *Testing the sensitivity of the results*

Figure 9.13 provides a test of how sensitive the results are to the choice of the structure imposed on the 'who acquires infection from whom' matrix. The figure is essentially a slice across the surface depicted in Fig. 5.12, showing the number of cases of CRS at equilibrium under policy 2, as a ratio, *w*, to the number before any vaccination. The proportions of children vaccinated at age 2 years are as shown, while the proportion of girls vaccinated between the ages of 10 and 15 years are as recorded in the UK in 1983 (roughly 85 per cent). The predictions under the three WAIFW structures whose underlying biological and social assumptions are summarized in Table 9.6 are virtually identical; WAIFWs B and C are simply indistinguishable.

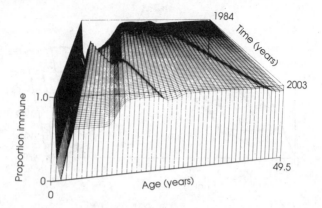

Fig. 9.12. As for Figs. 9.9 and 9.10, except now we show only the predicted age-specific serological profiles for rubella for females, assuming a three-stage policy (policy 4 of Table 9.5) which, beginning in 1985, immunizes 60 per cent of all 2-year-olds, 50 per cent of 25-year-old females, and the proportion of girls between 10 and 15 years of age that actually prevailed in 1984. The basic model, and the parameter estimates, are again as for Figs. 9.9 and 9.10; for further details see Anderson and Grenfell (1986).

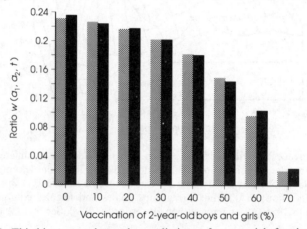

Fig. 9.13. This histogram shows the predictions of our models for the average value of the ratio w (rubella cases (in the age-range 16–40 years) after, divided by cases before, immunization), over the time interval 1985–2020, under the impact of a two-stage programme (policy 2 of Table 9.5) for different levels of coverage among 2-year-olds; the coverage levels among 10 to 15 years old girls are held constant at the actual UK levels for 1983. The figure clearly shows the benefits that could come from a change in the UK policy to a two-stage 'UK–USA' policy, provided levels of coverage were high enough. The figure also shows that these theoretical predictions are insensitive to the choice of the form of the WAIFW matrix among reasonable alternatives; for each level of coverage, the left-hand value of the histogram comes from a computation based on WAIFW A of Table 9.6, while WAIFWs B and C of Table 9.6 lead to indistinguishable results that are shown as the right-hand value. For further discussion see Anderson and Grenfell (1986).

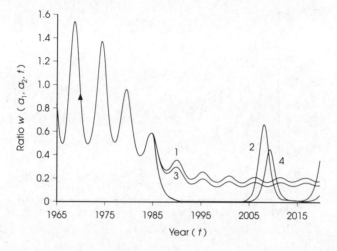

Fig. 9.14. The number of cases of CRS (expressed as a ratio to the yearly average before any immunization, w) is shown as a function of time, under the four different assumptions about immunization policy after 1985 that are listed in Table 9.5. The triangle in 1970 denotes the start of the single-stage UK policy (girls only, in the age range 10 to 15 years). Before 1970, the ratio w oscillates (with a four- to five-year period) around the average pre-immunization value of unity; over the interval 1970–84, recorded immunization rates in the UK were used in the numerical calculations. For further details about the computational procedure see Anderson and Grenfell (1986). The age-dependent forces of infection, λ_i, were taken from the serological data summarized in the top row of Table 9.7. It will be seen that the different policies can lead to significantly different patterns in the incidence of CRS over time; these patterns are not easy to intuit.

Figures 9.14 and 9.15 indicate some of the dynamical properties of the system under the different vaccination policies listed in Table 9.5. In these two figures, the number of CRS cases at time t is computed, by the procedure described earlier, as a ratio, $w(t)$, to the number at equilibrium before vaccination. The pre-vaccination system is set oscillating (so that it exhibits its basic inter-epidemic cycles with periods of 4–5 years) by an initial perturbation, and vaccination is initiated in 1970.(as denoted by the triangle) and maintained at the age-specific rates actually recorded in the UK over the 15-year span 1970–84. After 1985, Figs. 9.14 and 9.15 show the predicted dynamics following implementation of each of the four policies listed in Table 9.5; in these projections, the coverage levels are taken to be 60 per cent for children of age 2, 50 per cent for still-susceptible women of age 25, and the observed 1983 levels among girls between the ages of 10 and 15 years.

For the serologically based estimates of λ_i in Fig. 9.14, introducing vaccination of 60 per cent of 2-year-olds (policies 2 and 4) results at first in a very marked decrease in CRS compared with continuing the present UK policy or a slight modification of it (policies 1 and 3). As seen in the earlier, simpler models in Chapter 7 (Figs. 7.4(a, b)), however, there are likely to be pronounced up-swings

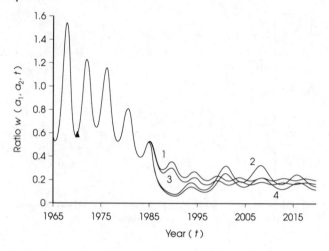

Fig. 9.15. As for Fig. 9.14, except here the age-dependent forces of infection, λ_i, upon which the computations are based, are estimated from case records (the second row in Table 9.7). These data—which we think may be less reliable than the serological data—lead to patterns of dynamical behaviour which are similar to, but for policies 2 and 4 less severely oscillatory than, those shown in Fig. 9.14.

in the incidence of CRS in later years, evoked by the intrinsically oscillating response of the system to perturbations of this kind; the reduction in the average transmission of rubella virus has here lengthened the inter-epidemic period to around 20–22 years. Comparing policy 4 with policy 2, we see that the three-stage policy, by adding vaccination of older women, substantially reduces the amplitude of the later up-swings.

Figure 9.15 repeats the computations in Fig. 9.14, but now employing the case-notification data to estimate λ_i (that is, using the second, instead of the first, row in Table 9.7). The basic trends in Fig. 9.15 are similar to those in Fig. 9.14, except that the excursions about the long-term average achievements under policies 2 and 4 are much less dramatic. The differences between Figs. 9.14 and 9.15 derive from the differences in age dependence of the forces of infection inferred from serology and from case records in Table 9.7: the serologically based estimates show a marked decrease in transmission at older ages, so that most virus transmission occurs in the 5–15 age band and oscillatory effects are promoted by recruitment and depletion of susceptibles in this relatively narrow range of ages; in contrast, the case-notification estimates of λ_i are relatively constant, which makes for less volatile dynamics. We have chosen to estimate λ_i from the serological data in most of the calculations reported above, partly because these data are free from some of the biases that afflict age-specific case records. The possibility that genetic and other hetero-geneities may complicate the analysis of serological information must, however, be kept in mind.

Overall, our numerical studies suggest that levels of herd immunity around 85–88 per cent should be sufficient to eradicate rubella; this estimate rests fairly robustly on the observation that the average age at infection before any vaccination was around 9–10 years. Such levels of herd immunity are attained by 90 per cent coverage in vaccination of children between the ages of 15 months and 2 years. This critical level has been exceeded in the USA, where rubella seems well on the way to eradication. In the UK, our calculations lead us to conclude that rubella could be eradicated within 40 years or so if 80–85 per cent of children were to be vaccinated at age 2 years in addition to maintaining present levels of vaccination of girls between the ages of 10 and 15 years.

9.6 A simple model with transmission concentrated within age cohorts

We conclude this chapter by discussing an analytic model that captures many of the essential aspects of situations in which transmission is concentrated within age cohorts (for instance, among school class-mates) along with a homogeneous background of transmission among all ages. This model is presented partly because the analytic solutions permit insight into the way the age-dependent epidemiological processes work, and partly because the model can exhibit the interesting property that its equilibrium state can be a mixture of epidemics within age cohorts, superimposed on an endemic background.

Specifically, we assume the age-dependent transmission rates $\beta(a, a')$ in eqn (9.5) have two components: a constant component, corresponding to a degree of homogeneous mixing, and a component representing transmission between infectors and infectees who are in the same age class. This situation is essentially that described by the matrix WAIFW 4 in Section 9.2, and by WAIFW B in the study of vaccination policies for rubella in Section 9.5.1. As the limiting case of this assumption, we may write (May 1986)

$$\beta(a, a') = \beta_b + \alpha\beta_a g(a)\delta(a - a'). \tag{9.14}$$

Here β_b measures the magnitude of the age-independent background transmission rate; β_a measures the characteristic strength of transmission within an age class; $g(a)$ describes the variation of the concentrated component with age; and α essentially measures the characteristic width of the age band of concentrated transmission. The quantity $\delta(a - a')$ is the Dirac δ-function, which is zero if $a \neq a'$ and infinite if $a = a'$, in such a way that its integral over all ages is unity (which is why we need the parameter α, with the dimensions of age, to keep the units consistent in eqn (9.14)). Substituting eqn (9.14) into (9.5), we get

$$\lambda(a) = \beta_b \bar{Y} + \alpha\beta_a g(a)Y(a). \tag{9.15}$$

The first term on the right-hand side is as for homogeneous mixing, with $\bar{Y}$ the total number of infectives. The second term in practice represents an approximation to transmission at a rate β_a (modified by the factor $g(a)$) from infectious individuals who are roughly in a relatively narrow age band, of width α, around the age of the susceptible individual.

To get a clear idea of how this model behaves, we begin by outlining its solution when $g(a) = 1$; that is, when the within-cohort transmission operates equally at all ages. We then extend this to the somewhat more realistic case where $g(a) = 1$ between the ages a_1 and a_2 (say, between 5 and 15 years) and zero elsewhere. We restrict attention to equilibrium situations, first calculating the age-specific susceptibility and force of infection, $X(a)$ and $\lambda(a)$, at equilibrium before vaccination, and then determining the critical level of coverage for eradication, p_c.

9.6.1 *Formal solution of the model*

For convenience, we repeat the equations for the changes in the age-specific number of susceptibles and infectives, at equilibrium (see Chapter 4):

$$dX(a)/da = -\lambda(a)X(a), \tag{9.16}$$

$$dY(a)/da = \lambda(a)X(a) - vY(a). \tag{9.17}$$

Here the initial conditions are $X(0) = N(0) = \bar{N}/L$ and $Y(0) = 0$; we have assumed Type I survival in a population of size $\bar{N}$ in which birth and death rates are equal. The force of infection, $\lambda(a)$, is related to $Y(a)$ by eqn (9.15). Equation (9.16) can be integrated immediately, to get

$$X(a) = N(0)\exp(-\Psi(a)). \tag{9.18}$$

The quantity $\Psi(a)$ is defined as

$$\Psi(a) \equiv \int_0^a \lambda(s)\,ds. \tag{9.19}$$

Substituting eqn (9.18) into eqn (9.17), we have a system of two equations— eqns (9.15) and (9.17)—for the two variables $\lambda(a)$ and $Y(a)$; this system can easily be integrated numerically for any specified function $g(a)$.

For simplicity, we put $g(a) = 1$ at this point. Then eqn (9.15) can be used to re-write eqn (9.17) in terms of $\lambda(a)$:

$$d\lambda(a)/da = v\lambda_0 - \lambda(a)(v - \alpha\beta_a N(0)\,e^{-\Psi(a)}). \tag{9.20}$$

This equation can be re-expressed as a second-order differential equation in the variable $\Psi(a)$, by using eqn (9.19) to write $\lambda(a) = d\Psi/da$:

$$\frac{1}{v}\frac{d^2\Psi}{da^2} = \lambda_0 - \frac{d\Psi}{da}(1 - R_a\,e^{-\Psi(a)}). \tag{9.21}$$

The initial conditions are $\Psi(0) = 0$, $d\Psi(0)/da = \lambda_0$. The quantities R_a and λ_0

are defined as

$$R_a \equiv \frac{\alpha \beta_a N(0)}{v} = \frac{\alpha}{L} \frac{\beta_a \bar{N}}{v}, \tag{9.22}$$

$$\lambda_0 = \beta_b \bar{Y}. \tag{9.23}$$

Finally, to complete this frenzy of defining things, we observe that eqns (9.16) and (9.17) can be added together (to get rid of the λX term) and integrated over all ages to obtain

$$v\bar{Y} = X(0) - X(L) = N(0)(1 - e^{-\Psi(L)}). \tag{9.24}$$

Here we have used Type I survival, and have ignored $Y(L)$. Moreover, $\Psi(L)$ will be of the order of L/A, where A is the average age at infection before vaccination; as L/A is usually quite large, $\exp(-\Psi(L))$ can be neglected compared with unity, whence $\bar{Y} \simeq N(0)/v$ and eqn (9.23) becomes

$$\lambda_0 \simeq R_b/L, \tag{9.25}$$

$$R_b \equiv \beta_b N/v. \tag{9.26}$$

As will emerge more clearly below, the quantities R_a and R_b defined by eqns (9.22) and (9.26) are essentially the basic reproductive rates of the microparasite within an age cohort ('a' for 'among') and within the background population ('b' for 'background'), respectively.

Once the parameters R_a and R_b (along with v and L) have been specified, eqn (9.21) can obviously be integrated to get $\Psi(a)$ and thence $X(a)$ and $\lambda(a)$ via eqns (9.18) and (9.19), respectively. But we can do better than that.

9.6.2 $R_a < 1$: *endemic equilibrium*

As argued more generally in Appendix D, the duration of infection will usually be very much shorter than other time-scales in equations like eqn (9.21); $1/v \ll A, L$. In this case, we may usually assume $1/v \to 0$, and simply drop the term on the left-hand side in eqn (9.21). This leads to the simpler equation:

$$\int_0^\Psi [1 - R_a \exp(-\Psi')] \, d\Psi' = \lambda_0 \int_0^a da'. \tag{9.27}$$

The approximation of dropping the term involving $1/v$ is, however, only sensible if the two sides of eqn (9.27) can indeed balance each other for all values of a and $\Psi(a)$. If $R_a < 1$, the term inside the square brackets in eqn (9.27) is indeed always positive, and the approximation works. Using eqn (9.18) to rewrite eqn (9.27) as an equation in $x(a) = X(a)/N(0) = \exp(-\Psi(a))$, we get

$$\int_x^1 (1 - R_a x') \, dx'/x' = \lambda_0 a. \tag{9.28}$$

Integration of eqn (9.28) leads to an implicit equation for x as a function of

a and the parameters R_a and λ_0 (with $\lambda_0 = R_b/L$):

$$x \exp[R_a(1 - x)] = \exp(-\lambda_0 a). \qquad (9.29)$$

As $a \to 0$, $x \to 1$, as it should. For $a \to L$, x becomes small: $x(L) \simeq \exp[-(R_a + R_b)]$. In Appendix D, we present a graphical way of solving eqn (9.29), which helps further to illuminate the difference between $R_a < 1$ and $R_a > 1$.

The age-specific force of infection, $\lambda(a)$, is determined from the definition (9.19), which gives $\lambda(a) = \mathrm{d}\Psi/\mathrm{d}a$. Applying this to eqn (9.27) gives immediately

$$\lambda(a) = \lambda_0/(1 - R_a x(a)). \qquad (9.30)$$

Notice that in the limit $a \to 0$, $x(0) \to 1$ and eqn (9.30) gives $\lambda(0) \to \lambda_0/(1 - R_a)$. But $Y(0) = 0$ by our initial assumptions, so from eqn (9.15) we expect $\lambda(0) \to \lambda_0$! The inconsistency comes from the neglect of the $(1/v)(\mathrm{d}^2\Psi/\mathrm{d}a^2)$ term on the left-hand side of eqn (9.21). For very small ages, around $a = 0$, λ changes very rapidly in this model (on the epidemic time-scale, $1/v$) and the factor $\mathrm{d}^2\Psi/\mathrm{d}a^2 = \mathrm{d}\lambda/\mathrm{d}a$ is large enough to compensate for the very small value of $1/v$; during this short period λ changes from λ_0 to $\lambda_0/(1 - R_a)$. In other words, the approximation of discarding the left-hand side of eqn (9.21) also reduces the order of the differential equation, and throws away a boundary condition; but all this happens on the epidemic time-scale, $1/v$, which is much shorter than all other time-scales of interest in the endemic situation, and we may simply regard $\lambda(a)$ as jumping discontinuously to start at $\lambda(0) = \lambda_0/(1 - R_a)$. This approximation technique rejoices in the name of 'singular perturbation theory', and is much used in fluid mechanics. As we shall now see, these 'singularities' obtrude themselves more vigorously when $R_a > 1$.

9.6.3 $R_a > 1$: a mixed endemic and epidemic situation

If $R_a > 1$, the term inside the brackets on the right-hand side of eqn (9.21) is initially negative ($\Psi \to 0$ when $a \to 0$). As $\mathrm{d}\Psi/\mathrm{d}a$ is necessarily positive, this means the entire right-hand side of eqn (9.21) is positive, and so the left-hand side cannot be ignored. As shown in more detail in Appendix D, the result is essentially an epidemic among new-borns, during which λ attains the high values characteristic of an epidemic and the fraction susceptible, x, falls very fast from its initial value $x(0) = 1$ to a lower value $x(0+) = 1/R_a$. All this happens on the time-scale, $1/v$, that characterizes epidemic processes (see the beginning of Chapter 6 and Fig. 6.1); by 'age $0+$' we mean an age of the order of $1/v$.

Once x has fallen to a value just below $1/R_a$, the term $1 - R_a x$ becomes positive, and we may now drop the term on the left-hand side in eqn (9.21) (that is, let $1/v \to 0$). The calculation now proceeds exactly along the lines laid down above, for $R_a < 1$. The equation determining $x(a)$ is, as before, given by eqn (9.28), with the one difference that the initial value of x is effectively

$x(0+) = 1/R_a$:

$$\int_x^{1/R_a} (1 - R_a x') \, dx'/x' = \lambda_0 a. \tag{9.31}$$

Equation (9.31) reduces to an implicit equation for $x(a)$:

$$(R_a x) \exp(1 - R_a x) = \exp(-\lambda_0 a). \tag{9.32}$$

A graphical way of solving this equation, which helps both to make clear the differences between the cases $R_a < 1$ and $R_a > 1$, and to illustrate the basic nature of the singular perturbation method, is given in Appendix D.

Again, $\lambda(a)$ is given by eqn (9.30), once $x(a)$ is given by eqn (9.32). Thus eqn (9.30) implies that $\lambda \to \infty$ as $a \to$ '0+' and $x \to 1/R_a$; what happens, of course, is that λ rises to high (epidemic) values and then falls back to the value λ_0 set by the boundary conditions, as a decreases to zero through the epidemic 'boundary layer' whose width is of order $1/v$. This singular region of λ is integrable, and we may define the summed values of λ over this boundary window (of width $\sim 1/v$) as $\Delta\lambda$:

$$\Delta\lambda \equiv \int_0^{0+} \lambda(a) \, da. \tag{9.33}$$

Using eqn (9.16) to write $\lambda = -(1/x)(dx/da)$, we have

$$\Delta\lambda = \int_{1/R_a}^{1} dx/x = \ln R_a. \tag{9.34}$$

That is, around $a \sim 0$, λ is essentially infinite (actually, $\lambda \sim v$) in an age range whose width is essentially zero (actually, $\sim 1/v$), in such a way that the integral over this age range, $\Delta\lambda$, is finite (given by eqn (9.34)). In commonsense terms, this means that in the initial age class, 0–1 years of age, the force of infection in this model has the average value $\Delta\lambda \simeq \ln R_a$, superimposed on the background value of λ_0.

9.6.4 *Within-cohort transmission restricted to ages a_1 to a_2*

A closer approximation to reality is obtained by assuming that the concentrated, within-cohort transmission is restricted to school ages. That is, we now put $g(a) = 1$ for $a_2 > a > a_1$, and $g(a) = 0$ otherwise.

For $a < a_1$, we now have a constant force of infection, $\lambda = \lambda_0$. The fraction susceptible decreases exponentially,

$$x(a) = \exp(-\lambda_0 a) \qquad \text{for } a < a_1. \tag{9.35}$$

This is also the case for $a > a_2$, where $x(a) = x(a_2) \exp[-\lambda_0(a - a_2)]$.

In the intermediate region, $a_2 > a > a_1$, we simply repeat the analysis just outlined, with two changes: the age variable is to be read as $a - a_1$; and R_a is replaced by its discounted value, $\rho_a = R_a x(a_1) = R_a \exp(-\lambda_0 a_1)$. For $\rho_a < 1$, we have the situation discussed above as 'endemic equilibrium', where $x(a)$ behaves continuously and the only singular behaviour is the jump in $\lambda(a)$ from λ_0 to $\lambda_0/(1 - \rho_a)$ at $a = a_1$. For $\rho_a > 1$, the situation is again a mixture of an endemic background, with an epidemic jump in λ and consequent very fast fall in x, at age a_1 when the within-cohort transmission effects are 'turned on'.

Figures 9.16(a, b) and 9.17(a, b) illustrate this behaviour. Figures 9.16(a, b) show $x(a)$ and $\lambda(a)$, respectively, for an 'endemic equilibrium' situation in which things happen in a continuous way. In contrast, Figs. 9.17(a, b) show $x(a)$ and $\lambda(a)$ for the mixed endemic/epidemic situation, in which the consequences of the epidemic that sweeps through each age cohort at age a_1 are clearly seen.

In practical applications, the population would usually be divided into one-year or coarser age blocks, and the discontinuous changes in Figs. 9.17(a, b) would be replaced by the kind of marked fall in susceptibility and rise in λ seen in much of the data in Chapter 8. In short, this artificially simple model is likely to embody many of the essential processes that govern the age dependence observed in the transmission of childhood infections in developed countries.

9.6.5 *Eradication criterion*

We conclude by finding the critical level of coverage, p_c, required to eradicate the infection. The actual level is then compared with the approximation obtained by treating the population as if it were homogeneously mixed: $\hat{p}_c = 1 - x^*$.

Suppose a fraction of each cohort is immunized essentially at birth. We may now repeat all the above calculations, but with primes on all the variables denoting their post-immunization equilibrium values and with $N(0)' \rightarrow (1 - p)N(0)$.

The eradication criterion is obtained in the limit $\lambda'(a) \rightarrow 0$ for all a. In this limit, we can show that the approximation of discarding the left-hand side in eqn (9.16) or (9.21) can always be made (there are no within-cohort epidemics), and eqn (9.17) gives us generally that

$$Y'(a) \simeq \lambda'(a)(1 - p_c)N(0)/v. \tag{9.36}$$

Here we have also used $X'(a) \rightarrow (1 - p_c)N(0)$ as $\lambda' \rightarrow 0$. Substituting eqn (9.36) into the basic eqn (9.15) for $\lambda'(a)$, and rearranging, we get

$$\lambda'(a) = \lambda_0'/[1 - g(a)R_a(1 - p_c)]. \tag{9.37}$$

As before, R_a is defined by eqn (9.22). Integrating over all ages, and recalling the definition of Ψ, eqn (9.19), we have

$$\Psi'(L) = \lambda_0' \int_0^L \frac{da}{1 - g(a)R_a(1 - p_c)}. \tag{9.38}$$

In the limit $\lambda' \rightarrow 0$, eqn (9.24) gives us another equation for $\Psi'(L)$, namely

$$\lambda_0' \rightarrow \Psi'(L)R_b(1 - p_c)/L. \tag{9.39}$$

Here we have used the definitions, eqns (9.23) and (9.26), for λ_0' and R_b,

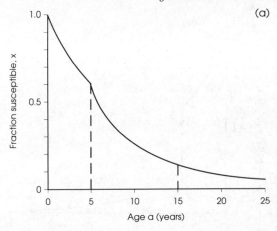

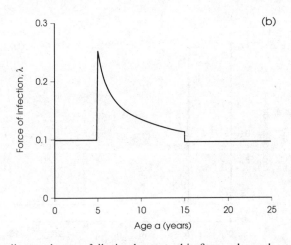

Fig. 9.16. (a) As discussed more fully in the text, this figure shows how the fraction susceptible to a particular infection decreases with age, assuming that the force of infection is a mixture of an age-independent component (derived from homogeneous mixing among all age groups) and a within-cohort component (derived from contacts strictly within each age cohort) in the school years, here taken to be from $a_1 = 5$ to $a_2 = 15$ years. In this figure, the within-cohort transmission does not result in an effective reproductive rate in excess of unity ($\rho_a = R_a \exp(-\lambda_0 a_1) < 1$), so there is only an enhancement of the spread of infection in the age range a_1 to a_2; this shows up here as a faster rate of decrease in the fraction susceptible, with age. Specifically, this figure is for the model discussed in the text, eqns (9.14) *et seq.*, with the parameter choices $R_b = 7.5$, $R_a = 1$, and Type I survivorship with $L = 75$ years (whence $\lambda_0 = 0.1\,\mathrm{yr}^{-1}$). (b) The force of infection, $\lambda(a)$, as a function of age, a, corresponding to Fig. 9.16(a). Under the assumption that the duration of infectiousness, $1/v$, is much shorter than all other time-scales, there is an effectively discontinuous upward jump in the magnitude of λ when the within-cohort effects switch on at age a_1.

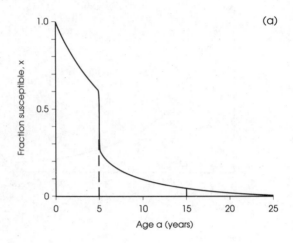

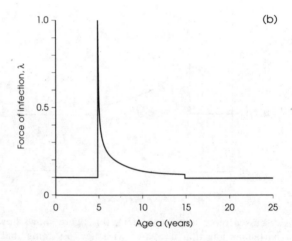

Fig. 9.17. (a) As for Fig. 9.16(a), except now $R_a = 3$, so that the effective reproductive rate of the infection from within-cohort effects exceeds unity, $\rho_a = R_a \exp(-\lambda_0 a_1) = 1.8$. As discussed in the text, there is consequently a mini-epidemic, which is superimposed on the endemic background of infection, showing up as a discontinuous decrease in the fraction susceptible; 'singular perturbation' theory shows how this apparent discontinuity actually corresponds to finite rates of change on time-scales of order $1/v$. (b) The age-specific force of infection, $\lambda(a)$, that corresponds to Fig. 9.17(a) is shown as a function of age, a. There is now an apparent singularity in λ at age a_1; this integrable singularity corresponds to the mini-epidemic among the cohort entering the age class at a_1. For a fuller account of this fascinating combination of endemic and epidemic effects at equilibrium, see the text.

respectively. Comparing eqns (9.38) and (9.39), we arrive at last at an equation which gives the eradication coverage value, p_c, implicitly:

$$1 = \frac{R_b(1 - p_c)}{L} \int_0^L \frac{da}{1 - g(a)R_a(1 - p_c)}. \tag{9.40}$$

In the simple case when $g(a) = 1$ for all a, this reduces to a familiar expression:

$$p_c = 1 - 1/(R_a + R_b). \tag{9.41}$$

More generally, for the case when $g(a) = 1$ for $a_2 > a > a_1$ and zero otherwise, as illustrated in Figs. 9.16 and 9.17, we obtain the expression for p_c that is given explicitly in Appendix D.

For the explicit examples illustrated in Figs. 9.16 and 9.17 we may compare the exact values of p_c with the estimates obtained (via $\hat{p}_c = 1 - x^*$) by finding the fractions susceptible before immunization. For the situation corresponding to Fig. 9.16 (where $a_1 = 5$ and $a_2 = 15$ years, $L = 75$ years, $R_a = 1$, and $R_b = 7.5$), numerical integration of the results for $x(a)$ gives $x^* = 0.11$ and $\hat{p}_c = 0.89$. The critical coverage, from eqn (9.40), is in fact $p_c = 0.87$. For the mixed endemic and within-cohort epidemic model depicted in Fig. 9.17 (where $R_a = 3$ and the other parameters are as for Fig. 9.16), we find $x^* = 0.075$; thus $\hat{p}_c = 0.93$ in comparison with the exact value $p_c = 0.88$.

As was the case in the much more empirically oriented computations that form the bulk of this chapter, the assumption of homogeneous mixing leads to estimates of p_c that are somewhat too high. The discrepancies are more pronounced, although still modest, when there is relatively intense transmission within age cohorts among schoolchildren (amounting to mini-epidemics super-imposed on a more homogeneous background of infection).

9.7 Summary

Motivated by the evidence presented in Chapter 8, we develop a theoretical framework in which the transmission rates, $\beta(a, a')$, depend on the ages of infectee and infector. These techniques are then applied to detailed analyses of the programmes of vaccination against measles and rubella in the UK. In both cases, we use serological and case-notification data about age-specific forces of infection before vaccination to infer the underlying coefficients in the matrix of transmission rates. Then, using the age-specific vaccination rates recorded for measles and for rubella in the UK, we use the mathematical models to predict the impact of vaccination; these predictions are in excellent agreement with observed data. In the case of rubella, the models are further used to evaluate the probable effects of various changes from the '12-year-old-girls-only' vaccination policy. The chapter ends by discussing the analytic solutions of a model which has transmission concentrated within age cohorts along with a background of homogeneous mixing; this model has some of the main features of real situations, and its properties are interesting and easily understood.

10

Genetic heterogeneity

In Chapter 8, we mentioned that the apparent decrease in the force of infection at older ages, seen in so many of the data, could in part by caused by genetic heterogeneity in response to infection. The importance of this issue was seen in Chapter 9, where we found that estimates of the level of herd immunity required for eradication of infection depend significantly on the degree to which intrinsic transmissibility really does decline among older age groups. Although there has been, in recent years, a growing amount of work on age-related, social, and other heterogeneities in host populations, the possibility of genetic hetero- geneity continues to be neglected in most epidemiological studies involving microparasites. This is understandable, because there is not much concrete evidence on which to base such studies.

In this chapter, we first explore a simple model in which some host genotypes are more susceptible than others. The model unfortunately involves no data; it is presented purely to show that the existence of such significantly different degrees of intrinsic susceptibility can have important implications for the design of immunization programmes, and can seriously complicate the estimation of transmission rates and eradication criteria. In the later part of the chapter, we consider other aspects of genetic heterogeneity within the host population, particularly the possibility that some individuals may be silent 'carriers' of infection.

10.1 Genetic heterogeneity and the interpretation of epidemiological data

The essence of the complication introduced by genetic heterogeneity can be appreciated in a qualitative way. In Chapters 8 and 9, any observed decline in the transmissibility of infections such as measles among older age groups (typically more than 10–15 years of age) was attributed to the intrinsic transmission rates being lower among such older age groups. But it could alternatively be that such apparent decline in transmissibility is simply because the most susceptible genotypes have largely been filtered out. If this is the case, then estimates of p_c based on pre-immunization values of the age-specific force of infection (as carried out in Chapter 9) will be too optimistic: as overall infection rates decline under an immunization programme, an increasing number of the more infectable genotypes will move into the older age classes of susceptibles, in effect causing the age-specific transmission rates to increase in the older age classes. In this way, genetic heterogeneity is in principle—and possibly in fact—capable of confounding the conventional assessments of the immunization coverage need for eradication.

10.1.1 *A simple model*

A simple model helps to make these ideas concrete. The genetic aspects of the model are admittedly greatly oversimplified, but the model has the compensating advantage that it illustrates the main points without distracting details. Consider a host population of constant magnitude, $\bar{N}$, in which a fixed proportion, $1 - f$, is of genotype A which is less resistant to a particular infection than is the remaining fraction, f, who are of genotype B. Apart from the genetic heterogeneity, the population is assumed to be homogeneously mixed, so that the force of infection for either genotype depends on the total number of infectives. For susceptibles of genotype A the transmission coefficient is β_A, and for genotype B it is β_B; the greater infectibility of genotype A is made specific by writing $\beta_A = \beta$ and $\beta_B = \varepsilon\beta$, with $\varepsilon < 1$. Thus we can write

$$\lambda_v = \beta_v(\bar{Y}_A + \bar{Y}_B). \tag{10.1}$$

Here the index v ($v = $ A, B) labels the genotypes, and $\bar{Y}_A$ and $\bar{Y}_B$ are the total number of infectives of genotype A and B, respectively, summed over all ages.

In this simple system, the two genotypes are essentially treated as two separate populations, with the densities of susceptible and infectious individuals of age a at equilibrium given by the standard equations

$$dX_v(a)/da = -\lambda_v X_v(a), \tag{10.2}$$

$$dY_v(a)/da = \lambda_v X_v(a) - vY_v(a). \tag{10.3}$$

Here v is the recovery rate, taken to be the same for both genotypes, and Type I survival is assumed. Integration of eqn (10.2) gives

$$X_v(a) = X_v(0)\exp(-\lambda_v a). \tag{10.4}$$

The above assumptions give the initial conditions $X_A(0) = (1 - f)\bar{N}/L$ and $X_B(0) = f\bar{N}/L$. The age-specific fraction of the population who are susceptible, $x(a)$, is thus

$$x(a) = (1 - f)\exp(-\lambda_A a) + f\exp(-\lambda_B a). \tag{10.5}$$

Here $\lambda_B = \varepsilon\lambda_A$, which follows from eqn (10.1) and our assumption about the relative magnitudes of β_A and β_B. Thus, if the more resistant genotype B is uncommon (f small), the fraction seropositive (estimated as $1 - x$) may saturate to around $1 - f$ relatively rapidly (at a characteristic age $\sim 1/\lambda_A$), but rise more slowly thereafter (on a characteristic time-scale $\sim 1/\varepsilon\lambda_A$). This process can mimic some of the features observed in age–serological profiles in Chapter 8.

10.1.2 *Criterion for eradication*

Suppose now that a fraction, p, of all new-borns is immunized, effectively at birth (as always, the analysis can be extended to include realistic complications such as more complex age-dependent immunization schedules). The critical fraction for eradication, p_c, can be found by the procedures explained in Chapter 5.

First, to calculate the reduction in the forces of infection as a result of the immunization programme, we find the underlying transmission rates, β_v, from the λ values before immunization in the usual way. As was done in obtaining eqn (9.24), we can add eqn (10.2) to eqn (10.3) and integrate from $a = 0$ to $a = L$ (ignoring $Y(L)$), to get

$$\bar{Y}_v = (X_v(0) - X_v(L))/v. \tag{10.6}$$

Substituting this into eqn (10.1), we obtain the desired relations between λ_v and β_v:

$$\lambda_v = (\beta_v \bar{N}/v)\xi. \tag{10.7}$$

Here eqn (10.5) for $x(a)$ has been used in eqn (10.6), so that ξ is defined as

$$\xi \equiv [(1 - f)(1 - e^{-\lambda L}) + f(1 - e^{-\varepsilon\lambda L})]/L. \tag{10.8}$$

In expressing ξ this way, we have used our assumption $\beta_B = \varepsilon\beta_A = \varepsilon\beta$ in conjunction with eqn (10.7), to write $\lambda_A = \lambda$ and $\lambda_B = \varepsilon\lambda$.

The immunization programme defined above has the effect of changing $\bar{N}$ to $\bar{N}(1 - p)$ throughout these equations, whence the reduced force of infection at the new post-immunization equilibrium (where $\lambda'_A = \lambda'$ and $\lambda'_B = \varepsilon\lambda'$) obeys

$$\lambda' = (1 - p)(\beta\bar{N}/v)\xi'. \tag{10.9}$$

Here ξ' is given by eqn (10.8) with λ' replacing λ throughout. Eradication corresponds to $\lambda' \to 0$, in which limit $\xi' \to \lambda'[1 - f(1 - \varepsilon)]$. Equation (10.9) then leads immediately to the eradication criterion

$$p_c = 1 - \frac{v}{\beta\bar{N}[1 - f(1 - \varepsilon)]}. \tag{10.10}$$

The condition (10.10) is similar to the criterion (5.2), $p_c = 1 - (1/R_0)$, for a homogeneously mixed population. Indeed eqn (10.10) reduces exactly to eqn (5.2) for a genetically homogeneous population, $f \to 0$ or $\varepsilon \to 1$ (for Type I survival, $R_0 = \beta\bar{N}/v$; see eqn (4.43)). If f is small, corresponding to the host genotype B being relatively rare, the critical immunization coverage required for eradication will not be very different from that estimated by assuming a homogeneous population, even though the force of infection may show a marked decline at older ages in the days before immunization. But if this genetically caused apparent decline in transmission at older ages is incorrectly attributed to intrinsically age-related effects in the transmission parameters, we could, for the reasons discussed in Chapter 9, come to misleadingly optimistic conclusions about the coverage, p_c, needed for eradication. A numerical example helps to make this plain.

10.1.3 *An explicit example*

Assume $f = 0.1$, $\lambda_A = 0.2$ yr^{-1}, $\lambda_B = 0.04$ yr^{-1} (that is, $\lambda = 0.2$ yr^{-1} and $\varepsilon = 0.2$), and $L = 75$. This corresponds to 90 per cent of the population being relatively susceptible, with an average age at infection of around 5 years, while the other 10 per cent are less susceptible to infection (by an intrinsic factor of one-fifth).

For this hypothetical population, $x(a)$ is shown as a function of a (from eqn (10.5)) in Fig. 10.1; this figure also shows how $x(a)$ would look for a population consisting wholly of genotype A ($f = 0$, $\lambda_A = 0.2$ yr^{-1}). Equation (10.8) gives $\xi = 0.0133$ and hence $\beta \bar{N}/v = 15.08$. It follows from eqn (10.10) that

$$p_c = 0.928. \tag{10.11}$$

The corresponding result for a population homogeneous in genotype A ($f = 0$ in eqns (10.8) and (10.10)) is $p_c = 0.933$. To put it another way, the approximate eradication criterion obtained by assuming the population is homogeneously

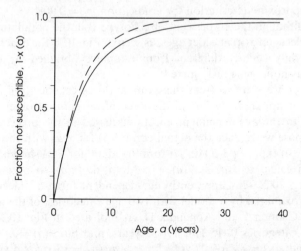

Fig. 10.1. The fraction of the host population that has lost susceptibility (as a result of infection), $1 - x(a)$, is shown as a function of age a for the population with two genotypes described by eqn (10.5). Specifically, the full curve is for eqn (10.5) with $f = 0.1$, $\lambda_A = 0.2$, and $\lambda_B = 0.04$; most of the relatively susceptible genotypes A have been infected by around age 10. Thereafter the total fraction susceptible decreases more slowly. The broken curve is for a population containing only the genotype A (i.e. $f = 0$).

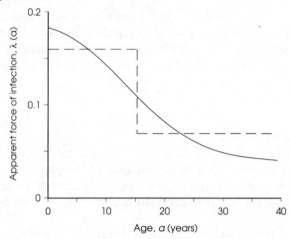

Fig. 10.2. The apparent force of infection, $\lambda(a)$, as a function of age a obtained by assuming (incorrectly!) that the solid susceptibility curve in Fig. 10.1 comes from a genetically homogeneous population with age-dependent transmission rates. The broken line segments illustrate the approximation used for the illustrative calculation in the text: $\lambda_1 = 0.16$, for $a < 15$ and $\lambda_2 = 0.07$ for $a > 15$.

mixed, $\hat{p}_c = 1 - x^*$, can be found by integrating eqn (10.5) to get x^* ($x^* = \int_0^L x(a)\,da/L$). With the parameters of this example, we get $x^* = 0.092$, and thence the approximate criterion for eradication, $p_c = 0.908$.

In short, although the 10 per cent of genotype B in the population produces significant effects on $x(a)$ at older ages, as seen in Fig. 10.1, the exact eradication criterion is only slightly different from estimates obtained by treating the population as homogeneously mixed.

But suppose we were to treat this population as genetically homogeneous, attributing the apparent decline in the force of infection at older ages shown in Fig. 10.2 to the age-dependent effects discussed in the preceding chapter. That is, suppose we replace the actual eqn (10.5) for $x(a)$ with the assumption that $x(a) = x(0) \exp(-\int \lambda(a')\,da')$. From the 'data' for $x(a)$ shown in Fig. 10.1, we will then calculate $\lambda(a)$ as $\lambda(a) = -(dx(a)/da)/x(a)$, to obtain the result shown in Fig. 10.2. This apparently age-dependent force of infection may in turn be approximated by a model with two age categories, of the general kind discussed in Chapter 9 and Appendix D. As indicated in Fig. 10.2, we choose the two age categories 0–15 and 15–75 years, and put $\lambda(a) = \lambda_1 = 0.16$ yr^{-1} for $a < a_1$ and $\lambda(a) = \lambda_2 = 0.07$ yr^{-1} for $a > a_1$ ($a_1 = 15$ years divides the two categories). We assume that the structure of the 2×2 WAIFW matrix is $\beta(a, a') = \beta_1$ if both a and $a' < a_1$, and $\beta(a, a') = \beta_2$ if either a or $a' > a_1$; this corresponds to one contact rate among children, and another (lower) rate when either or both of the individuals involved is above 15 years of age. The critical immunization coverage needed for eradication can then be calculated by the methods described in Chapter 9 (and Appendix D). The calculation gives the result (Anderson and May 1984)

$$\hat{p}_c = 0.823. \tag{10.12}$$

That is, if the genetically caused effects in Fig. 10.2 are wrongly attributed to age-related changes in intrinsic transmissibility, the ensuing estimate of the eradiction criterion, $\hat{p}_c$, can be significantly too optimistic (an estimated 82 per cent versus the true requirement of 93 per cent in this particular example). Other examples of this kind, and further discussion, are in Anderson and May (1985*d*).

In reality it is hard to distinguish genetic and age-related effects. More attention needs to be devoted to this task. Simply ignoring possible genetic heterogeneity, and treating all effects of the kind depicted in Fig. 10.2 as arising from age-related changes in basic transmission parameters may in many cases lead to serious errors.

10.2 Formal aspects of models with genetic and other heterogeneity

The approach outlined above may be generalized to the case where we have n distinct subgroups within the host population, each with its own particular set of epidemiological properties. The subgroups may be different genotypes, differing in their susceptibility to infection or in their clinical history once infected; some may exhibit symptoms and then recover, while others are asymptomatic yet transmit infection, possibly remaining 'carriers' for life. Alternatively, the subgroups may vary in social habits, with differences in nutritional state, hygiene, family size, and so on manifesting themselves as systematic differences in rates of infection and transmission. The average number of sexual partners per unit time, for example, is an important factor in the epidemiology of sexually transmitted diseases (STDs), and this quantity can vary widely among both heterosexual and homosexual individuals. Geographical setting can also affect maintenance and transmission of infection, with forces of infection being higher among groups in large cities than in remote villages.

We therefore pause at this point to construct a general framework for dealing with such heterogeneity within the host population. This framework can then be bent in various directions, to study the effects that genetic, social, spatial, and other kinds of heterogeneity have upon the transmission and maintenance of microparasitic infections. The paucity of factual information unfortunately makes much of this discussion more metaphorical than was the data-based discussion of age-related heterogeneities in Chapter 9.

10.2.1 *A model with n subgroups*
As was done earlier in this chapter, we regard the total host population as being made up of n distinct sub-populations, of sizes $\bar{N}_k$ ($k = 1, 2, \ldots, n$), in each of

which births balance deaths so that $\bar{N}_k$ is unchanging. The total population, of course, is $\bar{N} = \sum \bar{N}_k$. For each of the sub-populations, we may as before write down a set of partial differential equations describing the changes with time, t, and age, a, in the number protected by maternal antibodies, susceptible, latent, infectious, and immune: $I_k(a, t)$, $X_k(a, t)$, $H_k(a, t)$, $Y_k(a, t)$, $Z_k(a, t)$, respectively. The force of infection for members of the kth group at age a, $\lambda_k(a)$, is given by generalizing eqn (9.5):

$$\lambda_k(a, t) = \sum_{l=1}^{n} \int \beta_{kl}(a, a') Y_l(a', t)\, da'. \tag{10.13}$$

Here $\beta_{kl}(a, a')$ is the per capita transmission rate between infectives of age a' in group l and susceptibles of age a in group k.

As most of our conclusions are drawn in broad terms, we do not go into a lot of detail in the models that follow. Thus, for a start, we will ignore age-related differences in transmission from now on. Equation (10.13) then becomes

$$\lambda_k(t) = \sum_{l=1}^{n} \beta_{kl} \bar{Y}_l(t). \tag{10.14}$$

Here, as always, the 'bar' over $\bar{Y}_l$ denotes the total number of infectives, summed over all ages. In most of what follows we will, moreover, ignore the effects of maternal antibodies and latent periods, working with simple SIR models for the numbers in the various subgroups who are susceptible, infected-and-infectious, and recovered-and-immune.

10.2.2 *Age–serological profile at equilibrium*

At equilibrium ($\partial/\partial t = 0$), the number of susceptibles in the kth group as a function of age can be written down immediately:

$$X_k(a) = N_k(0)\ell_k(a) \exp(-\lambda_k a). \tag{10.15}$$

Here $N_k(0)$ is the net birth rate into the kth group, and $\ell_k(a)$ is the age-specific survival probability in the kth group (as defined by eqn (4.8); $\ell_k(a) = \exp(-\int_0^a \mu_k(s)\, ds)$).

If we assume that the age-specific death rate, and thence the survival probability, is the same for all groups, we can write a simple expression for the fraction of the population of age a who remain susceptible:

$$x(a) = \sum_{k=1}^{n} f_k \exp(-\lambda_k a). \tag{10.16}$$

Here f_k is the fraction of the total population in the kth group (for $\ell_k(a)$ independent of k, $f_k = N_k(a)/N(a) = \bar{N}_k/\bar{N}$). More generally, if essentially all new-borns are protected by maternal antibodies, for a period of characteristic duration $M \sim 1/d$, the age-specific fraction susceptible is

$$x(a) = \sum_{k=1}^{n} \frac{d f_k}{d - \lambda_k} [\exp(-\lambda_k a) - \exp(-da)]. \qquad (10.17)$$

10.2.3 *Equilibrium relationships among variables*

For simplicity, we now assume Type II survival, with the constant mortality rate, μ, being common to all groups. Integrating the partial differential equations over all ages, we arrive at the basic set of equations for the dynamics of the system:

$$d\bar{X}_k/dt = \mu \bar{N}_k - (\mu + \lambda_k)\bar{X}_k(t), \qquad (10.18)$$

$$d\bar{Y}_k/dt = \lambda_k \bar{X}_k - (\mu + v_k)\bar{Y}_k(t), \qquad (10.19)$$

$$d\bar{Z}_k/dt = v_k \bar{Y}_k - \mu \bar{Z}_k(t). \qquad (10.20)$$

As seen in Appendix C, the corresponding equations for Type I survival (everyone dies at exactly at L) lead to similar results, but the details are a bit messier.

The equilibrium values of λ_k, $\bar{X}_k$, and so on, are found by putting $d/dt = 0$ in eqns (10.18)–(10.20), and using eqn (10.14) to relate λ_k to $\bar{Y}_l$. As shown in Appendix E, the overall fraction of the population who are susceptible at equilibrium, x^*, is

$$x^* = \sum_{k=1}^{n} f_k \mu/(\mu + \lambda_k). \qquad (10.21)$$

The equilibrium values of the forces of infection are related to the inter-group transmission rates β_{kl} by the equation

$$\lambda_k = \sum_{l=1}^{n} \left(\frac{\mu \beta_{kl} \bar{N}_l}{\mu + v_l} \right) \left(\frac{\lambda_l}{\mu + \lambda_l} \right). \qquad (10.22)$$

The average age of infection, as defined and discussed earlier, is

$$A = \left(\sum_k f_k \lambda_k/(\mu + \lambda_k)^2 \right) \left(\sum_k f_k \lambda_k/(\mu + \lambda_k) \right)^{-1}. \qquad (10.23)$$

Before mass vaccination, the death rate is usually significantly smaller than rates of acquisition of infection, $\lambda_k \gg \mu$, so that the rather complicated eqn (10.22) takes the simpler form

$$\lambda_k \simeq \sum_l \mu \beta_{kl} \bar{N}_l/(\mu + v_l). \qquad (10.24)$$

10.2.4 *Eradication criterion*

Suppose a proportion $p(k)$ of children in the group k are immunized, essentially at birth (the generalization to immunization at age b is routine, but again makes for less transparent conclusions). The new force of infection in the kth group, λ'_k, follows from eqn (10.22) with $\bar{N}_k$ replaced by $\bar{N}_k(1 - p(k))$. The critical coverage for eradication, $p_c(k)$, corresponds to the limit $\lambda'_k \to 0$ for all k, which gives condition (see Appendix E)

$$\det \|A_{kl}\| = 0. \tag{10.25}$$

Here the matrix whose determinant must vanish has the elements

$$A_{kl} = (1 - p_c(l))\beta_{kl}\bar{N}_l/(\mu + v_l) - \delta_{kl}. \tag{10.26}$$

The quantity $\delta_{kl} = 1$ if $k = l$, and $\delta_{kl} = 0$ otherwise. In particular, if immunization is applied uniformly to all groups (so that p_c is the same constant for all groups), $1 - p_c$ is determined simply as the reciprocal of the dominant eigenvalue of the matrix whose elements are $\beta_{kl}\bar{N}_l/(\mu + v_l)$.

If we are given the set of quantities λ_k, we can now—at least in principle—calculate x^* from eqn (10.21), and thence estimate the eradication criterion under uniform coverage (from $\hat{p}_c = 1 - x^*$). More precisely, we may constrain the structure of the β_{kl} matrix (essentially as discussed in Chapter 9) so that its elements can be deduced from λ_k via eqn (10.22), and then evaluate critical levels of coverage from eqn (10.25). Conversely, if the transmission matrix elements β_{kl} were revealed unto us, we could compute the critical coverage levels directly from eqn (10.25); in this event, λ_k would be derived exactly from eqn (10.22) or approximately from eqn (10.24), and thence x^* from eqn (10.21). Before making some general remarks about the outcome of such calculations, we note the simplifications that ensue if the elements of the transmission matrix can be factored.

10.2.5 *Transmission matrix factorizes: equilibrium state*

The matrix element β_{kl} measures the probability, per unit time, that an infectious individual in group l will infect a susceptible individual in group k. There will be many circumstances in which this is a product of a probability, h_l, describing the production of transmission stages by infectives in group l, and another probability, g_k, describing the propensity of members of group k to acquire infection once exposed. That is, we often have $\beta_{kl} = g_k h_l$.

For instance, in the earlier part of this chapter, we assumed different genotypes differed only in their susceptibility to infection: $\beta_{kl} = \beta_k$. We conclude the chapter by discussing silent 'carriers', and for simplicity we assume transmission differs among infectives of various groups, but that all are equally susceptible to infection: $\beta_{kl} = \beta_l$. For many STDs, both the rates of spreading and of acquiring infection are roughly proportional to the number of sexual partners per unit time; in the simplest case this gives $\beta_{kl} = g_k g_l$. In short, we have sensible motives for studying the special case $\beta_{kl} = g_k h_l$, beyond the fact that it makes the analysis easier.

One consequence of the transmission matrix factoring in this way is that λ_k can be written as

$$\lambda_k = g_k \lambda. \tag{10.27}$$

Here g_k measures the intrinsic infectibility of members of group k, and λ is given by the relation

$$1 = \sum_{k=1}^{n} \left(\frac{\beta_{kk}\bar{N}_k}{\mu + v_k} \right) \left(\frac{\mu}{\mu + g_k\lambda} \right). \tag{10.28}$$

For the infection to be able to maintain itself in the population, we require $\lambda > 0$. The limiting condition for persistence is obtained by putting $\lambda \to 0$, which gives the requirement

$$R_0 \equiv \sum_{k=1}^{n} \beta_{kk}\bar{N}_k/(\mu + v_k) > 1. \tag{10.29}$$

This is the extension to these heterogeneous circumstances of the persistence criterion $R_0 = \beta\bar{N}/(\mu + v) > 1$, which was obtained earlier for a homogeneously mixed population (eqn (4.40), for Type II survival).

The eradication criterion, eqn (10.25), simplifies considerably when the transmission matrix can be factored. As shown in Appendix E, the critical levels of coverage now obey the relation:

$$1 = \sum_{k=1}^{n} (1 - p_c(k))\beta_{kk}\bar{N}_k/(\mu + v_k). \tag{10.30}$$

For uniform coverage, eqn (10.30) in conjunction with eqn (10.29) for the definition of R_0 in this situation gives the familiar result $p_c = 1 - (1/R_0)$.

10.2.6 *Transmission matrix factorizes: epidemic state*

In Chapter 6 we sketched some results for the initial rate of rise in infection, and for the fraction ever infected, for epidemics in a homogeneously mixed population. Bailey (1975) gives a more extensive review of this topic. There has, however, been very little work on epidemics in heterogeneously mixed populations. We summarize some new results here, as a preliminary to the discussion of AIDS in the next chapter.

As a description of an epidemic in a closed population, we use eqns (10.18)–(10.20) with $\mu = 0$; the epidemic rises and falls in a time short enough for births and deaths to be negligible. We further assume that λ_k is related to the quantities $\bar{Y}_l$ ($l = 1, 2, \ldots, n$) by eqn (10.14), with the transmission matrix factoring as discussed above, $\beta_{kl} = g_k h_l$.

We can then show the total fraction of the kth group to have been infected during the course of the epidemic, I_k, is given by

$$I_k = 1 - \exp(-g_k\alpha). \tag{10.31}$$

The parameter α is determined from the implicit equation

$$\alpha = \sum_{k=1}^{n} (h_k \bar{N}_k/v_k)[1 - \exp(-g_k\alpha)]. \tag{10.32}$$

These results are derived in Appendix E. Equation (10.32) has a non-trivial solution only if $\sum_k g_k h_k \bar{N}_k/v_k > 1$. This is identical (given that $\mu = 0$ here) with the criterion (10.29) for endemic persistence that was obtained above. If this requirement is not met, the epidemic simply cannot spread. As we shall see in the next chapter, the epidemic described by eqns (10.31) and (10.32) can end up infecting very different fractions within the different groups.

In the initial phase of the epidemic, the incidence of infection in each group, and other such quantities, will tend to increase exponentially at a rate Λ given by the set of homogeneous linear equations

$$\sum_{l=1}^{n} [\beta_{kl} \bar{N}_k - (v_k + \Lambda) \delta_{kl}] \bar{Y}_l(t) = 0. \tag{10.33}$$

Thus the rate Λ will correspond to the solution with the largest real part of the equation

$$\det\|\beta_{kl}\bar{N}_k - (v_k + \Lambda) \delta_{kl}\| = 0. \tag{10.34}$$

Again, this reduces to a much simpler expression if the transmission matrix factors. In this event, $\beta_{kl} = g_k h_l$, we have Λ as the dominant solution of the polynomial (see Appendix E):

$$\sum_{k=1}^{n} \frac{\beta_{kk}\bar{N}_k}{v_k + \Lambda} = 1. \tag{10.35}$$

We can identify this result for the heterogeneous population with the earlier result $\Lambda = v(R_0 - 1)$ for homogeneous mixing, using eqn (10.29) to define R_0 (and putting $\mu = 0$), but only if all the recovery rates v_k are equal. Do notice, however, that the condition for an epidemic to be possible is now $\Lambda > 0$, which again leads to the criterion of eqn (10.29) when $\mu = 0$.

10.2.7 *General remarks*

In the remainder of this chapter, we apply the above formulae to study the effect which silent 'carriers' can have on the transmission and maintenance of infection. The next two chapters use the formulae in other ways, to explore the epidemiological consequences of various kinds of social, cultural, and spatial heterogeneity. In all this work, there is one recurrent theme, which we end this overture by sounding.

Suppose we treat the population as if it were homogeneously mixed, and *estimate* the critical coverage for eradication from $\hat{p}_c = 1 - x^*$ (with x^* measured by serological studies or otherwise). This almost invariably results in an estimate that is lower than the coverage actually required for a *uniformly applied* immunization scheme in a heterogeneous population. That is, eqn (10.21) for x^* and eqn (10.25) for p_c lead to $p_c \geqslant 1 - x^*$ (unless β_{kl} behaves very oddly). We may, however, alternatively define the optimal coverage as that which eradicates infection by *targeting* immunization in such as way as to minimize the number of individuals treated. The overall coverage required by the optimal scheme, p_{opt}, is almost always lower than that estimated or actually needed under randomly applied immunization. That is, with the definitions given above, we virtually always have $p_c > \hat{p}_c > p_{opt}$ in a population that is genetically, culturally, or spatially heterogeneous.

10.3 Carriers of infection

The epidemiology and the control of many diseases is made complicated by chronic infection in immunodeficient individuals, who become 'silent' or inapparent carriers of the virus or bacterium, sometimes essentially for life.

Hepatitis B virus (HBV) is a case in point. The virus infects people everywhere in the world, with the highest rates of infection in sub-Saharan Africa and east Asia. Although the majority of cases are not serious in developed countries, a minority lead to acute hepatitis with jaundice, causing some deaths. Francis (1983) estimates there are about 200 000 new HBV infections in the USA each year, of which about 25 per cent experience acute hepatitis, leading to around 10 000 hospitalizations and 250 deaths. More generally, the outcome of HBV infection depends on the immune response of the individual. An adequate immune response will lead to the production of antibodies that clear the infection (possibly with the complications just mentioned) and produce lifelong immunity. An inadequate immune response allows continued viral replication; if maintained for six months or longer, such viral production usually persists indefinitely, and the infected individual becomes an asymptomatic carrier of infection. Such carriers are at risk to two types of slow-developing diseases later in life (one associated with liver inflammation and the other cancer of the liver), but in the intervening years they can transmit HBV infection. Transmission itself is via blood or blood products, and can occur during sexual intercourse, in the sharing of needles by drug abusers or as a misguided economy in vaccination programmes in some developed countries, or even (to cite a study that cuts across stereotypical views about HBV transmission) when bramble-scratched cross-country runners share a sauna.

The fraction, $1 - f$, of HBV infections which lead to illness followed by recovery and immunity, versus the fraction, f, which lead to persistent viraemia in the carrier state, varies greatly among countries. In the USA and most European countries, f appears to be around 0.1 to 2 per cent, ranging through significantly higher values in Africa and Asia, to as high as 50 per cent in some Pacific islands. The probability of becoming a carrier appears to be greater in children than in adults, which could explain a tendency to higher ratios in countries where infection is typically at younger ages, but part of the observed variability is documented as arising from genetic differences (in immune responses) among populations.

These carriers constitute an important reservoir of HBV infection. Their presence represents a complication for proposed programmes of immunization with new vaccines (derived from natural or genetically engineered antigen) in places like Taiwan, where the proportion of carriers is appreciable. It is unlikely that carriers can be removed by immunization, and it is possible that people predisposed to becoming carriers cannot be effectively protected by vaccination. An additional complication arises from the fact that HBV infection is transmitted vertically by infected mothers, with most of the children thus infected becoming carriers.

We have dwelt on the phenomenon of the carrier state for HBV, partly because it is well documented, and partly because it has a genetic aspect (which places it in this chapter). There are, however, other infections where carriers play a significant part in maintenance and transmission. Typhoid is one, with the historical episode of 'Typhoid Mary' giving an alternative name to the phenomenon. Cholera, tuberculosis, and possibly poliomyelitis may provide other examples. Table 10.1 attempts to summarize the essential aspects of these examples.

Table 10.1 Estimates of epidemiological variables for infections where carriers may play an important role in transmission

Infection	Normal infectious period, $1/v_1$	Carriers' infectious period, $1/v_2$	Proportion who are carriers, f	Infectivity of carrier relative to others, β_2/β_1	Source
HBV	~ 20 days	Lifelong	$\sim 1\%$ (USA, Europe) $\sim 5–10\%$ or more (Asia, Africa)	?	Francis (1983), Anderson and May (1985c)
Typhoid	~ 30 days	Lifelong	$\sim 3\%$	1[a]	Cvjetanovic et al. (1978)
Cholera	3–6 days[b]	Lifelong	10^{-5}	0.05	Cvjetanovic et al. (1978)

[a] Cvjetanovic et al. (1978) implicitly assume carriers and others are equally infective.
[b] Cvjetanovic et al. (1978) assume 4 per cent of cases are symptomatic and infectious for 3–6 days. A larger fraction, 96 per cent, became asymptomatic 'constant carriers', being 0.05 times as infective as symptomatic cases, for about 5–7 days. There are other, minor, complications, but these two categories determine R_0 for all practical purposes (making roughly equal contributions: the relevant ratio is $[(3 \text{ to } 6)/(5 \text{ to } 7)](4/96)(1/0.05) \simeq 0.6$).

We now present a simple model that illuminates aspects of endemic infection and its eradication. Bailey (1975) has given a comprehensive review of the mathematical literature dealing with the effects that carriers can have on epidemic outbreaks of infection.

10.3.1 *A model with carriers*

Applying the general formulae above, we assume that the population is made up of two distinct groups: a 'normal' fraction, $1 - f$, who recover from infection (at a rate v_1, or after a characteristic time $1/v_1$) and are immune thereafter; and a 'carrier' fraction, f, who recover much more slowly ($v_2 \ll v_1$) or never ($v_2 = 0$). We further assume that both groups are equally infectible, but that carriers are significantly less infectious than normal infectives (because they are producing HBV at lower rates); this corresponds to assuming $\beta_{kl} = \beta_l$ in eqn (10.14).

Equation (10.14) now gives

$$\lambda = \beta_1 \bar{Y}_1 + \beta_2 \bar{Y}_2. \tag{10.36}$$

Here the subscript 1 refers to normal infectives, and 2 to carriers. The assumption that λ is the same for both groups (which follows from $\beta_{kl} = \beta_l$) leads to a simple expression for the age–serological profile at equilibrium, $1 - x(a)$, where

$$x(a) = d(e^{-\lambda a} - e^{-da})/(d - \lambda). \tag{10.37}$$

This formula ignores vertical transmission and assumes that all are born protected by maternal antibodies (for a time of characteristic duration $1/d$); the formula is not likely to be reliable if f is large. Nevertheless, eqn (10.37) gives a good fit to the serological data for HBV in Senegal, shown in Fig. 10.3. The theoretical curve is for the parameters $d = 0.25 \, \text{yr}^{-1}$ and $\lambda = 0.11 \, \text{yr}^{-1}$, corresponding to an average age at infection of $A = 9$ years.

Integrating over all ages, and ignoring maternal antibodies, we describe the dynamics of the system by the appropriately particular versions of eqns (10.18) and (10.19):

$$d\bar{X}/dt = \mu \bar{N} - (\mu + \lambda)\bar{X}(t), \tag{10.38}$$

$$d\bar{Y}_1/dt = (1 - f)\lambda \bar{X} - (\mu + v_1)\bar{Y}_1(t), \tag{10.39}$$

$$d\bar{Y}_2/dt = f\lambda \bar{X} - (\mu + v_2)\bar{Y}_2(t). \tag{10.40}$$

Cooke (1982) has studied the formal properties of a closely similar set of equations.

The equilibrium solutions of these equations are easy to get. In particular, λ can be written (from eqn (10.28) with $g_k = 1$) as

$$\lambda = \mu(R_0 - 1). \tag{10.41}$$

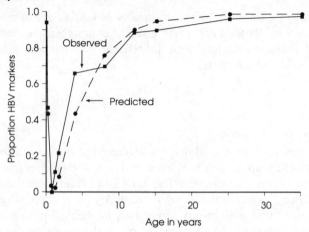

Fig. 10.3. The fit of eqn (10.37) to data acquired from a serological survey for antibodies to the hepatitis B virus (HBV) in a population in Senegal (Francis 1983). The predicted curve has parameter values $d = 0.25 \text{ yr}^{-1}$, $\lambda = 0.11 \text{ yr}^{-1}$, corresponding to an average age at infection of $A = 9$ years.

Here we have identified R_0 as

$$R_0 = \frac{(1-f)\beta_1\bar{N}}{\mu + v_1} + \frac{f\beta_2\bar{N}}{\mu + v_2}. \tag{10.42}$$

This result has an intuitive explanation. The coefficient of $1 - f$ in the first term on the right-hand side in eqn (10.42), $R_{01} \equiv \beta_1\bar{N}/(\mu + v_1)$, would be the R_0 of eqn (4.40) were the population entirely composed of individuals of group 1. Likewise, the coefficient of f in the second term, $R_{02} \equiv \beta_2\bar{N}/(\mu + v_2)$, would be R_0 if the population were all carriers. Since both groups are equally infectible, the actual R_0 is the weighted average of the individual R_0 values for normals and carriers.

The same point emerges in the eradication criterion, which (from eqn (10.30)) is

$$(1-f)R_{01}(1 - p_c(1)) + fR_{02}(1 - p_c(2)) = 1. \tag{10.43}$$

Again, R_{01} and R_{02} are as defined in the preceding paragraph. If vaccination is applied uniformly, and if it is equally effective for both normals and carriers, eqn (10.43) gives the familiar result $p_c = 1 - (1/R_0)$, with R_0 defined by eqn (10.42).

It is possible, however, that those in the carrier group may not be able to be protected by immunization, by reason of the lack of immunocompetence that places them in the carrier state following natural infection. If this is the case, then effectively $p_c(2) = 0$ in eqn (10.43), and eradication is impossible (even with 100 per cent coverage of the normal group) if $f\beta_2\bar{N}/(\mu + v_2) > 1$. Of course, HBV infection could be essentially eliminated from the non-carrier group by such a programme; the problem is that the vaccination programme would have to be perpetuated indefinitely, were the infection to be maintained in the population by an unimmunizable carrier group.

It is not easy to make an estimate of the relevant second term, fR_{02}, on the right-hand side of eqn (10.42). Using the Senegalese data in Fig. 10.3, we obtain $A \sim 5$–7 years, which is a fairly representative value. With the reciprocal of the average per capita birth rate, B, being around 35–50 years in Asian and African countries, we thus have the crude estimate $R_0 \sim 5$–10 for HBV (using $R_0 \simeq B/A$). An estimate of the relative contributions made to this number by the two terms in eqn (10.42) is harder. For normal HBV infections, the duration of the infectious period may typically be around 20 days. Carriers, however, may remain infectious for life; since infection is usually acquired in childhood, this means the duration of infectiousness is 30–50 years or more. Thus the ratio $(\mu + v_1)/(\mu + v_2)$ contributes a factor of roughly 500–1000 'favouring' the carriers. The ratio $f/(1-f)$ varies from country to country as noted above. In most Western countries it is typically around 1 per cent, which reduces the carriers 'advantage' to something like a factor of 5–10; but in Asian and African countries, f can be 5–10 per cent or more, so that the carriers' advantage stays up around a factor 50 or so. The ratio β_1/β_2, which measures the relative infectiousness of normal and carrier infectives, is most uncertain of all: a reasonable assumption may be that β is an order of magnitude less for carriers than for normal infectives. Putting all this together, we arrive at the tentative conclusion that the two terms on the right-hand side of eqn (10.42) may be roughly comparable in magnitude for HBV in western countries, but that the second term (corresponding to transmission by carriers) probably predominates in many Asian and sub-Saharan African countries. In either case, it seems unlikely that HBV can be eradicted by a vaccination programme if those who are predisposed to becoming carriers cannot be protected. There is a clear need for more work here, both on the question of whether potential carriers can be immunized, and on determining the parameter ratios estimated so crudely above.

In their numerical studies of the effects of various schedules of immunization against typhoid, Cvjetanovic *et al.* (1978) use the parameter estimates summarized in Table 10.1. For these values, the contribution to the basic reproductive rate by carriers is roughly ten times that from other individuals (in part because it is assumed $\beta_1 = \beta_2$). Cvjetanovic *et al.* assume immunization affects carriers and others equally, and they also restrict their numerical studies to a range of values of R_0 that are relatively low (in effect, though it is not put this way, they explore a range from $R_0 \simeq 1.06$ to $R_0 \simeq 2.4$).

For cholera, Cvjetanovic *et al.* assume that lifelong carriers comprise a fraction of about 10^{-5} of the population, which makes them epidemiologically negligible. The 'convalescent carriers' of Cvjetanovic *et al.* have a duration of infectiousness of around 14–21 days, and so their models for cholera are, in effect, of the basic kind discussed earlier.

10.3.2 *Vertical transmission*

The fact that HBV can be transmitted vertically to the offspring of mothers who are infected carriers represents an additional complication. To a rough approximation, such vertical transmission can be incorporated in the model defined by eqns (10.38)–(10.40) by assuming that a proportion v of births to infected carriers are themselves infected carriers (while the remaining fraction of these births give susceptibles in the carrier group). The approximation is undoubtedly too extreme in its assumption that the 'carriers' and 'normals' represent two closed sub-populations, but the modification does serve to illuminate the essential effects of vertical transmission.

With this modification, eqns (10.38)–(10.40) become

$$\mathrm{d}\bar{X}_1/\mathrm{d}t = (1 - f)\mu\bar{N} - (\mu + \lambda)\bar{X}_1(t), \tag{10.44}$$

$$\mathrm{d}\bar{X}_2/\mathrm{d}t = f\mu\bar{N} - v\mu\bar{Y}_2 - (\mu + \lambda)\bar{X}_2(t), \tag{10.45}$$

$$\mathrm{d}\bar{Y}_1/\mathrm{d}t = \lambda\bar{X}_1 - (\mu + v_1)\bar{Y}_1(t), \tag{10.46}$$

$$\mathrm{d}\bar{Y}_2/\mathrm{d}t = \lambda\bar{X}_2 + v\mu\bar{Y}_2 - (\mu + v_2)\bar{Y}_2(t). \tag{10.47}$$

It is now necessary to keep track of the susceptibles in the two groups separately. The equilibrium properties of these equations are straightforward, and will not be given in detail. Of interest is the eradication criterion corresponding to eqn (10.43) above:

$$(1 - f)R_{01}(1 - p_c(1)) + fR_{02}(1 - p_c(2)) = 1. \tag{10.48}$$

As before, $R_{01} = \beta_1\bar{N}/(\mu + v_1)$, but the basic reproductive rate for the carrier-only population is now

$$R_{02} = \beta_2\bar{N}/[v_2 + \mu(1 - v)]. \tag{10.49}$$

The effect of vertical transmission is to increase the value of R_{02}, thus requiring higher levels of coverage (if carriers can indeed be protected by immunization). In the artificial extreme where vertical transmission always occurs ($v = 1$) and carriers remain infectious for life ($v_2 = 0$), with no selective disadvantages occurring to the carrier state, we see that $R_{02} \to \infty$. This corresponds, understandably enough, to an equilibrium state in which the entire sub-population of carriers are infected ($\bar{Y}_2 = f\bar{N}$, $\bar{X}_2 = \bar{Z}_2 = 0$); even with an effective vaccine, infection can be eradicated only by 100 per cent coverage.

10.3.3 *Carriers and the inter-epidemic period*

Chapter 6 began by describing the dynamical properties of the basic SIR model. We noted the tendency of this simple system to oscillate about the endemic equilibrium state, with the cycles having a damping time ($T_d \sim 2A$) significantly greater than their basic period ($T \simeq 2\pi[A(D + D')]^{1/2}$). As catalogued in Table 6.1, this period agrees well with the observed inter-epidemic periods for a variety of infections.

A similar study of the sets of eqns (10.38)–(10.40), with λ defined by eqn (10.36), is easy in principle (although the linear stability analysis is made complicated in detail by having a cubic, rather than a quadratic, for the eigenvalues). If often happens, however, that the carrier group is primarily responsible for maintenance and transmission of infection within the population; as we have been, this occurs when $fR_{02} \gg (1 - f)R_{01}$ in eqn (10.42) or (10.43). In this event, $\lambda \simeq \beta_2 \bar{Y}_2$, and the dynamics are essentially described by the two differential equations for $X(t)$ and $\lambda(t)$, eqns (6.5) and (6.6), that were discussed in Chapter 6; as before, A is to be interpreted as the average age at infection (~ 5 to 7 years for HBV), but $D + D'$ is now the average duration of infectiousness in the carrier state ($1/(\mu + v_2)$), which can be virtually lifelong ($D + D' \sim 50$ years). In this limiting situation, $\bar{Y}_1(t)$ 'tracks' the dynamics determined by $\bar{X}(t)$ and $\lambda(t) \simeq \beta_2 \bar{Y}_2(t)$.

As can be seen from the analysis of eqns (6.5) and (6.6) given in Appendix C, once the duration of infectiousness significantly exceeds the average age at infection, the system no longer tends to oscillate. Disturbances from equilibrium simply damp out smoothly, with a fast damping time set by A and a slow one set by $1/(\mu + v_2)$. Figure 10.4 illustrates this, showing a numerical solution for a disturbance about an equilibrium state for the equations (10.38)–(10.40), with parameters chosen to be representative of HBV. In this case carriers and non-carriers contribute roughly equally to transmission, and so we do not have the limiting situation just described; the essential dynamical features are, however, as suggested by the approximate analysis. The numerical studies of temporal trends following vaccination against typhoid, by Cvjetanovic *et al.* (1978), can be read as illustrating these same points.

Figure 10.4 stands in vivid contrast to the marked oscillations seen in Fig. 7.1 for a typical microparasitic infection. It is intuitively sensible that the long duration of infectiousness in the carrier state should smooth over the lags involved in replenishing the pool of susceptibles, doing away with the boom-and-bust tendencies that arise when infection is short compared with recruitment times. We believe this is why infections like HBV and typhoid do not exhibit the pronounced non-seasonal cycles that are so often a characteristic feature of measles, pertussis, mumps, rubella, smallpox, and other infections where carriers play no role.

10.4 Summary

We begin with a simple model, demonstrating that genetic heterogeneity in susceptibility to infection can generate the illusion that transmission is intrinsically lower at older ages. Treating such genetically caused apparent decreases

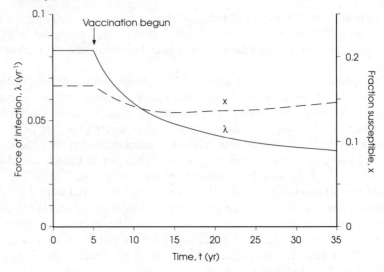

Fig. 10.4. The dynamical behaviour described by the epidemiological eqns (10.38)–(10.40), following the introduction (in year 5) of a programme that successfully immunizes 50 percent of all new-borns. For this illustrative calculation of the dynamical effects that 'carriers' can produce, the parameters are chosen to be roughly representative of HBV: $\mu = 1/60$ yr^{-1} ($L = 60$ years), $v_1 = 20$ yr^{-1} (non-carriers infectious for about 18 days), $v_2 = 1/30$ yr^{-1}, $f = 0.01$ (1 per cent of the population are carriers, typically being infectious for around 30 years), $\beta_2/\beta_1 = 0.1$ (non-carriers are ten times more infectious than carriers), and $R_0 = 6$ (resulting in the pre-immunization force of infection having the value $\lambda = 5\mu$, which corresponds to an average age at infection around $A = 12$ years). In marked contrast to the oscillations shown in Fig. 7.1, the effect of the long-lived infectiousness of carriers results in smooth changes: the force of infection, λ (the full curve), moves monotonically to its asymptotic value ($\lambda = 2\mu$); the fraction susceptible, x (the broken line), at first falls—as always—and then monotonically moves back to its original value. For further discussion, see the text.

in λ as if they derived from reduction in transmission at older ages could lead to excessively optimistic estimates of the critical coverage needed for eradication.

Next, we present some formal machinery for discussing various kinds of heterogeneity—genetic, social, cultural, spatial, and so on. This apparatus embraces formulae for the fraction infected and force of infection in the endemic equilibrium, criteria for eradication, and expressions for the fraction ever infected by an epidemic in a heterogeneous population.

The chapter ends by applying these formulae to discuss the influence that carriers—individuals with long-lived inapparent infections—can have on the maintenance and transmission of microparasites. The effects of carriers upon eradication criteria are examined, with particular reference to hepatitis B virus; the further complications attendant on vertical transmission are also considered.

If carriers with long-lived infections play a major part in transmission, there is no longer the tendency to non-seasonal oscillations of the kind remarked in Chapter 6; we suggest this is why carrier-borne infections like HBV and typhoid do not show the pronounced oscillations characteristic of so many childhood infections.

11

Social heterogeneity and sexually
transmitted diseases

A central theme in this chapter is that most sexually transmitted diseases (STDs) cannot be understood without acknowledging the marked heterogeneity in degrees of sexual activity within the overall population. We first consider the endemic maintenance of STDs, with particular attention to gonorrhoea. The second (and larger) part of the chapter focuses on the epidemic dynamics of STDs, using AIDS as an example.

11.1 Endemic infection: gonorrhoea and 'superspreaders'

Most STDs have characteristics that cause their epidemiology to be rather different from infections such as measles and rubella, which have received the bulk of our attention so far.

First, for STDs such as gonorrhoea, genital herpes, and non-gonococcal urethritis (often caused by *Chlamydia trachomatis*), only sexually active individuals who could be infected by their contacts need to be considered as candidates in the transmission process. In contrast with simple models for infections like measles or the common cold, a doubling of the population density does not increase the rate at which new infections are produced by infected individuals (unless we assume that social changes, induced by greater crowding, indirectly result in greater promiscuity).

Second, the carrier phenomenon is important for many STDs. Thus many people infected with gonorrhoea, especially women, are virtually asymptomatic and so do not seek treatment. Since individuals recover spontaneously from gonorrhoea only after a long time has elapsed, such asymptomatic carriers may be regarded as remaining infectious until they do receive antibiotic treatment. In so far as HBV can be simply regarded as a sexually transmitted disease, it also illustrates the importance of asymptomatic carriers. So, probably, does AIDS, as we shall see.

Third, many STDs result in little or no acquired immunity following recovery, so that most individuals who have been treated or who have spontaneously recovered rejoin the susceptible class. This is the case for gonorrhoea and for chlamydial infections, though not for HBV (where acquired immunity is manifested) nor for AIDS (where remission of infection appears not to occur).

This suite of properties—virtual absence of a threshold density of hosts, long-lived carriers of infection, absence of lasting immunity—adds up to microparasites that can be well adapted to persisting in small, low-density aggregations of humans.

Cooke and Yorke (1973) were the first to develop a mathematical model that catered specifically to these features of the epidemiology of gonorrhoea, which may be regarded as a canonical STD. Subsequent studies by Reynolds and Chan (1975), Constable (1975), Hethcote (1976), Nold (1980), and others are reviewed by Yorke *et al.* (1978) and in the monograph by Hethcote and Yorke (1984). These last two works are exemplary for the way in which the mathematical models are grounded on data, and the conclusions are aimed at public health workers in a way that emphasizes the ideas and is not cluttered with mathematical details. What follows is an abstract of this work on modelling the transmission and control of gonorrhoea.

In the USA, roughly one million cases of gonorrhoea are reported each year, and the Center for Disease Control suggests that between two and three million new cases may actually arise annually. One of the more serious consequences is the estimated 10–17 per cent of women with gonorrhoea who develop pelvic inflammatory diseases (PID) which is the leading cause of female sterility. Estimates of the direct and indirect costs related to PID and associated ectopic pregnancies exceeded 1.3 billion dollars in the USA in 1979.

For most of the infections we have studied so far, the 'density-dependent' factor that ultimately limits the prevalence of infection is acquired immunity; prevalence saturates at a level such that most contacts made by an infected person are 'wasted' on immune individuals. For gonorrhoea, however, there is no acquired immunity, and saturation effects instead arise when infectious individuals contact individuals who are already infected from some other source. Yorke *et al.* (1978) call this 'preemptive saturation', and emphasize that it is the only density-dependent mechanism capable of affecting a disease like gonorrhoea which does not evoke lasting immunity.

Turning to the data for gonorrhoea in the USA, Yorke *et al.* (1978) estimate the incidence to be around 2.6 million cases each year, and the average duration of infection (before treatment) to be 55 days for both sexes. This corresponds to a prevalence of about 400 000 cases at any given moment. By further assuming the population of sexually active people who are at risk to be around 20 million, Yorke *et al.* (1978) arrive at the conclusion that roughly 2 per cent of the at-risk population is infected at any one time. Changing the estimated size of the population at risk to 10 or 50 million does not affect the essentials of the subsequent argument.

Given that only 2 per cent or so of the contacts of an average infective person are themselves already infected, 'preemptive' saturation cannot be a significant factor if the population at risk is regarded as a single, homogeneous, freely mixing group. One possibility is that gonorrhoea is currently far from equilibrium, with its prevalence growing rapidly in the USA. This does not appear to be the case. The more likely reason for the observed discrepancy is that there are many distinct subgroups within the at-risk population, differentiated according to number of sexual partners, sexual practices, age, and other factors. Yorke *et al.* (1978) show, for example, that a 'core' population of around 500 000 individuals who are sexually very active, and who therefore have high prevalence (of the order of 20 per cent), would have pre-emptive effects substantial enough to explain the observed data. What is happening is essentially that each infective in the core population infects, on average, more than one susceptible person during the course of the infection, while each infective outside the core infects, on average, less than one susceptible; at equilibrium, these two rates combine to produce an overall average of one new infectee for each current infection.

11.1.1 *Implications for control*

The presence of such a core of 'superspreaders' has implications for the design of control programmes. If the core individuals could all be identified and kept free of gonorrhoea (by persistent surveillance and treatment, or by use of an as-yet hypothetical vaccine), the disease would die out, because its basic reproductive rate in the remaining non-core population is less than unity.

In the work drawn together by Hethcote and Yorke (1984), the population at risk is subdivided according to sex, the level of sexual activity (core and non-core), and whether the infection is symptomatic or asymptomatic. A set of eight ($2^3 = 8$) differential equations is used to model the dynamic interplay among the groups, and the consequences of various control strategies are explored.

In these studies, the probability of transmission from an infectious female to a susceptible male during sexual intercourse is estimated by Hethcote and Yorke to be 0.2–0.3, while the corresponding probability of transmission from an infectious male to a susceptible female is around 0.5–0.7. Because a new sexual encounter typically involves more than one act, the net female-to-male transmission probability may be around 0.5, and the male-to-female around 0.9, per encounter. These detailed values are of less significance in the models than is their ratio, namely 1:2 (female-to-male versus male-to-female; gonorrhoea does not obey Title IX).

Three general kinds of control strategies are considered by Hethcote and Yorke (1984; see also Hethcote *et al.* (1982)). Strategy AW involves the general screening of females, by testing cultures taken from women who use certain designated health facilities. The corresponding strategy AM does the same thing for males. Strategies BW and BM trace females and males, respectively, to whom an infection has been spread by an individual diagnosed as infected. Strategy CW identifies infectious females from the men they have infected, and strategy CM correspondingly identifies infectious males from their female infectees. In short, strategy A takes a slice in time, strategy B pursues the chain downstream, and C pursues it upstream.

Although the quantitative details depend on the specific parameters chosen in the various models, strategy C is always more effective than A, which in turn is markedly superior to B. This conclusion can be understood qualitatively, by noting that asymptomatics are more important transmitters than symptomatics (because they are infectious for a longer time), and that core individuals are more important transmitters than non-core (because they contact more people while they are infectious). Strategy C, by pursuing the chain of infection upstream, has a high likelihood both of identifying very active core individuals and of identifying asymptomatics. Strategy A, although relatively ineffective in finding core people, tends to locate asymptomatics. Strategy B is not particularly effective in finding either core individuals or asymptomatics.

Within any one strategy, finding infectious males by M controls tends to be more effective at reducing prevalence levels than is finding infectious females by W controls. This feature stems basically from the above-noted fact that transmission from males to females is roughly twice as efficient as the converse.

In practice, the relative merits of the various control programmes depend not just on how effective the finding of infectives is in decreasing prevalence, but also on the cost of discovering infectives by the method in question. As always, the biology and epidemiology is only part of the larger economic and political picture.

11.2 Some formal aspects of endemic STDs

The formal expressions describing the epidemiological effects of heterogeneity within the host population can be applied to STDs, with the main heterogeneity being the different degrees of sexual activity found among the various subgroups. These expressions were derived in Chapter 10 for infections with an immune class, which of course embraces lifelong infection with no recovery as a special case ($v_1 = 0$). In what follows we also indicate straightforward extensions to the case where there is no immune class, and individuals recover directly back into the susceptible class (as for gonorrhoea).

In our subsequent discussion, we use a subscript 'i' to label that group of individuals who have, on average, i sexual partners per unit time. We make no other discriminations among the host population; that is, we do not partition the population by age, sex, social class, or other variables that could be relevant in particular contexts. In partitioning the population according to a continuous measure of the rate of acquisition of sexual partners, we are effectively assuming that we know the probability distribution function, $P(i)$, which tells us the fraction of the population who are in the ith class. Often, however, all we will have is rough knowledge of the relative numbers of individuals in different, coarsely divided groups: for instance, those with 1–2, 3–5, 6–20, 20+ sexual partners per unit time. In this event, i will label the groups.

We assume the force of infection for a susceptible in the ith class, λ_i, is linearly proportional to the average number of sexual partners per unit time, i:

$$\lambda_i = i\lambda. \tag{11.1}$$

Here λ is the probability that a randomly chosen partner will produce infection, which in turn depends on a transmission parameter β and on the probability, π, that a given partner is infectious. β corresponds to the quantity estimated by Yorke *et al.* (1978) as being around 0.5 for female-to-male contact and around 0.9 for male-to-female for gonorrhoea, and π is obtained by weighting potential partners by their degree of sexual activity. We thus obtain

$$\lambda = \beta \sum_i i Y_i \left(\sum_i i N_i \right)^{-1}. \tag{11.2}$$

In effect, this assumption that $\lambda_i = i\lambda$, with λ defined by eqn (11.2), amounts to putting

$$\beta_{ij} \to ij\beta \left(\sum_i i N_i \right)^{-1} \tag{11.3}$$

in the formal expressions developed in Chapter 10 (see eqn (10.14)). The assumption that the transmission matrix β_{ij} is bilinear, being linearly proportional to the average rate of acquisition of sexual partners by both infector and infectee, in some respects overestimates and in some respects underestimates the net effects of heterogeneity in sexual habits. On the one hand, the bilinear form could underestimate the spread of infection by those who are in the less active classes, because the effective value of β—the transmission probability per relationship—could (for some STDs) be higher for the longer-sustained partnerships that may characterize less active individuals than for the brief encounters that may characterize the very active singles-bar/bathhouse set. On the other hand, the bilinear form assumes no correlations among individuals in different classes of sexual activity in their search for partners. In reality, it is likely that less active people may tend, other things being equal, to interact with other less active people, and highly active individuals may tend to interact within their own high-activity classes to a greater extent than captured by the factor ij. Since the highly active individuals are more likely to be infected, correlations of this kind could result in eqns (11.1) and (11.2) overestimating λ_i for individuals in the low-activity groups. In short, the assumption $\beta_{ij} \sim ij$ has potential faults that cut in both directions, and whose relative magnitudes are uncertain. This is one of the many areas where more factual information is needed.

Substituting eqns (11.1)–(11.3) for λ_i and β_{ij} into eqn (10.22) which determines the equilibrium value of the force of infection in the basic SIR model, we have

$$1 = \sum_i \frac{i^2 \mu \beta \bar{N}_i}{(\mu + v)(\mu + i\lambda)} \left(\sum_i i \bar{N}_i \right)^{-1}. \tag{11.4}$$

Here we have assumed the recovery rate is the same for all classes, $v_i = v$. This eqn (11.4) now determines the force of infection per partner, λ, implicitly.

A similar expression for λ can be obtained for the case where infectives recover directly into the susceptible class, with no immune class (as for gonorrhoea).

Here the basic model of eqns (10.18)–(10.20) can be replaced by

$$d\bar{X}_i/dt = \mu\bar{N}_i + v\bar{Y}_i - (\mu + \lambda_i)\bar{X}_i(t), \qquad (11.5)$$

$$d\bar{Y}_i/dt = \lambda_i\bar{X}_i - (v + \mu)\bar{Y}_i(t). \qquad (11.6)$$

The sum $\bar{X}_i(t) + \bar{Y}_i(t) = \bar{N}_i$, where $\bar{N}_i$ is the constant number of hosts in the ith group, so that eqns (11.5) and (11.6) give, in effect, only one dynamical equation. The force of infection, λ_i, is as defined above by eqns (11.1)–(11.3). The same analysis that led from eqns (10.18)–(10.20) to eqn (10.22) can be applied to eqns (11.5) and (11.6) to get (see Appendix E):

$$1 = \sum_i \frac{i^2\beta\bar{N}_i}{\mu + v + i\lambda}\left(\sum_i i\bar{N}_i\right)^{-1}. \qquad (11.7)$$

Equation (11.7) is the analogue of eqn (11.4), for an infection that does not evoke immunity.

11.2.1 *Basic reproductive rate, R_0*

The condition for the microparasite to be able to maintain itself within the host population (corresponding to $R_0 > 1$) is found by taking the limit $\lambda \to 0$ in expressions such as eqn (11.4) or (11.7). Whether or not there is acquired immunity, we obtain from eqn (11.4) or (11.7) the criterion for persistence:

$$R_0 \equiv \beta c/(\mu + v) > 1. \qquad (11.8)$$

Here we have defined c as the appropriately averaged number of sexual partners per unit time,

$$c \equiv \langle i^2\rangle/\langle i\rangle, \qquad (11.9)$$

with $\langle i^n\rangle$ being the nth moment of the distribution in the number of sexual partners, $P(i)$, within the population in question. The mean number of partners is $m = \sum_i iP(i) \equiv \langle i\rangle$, and the variance is $\sigma^2 = \sum_i (i - m)^2 P(i) \equiv \langle i^2\rangle - \langle i\rangle^2$. Incidentally, it is not surprising that the presence or absence of an immune class is irrelevant to the expression (11.8) for the basic reproductive rate of the infection, because R_0 pertains to the limit when virtually all hosts are susceptible.

As discussed more generally at the beginning of this chapter, this expression (11.8) for R_0 for a typical STD differs from that for most microparasites in not depending on the population density of the host. In the heterogeneous situation described above, R_0 depends only on the transmission probability per partner, β, the typical time spent in the infectious state, $1/(\mu + v)$, and a measure of the number of partners per unit time, c. Notice, however, that c is not simply the mean, m, of the $P(i)$ distribution, but rather can be written (using eqn (11.9) and the definition of σ^2)

$$c = m + \sigma^2/m. \qquad (11.10)$$

Thus the effective value of the average number of sexual partners for epidemiological purposes can be significantly larger than the simple mean, if the variance is high (May and Anderson 1987; Anderson *et al.* 1986). This really is another way of saying that 'superspreaders' play a disproportionate role in the maintenance and transmission of infection; their importance scales effectively as i^2, not simply as i.

An approximation that neglected heterogeneities in sexual habits, and estimated c as just the simple mean number of partners, could result in a serious underestimate of R_0. For example, suppose we could crudely divide a population into a core group, comprising 10 per cent of the population, with on average 20 partners per unit time, and a non-core group, comprising 90 per cent, with on average 2 partners: the mean number of partners per unit time is $m = 3.8$, but the epidemiologically relevant moment of the distribution is $c = 11.5$.

11.2.2 *Eradication criterion*

Suppose we could immunize a fraction $p(i)$ of the ith group, essentially before they entered the pool of people transmitting infection. In practice, this might for example correspond to identifying a proportion $p(i)$ of gonorrhoea patients in group i by one of the strategies described by Hethcote and Yorke (1984), and then keeping them free from infection by surveillance and treatment. The infection could in this way be eradicated, if the proportions exceeded a critical set of values given (from eqn (10.30) with eqn (11.3) for β_{ij}) by:

$$1 = \left(\sum_i \frac{i^2 \beta \bar{N}_i (1 - p_c(i))}{\mu + v} \right) \left(\sum_i i \bar{N}_i \right)^{-1}. \qquad (11.11)$$

Again, this formula applies equally to those infections that do evoke immunity and those that do not.

If the immunization or equivalent control measure is applied uniformly to all groups, the critical level of coverage, p_c, has the familiar form:

$$p_c = 1 - (1/R_0), \qquad (11.12)$$

with R_0 defined by eqn (11.8).

It is evident, however, that greater gains are to be realized (for a specified level of overall coverage) by targeting control measures to individuals in the more active groups. Commonsense makes this result plain, but it can be buttressed by formal evaluation of the optimal eradication strategy, which was defined earlier as that which eliminates infection with the minimum level of overall coverage, p_{opt}. In these terms, the problem is to choose a set of group-specific coverage levels, $p(i)$, such as to *minimize* the overall coverage,

$$p = \sum_i p(i) P(i), \qquad (11.13)$$

subject to the *constraint* set by eqn (11.11):

$$R_0 \sum_i i^2 [1 - p(i)] P(i) \left(\sum_i i^2 P(i) \right)^{-1} = 1. \tag{11.14}$$

Here $P(i)$ is the proportion of the population in the ith group, and eqn (11.8) has been used to rewrite eqn (11.11) in terms of R_0. As $p(i)$ enters in a simple linear way into both the quantity to be minimized and into the constraint, the solution to this optimization problem is a 'bang-bang' strategy: the optimal coverage is attained by immunizing or otherwise treating 100 per cent of individuals in the groups above a certain level of sexual activity, i_c, and not treating anyone in groups below that level; the critical level i_c is chosen such that the constraint (11.14) is satisfied,

$$R_0 \sum_{i=0}^{i_c} i^2 P(i) = \sum_{\text{all } i} i^2 P(i). \tag{11.15}$$

Obviously such a 'bang-bang' extreme is not feasible in practice, but the formal result helps to illuminate the essentials.

We conclude this discussion by returning to the artificially simple example of a population in which 10 per cent of the sexually active individuals have on average 20 sexual partners per unit time, and 90 per cent have on average 2. We further assume $R_0 = 5$ for a hypothetical STD in this obligingly simple population. By regarding this population as homogeneously mixed—which it clearly is not—we could estimate the coverage needed for eradication by $p_c = 1 - x^*$ (under homogeneous mixing, it makes no sense to think of other than uniform coverage). But, for an infection like gonorrhoea where there is no immune class, x^* can be calculated from eqns (11.5) and (11.6) to be

$$x^* = \sum_i P(i)(\mu + v)/(\mu + v + i\lambda). \tag{11.16}$$

In turn, λ can be calculated from eqn (11.7). Thus, for the numerical example given above, we find $x^* = 0.605$, which leads to the very rough estimate $p_c = 40$ per cent. The true level of coverage under a uniformly applied scheme, however, follows immediately from eqn (11.12) and is $p_c = 80$ per cent. In contrast, the optimal strategy, as defined in detail above, requires that we protect 87.2 per cent of the people in the very active 10 per cent of the population, and no one else, for an overall average level of coverage of only 8.7 per cent. This artificially extreme example illustrates the general theme we have already alluded to: in heterogeneous situations, the critical level of coverage required for eradication under a uniformly applied programme is higher than estimated by assuming the population is homogeneously mixed and determining x^* from serological or other data ($p_c \sim \hat{p}_c = 1 - x^*$); but a targeted programme can lead to eradication at coverage levels lower than estimated from $1 - x^*$.

11.3 Epidemic aspects of sexually transmitted diseases: acquired immunodeficiency syndrome

Many of the same points about the importance of heterogeneity in sexual habits, and its effects on estimates of epidemiological parameters such as R_0, also arise in considerations of epidemics of STDs. In this section, we give an account of some of these issues, particularly as they may apply to understanding the current epidemics of AIDS in developed and in developing countries. More generally, this section shows how mathematical models can be used to clarify thinking about the kinds of information needed to anticipate the future course of an epidemic.

11.3.1 *Biological background*

Between October 1980 and May 1981, five young homosexual men were treated for *Pneumocystis carinii* pneumonia in hospitals in Los Angeles. The cases attracted attention because *P. carinii* pneumonia was known to be a disease associated with immunodepression (CDC 1981*c*). Around the same time Kaposi's sarcoma was being diagnosed with increasing frequency in young men in New York City and in California (Peterman *et al.* 1985; CDC 1981*d*). These observations heralded the early stages of the emergence in the USA of an apparently new disease, subsequently termed Acquired Immune Deficiency Syndrome or AIDS (CDC 1982).

By the autumn of 1981 the United States Public Health Service had begun its efforts to try to define and understand this new disease. Three major lines of inquiry were initiated. The first was directed at the epidemiological characterization of the disease, the second at definition of the aetiology and pathogenesis, and the third at development of a treatment. By early 1982 the epidemiological evidence clearly pointed to a sexual route for transmission, especially through semen. In 1982, however, cases of AIDS began to be reported in people suffering from haemophilia, persons receiving blood transfusions, intravenous drug abusers, and children born to mothers who were at a high risk of AIDS. These observations clearly implicated blood as a route of transmission and confirmed the suspicion that an infectious agent was involved.

The hunt for a transmissible agent rapidly narrowed down to a search for a virus. In 1983 the isolation and cultivation of a retrovirus was announced by a research team at the Pasteur Institute in France (Barre-Sinoussi *et al.* 1983). This virus was named the lymphadenopathy-associated virus (LAV). Shortly after this announcement, a group of scientists at the National Institutes of Health in the USA identified a virus in patients with AIDS which they named the human T-cell lymphotrophic virus type III (HTLV-III) (Gallo *et al.* 1984). The French and American viral isolates proved to be of the same strain and an International Committee for the Taxonomy of Viruses named the human immunodeficiency virus (HIV) the aetiological agent of AIDS. Since the

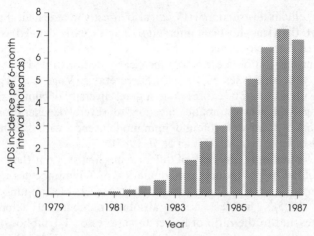

Fig. 11.1. The incidence of reported cases of AIDS in the United States, per six-month period. Note that the apparent decline in incidence, from the end of 1986 to the beginning of 1987, is an artefact created by the delay between diagnosis of AIDS and reporting to the Centers of Disease Control.

identification of the disease AIDS in 1981 and the discovery of the aetiological agent HIV in 1984, major epidemics of the infection and the disease have emerged in most developed and many developing countries. In the United States, for example, since the beginning of the epidemic approximately 39 000 cases of AIDS had been reported to the Centers of Disease Control by the end of June 1987 (Fig. 11.1).

HIV is a retrovirus with morphological, molecular, and biological character-istics that have led to its proposed classification with the pathogenic animal lentiviruses. Recent work has demonstrated that other primate species, notably the African green monkey, may be symptomless carriers of a related retrovirus that can also infect humans, apparently without causing disease (Kanki *et al.* 1985). Further investigation of such viruses in primates may provide clues to the possible origins of HIV in human communities.

HIV is a single-stranded RNA virus which selectively infects and is cytotoxic for the sub-population of T-lymphocytes with helper/inducer phenotype. After attaching to the T4 receptor molecule on the cell surface, HIV penetrates the cell membrane and initiates the process of replication by means of an enzyme, reverse transcriptase. This RNA-dependent DNA polymerase permits transcrip-tion of viral RNA into DNA. Double-stranded proviral DNA sequences are incorporated into the host genome and the normal replication cycle of the host cell produces viral subunits which are subsequently assembled into mature retroviral particles that bud and are extruded from the cell surface. The viral genetic material remains latent in some infected T-cells, while in those that are immunologically active, viral replication dominates host cell activity, leading ultimately to cellular destruction. HIV can also directly invade neural microglial cells, although the virus–host cell interaction is not clearly defined as yet. HIV can be isolated from blood, semen, saliva, tears, urine, and cervical secretions. However, transmission of infection can be clearly demonstrated to occur only after contact with blood, semen, or cervical secretions (Vogt *et al.* 1986).

Infection with HIV can be expressed in a great diversity of clinical manifestations, ranging from asymptomatic infection to severe degenerations of the central nervous system or profound immunodeficiency with life-threatening secondary diseases or cancers (Fauci *et al.* 1985).

HIV causes disease by a variety of different mechanisms but the cumulative destruction of the helper/inducer subpopulation of T-lymphocytes leads in its severest form to a progressive and ultimately irreversible immunodeficiency (Montagnier 1985). The decrease in absolute numbers of helper/inducer T-lymphocytes and in the ratio of helper to suppressor T-lymphocytes results in depressed cell-mediated immunity. This manifests itself by the failure to respond to antigenic and mitogenic stimulation *in vitro*, partial or complete absence of delayed hypersensitivity to skin-test antigens, decreased lymphokine production, depressed helper function, decreased lymphocyte cytotoxicity, and diminished response to interleukin-2 (Bowen *et al.* 1985). These immunological abnormalities interact to predispose the most severely affected patients to repeated opportunistic infectious and neoplasms, which are characterized as the acquired immunodeficiency syndrome, AIDS. A list of the diseases considered by the United States Centers for Disease Control (CDC) to be at least moderately predictive of underlying immunodeficiency associated with AIDS is presented in Table 11.1.

Since the discovery of HIV in 1983, the progress of research at the molecular and the cellular levels of study has been very rapid indeed. A good illustration of the pace of discovery is provided by a paper by Hahn *et al.* (1986) that describes genetic variation in HIV via genomic analysis, molecular cloning, and nucleotide sequencing. These authors compared the nucleotide sequences, and deduced amino acid sequences of the gene encoding the extracellular envelope glycoprotein of the virus (the gene is called *env*) in four to six isolates obtained from each of three patients over a one-year to two-year period. The study highlights the hypervariability of *env* relative to the remainder of the viral genome and pinpoints localized regions of hypervariability within the gene. Genetic changes among different viruses result largely from duplications, insertions, or deletions of short stretches of nucleotides, as well as from an accumulation of nucleotide point mutations. The detail of this research is impressive when viewed in the context of the short time period that had elapsed since the virus was first isolated in 1983.

In sharp contrast to our current understanding of the genetic structure and function of the virus, and of the pathology induced by infection, is the present state of knowledge concerning the epidemiology and the transmission dynamics of HIV (May and Anderson 1987). Public health planning continues to be

Table 11.1 Diseases considered by CDC to be at least moderately predictive of underlying cellular immunodeficiency associated with AIDS

Protozoan and helminth infections	Intestinal cryptosporidiosis causing chronic diarrhoea. *Pneumocystis carinii* pneumonia. Strongyloidosis (of the lung, central nervous system, or disseminated beyond the gastrointestinal tract). Toxoplasmosis (of internal organs besides the liver, spleen, or lymph nodes). Isosporiasis causing chronic diarrhoea
Fungal infections	*Candida* oesophagitis. Bronchial or pulmonary candidasis. Cryptococcus (of central nervous system or disseminated in the lungs and lymph nodes). Histoplasmosis (disseminated)
Bacterial infections	*Mycobacterium avium* complex or *M. kansasii* (disseminated beyond lungs, lymph nodes)
Viral infections	Cytomegalovirus (of internal organs besides liver, spleen, or lymph nodes). Herpes simplex virus (chronic mucocutaneous, pulmonary, gastrointestinal tract, disseminated). Progressive multifocal leukoencephalopathy (presumed due to papovirus)
Cancers	Kaposi's sarcoma. Central nervous system lymphoma. Non-Hodgkin lymphoma (plus positive HIV test)

hampered by uncertainties about key epidemiological parameters such as the typical duration and intensity of infectiousness, and the fraction of those infected who will go on to develop AIDS and after how long a time period. In the absence of such information, mathematical models of the transmission dynamics of HIV cannot be used at present to make accurate predictions of future trends in the incidence of AIDS. However, they can facilitate the indirect assessment of certain epidemiological parameters, clarify what data are required to predict future trends, make predictions under specified assumptions about the course of infection in individuals and patterns of sexual activity within defined populations (or changes therein), and, more generally, provide a template to guide the interpretation of observed trends (Anderson *et al.* 1986, 1987*b*; May and Anderson 1987; Medley *et al.* 1987).

Before turning to the description and analysis of simple models of transmission we first present a summary of what is, and is not, known about the basic epidemiological characteristics of HIV infection and the disease AIDS.

11.3.2 *Epidemiological characteristics*

11.3.2.1 *Risk groups*   In the United States, where to date the largest number of cases of AIDS have been reported (see Fig. 11.1), 95 per cent of all AIDS patients can be placed into groups that suggest a possible means of acquisition of infection. As of January 1986 in the United States, 74 per cent of all patients are homosexual or bisexual men (8 per cent are both homosexual and have a history of intravenous drug use), 17 per cent are heterosexual intravenous (IV) drug abusers, 1 per cent are haemophiliacs, 1 per cent are heterosexual partners of persons with AIDS or persons at risk of AIDS, and 2 per cent are recipients of infected blood or blood components. Of the 5 per cent for whom recognized risk factors for AIDS cannot be identified, a majority were born outside the US. As illustrated in Fig. 11.2, despite the steady rise in the incidence of AIDS in the mid-1980s, the relative proportion of AIDS cases in the different risk groups has remained fairly stable. Similar patterns have emerged in most European countries (Fig. 11.3(b)).

11.3.2.2 *Distribution by age and sex*   The majority of cases reported so far in developed countries are male homosexual/bisexual patients in the age range 20–49 years (90 per cent of adult patients in the US) (Fig. 11.3(d)). In the

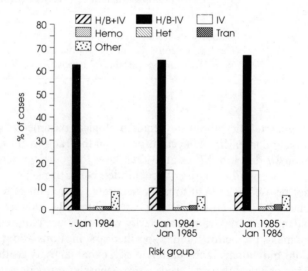

Fig. 11.2. The percentage of the total number of cases of AIDS reported over the interval 1984–5 in the United States in each risk group. H/B + IV denotes male homosexuals and bisexuals who are IV drug abusers; H/B − IV denotes male homosexuals and bisexuals who are not IV drug abusers; IV denotes intravenous drug abusers who are not homosexual or bisexual; Hemo denotes haemophiliacs; Het denotes heterosexuals; Tran denotes transfusion recipients; Other denotes other unidentified risks.

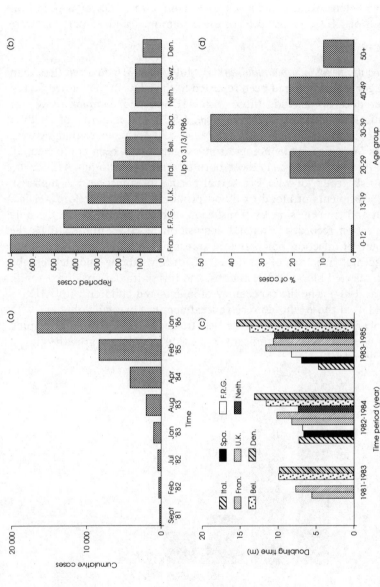

Fig. 11.3. (a) Cumulative number of AIDS cases reported to the Centers of Disease Control in the United States up to the end of January 1986. (b) Reported cases of AIDS up to the end of March 1986 in various European countries (Fran, France; FRG, Federal Republic of Germany; UK, United Kingdom; Ital, Italy; Bel, Belgium; Spa, Spain; Neth, The Netherlands; Swz, Switzerland; Den, Denmark). (c) Doubling times, t_d, in months, estimated from case reports of AIDS in various European countries (see legend to graph (b) for abbreviations) over three time intervals; 1981–3, 1982–4, and 1983–5. (d) Percentage of reported cases of AIDS in the United States as of January 1986 in different age classes of the population.

United Kingdom, for example, of the 616 cases reported by the end of 1986, 598 were male patients and 18 were female patients. In the United States, as of 10 March 1986, of the 242 patients with AIDS reported from the risk group designated as heterosexual contact with a person with AIDS or a person at increased risk of AIDS, 17 per cent of these were men and 83 per cent were women.

11.3.2.3 *Infection in infants and children*　By July 1986, 316 children (less than 13 years of age) with AIDS had been reported to the CDC in the United States. This number does not include those with AIDS-related complex (ARC) or asymptomatic HIV infection (Connor *et al.* 1987). The majority of children with AIDS are less than 2 years old, and 79 per cent are younger than 5 years. Among cases for which epidemiological investigation has been completed, all children fall into two groups: (1) those born to a mother who has AIDS, who is in a high-risk group, or who is a sexual partner of someone in a high-risk group; or (2) recipients of blood or blood products. So far, therefore, vertical transmission and transmission by transfusion of blood products are the only routes of infection recorded. Prenatal acquisition of HIV appears to be the principal route of infection but perinatal transmission may occur (i) *in utero* via transplacental infection of the fetus, (ii) during labour and delivery by contact with infected blood and secretions, and (iii) postnatally via breast milk (Connor *et al.* 1987). The life expectancy of infants and children with AIDS is short (Fig. 11.4) in those who do receive treatment (e.g. with γ-globulins), with an average of around 10–11 months. Vertical transmission of HIV in developing countries is likely to have a significant impact on population growth rates in the coming decades.

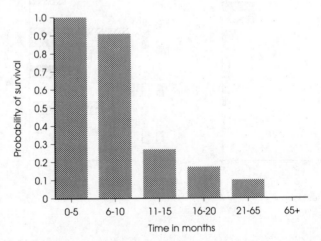

Fig. 11.4. AIDS in infants: the figure shows the probability of surviving to a given age following infection at or before birth (data from Connor *et al.* 1987).

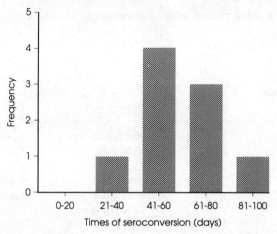

Fig. 11.5. Frequency distribution of observed time intervals between infection with HIV and the point of seroconversion. The distribution is based on studies of nine patients (data from Cooper *et al.* 1985, Ho *et al.* 1985, and Wall *et al.* 1987).

11.3.2.4 *Seroconversion*   The detection of antibodies specific to HIV antigens, which are expressed as a result of viral infection, is of central importance in the epidemiology of HIV and AIDS. A variety of accurate serodiagnostic tests for HIV antibodies are now available and they have been used extensively to screen blood and blood product donations and samples from people belonging to various groups at high risk of infection.

Current knowledge of retroviral infections suggests that once a host is infected the virus persists for the life of that host (Weiss 1982). HIV, for example, has a complex life cycle that includes a chromosomally integrated proviral DNA stage that has the potential for indefinite persistence. As such the presence of antibodies specific to HIV antigens indicates the presence of virus in the body of the host.

Data recording the time interval between infection and the point at which antibodies to HIV antigens can be detected are limited at present. The most detailed studies concern patients infected via transfusion or via parental exposure. On average the interval between infection and seroconversion is around six to ten weeks, with an average of approximately 65 days (Fig. 11.5). However, different HIV-specific antibodies are expressed as a result of viral infection and some appear earlier than others. Published studies suggest that after seroconversion the antibody titre continues to rise for at least seven to nine months after initial antibody detection (Esteban *et al.* 1985).

11.3.2.5 *Primary HIV infection and ARC/PGL*   In order to understand the complex relationship between HIV infection and the manifestation of symptoms of disease it is important to distinguish clearly between primary or initial

Table 11.2 Incubation period of the disease syndrome associated with primary HIV infection

Incubation period from the time of presumed exposure (days)	Sample size	Comment	Reference
6	1	Homosexual male	Cooper *et al.* (1985)
13	1	Needle stick transmission	Gaines *et al.* (1987)
11–28	8	Homosexual males	Gaines *et al.* (1987)
21	1	Heterosexual IV drug using male	Ho *et al.* (1985)
42	1	Homosexual male	Ho *et al.* (1985)

infection and later symptoms of the disease as a patient moves towards the state classified as AIDS. Primary or initial infection with HIV may be asymptomatic in some patients or, more typically, may manifest itself as a self-limited febrile illness. A mononucleosis-like syndrome occurs in primary HIV, characterized by fever, arthralgias, myalgias, diarrhoea, and/or maculo-papular rash. The incubation period of the disease syndrome arising from primary HIV infection is variable among patients, being in the range of 2–6 weeks (i.e. shorter than the seroconversion period) (Table 11.2). The duration of symptoms of primary HIV infection is also variable, with a range of between 5–24 days and a mean of around 8 days (Cooper *et al.* 1985). Virus may be isolated from blood during primary HIV infection.

Following this initial phase, there may follow a short or long period of asymptomatic HIV infection where the cells and body fluids harbour the virus. Patients with asymptomatic HIV infection may be found to have some of the abnormalities characteristic of overt disease, including depressed T-helper cell of number and function, and raised immunoglobulin levels.

Patients may convert from asymptomatic infection to a state categorized as persistent generalized lymphadenopathy (PGL). This state is a common sign of HIV infection and—although observed in all groups at risk of the infection—it has been most extensively studied in homosexual men (Mildvan and Soloman 1987). PGL is defined as palpable lymphadenopathy at two or more extra-inguinal sites for more than three months in the absence of an identifiable cause other than HIV infection. The observation that PGL can persist in some patients for many years without progression of illness may suggest that PGL denotes a host immune response that is effective in suppressing viral abundance and replication. However, many patients with PGL progress to develop AIDS after a variable time period. The syndrome of chronic unexplained lymphadenopathy and persistent depletion of T-helper cells is often termed

Sequence of states

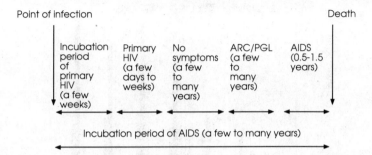

Fig. 11.6. Schematic diagram of the sequence of disease and incubation states for primary HIV infection and AIDS.

AIDS-related complex or ARC for short. This syndrome is equivalent to PGL. A schematic representation of these various states of disease during the course of HIV infection from the acquisition of the virus to the development of AIDS is presented in Fig. 11.6.

11.3.2.6 *The incubation period of AIDS* A crucial aspect of the relationship between the incidence of HIV infection and the incidence of AIDS is the probability distribution of the incubation period of the disease, with this period defined as the time interval from infection to diagnosis. Data from individual patients recording the time of infection and disease diagnosis are limited at present. However, there is one set of data from the United States in which a good approximation to the time of infection has been found retrospectively in AIDS patients who received a single transfusion or short course of transfusions of infected blood or blood products (Curran *et al.* 1984; Peterman *et al.* 1985; Lui *et al.* 1986; Medley *et al.* 1987). These data are summarized in Fig. 11.7.

Many problems surround the interpretation of these data. The number of patients infected by this route who have not yet developed AIDS is unknown, so that the data give no information whatever about the proportion of infected individuals who will ultimately develop AIDS. Moreover, individuals transfused later have been at risk of developing AIDS for a much shorter length of time so that the frequency distribution of incubation periods as directly observed is misleading (Fig. 11.7).

A paper by Medley *et al.* (1987) describes a statistical analysis of the data on AIDS cases in transfusion recipients in the United States up to the end of 1986 (the total size of this sample of patients, whose dates of transfusion and diagnosis of disease are substantiated, is 297). The analysis involves the postulation of simple mathematical forms (e.g. exponential) for the growth in the number of infected individuals who will ultimately develop AIDS, and for the distribution (Weibüll or gamma) of incubation period of those individuals.

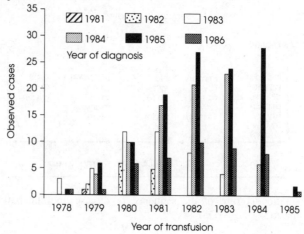

Fig. 11.7. Data on the distribution of the incubation period of AIDS derived from studies of transfusion recipients in the United States (data from Dr T. Peterman, Centers for Disease Control, USA). Observed cases of AIDS are recorded as a function of the year of transfusion (the assumed point of acquisition of infection) and the year of diagnosis.

In certain of the models a time-dependent probability of diagnosis was included, of probit form. Explicit expression for the log-likelihood of the data, based on different models, were obtained and sensitiveness to assumptions tested by the comparison of the maximized log-likelihoods achieved via different models (Medley *et al.* 1987).

The data are such that there is relatively direct information on the distribution of incubation times up to 4–5 years, but beyond that one is extrapolating on the basis of the assumed mathematical form of the distribution. As noted by Medley *et al.* (1987), this implies that the mean, which depends critically on the upper tail of the distribution, is not a good indication of the information in the data. The principal conclusions of the Medley *et al.* (1987) analyses are that the incubation period is long and variable, depends on patient age and sex, and its distribution is equally well described by the Weibüll and gamma distributions. Divisions of the data by sex showed the incubation times for females to be longer than for males. Notional means (and medians) for the females and males are 8.8 years (8.4 years) and 5.6 years (5.5 years), respectively, on the basis of a model that assumes exponential growth in incidence of infected transfusions and a Weibüll distribution for the incubation period. Interestingly, the Weibüll distribution is widely used in survival studies; it is equivalent to supposing that the risk of converting to AIDS increases as the time from HIV infection increases (Cox and Oates 1984; Anderson *et al.* 1986).

The same model suggested that the mean (median) incubation time for children (0–4 years at transfusion) is much shorter, being 2.0 years (1.9 years), than for older patients. The incubation period for patients older than 59 years is less than that for the 5–59 years age groups with means (and medians) of 5.5 (5.4) and 8.2 (8.0) years, respectively. The differences between the mean incubation periods of young children, older children and adults, and elderly patients, along with the differences between females and males, are in accord with age- and sex-related differences in immunocompetence.

Medley *et al.* (1987), note that, in the interpretation of these results, a number of caveats must be borne in mind. First, the distribution of incubation times in patients infected by blood transfusions is not necessarily the same as that in patients infected via other routes, such as sexual intercourse. Second, as more data become available it is important continually to up-date these estimates. Third, it appears likely that as more data are collected, the estimate of the average incubation period is likely to rise further. Before the study of Medley *et al.* (1987), widely quoted figures from early data were in the range of 4–5 years as an average (Lui *et al.* 1986). Finally, it is unknown how these results from an industrialized nation pertain to the developing world, where individuals are typically exposed more frequently and to a larger range of infectious agents. However, with the advent of mandatory screening of blood donations for HIV infection in the USA and Europe, the USA transfusion-related AIDS cases are likely to remain a prime source of information on the incubation period for some time (Table 11.3).

11.3.2.7 *Infectious and latent periods* In studying the transmission dynamics of HIV infection it is important to ascertain the relationship between the incubation period of the disease AIDS, and the duration and intensity of infectiousness over the incubation period. There are many different approaches to the study of this problem, but few have been undertaken at present. One approach is to study susceptible sexual partners of HIV infected patients (in both homosexual or heterosexual relationships), or susceptible persons who share needles with infected IV drug users, in a longitudinal manner so as to ascertain if and when seroconversion of the susceptible partner occurs. Ideally such studies should also record, in a quantitative manner, changes in viral abundance in the infected patient through time. Unfortunately, however, in such a study design it is essential to know precisely when each partner seroconverted and, in addition, to acquire information on the frequency and type of sexual activity between partners or the frequency of needle sharing among drug abusers. To date little information of this kind has been collected.

An alternative, but less rigorous, approach is to assume that the infectiousness of an infected person is in direct proportion to a quantitative score of viral abundance in blood sera, secretions (e.g. semen), or excretions (e.g. urine or saliva). If this assumption is reasonable, then longitudinal changes in viral abundance in individual patients will reflect longitudinal changes in infectiousness over the long incubation period. Data recording such changes in viraemia are limited, and again subject to the restriction that for each patient studied the approximate data of infection or seroconversion should ideally be known.

Table 11.3 The incubation period of AIDS. Observed and expected numbers of patients with AIDS by year of transfusion and diagnosis. The observed numbers are from studies of transfusion recipients of infected blood in the USA and the expected numbers are generated by a model of the incubation period of the disease that assumes a Weibüll distribution for the period and an exponential rise in the incidence of infected transfusions over time (see Medley *et al.* 1987). (The years 1978 and 1986 extend from April to December, and January to June respectively.)

Year of diagnosis		Year of transfusion								
		1978	1979	1980	1981	1982	1983	1984	1985	1986
1978	Expected	0.01								
	Observed	0								
1979		0.19	0.07							
		0	0							
1980		0.56	0.66	0.14						
		0	0	0						
1981		0.97	1.69	1.34	0.28					
		0	0	0	0					
1982		1.34	2.81	3.43	2.71	0.57				
		0	2	2	5	1				
1983		1.58	3.77	5.70	6.97	5.50	1.15			
		1	2	10	7	7	3			
1984		1.67	4.38	7.64	11.56	14.13	11.15	2.33		
		0	5	7	15	18	20	2		
1985		1.58	4.54	8.88	15.49	23.44	28.66	22.61	4.73	
		1	5	8	16	25	23	26	5	
1986		0.72	2.19	4.62	8.80	14.86	21.49	24.24	15.04	0.83
		0	3	3	16	13	23	14	7	1

An analysis of the available data on longitudinal changes in viraemia (recorded as HIV antigen concentration in nanograms per millilitre of blood sera) in HIV infected patients reveals some interesting patterns. Broadly, antigen concentrations appear to be very low, if at all detectable, in the first few days to weeks following infection, to rise to high levels following primary HIV infection (hence after seroconversion) and remain high for a number of months, to fall to low levels during the asymptomatic (see Fig. 11.7) phase of infection, and then to begin to rise in patients with ARC/PGL again attaining high levels in AIDS patients. Two illustrative examples are presented in Figs. 11.8 and 11.9. Figure 11.8 records antigen concentration in blood sera drawn from samples of infected patients (homosexual males) at various time points after seroconversion. This figure illustrates changes in the early stages of infection. Figure 11.9 records changes in antigen concentration in a single patient

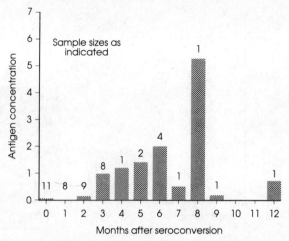

Fig. 11.8. HIV antigen concentration (ng/ml) in the serum of infected patients as a function of the time (or presumed time) since seroconversion (detectable levels of antibodies specific to HIV antigens). The numbers above the bars denote sample sizes (data from Goudsmit *et al.* 1986).

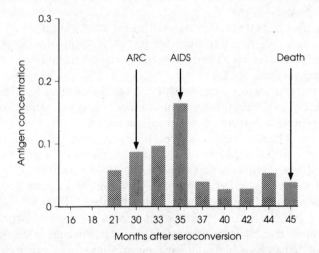

Fig. 11.9. HIV antigen concentration (ng/ml) in the serum of an infected male homosexual patient as a function of months after seroconversion (data from Lange *et al.* 1986).

(homosexual male) as he progressed from the asymptomatic stage, to ARC, and finally to AIDS and subsequent death (Goudsmit *et al.* 1986; Lange *et al.* 1986). A further illustration of antigen concentrations in samples of children and adults either with AIDS or infected but asymptomatic is presented in Fig. 11.10 (Goudsmit *et al.* 1986; Anderson and May 1988*a*).

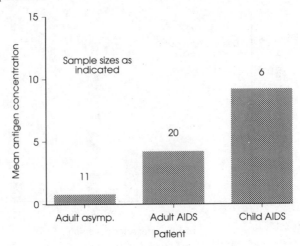

Fig. 11.10. HIV antigen concentrations (means in ng/ml) in adults (asymptomatic and AIDS patients) and children (with AIDS) (data from Goldsmit *et al.* 1986). The numbers above the bars denote sample sizes.

A tentative hypothesis deriving from such studies, keeping in mind the limited nature of the data, is that there are two phases of peak infectivity during the long incubation period of AIDS, one lasting for a few months to a year or more following initial infection, and the other just prior to the onset of AIDS. In the intervening period between these peaks in viraemia, infectiousness of the patient may well be very low (or zero).

One problem in the interpretation of average trends in antigen concentration (and hence assumed infectiousness) in samples of infected patients derives from the highly variable nature of the incubation periods of both primary HIV infection and AIDS. Consider a hypothetical example in which five infected patients are monitored at six-monthly intervals, over a 10-year period, for HIV antigen concentration in serum samples. Suppose patients 1, 3, 4, and 5 are diagnosed as having AIDS at years 7, 3, 9, and 5 respectively (an average incubation period of 6 years) while patient number 2, although infected, does not develop AIDS over the 10-year study period. An invented series of antigen concentrations at each six-month interval for each patient is displayed in Fig. 11.11. Note that all have high antigen concentrations in the primary HIV phase, while the interval between this peak and a further peak in antigenicity is determined by the different rates at which they convert to AIDS. The patient (number 2) who does not develop AIDS has no second peak in antigen concentration. If we average the concentration at each six-month time point over the five patients in the study a pattern emerges of fluctuating but persistent abundance of antigens, over the 10-year period. In short, taking averages in this hypothetical study would reveal a relatively constant pattern of antigen abundance (hence assumed infectiousness) over a period of 10 years. The true

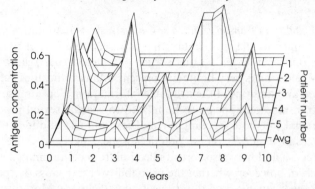

Fig. 11.11. A hypothetical illustration of bimodality in antigen concentration in five patients during the incubation period of AIDS. See text for further details. The patients are numbered 1 to 5, and the average antigen concentration (ng/ml) is displayed for each time point (labelled AVG). The incubation periods of AIDS in patients numbered 1, 3, 4, and 5 were set at 7, 3, 9, and 5 years, respectively. Over the 10-year observation period AIDS was assumed not to develop in patient number 2.

picture that emerges over the coming years will undoubtedly be more complex than this simple illustrative example (Anderson and May 1988a). However, as a first approximation, it may not be too unreasonable to assume for population-based studies of transmission that, on average, there is a roughly constant level of infectiousness over the entire duration of the average incubation period of AIDS.

A second problem that emerges in studies of infected patients concerns those who have not as yet developed AIDS, despite a long duration of infection. It may be that such individuals are only infectious to others during the phase of primary HIV infection. This is obviously an optimistic view and, until knowledge improves, it is certainly safer to assume—in the treatment of patients and the development of public health measures along with educational campaigns—that all infected persons are infectious.

A final point about infectiousness relates to the latent period of infection. In earlier chapters that considered the transmission of common childhood infections such as measles, it was observed that the latent period (defined as the interval between the point of infection and the beginning of the state of infectiousness) had an important influence on the dynamics of transmission. This was particularly so if the length of this period was similar in magnitude, or greater than, the length of the infectious period. It will be clear from the earlier contents of this section that, in the case of primary HIV infection, the latent period is probably of short duration in comparison with the length of the period during which antigen concentration in blood serum is at measurable levels. The duration of the latent period is probably (although data are limited at present) in the region of a few days to a few weeks. As such, the latent period is of limited significance to the dynamics of HIV transmission.

11.3.2.8 *Probability of transmission via sexual activity*   Quantitative information on average values of the probability that a susceptible sexual partner of an infected person, whether in a homosexual or heterosexual relationship, will acquire HIV infection is very limited at present. Many difficulties surround the interpretation and analysis of the available information. For homosexual males the risk of transmission appears to be related to specific sexual practices such as receptive anal intercourse, manual-rectal sex, and use of dildos (Goedert *et al.* 1984; Moss *et al.* 1987). These practices appear likely to cause trauma to the rectal mucosa and may also spread infection from contaminated equipment. It is still unclear, however, whether the probability of transmission (per partner) is related to the frequency and duration of sexual activity. Moreover, attempts to dissect out 'low-risk' and 'high-risk' activities have proved difficult, owing to the need for very precise quantitative information on type, frequency, and duration of sexual activity. In addition, as was discussed in the previous section, the infectivity of a seropositive appears to vary as a function of the time interval since the acquisition of infection. Current estimates of the transmission probability (per partnership) vary widely, from 0.05 to 0.5 per partner (May and Anderson 1987).

In the case of intravenous drug users the likelihood of transmission appears to correlate with the number of injections involving sharing of unsterilized needles (Mortimer *et al.* 1985).

Although heterosexual transmission at present in developed countries appears to be important in only a small proportion of the reported cases (see Fig. 11.2), it is beyond doubt that heterosexual activity can result in transmission. Anal intercourse may facilitate the entrance of the virus, but vaginal intercourse alone appears to account for most heterosexual transmission, whether from male to female or vice versa (Harris *et al.* 1983; van de Pierre *et al.* 1985; Redfield *et al.* 1985; Stewart *et al.* 1985). Studies of the heterosexual partners of AIDS patients have provided firm evidence of transmission. For example, in a study reported by Fischl *et al.* (1987), of 45 spouses of AIDS patients, 13 had antibodies to HIV on enrolment in the study (9 males and 4 females). During the course of the study 3 males and 10 females seroconverted. Absence of the use of barrier contraceptives, and oral sex, were both associated with sero-conversion. In those seropositive there was, however, no significant correlation between infection and the duration of the sexual association with their diseased partners. A detailed study, by Peterman *et al.* (1988), of the risk of HIV transmission within monogamous heterosexual relationships in which one partner was infected via transfusions revealed that 2 of 25 husbands and 10 of 55 wives who had had sexual contact with infected spouses were seropositive for HIV. Surprisingly, compared with seronegative wives, the seropositive wives were older (median ages 54 and 62 respectively) and reported somewhat fewer sexual contacts with the infected husbands. Peterman *et al.* (1988) found no difference in types of sexual contact or methods of contraception between those

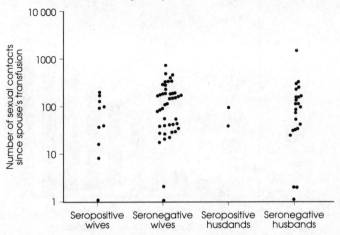

Fig. 11.12. For each of 80 individuals, this figure shows the number of sexual contacts with a spouse, after the spouse was (unknowingly) infected with HIV by blood transfusion. The 25 husbands and 55 wives of infected individuals are divided according to current serological status. The figure shows that, in this study group, transmission probability is uncorrelated with number of sexual contacts (after Peterman *et al.* 1988).

spouses who did, and did not, acquire infection. Many husbands and wives in this study remained uninfected, despite repeated sexual contact without protection, while others acquired infection after only a few contacts. These results are summarized in Fig. 11.12.

The work of Fischl *et al.* (1988) and Peterman *et al.* (1987) clearly illustrate the problems in understanding what determines the risk of transmission in a heterosexual partnership. In part, the problems are associated with the paucity of carefully designed longitudinal studies of the partners of infected persons. Equally important, however, is the problem addressed in the previous section, namely great variability in infectiousness both between infected individuals and through time in an individual. Much remains to be explained concerning differences in susceptibility and infectivity among people (May 1988).

11.3.2.9 *Proportion of infected persons who will develop AIDS* The proportion of infected individuals who will eventually develop AIDS is unclear at present. Early studies of seropositive homosexual men in Denmark and New York City suggested that of the order of 9–14 per cent developed the disease over a two-year period (Melbye *et al.* 1984; Goedert *et al.* 1984). More recent studies in homosexual men from Manhattan indicate a figure in the region of 35 per cent (see Fig. 11.13) over a three-year study period (Goedert *et al.* 1986). Studies by Hunter and De Gruttola (1986) employing statistical models of time-dependent survival rates of infected homosexual men from San Francisco indicate figures of 8 per cent after one year, 24 per cent after two years, and

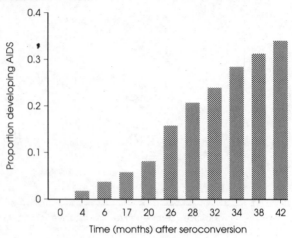

Fig. 11.13. Actuarial incidence of AIDS in a cohort of homosexual/bisexual men in Manhattan, New York (data from Goedert *et al.* 1986).

43 per cent after three years. Given the long incubation period of the disease, as discussed in a previous section, the eventual percentage derived from decade-long studies of seropositives is likely to be much higher than current estimates. The progressive sequence of steps which eventually impair the ability of the immune system to respond to opportunistic infection seem not to be reversible. But whether all those infected with HIV are moving towards AIDS at different rates, or whether some will develop AIDS while others never will, remains uncertain. Variability in the incubation period, and whether or not an infected person develops AIDS, could be accounted for by genetic heterogeneity within the host population (perhaps HLA-linked, see Scorza Smeradli *et al.* (1986)), or could be associated with infection by specific strains of the antigenically variable HIV (Hahn *et al.* 1986), or could arise from other causes (such as presence or absence of other infections).

11.3.2.10 *Life expectancy of AIDS patients*   Once AIDS is diagnosed, the life expectancy of patients is relatively short, although it depends on factors such as age, risk group, and the nature of the opportunistic infection or cancer that triggered the diagnosis of the disease. The average survival period is commonly quoted as being between 9 months to 1.5 years (Peterman *et al.* 1985). In the United Kingdom, data collected up to the end of 1986 reveal a short life expectancy of around 1 year (see Fig. 11.14). Patients in the UK with Kaposi's sarcoma have a better prognosis than patients with opportunistic infection (Marasca and McEvoy 1986). The median survival from diagnosis was 21 months for 44 cases presented with Kaposi's sarcoma, and 12 months for 124 cases with other diseases.

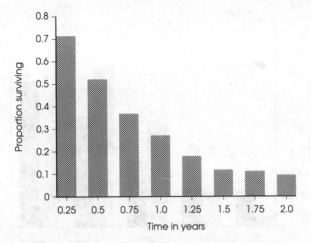

Fig. 11.14. Time-dependent survival of AIDS patients (from the date of diagnosis of AIDS) in the United Kingdom. The data are from diagnosed cases up to the end of 1986.

11.3.2.11 *Sexual activity* In both homosexual and heterosexuals one of the principal factors that determines the likelihood of acquiring HIV infection is the rate at which sexual partners are changed (defined per unit of time). A clear illustration of this point is provided by a study of Winkelstein *et al.* (1987) of the relationship between sexual activity (number of different male partners over a two-year period), and the percentage of each sexual activity group who were seropositive for HIV antibodies (Fig. 11.15).

Data on rates of sexual partner change are limited at present, particularly for heterosexual communities. Two studies of sexual activity amongst homosexual males in London, and one study of a similar risk group in San Francisco, provide some information on the frequency distribution of the number of different sexual partners per unit of time (McKusick *et al.* 1985*a*; McManus and McEvoy 1987; C. Carne and I. Weller, personal communication). These data are presented in Fig. 11.16 (graphs a, b, and c). Striking features of these studies of male homosexuals are the high means of the frequency distributions and the very large variances (variance ≫ mean). For example, in the unpublished study of Weller and Carne of a sample of homosexual males attending a London STD clinic in January 1986, the mean number of partners per month was 4.3 and the variance was 57.9. The data were collected, however, from a highly selected sample of patients with PGL or AIDS, partners of patients with PGL or AIDS, or homosexual men with more than 10 partners in the last three-month period. As such, the mean is probably much higher than the mean of a randomly drawn sample from the total homosexual population of London. However, high means were also recorded in the London study of McManus and McEvoy (1987) and the San Francisco study of McKusick *et al.* (1985*a*).

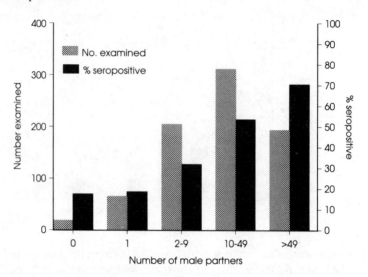

Fig. 11.15. The relationship between sexual activity amongst a sample of homosexual/bisexual males in San Francisco (as measured by the number of male partners over a 2-year period) and the percentage of each group who were seropositive for HIV antibodies (data from Winkelstein *et al.* 1987).

In the former, the mean rate of partner change was of the order of 20–30 partners per year while in the latter (in November 1982) it was 6.8 per month.

Similar studies of heterosexual activity are rare at present. The data from one small study carried out in England in November 1986 are presented in Fig. 11.16(d). This sample of 823 people drawn from the 18–44 year age groups (stratified by age and sex) had a mean (number of different partners per year) of 1.4 and a variance of 4.4. Both the mean and the variance were related to the age and the sex of the individual (Anderson and Medley, unpublished data). For example, the 18–24-year-old group in this study has a higher rate of sexual partner change than older age groups (Fig. 11.17(a)) (mean number of partners per year of 1.9, 1.5, and 1.1, variances of 9.3, 5.4, and 1.2, respectively, in the 18–24, 25–34, and 35–44 age groups). A recent study which provides a direct comparison between rates of partner change in homosexual and heterosexual groups is documented in Fig. 11.17(b). Here again marked differences between the groups are apparent (BMRB 1987).

These studies of heterosexual and homosexual communities reveal an important difference between the two risk groups. There appears to be an eight- to twentyfold difference in the average rate of acquisition of sexual partners between heterosexuals and homosexuals. Irrespective of the relative magnitudes of other factors that determine the rate of transmission of HIV, this factor by itself suggests that the spread of HIV in heterosexual communities in developed countries will be much slower than that observed in homosexual

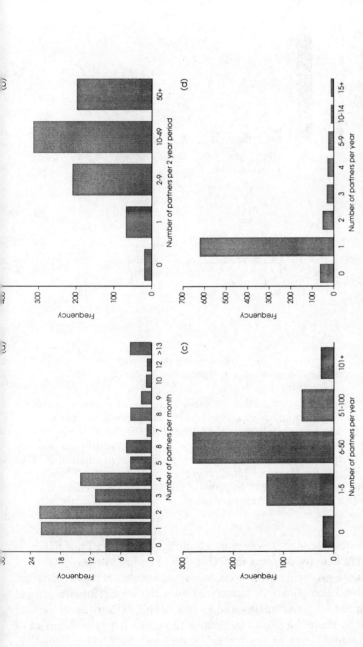

Fig. 11.16. Studies of sexual activity amongst male homosexuals (a, b, and c) and heterosexual communities (d). The graphs show frequency distributions for the number of sex partners per defined time period in samples of homosexual/bisexual males and heterosexual males and females. (a) Homosexual/bisexual males resident in London and surveyed in 1986 (unpublished data, C. A. Carne and I. V. Weller) ($m = 4.7$ per month, $\sigma^2 = 57$). The data denote male partners per month. (b) Homosexual/bisexual males resident in San Francisco and surveyed in 1984–5 (data from McKusick *et al.* 1985*a*). The data denote male partners per 2-year period. (c) Homosexual/bisexual males resident in London and surveyed in 1984 (McManus and McEvoy 1987). The data denote male partners per year. (d) Heterosexuals between the ages of 18 and 44 years in England, surveyed in November 1986 (unpublished data, R. M. Anderson and G. F. Medley). Data denote partners of the opposite sex per year (sample size $= 823$, $m = 1.4$, $\sigma^2 = 4.4$).

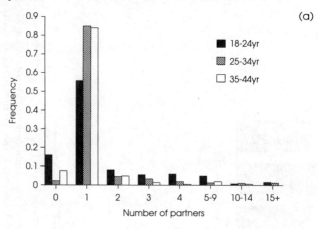

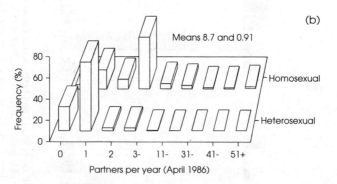

Fig. 11.17. (a) Sexual activity amongst heterosexuals in England. The graph records the frequency distribution of the number of sex partners of the opposite sex per one-year period, stratified by age group. Data source as defined in Fig. 11.16(d); see text for further details. (b) Patterns of sexual behaviour, as reflected by reported rates of sexual partner change, in heterosexuals and male homosexuals sampled in England in April 1986. The graph records the frequency distributions of the number of different sexual partners per person over the past year. Samples of people were obtained via a quota sampling method (see BMRB 1987; Anderson 1988*b*).

communities. More generally, however, much more quantitative information is required on sexual activity patterns in both types of communities.

In addition to the problem of limited data on rates of sexual partner change, there are additional complications associated with the impact of educational campaigns mounted by governments and public health authorities in various countries, aimed at changing sexual behaviour to reduce the rate of spread of HIV. Such campaigns, both in the United States and the United Kingdom, have had a measurable impact of rates of sexual partner change in homosexual

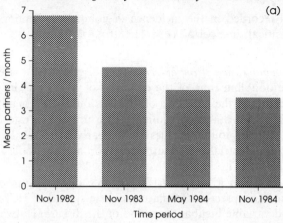

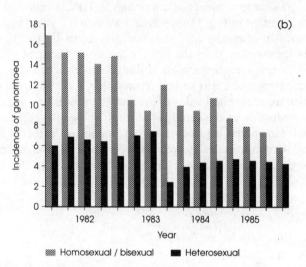

Fig. 11.18. Changes in sexual behaviour. (a) The mean number of partners per month for homosexual/bisexual men surveyed in San Francisco over the period November 1982 to November 1984 (data from McKusick *et al.* 1985*b*). The mean declined from 6.8 to 3.5 partners per month. (b) Changes in the rate of gonorrhoea (numbers of patients with gonorrhoea/total number of patients with and without gonorrhoea) among homosexual/bisexual and heterosexual men attending a London STD clinic, by quarterly periods from 1982 to 1985 (Carne *et al.* (1985)).

communities (Fig. 11.18). In a study by McKusick *et al.* (1985*b*) in San Francisco, for example, the mean rate of partner change amongst male homosexuals (defined per month) fell from 6.8 to 3.5 over the interval November 1982 to November 1984 (Fig. 11.18(a)). Similarly, a study by Carne *et al.* (1987) in London revealed a sharp decline in the incidence of gonorrhoea amongst male homosexuals over the interval 1982 to 1985. In the same study, little change was recorded in the incidence of gonorrhoea amongst heterosexuals over the identical time period (Fig. 11.18(b)).

11.3.2.12 *Doubling time of the epidemic*   As discussed in a later section of this chapter, the doubling time of the epidemic of AIDS (t_d, defined as the time interval over which the incidence of disease doubles in magnitude), during its early stages, provides a good summary measure of the rate of spread of the infection. Recorded doubling times for the early stages of the AIDS epidemic in a variety of industrialized countries tend on average to lie in the range of 8 months to 1 year (Fig. 11.3(c)).

Changes in the incidence of AIDS provide one measure of this summary statistic, but more precise information on the spread of HIV infection (given the long and variable incubation period of the disease) is revealed by longitudinal studies of seroprevalence of antibodies to HIV infection. A series of such studies are recorded in Fig. 11.19, which draws from a variety of countries and focuses on different risk groups (e.g. homosexual males or IV drug abusers). The similarities, rather than the differences, in the rates of increase of seropositivity through time is the most striking feature recorded in Fig. 11.19. As the epidemic progresses, it is to be expected that, over time, the doubling time will lengthen from its initial value of around 10 months to 1 year, as saturation effects (the reduction in the supply of susceptible people) come into play or as educational campaigns begin to have an impact on rates of sexual partner change and sexual practices. As yet, however, there is no clear indication from reports of AIDS cases that the epidemic is slowing in the United States.

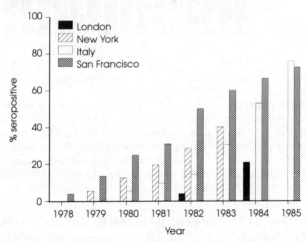

Fig. 11.19. Examples of the observed rise in seropositivity to HIV antigens in samples of patients over the period 1978–85. The studies in San Francisco, London, and New York were of homosexual/bisexual males. The study in Italy is of drug addicts (data sources given in May and Anderson (1987)).

In contrast, serological studies of cohorts of homosexual/bisexual men in cities such as San Francisco, New York, and London indicate that changes in behaviour, and the depletion of the supply of susceptible individuals, are beginning to decrease the rate at which new infections arise in specific at-risk groups.

11.3.2.13 *AIDS in the developing world* It has recently become apparent that AIDS is not simply a problem in wealthy industrialized societies. Over the past five years cases of AIDS have been identified in over 80 countries on five different continents, including Africa with several thousand cases suspected and many more unrecognized, and the Americas, particularly the Caribbean and South America, with over 4000 cases reported to the Pan American Health Organization (CDC 1986; Francis and Quinn 1987). AIDS has become a global epidemic, threatening the health of human communities throughout the world.

The epidemiology and clinical features of HIV infection and AIDS vary in different countries, depending on cultural differences (e.g. sexual behaviour and practices), the presence of other endemic diseases, and other unidentified risk factors. The most striking differences between many tropical countries and the United States or Europe is the rapid spread of infection among heterosexuals and the various clinical presentations of AIDS. The failure to identify risk factors traditionally associated with AIDS, such as homosexuality and intravenous drug abuse (which have been found in over 90 per cent of AIDS patients in the United States), has raised many questions about the factors that cause the spread of HIV in tropical regions.

The finding of AIDS among African residents in Europe prompted a series of investigations to determine the presence of HIV and AIDS in Central Africa. During a three-week period in 1983, 38 cases of AIDS and 20 cases of AIDS-related diseases were identified in patients in a hospital in Kinshasa, Zaire (Piot *et al.* 1984). The male:female ratio was 1:1, and the annual case rate for Kinshasa was estimated to be at least 17 per 100 000 population. The female AIDS patients were younger than the male patients with AIDS (mean age 28 and 41 years, respectively) and were more often unmarried. Furthermore, several clusters of AIDS among males and females with frequent heterosexual contact provided some evidence for heterosexual activity as a primary risk factor. At the same time, another study in Kigali, Rwanda, revealed, over a four-week surveillance period, 26 patients (17 males and 9 females) with AIDS (van de Pierre *et al.* 1985).

Subsequent studies in Zambia, Uganda, Central African Republic, Kenya, and Tanzania, have confirmed these initial findings of endemic AIDS primarily among heterosexual men and women (Melbye *et al.* 1984; Serwadda *et al.* 1985; Kreiss *et al.* 1986). Heterosexual transmission has been further confirmed by recent serological studies of HIV infection which have demonstrated high seroprevalence rates among both African prostitutes and men exposed to these prostitutes (van de Perre *et al.* 1985; Quinn *et al.* 1986). Other serological studies

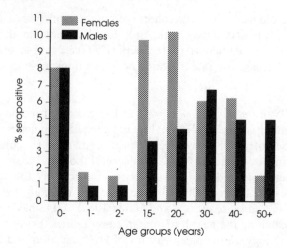

Fig. 11.20. HIV seroprevalence among 5099 healthy individuals as a function of age, in Kinshasa, Zaire, 1984–5 (data from Quinn *et al.* 1986). The sample population consisted of 2982 men and 2117 women. Positive patients had sera that were repeatedly reactive on a commercially available ELISA and were Western-blot positive.

have also suggested the possibility of transmission via contaminated needles used in medical treatment and blood transfusions, and of vertical transmission from mothers to infants (Quinn *et al.* 1986). The most striking features of these studies are the 1:1 male:female ratio of cases (which is to be compared with a ratio of around 16:1 in developed countries) and the high incidence of HIV infection in certain heterosexual communities. These aspects of the epidemiology survey from Kinshasa, Zaire are presented in Fig. 11.20. The age and sex distributions of seroprevalence provides strong evidence that heterosexual activity is a major determinant of the spread of infection. They also contradict unconfirmed reports that insect vectors, such as mosquitoes, are a factor in the transmission of HIV in tropical regions.

The rapid spread of HIV infection in certain developing regions of the world, such as Africa, present international aid agencies and national public health authorities with enormous problems in the supply of resources and trained personnel. There seems little doubt that the epidemic will have a very substantial impact on population sizes and structure in many regions of the world over the coming decades.

11.3.2.14 *The origin of HIV*   Examination of stored sera suggests that HIV appears to have been present in the United States only since 1976–7 (Melbye *et al.* 1984). Similar studies in Europe suggest that HIV was introduced around 1978–80 and that it came from the United States. Haitians were among the first to be diagnosed as having AIDS in the Americas, although there are no data to indicate whether HIV was brought to Haiti from the USA or vice versa.

It is possible that the virus was brought to Haiti from Central America as a consequence of immigration and commercial links between Haiti and Zaire in the early 1960s.

Melbye *et al.* (1984) suggest that there is no conclusive evidence that HIV originated in Africa. They do, however, point out that there is evidence to suggest the occurrence of case reports of a disease consistent with AIDS among residents in Africa in the mid-1970s, as well as seropositivity to what may be a virus closely related to HIV in sera from Ugandan children in 1972–3 and the isolation and identification of related retroviruses both in humans and in non-human primates. They suggest that if the virus is new in Africa in its present form, it probably had existed as a non-pathogenic virus in humans or it had come from other primate populations. What is becoming clear is that African HIV isolates appear to have a higher degree of genetic diversity than those obtained in the United States and Europe (Kanki *et al.* 1987).

Recent studies of the molecular sequence of human HIV viruses and of related viruses in other primates suggest that HIV may have first appeared in human populations as long as 150 years ago. Why did HIV prevalence and associated AIDS disease not rise to noticeable levels sooner? These molecular studies, and some ideas about how the initial spread of HIV may have been very slow, are discussed elsewhere (May and Anderson 1990).

11.3.3 *A simple model for homosexually transmitted HIV*

Faced with the many uncertainties that surround the key epidemiological parameters determining the transmission of HIV, we begin by restricting attention to transmission among homosexuals; such infections, as we have seen, constitute roughly three-quarters of known cases in the USA (Fig. 11.2). As a very crude first approximation, we divide the host population into two epidemiological types, along the lines followed for hepatitis B and other carrier-borne infections in the preceding chapter. We assume that both types are equally susceptible to infection with HIV. A proportion, f, of those infected move at a rate v_1 (that is, after a characteristic time $1/v_1$) into the class with clinical AIDS. These infected individuals are assumed to be infectious, with a probability β_1 of infecting any one sexual partner, up to the point where they manifest overt symptoms of AIDS; thereafter, they are assumed not to contribute to virus transmission within the population. The remaining fraction, $1 - f$, of those infected are seropositive, but do not go on to develop full-blown AIDS. Infected individuals of this second type are also infectious, with a transmission probability β_2 per sexual partner; they are assumed to move into a non-infectious state at a rate v_2 (that is, after a characteristic time $1/v_2$).

The deliberately oversimplified assumptions in this model make it a very rough caricature of the epidemiology of AIDS. It does serve, however, to illuminate some of the essential dynamical properties of the system. As such, the model gives basic insights and understanding, which can be used as a point of departure for numerical studies of more complicated and more realistic models. Simple though it is, the model defined by eqns (11.17)–(11.21) does embrace a range of possibilities, which future research can narrow. If there do exist type 2 individuals (those who do not develop overt AIDS), they might remain infectious for life ($v_2 = 0$), although this seems unlikely. As just reviewed, the evidence increasingly indicates that the distribution of incubation periods in different individuals is quite wide, so that f is considerably higher than suggested by early estimates, which took $1/v_1$ to be around 3–5 years, on the basis of early case records; possibly $v_1 = v_2$. Such a wide distribution in the duration of infectiousness, and the consequent appearance of many classes of infected individuals, could conceivably arise from clinical AIDS being produced when some other stress is superimposed on non-clinical AIDS infection. By the same token, it may be that those destined to develop full-blown AIDS are more infectious beforehand than are type 2 infectives ($\beta_1 > \beta_2$), or it may not.

In this first, simplest, model we have assumed that those who develop full-blown AIDS remain infectious until they do so, and then abruptly cease to be infectious. More generally, it may be that infectiousness is high initially, declines to a low level, and then rises again as the disease state is approached. This is another aspect of the imprecision inherent in our assumption that individuals move out of the infectious state at constant rates, v_1 and v_2, giving rise to a simple exponential spread in the duration of infectiousness (with the probability that any one infected person will remain infectious for a period of duration t or more being $\exp(-v_k t)$; see Fig. 3.1 and the accompanying discussion). The indications seem to be that for AIDS this is a more accurate approximation than the opposite extreme of assuming an infectious interval of duration exactly $1/v_k$. Best, of course, would be enough information to define the actual distribution of intervals of infectiousness, along with the corresponding transmission probabilities per partner at various stages; we will return to this below.

On the basis of the above discussion, we have a model in which the total host population, $N(t)$, is divided into five categories: susceptibles, $X(t)$; infectious individuals of types 1 and 2, $Y_1(t)$ and $Y_2(t)$, respectively; those with clinical AIDS, $A(t)$; and non-infectious individuals of type 2, $Z(t)$:

$$dX/dt = B - (\mu + \lambda)X, \tag{11.17}$$

$$dY_1/dt = f\lambda X - (\mu + v_1)Y_1, \tag{11.18}$$

$$dY_2/dt = (1 - f)\lambda X - (\mu + v_2)Y_2, \tag{11.19}$$

$$dA/dt = v_1 Y_1 - (\mu + \alpha)A, \tag{11.20}$$

$$dZ/dt = v_2 Y_2 - \mu Z. \tag{11.21}$$

Here we have again, as in Chapter 6, departed from the practice of placing bars over the top of variables referring to total populations, summed over all ages. As earlier, the set of eqns (11.17)–(11.21) assumes a Type II, constant mortality rate, μ; the conclusions are very similar to those obtained using more realistic death rates (partly because $L = 1/\mu$ is significantly longer than other time-scales in the system).

The term B in eqn (11.17) represents the rate of input of new susceptibles into the homosexual population. The death rate for those with clinical AIDS is determined by α in eqn (11.20). Unlike most of the systems we have studied up to now, this system has a mortality explicitly associated with the disease, and so the total population can change over time. Adding eqns (11.17) through (11.21), and noting $N = X + Y_1 + Y_2 + A + Z$, we have

$$dN/dt = B - \mu N - \alpha A. \tag{11.22}$$

The force of infection, λ, in these equations is given by

$$\lambda = c(\beta_1 Y_1 + \beta_2 Y_2)/N. \tag{11.23}$$

Here β_k is the probability that infection will be acquired from an infected sexual partner of type k, and Y_k/N is the probability that a randomly chosen partner will in fact be an infective of type k $(k = 1, 2)$. This assumes homogeneity in the sexual habits within this population, ignoring for the moment the heterogeneities dealt with (for gonorrhoea and other STDs) earlier in this chapter. Under this assumption, c represents the average number of sexual partners per unit time; we shall discuss the interpretation of c further, below.

Finally, we note that eqns (11.17)–(11.21) take no account of a latent class. As discussed earlier, this seems sensible, because the data suggest that the latent period, between becoming infected and becoming infectious, is much shorter than other time-scales in this system, being of the order of a few weeks at most.

11.3.4 *Properties of the simple model*

In the early stages of the epidemic, essentially all hosts are susceptible ($X \simeq N$), and the effect of deaths from AIDS is negligible. We may also, to a first approximation, neglect inputs of new susceptibles and natural deaths, regarding the population as roughly closed and constant on the time-scale of the initial phase of the epidemic. In the absence of precise knowledge about the characteristic duration of infection in those who do go on to develop clinical AIDS and those who do not, we start by assuming that the two times are equal: $v_1 = v_2 = v$. We also start by putting $\beta_1 = \beta_2 = \beta$. Then we can add eqns (11.18) and (11.19), to get a simple expression for the initial rise in infection:

$$dY/dt \simeq (\beta c - v)Y. \tag{11.24}$$

That is, the number of seropositives initially rises exponentially, $Y(t) \simeq Y(0) \exp(\Lambda t)$, with the growth rate Λ given by

$$\Lambda = \beta c - v. \tag{11.25}$$

The initial doubling time, t_d, is given by $\Lambda t_d = \ln 2 \simeq 0.7$, whence

$$t_d \simeq 0.7/(\beta c - v). \tag{11.26}$$

All this has a very simple intuitive explanation. In the early stages of the epidemic, before any saturation effects occur, the number of new infections produced by an infected individual, per unit time, is equal to the effective average number of sexual partners (c) times the probability of infecting any one partner (β). On the other hand, infected individuals are removed at the rate v. Hence the rate at which the epidemic initially grows exponentially is given by $\Lambda \simeq \beta c - v$.

The approximation of eqn (11.24) for $Y(t)$ may now be used in eqn (11.20), to obtain an expression for the growth in the number of people with clinical AIDS in the early stages of the epidemic:

$$A(t) \simeq \frac{fvY(0)}{\Lambda + \mu + \alpha} (e^{\Lambda t} - e^{-(\mu + \alpha)t}). \tag{11.27}$$

Here it is as well to include the terms of order α and μ. After a brief interval, of the order of one doubling time, the first of the two exponential terms inside the brackets will predominate, and the number of diagnosed cases of AIDS will also increase exponentially at the rate Λ in these early stages of the epidemic.

More generally, if we allow v_1 and v_2, and β_1 and β_2, to have unequal values, the initial phase of the epidemic in this otherwise homogeneous population will still see the number seropositive and the number of diagnosed cases of AIDS rising exponentially at a rate Λ, which now is the dominant root of the equation (see eqn (10.35) and the surrounding discussion):

$$\frac{f\beta_1 c}{\Lambda + v_1} + \frac{(1-f)\beta_2 c}{\Lambda + v_2} = 1. \tag{11.28}$$

Notice that if we knew v_1, v_2, f, and the ratio of β_1 to β_2, we could use this equation in conjunction with data for the initial rate of rise, Λ, to infer $\beta_1 c$ and $\beta_2 c$; these quantities are hard to estimate by other means.

Our earlier results for the total fraction ever infected by an epidemic in a closed population, I, can be applied here, provided we retain the approximations of neglecting input of new susceptibles and AIDS-related deaths ($B = 0$ and $\alpha = 0$; in distinction with eqn (11.28), however, we no longer neglect deaths from causes other than AIDS, $\mu \neq 0$). In effect we put $\beta_k = \beta c/N$ in eqns (10.31) and (10.32), to obtain

$$I = 1 - \exp(-R_0 I). \tag{11.29}$$

Here R_0 for AIDS is defined by

$$R_0 = \frac{f\beta_1 c}{v_1 + \mu} + \frac{(1-f)\beta_2 c}{v_2 + \mu}. \tag{11.30}$$

The fraction seropositive saturates to I as the epidemic progresses. If R_0 is appreciably in excess of unity, eqn (11.29) gives $I \simeq 1 - \exp(-R_0)$, and seropositivity levels are close to 100 per cent.

Although the above results, eqns (11.24)–(11.28), represent an excellent approximation for the early stages of an epidemic described by the set of eqns (11.17)–(11.23), deaths from AIDS and (to a somewhat lesser extent) input of new susceptibles and other deaths come to be important as the epidemic progresses. Figures 11.21(a–d) show numerical solutions of the model for the number seropositive, number of new cases, and cumulative deaths from AIDS, as functions of time from the introduction of the first infectives. The parameter choices are dictated by our previous discussions of the equivocal evidence, and are defined in the captions. The key choices are, in Figs. 11.21(a) and (b), $1/v_1 = 1/v_2 = 8$ years, and $f = 0.2$ and 0.5, respectively. Figures 11.21(c) and (d) correspond to (a) and (b), respectively, except now $1/v_2 = 20$ years. In all four figures, we put $\beta_1 c = \beta_2 c = 1$, which is estimated from data on the initial rise in seropositivity in the USA and in London, as discussed more fully below. These parameter choices correspond roughly to $R_0 \simeq 7, 7, 13, 11$ in Figs. 11.21(a, b, c, d), respectively. The decrease in the fraction seropositive in the later stages of the epidemic (which is a feature not found in the formula (11.29) for the saturation level of seropositivity) derives from AIDS-related deaths removing an increasing fraction of seropositives as time goes on.

Despite the simplicity of the model and the crudity of the parameter estimates, the broad patterns displayed in Figs. 11.21(a–d) are similar to the tends observed in cities such as San Francisco (see Figs. 11.1–11.19), both in the timing of the epidemic (which reaches its maximum incidence 10–12 years from its first invasion) and in the proportion seropositive in the homosexual community at the peak incidence (around 80 per cent). In this simple model, the predicted trends are not particularly sensitive to assumptions about the duration of infectiousness of type 2 ('carrier') individuals, $1/v_2$, although the epidemic does peak somewhat sooner and at higher seropositivity levels for longer $1/v_2$ (essentially because they give larger values of R_0).

Data from New York City and San Francisco in the late 1980s suggest the incidence of AIDS among homosexual men is beginning to level off and even possibly show a slight decline. It has been argued that this is a consequence of changes in sexual habits in homosexual communities, both in average number of sexual partners per unit time and in the kind of sexual activity (Pickering *et al.* 1986). Such changes clearly do exist; see Fig. 11.18. However, the simple model whose behaviour is illustrated in Fig. 11.21 suggests that, even with no change in sexual practices, the epidemic will peak in the homosexual community somewhere around 10–12 years after the initial introduction of infection. This property of Figs. 11.21(a–d) can be understood by observing that the time taken to reach peak incidence is very roughly given by $t \sim t_d \ln[f(\text{population size})/(\text{early number of AIDS infections})]$; for factors inside the square brackets ranging from around 10^4 to 10^6, and the observed doubling time of around 9 months, this gives $t \sim 10$ years once logarithms are taken.

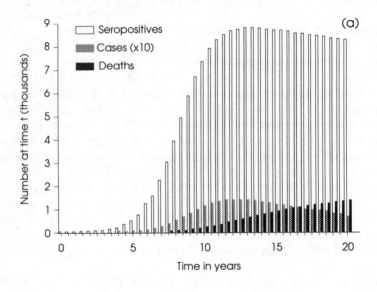

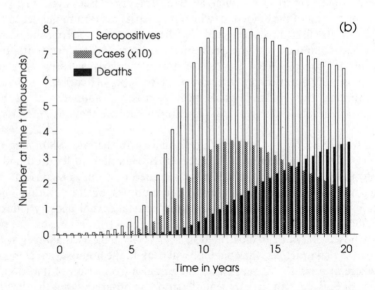

Fig. 11.21. Numerical solutions of the homogeneous mixing model defined by eqns (11.17)–(11.21). The four graphs ((a) to (d)) record changes, through time, in the number of seropositive individuals, the number of cases of AIDS ($\times 10$), and cumulative number of deaths from AIDS. Parameter values are as follows: (a) $N_0 = 10\,000$, $Y_1(0) = 5$,

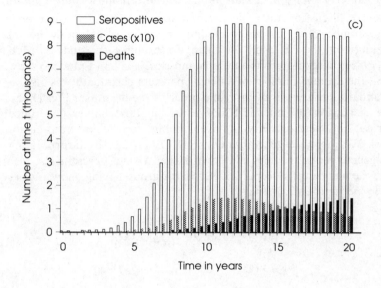

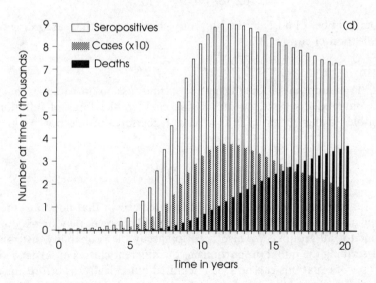

Fig. 11.21 (cont.). $\mu = 1/75 \text{ yr}^{-1}$, $1/v_1 = 1/v_2 = 8$ years, $f = 0.2$, $\alpha = 1 \text{ yr}^{-1}$, $\beta_1 c = \beta_2 c = 1 \text{ yr}^{-1}$, $B = N_0\mu$; (b) Same as for (a) except $f = 0.5$; (c) Same as for (a) except $1/v_2 = 20$ years; (d) Same as for (c) except $f = 0.05$.

11.3.5 *Heterogeneity in sexual habits within a homosexual population*

The above discussion takes no account of the substantial variation in the average number of sexual partners found among individuals in the homosexual communities in the USA and elsewhere. For example, the study by McKusick *et al.* (1985*a*) of sexual habits among homosexuals in San Francisco shows that in 1982 the average number of different partners per month was 5.9, but that the standard deviation is of the same order as the mean (see Fig. 11.15).

The discussion of endemic STDs earlier in this chapter underlined how important this heterogeneity in sexual habits can be for transmission and control. We therefore generalize eqns (11.17)–(11.23), by incorporating such heterogeneity along the lines laid down earlier. Using subscripts *i*, as before, to denote the number of susceptibles, etc., in the group having on average *i* sexual partners per unit time, we have:

$$dX_i/dt = B_i - (\mu + \lambda_i)X_i, \tag{11.31}$$

$$dY_{1i}/dt = f\lambda_i X_i - (\mu + v_1)Y_{1i}, \tag{11.32}$$

$$dY_{2i}/dt = (1 - f)\lambda_i X_i - (\mu + v_2)Y_{2i}, \tag{11.33}$$

$$dA_i/dt = v_1 Y_{1i} - (\mu + \alpha)A_i, \tag{11.34}$$

$$dZ_i/dt = v_2 Y_{2i} - \mu Z_i. \tag{11.35}$$

The total number of hosts in the *i*th group changes over time, according to the generalization of eqn (11.22):

$$dN_i/dt = B_i - \mu N_i - \alpha A_i. \tag{11.36}$$

Under the assumptions about the matrix of transmission probabilities that were spelled out and discussed earlier in this chapter, the force of infection for susceptibles in the *i*th group is $\lambda_i = i\lambda$, with the force of infection per partner being

$$\lambda = \sum_i i(\beta_1 Y_{1i} + \beta_2 Y_{2i})\left(\sum_i iN_i\right)^{-1}. \tag{11.37}$$

The parameters are all as for the simple model, except that now B_i is the rate of input of new susceptibles into the *i*th group (where B_i may or may not be the same for all groups). We also need to specify the probability distribution, $P(i)$, describing the initial proportions in the different classes of sexual activity.

This set of equations can now be integrated numerically, as before, once the parameter values and the initial conditions are specified. Before presenting such numerical results, it is illuminating to look at some limiting cases, as we did for the simple, sexually homogeneous, model.

Consider first the early stages of the epidemic, when essentially all are susceptible ($X_i \simeq N_i$), and when deaths and inputs can, to a good approximation, be neglected ($\mu \simeq \alpha \simeq B_i = 0$). If we make the further assumption, as before, that $v_1 = v_2 = v$ and $\beta_1 = \beta_2 = \beta$, we can obtain from eqns (11.32), (11.33), and (11.37) the analogue of the earlier eqn (11.24):

$$d\lambda/dt \simeq (\beta c - v)\lambda. \tag{11.38}$$

This is exactly the same expression as before, except that now c has the explicit interpretation $c = \langle i^2 \rangle / \langle i \rangle$, as for the endemic situation discussed earlier. That is, repeating eqn (11.10) for convenience,

$$c = m + \sigma^2/m. \tag{11.39}$$

Here m is the mean number of sexual partners per unit time, and σ^2 is the variance in the distribution of numbers of partners. In the simple approximations which treat the population as homogeneous in sexual habits, c should be interpreted as having the numerical value given by eqn (11.39), which can be significantly larger than the simple average, m (see Fig. 11.15).

As for the simple model, eqn (11.38) tells us that the force of infection, and thence the incidence of infection in the various groups, rises approximately exponentially in the early phase of the epidemic, at a rate Λ given by eqn (11.25). More generally, if $v_1 \neq v_2$ and $\beta_1 \neq \beta_2$, we still have exponential growth at a rate Λ in the initial stages of the epidemic, with Λ now given as the dominant root of eqn (11.28) (and c still defined by eqn (11.39)).

For the general case $v_1 \neq v_2$ and $\beta_1 \neq \beta_2$, but retaining the approximation of a closed population in which inputs of new susceptibles and disease-related deaths are neglected ($B_i = 0$, $\alpha = 0$), we can obtain an analytic expression for the total fraction ever infected in the ith group, I_i:

$$I_i = 1 - \exp(-i\alpha). \tag{11.40}$$

Here α (which is the integral of $\lambda(t)$ from $t = 0$ to $t \to \infty$) is determined from the implicit relation

$$\alpha = R_0 \sum_i iP(i)(1 - e^{-i\alpha}) \left(\sum_i i^2 P(i) \right)^{-1}. \tag{11.41}$$

This result is obtained by taking the appropriate form for β_{kl} in eqns (10.31) and (10.32) (see Appendix E). R_0 is as defined above by eqn (11.30), with c now given explicitly by eqn (11.39); this formula for R_0 is the appropriate special form of eqn (10.29).

In concrete illustrations of these ideas and results, we may choose the distribution in numbers of sexual partners, $P(i) = N_i/N$, to be given by actual data, such as that in Figs. 11.15 and 11.16. Alternatively, we may assume some particular statistical distribution in degrees of sexual activity, $P(i)$, whose characterizing mean and variance (and possibly other moments) are determined by the data. The latter approach sacrifices some detail, but has the compensating

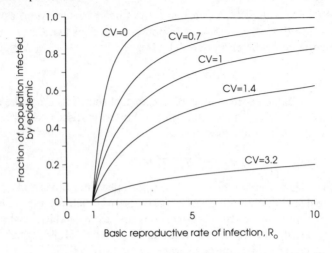

Fig. 11.22. The asymptotic fraction of people who are seropositive for HIV antibodies, as a function of the basic reproductive rate, R_0, for different amounts of variability in degrees of sexual activity within the population, as measured by the coefficient of variation, $CV = \sigma/m$. See text and eqns (11.44) and (11.45) for further details.

advantage of allowing us to see clearly how increasing variance in numbers of sexual partners affects the dynamics of the epidemic.

Specifically, in much of what follows we characterize $P(i)$ by a continuous gamma distribution:

$$P(i)\,di = (k^k/m^k\Gamma(k))i^{k-1}\exp(-ik/m)\,di. \tag{11.42}$$

Here m is the mean value of i, and the parameter k is an inverse measure of the coefficient of variation of the distribution:

$$\sigma^2/m^2 = 1/k. \tag{11.43}$$

Averaging over eqn (11.40) for this distribution function, we find the overall fraction of the host population ever to be infected—which corresponds to the saturation level of the fraction seropositive—is

$$I = 1 - (1 + \theta)^{-k}. \tag{11.44}$$

Here $\theta \equiv m\alpha/k$ is determined from eqn (11.41), which gives the implicit relation

$$R_0 = (k+1)\theta/[1 - (1 + \theta)^{-(k+1)}]. \tag{11.45}$$

In the limit of a community that is uniform in its sexual habits, $\sigma^2 \to 0$ and $k \to \infty$, eqns (11.44) and (11.45) reduce to the earlier and simpler expression (11.29). More generally, Fig. 11.22 shows the asymptotic fraction who are seropositive, as a function of R_0, for different amounts of variability in degrees of sexual activity within the population (as measured by the coefficient of variation, $CV = \sigma/m$). Equations (11.44) and (11.45), and other formulae giving analytic expressions for the dynamics of the epidemic in a population with a gamma distribution for levels of sexual activity (but with $B_i = 0$), are derived in Appendix F.

As in the simple model, AIDS-related deaths affect the trajectory of the epidemic in its later stages, and so (to a lesser extent) do other deaths and inputs of new susceptibles. Figures 11.23(a) and (b) therefore show results obtained

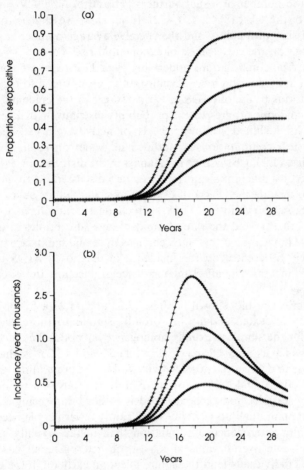

Fig. 11.23. Numerical solutions of an approximation to the heterogeneous-mixing model with recruitment of susceptibles (eqns (11.31)–(11.35)). The graphs show: (a) the proportion seropositive to HIV, and (b) the incidence of AIDS per year for four different coefficients of variation (CV) of the gamma distribution of sexual activity, namely 0.45 (top curve), 1.0, 1.4, 2.0 (bottom curve). The parameter values are: $R_0 = 5$, $1/v_1 = 1/v_2 = 5$ years, $f = 0.2$, $\alpha = 1\,\mathrm{yr}^{-1}$, $N_0 = 100\,000$, and $1/\mu = 50$ years. Six categories of sexual activity were defined in the discrete approximation to the gamma distribution: 0–1, 2–5, 6–9, 10–49, 50–100, and 100+ partners per year. The values of B_i and i were chosen from gamma distributions with the mean number of partners fixed at $5\,\mathrm{yr}^{-1}$ and variances of 5 (top curve), 25, 50, and 100 (bottom curve) (see Anderson *et al.* 1986).

numerically by integrating eqns (11.31)–(11.37), using a gamma distribution to characterize the distribution in degrees of sexual activity. Figure 11.23(a) shows the proportion seropositive, and Fig. 11.23(b) shows the incidence of newly-diagnosed cases of AIDS, as functions of time since the infection first appeared. Each figure shows the results for a range of assumptions about the coefficient of variation in number of sexual partners per unit of time, $CV = \sigma/m = 1/k^{1/2}$ (for values of the CV of 0.45, 1, 1.4, 2). In all cases we choose the product of the transmission probability and the effective average number of partners, βc, to fit the data on the early phase of exponential rise.

The numerical computations underlying Figs. 11.23(a, b) are complicated by the fact that individuals in more sexually active groups tend to become infected sooner, and thus to die of AIDS at earlier stages of the epidemic. This means that, as the epidemic progresses, the probability distribution in degrees of sexual activity is itself shifted to lower levels of activity. Formal machinery for expediting such computations is outlined in Anderson *et al.* (1986). All the results in Figs. 11.23(a, b) assume no changes in the distribution, $P(i)$, other than those created by differential mortality, as just discussed. More generally, it is necessary to include the effects of changes in sexual habits as a result of fears about AIDS. As shown in Fig. 11.18, such changes clearly have occurred. They will affect both $P(i)$ and the rate of input of new susceptibles into group i, B_i. Although we have argued that such changes in sexual habits are likely to have had relatively little effect on the incidence of diagnosed AIDS to date, they certainly will increasingly affect the incidence of infection and of clinical AIDS as time goes on.

The numerical results shown in Figs. 11.22 and 11.23(a, b) for models with heterogeneity in sexual activity are broadly similar to those shown in Figs. 11.21(a–d) for the simpler, sexually homogeneous, model. The most important difference, which is seen clearly in Figs. 11.22 and 11.23, is that significant heterogeneity in degrees of sexual activity within the population tends to result in fewer infections, and thus in lower asymptotic levels of seropositivity, than predicted by sexually homogeneous models (other things being equal).

We can explain qualitatively why significantly fewer people become infected in the sexually heterogeneous population than in the sexually homogeneous one, for the same overall value of R_0. In the heterogeneous case, the highly promiscuous individuals tend to acquire infection early on in the course of the epidemic, and they therefore tend to be removed from the infectious class during the first few years (either by acquiring full-blown AIDS or by moving into the seropositive but non-infectious class). As the sexually more active individuals are thus removed, the force of infection declines among the remaining, less active, individuals; many of these less active individuals may still be uninfected at the point when the effective reproductive rate of the virus drops below unity and the epidemic dies out. In this way, a substantial fraction of the at-risk population can remain uninfected, even for moderately large R_0, if variability in sexual habits is significantly high (CV sufficiently large). This is the mechanism underlying the patterns seen in Fig. 11.22. The figure is a striking illustration of the dangers of working with simple averages (the homogeneous model; $CV = 0$) in non-linear dynamical situations. Of course, as the duration of infectiousness in type 2 ('carrier') individuals is taken to be longer, the fraction ever infected increases; this corresponds to R_0 increasing in Fig. 11.22 (see eqn (11.30) for the relation between R_0 and $1/v_2$).

In short, comparison of Figs. 11.23(a, b) with Figs. 11.21(a–c) shows that heterogeneous models with a high degree of variability in levels of sexual activity predict that the epidemic peaks at roughly the same time as in the homogeneous models, but that it induces fewer AIDS cases, results in lower levels of seropositivity in the population, and has a longer 'tail' to the epidemic.

The data summarized in Fig. 11.16 suggest that indeed there is high variability in the levels of sexual activity within homosexual communities. Figures 11.22 and 11.23 show, however, that models with heterogeneous mixing have difficulty reconciling such high variance ($CV > 1$) with observed levels of seropositivity, which are currently around 60–70 per cent or more in some homosexual communities. Irritatingly, the homogeneously mixed models fit the epidemiological observations better. There are at least three factors that could help explain this discrepancy between reported variance in sexual habits and seropositivity levels, and the predictions of the heterogeneous model with currently accepted parameters. First, it may be that some individuals exaggerate and others play down their level of sexual activity, so that surveys (such as those recorded in Fig. 11.16) overestimate the variance. Second, it easily could be that the levels of seropositivity reported in the San Francisco study, Fig. 11.19, are a sample biased toward more active individuals, and that lower levels of seropositivity prevail among the homosexual community of San Francisco as a whole. Third, it may be that a very high proportion of those who become seropositive will eventually develop clinical AIDS, so that the incubation period ($1/v_1$) is significantly longer than the current estimate of 5–8 years; alternatively, it may be that those who acquire infection but never develop clinical AIDS remain infectious for a very long time ($1/v_2$ large). Either mechanism could produce a value of R_0 larger than usually estimated, and consequently a higher asymptotic level of seropositivity for specified CV in sexual habits (see Fig. 11.22). In practice, all three factors may be operating.

11.3.6 *Effects of distributed incubation periods and infectiousness*

In the preceding models, as throughout most of the discussion of microparasitic infections, we have assumed that infected individuals move through the incubation interval at a constant rate ($v = $ constant), and that they have a constant infectiousness or transmission coefficient during this period ($\beta = $ constant). But, as we saw in our review of the epidemiological characteristics of HIV/AIDS, the observations seem to be that the probability for an individual infected with HIV to manifest full-blown AIDS increases steadily as the time from infection lengthens. One simple way of describing the data is to assume that the probability of getting AIDS, at a time τ since the original HIV infection, increases as $v_0\tau^v$ (where v_0 and v are parameters to be fitted to the data); this leads to a Weibüll distribution for the distribution in incubation times, $f(\tau)$:

$$f(\tau) = v_0\tau^v \exp[-v_0\tau^{v+1}/(v+1)]. \tag{11.46}$$

That is, $f(\tau)$ gives the probability that an individual will fall ill with AIDS at a time τ since first acquiring HIV infection. The average incubation time, D, is given in terms of v_0 and v as

$$D = \Gamma\left(\frac{v+2}{v+1}\right)\left(\frac{v+1}{v_0}\right)^{1/(v+1)}. \tag{11.47}$$

A constant incubation rate corresponds to $v = 0$ (no dependence on time since infection), giving the familiar result $D = 1/v_0$. $\Gamma(z)$ is the Γ-function.

By the same token, Figs. 11.8 and 11.9 and the surrounding discussion suggest that the transmission probability is unlikely to be a constant, but rather that $\beta(\tau)$ will be relatively high for some characteristic time T_0 following the original HIV infection, and again for a characteristic time T_1 around the point where the immune system collapses and AIDS disease appears. Very roughly, for an individual who takes a time T to incubate AIDS, we might describe the time-dependent transmission probability $\beta(\tau)$ as

$$\beta(\tau) = \beta_0 \exp(-\tau/T_0) + \beta_1 \exp[-(T-\tau)/T_1]. \tag{11.48}$$

This gives the kind of temporal behaviour shown in the relevant Figs. 11.8 and 11.9.

These complications may be included, by extending the analysis given in Chapter 10 for heterogeneous systems. Defining $Y_i(t, \tau)$ to be the number of infectives at time t, in the sexual-activity class i, who have been infected for a time τ, we have the partial differential equation (May and Anderson 1988)

$$\partial Y_i(t, \tau)/\partial t + \partial Y_i(t, \tau)/\partial \tau = -(\mu + v(\tau))Y_i(t, \tau). \tag{11.49}$$

This equation has the boundary condition

$$Y_i(t, 0) = i\lambda(t)X_i(t), \tag{11.50}$$

corresponding to new infectives appearing at a rate $i\lambda(t)X_i(t)$ at time t. The force of infection, $\lambda(t)$, in turn is given by the appropriate extension of eqn (11.37).

$$\lambda(t) = \sum_j j \int \beta(\tau)Y_j(t, \tau)\, d\tau \left(\sum_j jN_j\right)^{-1}. \tag{11.51}$$

The other boundary condition in eqn (11.49) consists of the specification of $Y_i(0, \tau)$ at time $t = 0$.

By considering the endemic, equilibrium state (where $\partial/\partial t \to 0$), we can integrate eqn (11.49) for $Y_i^*(\tau)$. Substituting this result into the equilibrium (or static) version of eqn (11.51), and comparing with the earlier discussion in Chapter 4, we arrive at an expression for the basic reproductive rate:

$$R_0 = c \int_0^\infty \beta(\tau) \exp\left(-\int_0^\tau v(\tau') \, d\tau'\right) d\tau. \tag{11.52}$$

Here c is as defined by eqn (11.39), and we have neglected the natural mortality rate, $\mu = 1/L$, as being much smaller than other relevant rate parameters. This expression for R_0 reduces to the familiar $R_0 = \beta c/(\mu + v)$ if β and v are both constant. More generally, suppose the incubation time is exactly D (so that $v(\tau) = 0$ for $\tau < D$); then eqn (11.52) for R_0 becomes

$$R_0 = c \int_0^D \beta(\tau) \, d\tau. \tag{11.53}$$

If $\beta(\tau)$ is given by eqn (11.48), we then have for R_0 the explicit expression

$$R_0 = c\{\beta_0 T_0[1 - \exp(-D/T_0)] + \beta_1 T_1[1 - \exp(-D/T_1)]\}. \tag{11.54}$$

Figures 11.8 and 11.9 suggest that typically T_0 and T_1 may both be around 1 year, while D is around 6 years or so (giving an average of about 8 years between the original HIV infection and the onset of AIDS disease). In this event, R_0 is to an excellent approximation given by

$$R_0 \simeq c(\beta_0 T_0 + \beta_1 T_1). \tag{11.55}$$

Equation (11.55) is intuitively understandable: new infections are produced at a rate $\beta_0 c$ over an average interval T_0 early in the course of a typical HIV infection; later, further infections are produced at a rate $\beta_1 c$ over an average interval T_1.

More realistically, we have seen there is likely to be some distribution of incubation times, with the probability, $f(T)$, to observe an incubation time T being given by the Weibüll distribution (eqn (11.46)) or some other. In this event, eqn (11.52) is replaced by

$$R_0 = c \int_0^\infty f(T) \, dT \int_0^T \beta(\tau) \, d\tau. \tag{11.56}$$

Here $\beta(\tau)$ is described by eqn (11.48), or some other appropriate expression.

These complications can have an influence on estimates of the rate at which new infections appear in the early stages of the epidemic.

As usual, the dynamics of the initial phase of the epidemic can be elucidated by putting $X_i \simeq N_i$, whereupon the problem becomes a linear one. The solution of eqn (11.49), with the boundary condition given by eqns (11.50) and (11.51), is outlined in Appendix F. The force of infection, $\lambda(t)$, and the total number infected in each sexual-activity class, $Y_i(t) = \int Y_i(t, \tau) \, d\tau$, all grow exponentially (as $\exp(\Lambda t)$) in the early stages of the epidemic. The early growth rate, Λ (which is related to the doubling time by eqn (11.26)), is shown in Appendix F to be given by the 'dispersion relation'

$$1 = c \int_0^\infty \beta(\tau) \exp\left(-\Lambda\tau - \int_0^\tau v(\tau')\,d\tau'\right) d\tau. \qquad (11.57)$$

As usual, c is given by eqn (11.39). This eqn (11.57) is formally identical to the demographers' Euler equation that gives the growth rate of a population in terms of age-specific birth and death rates. Indeed, eqn (11.57) *is* the Euler equation for the demography of the infection within its host population: $c\beta(\tau)$ represents the 'age-specific birth' of new infections from an existing infection; $v(\tau)$ represents the 'age-specific death rate' at which infections are removed; and Λ is the (constant) growth rate of the population of infections in the early stages (before saturation effects start introducing density dependences into the vital rates). For a fuller discussion, see May *et al.* (1988*a*).

If we assume the incubation time is exactly D, and that $\beta(\tau)$ is given by eqn (11.48)—as we did in deriving eqn (11.54) for R_0—we find Λ to be given by the implicit expression

$$1 = \frac{c\beta_0 T_0}{1 + \Lambda T_0} [1 - \exp(-\Lambda D - D/T_0)] + \frac{c\beta_1 T_1}{1 - \Lambda T_1} [\exp(-\Lambda D) - \exp(-D/T_1)].$$

$$(11.58)$$

Let us again assume, for the reasons given above, that T_0 and T_1 are around 1 year and that D is around 6 years or so. Then if the doubling time in the early exponential phase is around 6–12 months, we also have $\Lambda \sim 1\,\mathrm{yr}^{-1}$ (remember $\Lambda = 0.7/t_d$). This means that ΛD is significantly in excess of unity, whence $\exp(-\Lambda D) \ll 1$ and eqn (11.58) reduces approximately to

$$\Lambda \simeq c\beta_0 - 1/T_0. \qquad (11.59)$$

This approximation is not sensible if $\beta_1 T_1$ is larger than $\beta_0 T_0$ by enough to compensate for the exponential discount factor (which is roughly $\exp(-\Lambda D)$ if ΛT_1 is significantly less than unity, roughly $[\exp(-D/T_1)]/(\Lambda T_1)$ if ΛT_1 is significantly greater than unity, and around $\Lambda D \exp(-\Lambda D)$ if $\Lambda T_1 \simeq 1$). Figure 11.24 illustrates the exact relationship, eqn (11.58), between $c\beta_0$ and Λ for several values of β_1/β_0 and with T_0, T_1, and D set at $T_0 = T_1 = 1$ year, $D = 6$ years.

At first glance, eqn (11.59) appears similar to our earlier result, eqn (11.25). The difference is that eqn (11.25) pertained to a model in which there was a single infectious period (of duration D and with transmission probability β); the approximate eqn (11.59) pertains to a situation in which the infected individuals are infectious in two intervals, one of duration T_0 (and intensity β_0) following the original infection, and a second of duration T_1 (and intensity β_1) a time roughly D later. Yet only the first episode enters into the approximate relation between the growth rate and the transmission parameters, eqn (11.59). The reason is that, in the early phases of the epidemic, the contribution to the

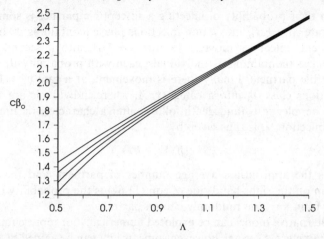

Fig. 11.24. The relationship between $c\beta_0$ and Λ as defined by eqn (11.58). Parameter values are set at $c = 10$ yr^{-1}, $T_0 = T_1 = 1$ year, $D = 6$ years, and $\beta_1 = 0.05$ (top curve), 0.1, 0.15, and 0.2 (bottom curve).

total number of infecteds or of AIDS cases from infections produced in the later episode of infectiousness ('β_1, T_1 infections', as it were) are effectively discounted—by a factor of the general order of $\exp(-\Lambda D)$—by virtue of the exponential growth of the population of infectives. Again, this phenomenon may be more familiar in conventional demographic contexts: in a fast-growing population, early births contribute significantly more to the population growth rate, r, than do later ones (to such an extent that age at first reproduction can be more important than is total family size). As we mentioned immediately below eqn (11.58), if $\beta_1 T_1$ is larger than $\beta_0 T_0$ by enough to compensate for the exponential 'discount factor', the approximate eqn (11.59) is invalid. The basic point, to which we will return in the next subsection, is that the existence of a transmission probability that depends significantly on time from first infection, $\beta(\tau)$, can complicate the analysis in ways that may not be intuitively obvious.

An alternative approach to describing the two distinct episodes of infectiousness is to add extra compartments to the model. In the simplest model, we can replace eqns (11.18)–(11.21) by the set

$$\mathrm{d}Y_1/\mathrm{d}t = \lambda X - v_0 Y_1, \tag{11.60}$$

$$\mathrm{d}Y_2/\mathrm{d}t = v_0 Y_1 - s Y_2, \tag{11.61}$$

$$\mathrm{d}Y_3/\mathrm{d}t = s Y_2 - v_1 Y_3, \tag{11.62}$$

$$\mathrm{d}A/\mathrm{d}t = v_1 Y_3 - \alpha A. \tag{11.63}$$

Here susceptibles, X, move into the first episode of infectiousness (containing Y_1 individuals) at a rate λ. Infected individuals move out of this first phase (in which their probability of infecting a susceptible partner is some constant, β_0) at a rate $v_0 = 1/T_0$, into a non-infectious phase (containing Y_2 individuals). These 'silent' infectives move, at a rate $s = 1/D$, into a second episode of infectiousness (containing Y_3 individuals, each with probability β_1 of infecting a susceptible partner). Finally there is movement, at a rate $v_1 = 1/T_1$, out of the infectious class Y_3 into a category, A, where individuals are too ill with AIDS to be infectious (and death follows after a characteristic time $1/\alpha$). The force of infection, λ, is thus given by

$$\lambda = c(\beta_0 Y_1 + \beta_1 Y_3)/N. \tag{11.64}$$

Here c is the appropriate average number of partners, and the rest of the expression on the right-hand side of eqn (11.64) is the probability of acquiring infection from any one randomly chosen partner.

This alternative model can be explored numerically for representative choices of the parameters. As usual, however, some insight can be gained by considering the early phase of the epidemic, in which essentially everyone is still susceptible, $X \simeq N$, so that the equations are approximately linear. With this linearization, the essential dynamics are given by eqns (11.60)–(11.63) in conjunction with the definition (11.64) for λ:

$$\mathrm{d}Y_1/\mathrm{d}t \simeq (c\beta_0 - v_0)Y_1 + c\beta_1 Y_3, \tag{11.65}$$

along with eqns (11.61) and (11.62) for $\mathrm{d}Y_2/\mathrm{d}t$ and $\mathrm{d}Y_3/\mathrm{d}t$, respectively. The solutions of this three-dimensional set of linear differential equations behave, after very early transients dependent on initial conditions have died away, as $\exp(\Lambda t)$, where Λ is the dominant root of the cubic equation

$$[\Lambda - (c\beta_0 - v_0)](\Lambda + s)(\Lambda + v_1) - c\beta_1 v_0 s = 0. \tag{11.66}$$

This result is derived and discussed more fully in Appendix F. Figure 11.25 displays $c\beta_0$ versus Λ, for various values of β_1/β_0 and for the particular choice $v_0 = v_1 = 1\,\mathrm{yr}^{-1}, s = 1/6\,\mathrm{yr}^{-1}$; Fig. 11.25 is the analogue, for the present model, of the earlier Fig. 11.24.

If we again assume D significantly greater than T_0 and T_1 (as 6 years are larger than 1 year)—which is to say if we assume s significantly less than v_0 and v_1—then eqn (11.66) gives us the approximate result $\Lambda \simeq c\beta_0 - 1/T_0$. This is the result, eqn (11.59), that we derived from our earlier model, and discussed above. Again, as can be seen from Fig. 11.25, this approximation will be invalid if β_1 is sufficiently larger than β_0.

Further insights into the influence of distinct episodes of infectiousness can be gained from numerical studies of the model defined by eqns (11.60)–(11.63). An example is presented in Fig. 11.26, where changes in the cumulative number of cases of AIDS, as a function of the time from the introduction of the infection, are recorded for various values of the parameters β_0 and β_1. These numerical solutions were calculated for a closed population of fixed size (10 000 people) where five infectious individuals ($Y_1(0) = 5$) were introduced at time

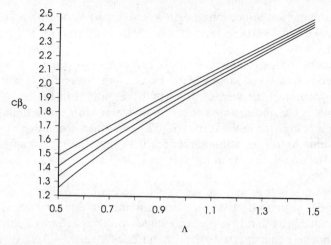

Fig. 11.25. The relationship between $c\beta_0$ and Λ as defined by eqn (11.66). Parameter values are set at $c = 10 \text{ yr}^{-1}$, $v_0 = v_1 = 1 \text{ yr}^{-1}$, $s = 1/6 \text{ yr}^{-1}$, and $\beta_1 = 0.05$ (top curve), 0.1, 0.15, and 0.2 (bottom curve).

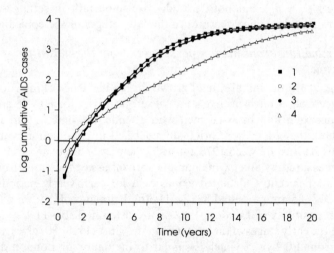

Fig. 11.26. Changes in the cumulative number of AIDS cases, as a function of time from the introduction of the infection, for various values of the parameters β_0 and β_1, as predicted by eqns (11.60)–(11.63); see the main text for further details. The numerical solutions were calculated for a closed population of size 10 000 where five infectious individuals ($Y_1(0) = 5$) were introduced at time $t = 0$. Four numerical projections are presented (curves 1–4): β_0 and $\beta_1 = 0.2$ (curve 1); $\beta_0 = 0.1$, $\beta_1 = 0$ (curve 3); and $\beta_0 = 0.1$, $\beta_1 = 0.3$ (curve 4). Curve 2 is for the case where infectiousness is assumed to be constant over an 8-year average incubation period. The parameters v_0, v_1, and s are set at 1 yr^{-1}, 1 yr^{-1}, $1/6 \text{ yr}^{-1}$, respectively.

$t = 0$. Four numerical projections are presented (lines 1 to 4), with $\beta_0 = \beta_1 = 0.2$ (line 1), $\beta_0 = 0.1$, $\beta_1 = 0$ (line 3), and $\beta_0 = 0.1$, $\beta_1 = 0.3$ (line 4). The parameters v_0, v_1, and s were set at $1\,\mathrm{yr}^{-1}$, $1\,\mathrm{yr}^{-1}$, and $1/6\,\mathrm{yr}^{-1}$, respectively, to yield an average incubation period $(1/v_0 + 1/v_1 + 1/s)$ of 8 years. Line 2 is for the case where infectiousness was assumed to be constant over the 8-year average incubation period of the disease. Note that the pattern in the early stages of the epidemic is curvilinear (on a logarithmic scale), with the doubling time of the epidemic being high in the very early stages and then decreasing to a roughly constant value until saturation effects begin to slow the rate of spread of the infection. The doubling time in the very early stages is most rapid for the cases in which $\beta_0 > \beta_1$.

Drawing all this together, we see that if there are two distinct episodes of infectiousness, separated by a non-infectious interval longer than either one, the exponential growth rate in the early stages will tend to be set approximately by the parameters characterizing the first episode $(\Lambda \simeq c\beta_0 - 1/T_0$, eqn (11.59)), while the expression for R_0 will involve both episodes of infectiousness $(R_0 \simeq c\beta_0 T_0 + c\beta_1 T_1$, eqn (11.55)). This makes sense: early 'births' count more than later ones toward population growth rates, but all 'births' are relevant to the total number of offspring. To put it yet another way, the early, exponential growth phase of the epidemic depends mainly on the first episode of infectiousness (unless $\beta_1 \gg \beta_0$), but both episodes are important in setting saturation levels and other dynamical features of the later stages of the epidemic.

11.3.7 *Estimating transmission parameters from the initial phases of the epidemic*

A rough guide to the initial rate of growth in the incidence of infection, Λ, can be obtained from a retrospective study of seropositivity for HIV in a cohort of 6875 homosexual and bisexual men who attended a clinic in San Francisco (CDC 1989); these data were originally collected in conjunction with a study of hepatitis B virus. Between 1978 and 1985 the prevalence of antibody to AIDS virus, as measured by an enzyme immunosorbent assay, increased from 4.5 per cent to 73.1 per cent. Calculated values of Λ for each yearly period over the interval 1978–85 are presented in Fig. 11.3(c). Estimates of Λ from data on the rise in seropositivity in London, 1982–5, are listed in Table 11.4.

Taking the early stages of the epidemic in the USA (1978–80) gives an average Λ value around $0.9\,\mathrm{yr}^{-1}$, which is similar to the figure for London during the early stages of the spread of AIDS. This estimate of Λ corresponds to a doubling time of about 9 months (see eqn (11.26)).

Under our simplest assumption of a constant rate of transition, v_1, from the infected state to full-blown AIDS disease (eqn (11.18)), we expect the number of diagnosed cases also initially to rise (after a few doubling times) exponentially at the rate Λ; see eqn (11.27) and the surrounding discussion. By contrast, if we assume a defined interval of duration exactly D between acquisition of infection and manifestation of disease, we expect the initial rise in cases to be

Table 11.4 Doubling time, t_d, from longitudinal serological studies of HIV infection in the early stages of the epidemic in various countries. Data from CDC (1989), Carne *et al.* (1985*a*), and Mortimer *et al.* (1985)

Country/city	Risk group	Period	Doubling time (months)
San Francisco, USA	Homosexual	1978–80	11.3
New York, USA	Homosexual	1982–3	10.7
London, UK	Homosexual	1982–4	9.9
London, UK	IV drug	1983–5	11.5
Switzerland	IV drug	1983–4	8.6
Italy	IV drug	1980–3	15.2

exponential at the rate Λ, only now lagging behind the rise in seropositivity by a time interval D. Intermediate between these two extremes is the assumption of a range of incubation times obeying a Weibüll or other such distribution; this also will lead to the number of AIDS cases initially rising (after the first few doubling times) as $\exp(\Lambda t)$. In any event, the early rise in the number of cases—although a less reliable estimate of Λ than is the rise in seropositivity—gives an independent estimate of Λ. Such data on reported cases are summarized in Table 11.3 and Fig. 11.3(c); the estimate of Λ is very roughly $1\,\mathrm{yr}^{-1}$, which is consistent with the $0.9\,\mathrm{yr}^{-1}$ obtained from serology.

For a population with $v_1 = v_2$ and $\beta_1 = \beta_2$ (so that there is no difference in transmission from those who do, and do not, develop clinical AIDS following infection) our simplest eqn (11.25) gives $\Lambda = \beta c - v$. This can be turned around to give a direct estimate of the combination of parameters, βc, in terms of the observed Λ and an estimate of v:

$$\beta c \simeq \Lambda + v. \tag{11.67}$$

In our original simple model, we assumed infectiousness was constant throughout the incubation period, leading to the estimate $v \simeq 1/8\,\mathrm{yr}^{-1}$. Since this estimate for v is significantly smaller than that for Λ, we have a fairly robust estimate $\beta c \sim 1\,\mathrm{yr}^{-1}$ on the basis of the above assumptions.

Staying with this simplest model, we acknowledge the possibility that there may be a fraction, f, who do develop AIDS (with parameters β_1 and v_1 in eqns (11.17)–(11.20)), and a fraction, $1 - f$, who remain asymptomatic carriers (with parameters β_2 and v_2). It remains likely that Λ is significantly bigger than either v_1 or v_2 in this case, whence $\Lambda \sim c[f\beta_1 + (1 - f)\beta_2]$. If $(1 - f)\beta_2$ is significantly smaller than $f\beta_1$, which could easily be the case if 'carriers' are substantially less infectious than those who will develop clinical AIDS, we have $c\beta_1 \sim \Lambda/f$. That is, such effects could result in $c\beta_1$ being significantly larger than the value $c\beta \sim 1\,\mathrm{yr}^{-1}$ (from $\Lambda \sim 1\,yr^{-1}$) that we found by assuming $\beta_1 = \beta_2$.

A more important and relevant complication arises if there are two distinct phases of infectiousness, as was just discussed at some length. For either the 'distributed model' or the model with three distinct categories of infecteds, we found the over-simple eqn (11.25) replaced by the approximate result $\beta_0 c \simeq \Lambda + 1/T_0$. But T_0 is much shorter than the average incubation time, possibly as short as 0.5 to 1 year. Thus, if $\Lambda \sim 1\,\mathrm{yr}^{-1}$, this leads to the estimate $\beta_0 c \sim 2\text{--}3\,\mathrm{yr}^{-1}$. Notice that this gives a significantly higher estimate of β_0 (which is the transmission coefficient in only the first episode of infectiousness) than the $\beta c \sim 1\,\mathrm{yr}^{-1}$ found earlier using the simplest model. More generally, if infectiousness is much greater in the second episode, at the onset of AIDS, we have $\beta_1 \gg \beta_0$ and Fig. 11.24 or 11.25 must be used to draw inferences about the magnitude of $\beta_0 c$ and $\beta_1 c$ for any specified set of guesstimates of Λ, T_0, T_1, D, and β_1/β_0.

Crude and contingent though these estimates of βc are, they are of use in providing an indirect assessment of the value of β, once c has been estimated from sociological surveys. As we discussed earlier, there are some direct estimates of β, but such estimates are understandably hard to come by and could be for groups that are not representative of risk groups in general (most of the estimates come from studies of partners of people infected by blood transfusions). Independent estimates of values of β are correspondingly useful.

11.3.8 *Numerical results for more realistic models*

To describe the full course of the epidemic, beginning with the initial invasion and following on through the approach to the equilibrium state, we require a more complicated model than those outlined in the preceding sections. Added realism, however, necessitates the use of numerical methods to generate trajectories of the incidences of infection and disease as functions of time.

We think that the two most important complications that must be incorporated in the model are a distributed incubation period and heterogeneity in sexual activity. In this section we consider the dynamics of a model with these refinements, and restrict our attention to a male homosexual community.

We define $X(t, s)$ and $Y_2(t, s)$ as the number of susceptibles, and the number of infectious people who do not develop AIDS, at time t with sexual activity s (where s is the number of different partners per unit of time), respectively. We again assume that a proportion f of infectious individuals proceed to 'fully fledged' AIDS and a proportion $1 - f$ moves to a non-infectious seropositive state. We define the variable $Y_1(t, s, \tau)$ as the number of infectious people at time t, in the sexual-activity class s, who will go on to develop AIDS and who have been incubating the infection for a time τ. The rate of leaving this class is assumed to be a function of the time period over which an individual has been harbouring the virus, $v_1(\tau)$ (see Anderson *et al.* 1986). We make a very simple assumption concerning the form of $v_1(\tau)$, namely, that the rate is directly proportional to the duration of incubation ($v(\tau) = \alpha\tau$). As discussed above (eqn (11.46)), this so-called 'hazard function' for the duration of stay in the Y_1 class results in a probability distribution for the incubation period that is Weibüll in form (Cox and Oates 1984; Anderson *et al.* 1986). As also discussed earlier, this particular probability model provides a good empirical description of observed data on incubation times for patients infected with HIV via blood transfusions in the USA (Medley *et al.* 1987, 1988; Lui *et al.* 1986). The rate of leaving the Y_2 class (infectious individuals who do not develop AIDS) is assumed to be constant, and independent of the duration of incubation, with an average period of stay in this class of $1/v_2$.

These assumptions lead to the following set of partial differential equations for X_1, Y_1, Y_2, A, and Z:

$$dX(t, s)/dt = B(s) - sX(t, s)\lambda(t) - \mu X(t, s), \tag{11.68}$$

$$\partial Y_1(t, s, \tau)/\partial t + \partial Y_1((t, s, \tau)/\partial \tau = -(v_1(\tau) + \mu)Y_1(t, s, \tau), \tag{11.69a}$$

$$d Y_2(t, s)/dt = (1 - f)sX(t, s)\lambda(t) - (v_2 + \mu)Y_2(t, s), \tag{11.69b}$$

$$dA(t)/dt = \int_0^t \left(v(\tau) \int_0^\infty Y_1(t, s, \tau)\, ds \right) d\tau - (d + \mu)A(t), \tag{11.70a}$$

$$dZ(t)/dt = v_2 \int_0^\infty Y_2(t, s)\, ds - \mu Z(t). \tag{11.70b}$$

The force of infection, $\lambda(t)$, is defined as

$$\lambda(t) = \left[\beta \int_0^\infty s\left(\int_0^t Y_1(t, s, \tau)\, d\tau + Y_2(t, s) \right) ds \right]\left(\int_0^\infty sN(t, s)\, ds \right)^{-1}. \tag{11.71}$$

Here $N(t, s)$ is the total number of people at time t, with sexual activity pattern s. For simplicity, the transmission probability, β, is assumed to be constant and independent of the duration of time that an infected person has been incubating the disease. The term $B(s)$ denotes total rate of recruitment to the homosexual population, of individuals with sexual activity s. The boundary condition for eqn (11.69a) is

$$Y_1(t, s, 0) = fsX(t, s)\lambda(t). \tag{11.72}$$

From eqn (11.68), the number of susceptibles, $X(t, s)$, is

$$X(t, s) = X_0(s)\exp\left(-\mu t - s \int_0^t \lambda(u)\, du \right)$$

$$+ B(s) \int_0^t \exp\left(-\mu(t - h) - s \int_h^t \lambda(u)\, du \right) dh. \tag{11.73}$$

Here $X_0(s)$ is the number of susceptibles of activity s, at time $t = 0$.

If we assume that the distribution of sexual activity is described empirically by the gamma distribution with mean m and variance m^2/k (see eqn (11.43)), then the model can be expressed in terms of the parameters of the distribution, m and k (Anderson *et al.* 1986).

The model is complex in structure and numerical methods are required to explore its properties. The scale of the computational problem can be reduced somewhat by employing a discrete approximation to the continuous gamma distribution of sexual activity. For example, a series of sexual-partner classes can be defined (i.e. those individuals who have 0–1, 2–5, 6–9, 10–49, 50–99, and 100+ partners per year), and the mean number of partners for the ith class, s_i, and the mean recruitment rate, B_i, of susceptibles into this class may be calculated from gamma distributions with defined means (averaged over all classes) and variances (Anderson *et al.* 1986, 1987*b*).

Numerical studies of this model with discrete sexual-partner classes provide some insight into the manner in which the degree of sexual activity amongst homosexuals influences the pattern of the epidemic. Predictions about the way in which changes in the coefficient of variation, CV, of the distribution of sexual activity can affect the incidence of AIDS and the proportions seropositive in the at-risk community are presented in Fig. 11.27.

The graphs in this figure show clearly that increasing degrees of heterogeneity decrease the magnitude of the epidemic of AIDS and reduce the maximum level of seropositivity for HIV infection attained during the course of the epidemic, for a given value of R_0. A very high coefficient of variation implies that the population contains a small fraction of highly sexually active individuals, who are removed rapidly from the infectious pool (either by death from AIDS or by passage into the non-infectious seropositive class). The rapid removal of these individuals reduces the magnitude of the epidemic. The magnitude of the coefficient of variation has little influence on the time period that elapses from invasion to the peak in cases of AIDS.

Any trajectory for the overall incidence of AIDS within the entire community, through time, for a fixed value of the coefficient of variation in sexual activity, can be dissected into trajectories for each individual class of sexual activity (in the discrete approximation to the gamma distribution). Figure 11.28 records an example which shows changes in incidence and in seropositivity, through time, for six categories of sexual activity (0–1, 2–5, 6–9, 10–49, 50–99, and 100+ partners per year). As one might expect, the epidemic moves rapidly through the high-activity classes, and the level of seropositivity in such classes attains a very high value. Since these individuals form only a small fraction of the total community, their direct contribution to the total number of cases of AIDS is small. Their indirect contribution, in terms of initiating the spread of infection throughout the lower-activity classes is, however, substantial.

The general pattern of the epidemic predicted by the more complex model is similar in shape, magnitude, and timing to that predicted by much simpler models (compare Fig. 11.27 with Fig. 11.23). The variable incubation period tends to make the epidemic more 'spikey' and to produce a longer tail, compared with the predictions of models in which those with infectious HIV

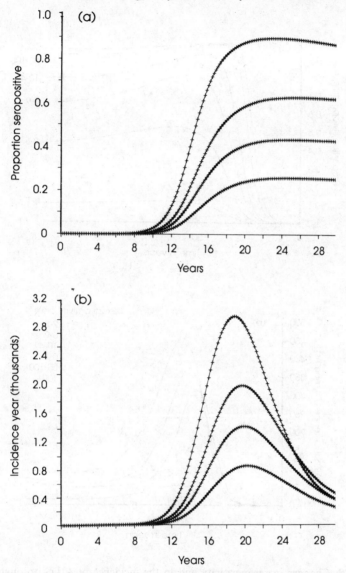

Fig. 11.27. Numerical solutions of the heterogeneous mixing model with recruitment of susceptibles (at a rate $B \, \mathrm{yr}^{-1}$) and a distributed incubation period (Weibüll distribution with the
mean set at 5 years), as defined by eqns (11.68)–(11.72) in the main text. The numerical methods
used to generate these solutions are discussed in Anderson *et al.* (1986) and the legend to Fig.
11.23, in which parameter values are defined. Graphs (a) and (b) record changes in: (a) the
proportion seropositive through time; and (b) the incidence of AIDS per year, for four different
values of the coefficient of variation (CV) of the distribution of sexual activity (defined as
partners per unit of time; the distribution is assumed to be a gamma distribution). The values
of CV are 0.45 (top curve), 1.0, 1.4, and 2.0 (bottom curve).

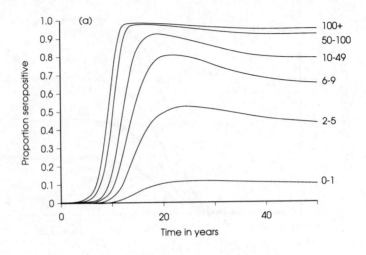

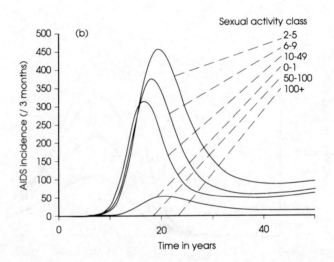

Fig. 11.28. Changes in seropositivity and in the incidence of AIDS, through time, as predicted by the discrete approximation to the heterogeneous mixing/variable incubation period model defined in eqns (11.68)–(11.72), stratified according to number of sexual partners. Graph (a) records seropositivity and graph (b) the incidence of AIDS (yr^{-1}). The six classes represent 0–1, 2–5, 6–9, 10–49, 50–99, and 100+ partners per year. Parameter values as for Figs. 11.23 and 11.27, with the mean incubation period set at 8 years (see Anderson *et al.* 1986, 1987*b*).

leave that class at some simple, constant rate. The differences, however, are minor.

One of the primary aims in the development and analysis of these more complex models is to refine attempts at predicting the likely course and magnitude of the current epidemic. The rationale behind such research is the urgent need to provide guidelines, no matter how crude, for future health planning. The depressing pictures provided by such projections add weight to publicity and educational campaigns that aim to encourage homosexuals and heterosexuals to change partners less frequently, to use condoms and otherwise engage in 'safer sex', and to discourage intravenous drug users from sharing needles.

There are many possible approaches to making predictions, ranging from the use of statistical procedures to fit simple functions (such as exponentials) to available incidence data, to the formulation of complex mathematical models of viral transmission within and between different risk groups. Statistical projections that reach more than two or three years ahead are unreliable, because there is no *a priori* reason to assume that extrapolation is valid. However, complex models are also unreliable because their predictions depend on the availability of detailed biological and epidemiological data. As we have repeatedly emphasized, such information is, as yet, very limited.

A good illustration of the problem is provided in a paper by Anderson *et al.* (1987*b*). This study attempts to predict the 'minimum' size of the AIDS epidemic in the United Kingdom under the extreme assumption that all transmission of the virus ceased at the beginning of 1987. The model defined by eqns (11.68)–(11.72) was employed to estimate the total number of cases of AIDS under two different assumptions concerning the mean incubation period of the disease. In one case, the mean incubation period was set at 4.3 years (Lui *et al.* 1986), and in the other cases it was set at 8 years (Medley *et al.* 1987). In both projections, the transmission probability β was estimated by fitting the projections over the interval 1978–86 to the observed data on the incidence of AIDS in the male homosexual population in the United Kingdom. The projections generated by the two different assumptions concerning the mean incubation period are recorded in Fig. 11.29. When the fraction who go on to develop AIDS was set at 0.5, with a 4.3 year mean incubation period, the prediction of the total number of deaths from AIDS was 7200 or so. In contrast, when the mean incubation period was set at 8 years, the total number of deaths was predicted to be around 19 000. This example illustrates well the way in which the predictions of models are sensitive to parameter values.

More generally, complex models for the spread of infectious disease can sometimes help in the emphasis and design of control programmes. In the case of AIDS, the only method of control currently available is education to promote safer sex practices, a reduction in prevailing levels of promiscuity, and the elimination of needle sharing among IV drug abusers. For sexual transmission, the model defined by eqns (11.68)–(11.72) can be used to assess the merits of

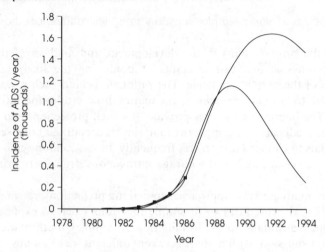

Fig. 11.29. Predicted changes in the incidence of AIDS (yr^{-1}), assuming that all transmission ceases at the beginning of 1987; this prediction is based on the numerical solution of eqns (11.68)–(11.72) (see Anderson *et al.* (1987*b*) for further details). The squares denote observed data for the incidence of AIDS among homosexual/bisexual men in the United Kingdom. The predictions are based on the assumption that $f = 0.5$ and that the average incubation period (Weibüll distribution) is either 8 years (top curve at 1992) or 4.3 years (bottom curve).

focusing such educational campaigns on specific groups within a community, such as those who change sex partners very frequently. The broad conclusion to emerge from numerical studies of this issue is that much is to be gained by reductions in the rate of change of sexual partners by those in the most active groups (i.e. the high-activity end of the distribution). This point is made much more explicitly in eqn (11.39), which is derived from the simple model of heterogeneity in transmission of HIV, defined by eqns (11.31)–(11.35). Reductions in the variance of sexual activity, σ^2, resulting from reductions in the rate of partner change in the high-activity tail of the distribution, have a much greater impact on c (the effective average rate of partner change) than do similar changes in the mean, m, of the distribution.

11.3.9 *Models for heterosexually transmitted HIV*

The accumulating evidence leaves no doubt that in sub-Saharan Africa AIDS has spread and is spreading by purely heterosexual transmission.

Figure 11.30 shows the distribution by age and sex of the first 500 cases of AIDS diagnosed in Kinshasa (the capital of Zaire, some aspects of whose social structure are captured in Naipaul's *The Bend in the River*) in the last half of 1985. There are roughly equal numbers of cases among males and females (45 to 55 per cent), and the age distributions correlate with probable levels of sexual activity (differently for males and females, as discussed below). The relatively

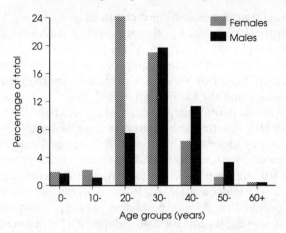

Fig. 11.30. Distribution by age and sex of the first 500 AIDS cases diagnosed in Kinshasa, Zaire, between August 1985 and December 1985 (data from Quinn *et al.* 1986).

low levels among those under 20 years of age seems to us to rule out any significant transmission from needle-sharing in public health programmes or from insect vectors.

Tests for HIV antibodies in blood sera stored from earlier studies (often for different purposes) show seropositivity levels among female prostitutes rising from 4 per cent in 1980–1 to around 51 per cent in 1983–4 and 59 per cent in 1985–6, and from 1 to 14 and 18 per cent at the corresponding times for males attending a clinic for sexually transmitted diseases, in Nairobi. Recent sero-prevalence levels among high-risk groups, such as female prostitutes, in Africa, have been reported to range from 27 to 88 per cent, depending on socioeconomic status and geographic location. In a general survey of pregnant women in Nairobi, seropositivity levels rose from 0 per cent in 1980–1 to 2 per cent in 1985–6. A similar survey of pregnant women in Kinshasa shows seropositivity levels rising from 0.2 per cent in 1970 to 3 per cent in 1980–1 and 8 per cent in 1985–6. More generally, the fraction seropositive among healthy populations (excluding diagnosed AIDS cases) appears to range from 0.7 per cent for blood donors in Zaire, to as high as 18 per cent for blood donors in Kigali, Rwanda (Quinn *et al.* 1986). A study of some 600 seronegative men and women working in a general hospital in Kinshasa, the capital of Zaire, from 1984 to 1985 found the annual incidence of HIV antibodies was around 0.8 per cent, a figure which Quinn *et al.* (1986) think may be representative of the annual incidence of new HIV infections in Central and East Africa.

Further evidence for heterosexual transmission as the dominant mode in Africa comes from a study of 2400 AIDS cases diagnosed in adults in Europe up to 31 March 1986. For the 2235 cases thought to originate in Europe or elsewhere other than Africa and the Caribbean, 92 per cent fall in the risk categories usual for adults in developed countries (homosexual/bisexual males, intervenous drug users, blood transfusions), with a male:female ratio of 16:1. For the cases thought to originate in Africa (177 cases) or the Caribbean (61 cases), only 10 per cent fell in these categories, and the male:female ratio was 1.6:1 (undoubtedly biased by the fact that more males than females travel to Europe from Africa and the Caribbean).

The kinds of mathematical analysis sketched earlier apply also to heterosexual transmission of HIV infection, except now we must deal with two reciprocating populations: males transmitting infection to females, and females transmitting infection to males. We need to consider separately the probability that an infected male will transmit infection to a susceptible female, β, and that an infected female will infect a male, β'. It seems likely that the male-to-female transmission probability, β, may be higher—possibly substantially higher—than the female-to-male transmission probability, β' (Peterman *et al.* 1988). For gonorrhoea, which is admittedly a weak analogy, β is roughly twice β'. Both transmission probabilities may, moreover, typically be higher in Africa than in developed countries owing to the widespread incidence of gonorrhoea, genital ulcers, syphilis, and other sexually transmitted diseases that often disrupt the integrity of the genital epithelia and thereby facilitate transmission of HIV during vaginal intercourse. In studies among prostitutes in Nairobi, HIV seropositivity was significantly correlated with the presence of other sexually transmitted diseases, and in another study in Zambia seropositivity in men was also correlated with the presence of genital ulcers; these may, of course, be correlation without causation.

Less obviously, we also need to know the two separate distributions in the rates of acquiring new sexual partners by males and by females. As before, the quantities that influence the dynamics of transmission are not simply the mean numbers of new sexual partners per unit time, but rather the ratio of mean-square to mean numbers, c for males acquiring female partners and c' for females acquiring male partners. Although the mean rate at which males acquire new female sexual partners must obviously be identical with the mean rate at which females acquire male partners, c and c' will not be identical if the variability in levels of sexual activity among males differs significantly from that among females. This point will be developed further below, using an illustrative numerical example which may be broadly representative of the situation in some parts of Africa.

11.3.9.1 *A simple model*   For a simple model which captures some of the essential dynamics of heterosexually transmitted HIV infection, we include the effects of heterogeneity in rates of acquiring new sexual partners but assume that the transmission coefficients (β, β') and rates of moving out of the infectious class (v) are constant; that is, we do not deal with the complications introduced by bimodal or other time-dependent transmission probabilities nor with the complications attendant upon distributed incubation times. We use primes to denote variables pertaining to the female population, so that the number of susceptible and infectious individuals in the ith category of sexual activity are X_i and Y_i for males, and X_i' and Y_i' for females, respectively. The basic equations in this simple model for HIV transmission within a closed population are then:

$$dX_i/dt = -i\lambda X_i, \tag{11.74}$$

$$dY_i/dt = i\lambda X_i - vY_i, \tag{11.75}$$

$$dX_i'/dt = -i\lambda'X_i', \tag{11.76}$$

$$dY_i'/dt = i\lambda'X_i' - vY_i'. \tag{11.77}$$

The quantity λ represents the probability that any one (randomly chosen) female partner will infect a susceptible male, and λ' correspondingly represents the probability that a male will infect a female. Under the assumptions discussed above for homosexual transmission, we may write

$$\lambda = \beta' \sum j Y_j' (\sum j N_j')^{-1}, \tag{11.78}$$

$$\lambda' = \beta \sum j Y_j (\sum j N_j)^{-1}. \tag{11.79}$$

Here β and β' are the male-to-female and female-to-male transmission probabilities, respectively, as discussed above. N_j and N_j' are the total number of males and females, respectively, in the class having j new sexual partners per unit time. This simple model deals with a closed population, and neglects mortality from causes other than AIDS. More accurate models—particularly if directed toward longer-term predictions—need to incorporate the effects of birth and death rates (especially in countries with rapidly growing populations), along with the effects of vertical transmission upon the effective birth rate. For the moment, however, we deal with some insights that can be gained from the simple model defined by eqns (11.74)–(11.79).

11.3.9.2 *Early stages of the epidemic*

In the early stages of the epidemic, we may assume, in the by-now familiar way, that essentially everyone is susceptible, so that $X_i \simeq N_i$ and $X_i' \simeq N_i'$. Substituting these approximations into eqns (11.75) and (11.77), respectively, and then multiplying by i and summing over all sexual-activity classes i in each equation, we obtain linear approximations for the dynamics of the forces of infection, λ and λ', in the early stages of the epidemic:

$$d\lambda/dt = \beta'c'\lambda' - v\lambda, \tag{11.80}$$

$$d\lambda'/dt = \beta c\lambda - v\lambda'. \tag{11.81}$$

Here c is the mean-square/mean number of female partners of males, $c = \langle i^2 \rangle / \langle i \rangle$ averaged over the distribution $\{N_i\}$; c' correspondingly is the mean-square/mean number of male partners of females, $c' = \langle i^2 \rangle / \langle i \rangle$ averaged over the distribution $\{N_i'\}$.

The solution to the pair of linear eqns (11.80) and (11.81) behaves, in the usual way, as a linear combination of the factors $\exp(\Lambda_k t)$, where the two eigenvalues, Λ_k ($k = 1, 2$), are given by the quadratic equation

$$(\Lambda + v)^2 - \beta c \beta' c' = 0. \tag{11.82}$$

The behaviour of λ and λ' in the very first stages of the epidemic depends on the details of the initial conditions, but these transients rapidly give way to a phase of approximately exponential growth, as $\exp(\Lambda t)$, where Λ is the dominant root of eqn (11.82):

$$\Lambda = (\beta c \beta' c')^{1/2} - v. \tag{11.83}$$

This phase of exponential growth lasts until saturation effects begin to be pronounced, with a significant fraction of those in the highest-risk groups (those with the highest rates of acquiring new sexual partners) being infected. In this exponential growth phase, $\lambda(t)$ behaves as

$$\lambda(t) \sim A \, e^{\Lambda t}. \tag{11.84}$$

Here the constant A is essentially set by the initial conditions. The corresponding behaviour of $\lambda'(t)$ follows from eqn (11.81), which gives $\lambda'(t) = [\beta c / (\Lambda + v)]\lambda(t)$. Using eqn (11.83) for Λ, we thus see that, in the early phase of approximately exponential growth, the quantities λ and λ' are related by

$$\lambda'(t) = (\beta c / \beta' c')^{1/2}\lambda(t). \tag{11.85}$$

In this simple model, new cases of AIDS appear at the rate vY_i or vY'_i; this is the rate at which males or females in the ith class of sexual activity pass into the 'AIDS disease' category, A_i or A'_i, respectively. It follows that the incidence of new cases among males in the ith group, $C_i = vY_i$, is given from eqn (11.75) approximately (in the exponential growth phase) as

$$C_i = \frac{i\lambda v N_i}{\Lambda + v} = iN_i B \, e^{\Lambda t}. \tag{11.86}$$

Here the constant B is related to the A of eqn (11.84) by $B = vA / (\beta c \beta' c')^{1/2}$. Similarly, using eqn (11.85), the incidence of AIDS cases among females in the ith category of sexual activity is

$$C'_i = iN'_i (\beta c / \beta' c')^{1/2} B \, e^{\Lambda t}. \tag{11.87}$$

The total incidence of AIDS cases among males, $C(t)$, is obtained by summing over all classes, $\{N_i\}$, to get

$$C(t) = mNB \, e^{\Lambda t}. \tag{11.88}$$

Here m is the mean rate at which new sexual partners are acquired; as remarked earlier, m must be the same for males and females. The corresponding expression for the total incidence of AIDS cases among females, $C'(t)$, is similarly obtained from eqn (11.87). We thus have the interesting result that, in the early phase of approximately exponential growth, the incidences of AIDS cases among males and females are in the ratio

$$C/C' = (\beta'c'/\beta c)^{1/2}. \tag{11.89}$$

Thus in the early, exponentially growing stages of such an epidemic of heterosexually transmitted HIV infection, we expect the ratio of seropositivity levels, or of AIDS cases, among males to that among females to be roughly constant, at around $(\beta'c'/\beta c)^{1/2}$. Notice that this result is in direct contradiction to the expectation—explicitly or implicitly stated in essentially all writing on this subject—that the ratio of HIV infections, and thence of AIDS cases, among males and females should be roughly equal if infection is transmitted hetero-sexually. Indeed, given the expectation that male-to-female transmission prob-ability, β, may be significantly larger than the female-to-male probability, β', we could regard the 1:1 sex ratio among cases more as a problem to be explained than as a confirmation of heterosexual transmission.

If we were heedless of variability in the degrees of sexual activity within male and female populations, c and c' would be identical, both being simply equal to the average rate, m, at which new sexual partners were acquired. But we have seen that $c \sim m + \sigma^2/m$, where σ^2 is the variance in the rates at which different males acquire new partners (with a parallel expression for c'). In much of Central Africa it may be that most females have relatively monogamous marriages or 'union libres' (persistent cohabitation without formal marriage), but that many of the male partners in such relationships may be less monogamous, with the books kept in balance by a cadre of young female prostitutes who are very sexually active. In this event, the variance term is likely to be greater among females than among males, $(\sigma')^2 > \sigma^2$, resulting in c' (the *effective* average rate at which females acquire new male partners) being significantly larger than c (the effective average rate at which males acquire new female partners). That is to say, such differences in the distributions of degrees of sexual activity among males and females in Africa probably leads to ratios of c'/c that are significantly above unity. This, in turn, can counterbalance the above-noted expectation that β'/β is likely to be significantly below unity. By the time one takes the square root of the product of these counterbalancing ratios in eqn (11.89), it would not be surprising to have a number around unity. We believe this is probably the real, and more complicated, explanation for the ratio of male to female cases of AIDS in Africa being around unity.

With the above assumptions about qualitative differences in male and female patterns of sexual activity in Africa, a more detailed analysis of the dynamics of heterosexual transmission leads us to expect the 'core group' of female prostitutes relatively rapidly to obtain high levels of seropositivity, accompanied by moderate levels among males and lower levels among the female population more generally. This accords with the observations about seropositivity levels in Africa among female prostitutes, men attending clinics, and pregnant women, that were discussed above. The theoretical analysis also matches Fig. 11.30, where the average age of female AIDS patients is significantly below that for males (30 years versus 37 years); in this study, females with AIDS were more likely than males to be unmarried (61 per cent versus 36 per cent). Another study, in Kigali in Rwanda, identified 43 per cent of female AIDS patients as prostitutes.

More generally, a growing number of data confirm the correlation between rates of acquiring new sexual partners and the probability of acquiring HIV infection or AIDS disease, both for heterosexual transmission in Africa and homosexual transmission in the developed world. Reviewing data from Africa, Quinn *et al.* (1986) report that 'case-control studies have shown that AIDS patients have a significantly higher number of heterosexual partners than controls (mean of 32 versus 3) ... and that the risk of seropositivity increases significantly with the number of different sexual partners per year'. Figure 11.15 earlier indicated a similar correlation between HIV seropositivity levels and numbers of sexual partners among homosexuals in San Francisco.

11.3.9.3 *An illustrative numerical example*   Purely for illustrative purposes, we consider a numerical example in which HIV infection is transmitted hetero-sexually within a population in which all males are moderately promiscuous, all having around five new (female) sexual partners per year, while the female population is more heterogeneous in its sexual habits with 90 per cent having one new (male) partner per year and the other 10 per cent having on average 41 new partners annually. Both male and female populations have the same average number of five new sexual partners per year, as they clearly must. For males, the epidemiologically relevant quantity is also $c = 5$ per year (because $\sigma^2 = 0$). But for females, the ratio of mean-square to mean number of partners is $c' = (0.9 \times 1 + 0.1 \times (41)^2)/5 \simeq 34$ per year. This example, although constructed artificially, may be broadly representative of the situation in some parts of Africa. We see that the female prostitutes have a disproportionate impact on the transmission of infection, with their greater sexual activity giving them a greater propensity both to acquire and to transmit infection; the overall effect is as if females, on average, acquired new sexual partners at a rate roughly seven times (34/5) that of males.

Suppose further that the male-to-female transmission probability is five times larger than the female-to-male one, with $\beta = 0.2$ and $\beta' = 0.04$. The ratio in the overall incidence of AIDS cases among males and females in the early stages of the epidemic would then, in this illustrative example, be given from eqn (11.89) as around 1.2. But we can see that this ratio of around unity has arisen in a complicated way, and is not a simple consequence of heterosexual transmission as such. Using eqn (11.87), we see in more detail that the incidence of AIDS among females in the ith sexual-activity class is proportional to i. Thus, in our illustrative example, the incidence of AIDS among female prostitutes is greater than among males in general by a factor $(41/5)(0.86) \simeq 7$, while AIDS incidence among the rest of the female population is lower than among the male population in general by a factor $(1/5)(0.86) \simeq 1/6$.

11.3.9.4 *Basic reproductive rate for HIV infection*

In the above model for heterosexually transmitted HIV infection, the basic reproductive rate, R_0, can be seen to be

$$R_0 = (\beta c \beta' c')^{1/2}/v. \qquad (11.90)$$

One way of obtaining this result is to apply the standard expression for the exponential growth phase, $\Lambda = v(R_0 - 1)$, to eqn (11.77) for Λ.

In analogy with our earlier analysis of the total fraction, I_i, of individuals in the ith category ever to be infected in an epidemic in a closed population, we can show from eqns (11.74)–(11.77) that for males

$$I_i = 1 - \exp(-i\alpha). \qquad (11.91)$$

The proportion of females in the ith class ever to be infected, I_i', is similarly given by

$$I_i' = 1 - \exp(-i\alpha'). \qquad (11.92)$$

Here the parameter α is defined as $\alpha = \int \lambda(t)\,dt$, with a corresponding definition for α'. The parameters α and α' are determined self-consistently from the appropriate analogues of eqn (11.41):

$$\alpha = \frac{\beta'c'}{v}\left(\sum i[1 - \exp(-i\alpha')]N_i'\right)\left(\sum i^2 N_i'\right)^{-1}, \qquad (11.93)$$

$$\alpha' = \frac{\beta c}{v}\left(\sum i[1 - \exp(-i\alpha)]N_i\right)\left(\sum i^2 N_i\right)^{-1}. \qquad (11.94)$$

It can be seen that non-trivial solutions for α and α' exist only if $R_0 > 1$, with R_0 defined by eqn (11.90).

11.3.10 *Possible future trends in the AIDS epidemic*

Predictions about the course of the epidemic past its early stages, and in particular predictions about the total number of cases, depend essentially on knowing the incubation period, the patterns of infectiousness, and the distribution in sexual habits (possibly characterized by the coefficient of variation in the number of partners). Some of the essential aspects of this information can be characterized by the parameters f and R_0 (see Fig. 11.23). If we assume that $\beta_1 = \beta_2$, R_0 is given crudely from eqn (11.30) as $R_0 = \beta c[f/(\mu + v_1) + (1 - f)/(\mu + v_2)]$. If βc can be roughly estimated, from early doubling rates, the remaining uncertainties are about f and about v_1 and v_2.

In a homogeneous population, the incidence of clinical AIDS cases around the point where the epidemic peaks is given very roughly by

$$\text{peak incidence} \sim f v_1. \tag{11.95}$$

This peak incidence is expressed as a fraction of the total population. An exact expression for the peak incidence of infection in a homogeneous population (which is equal to $v y_{max}$) is given by eqn (6.20), which can be seen to reduce to eqn (11.95) when R_0 is significantly in excess of unity. The presence of carriers and of heterogeneity in sexual habits produce complications, but eqn (11.95) remains a good back-of-an-envelope estimate (so long as R_0 is appreciably greater than unity), and is consistent with broad trends seen in Fig. 11.23. The result (11.95) arises essentially because a fraction f of those infected move into the class with full-blown AIDS at a rate v_1, following the initial stages of the epidemic in which (for R_0 large) most of the population is infected. Thus observations of the incidence of clinical AIDS as the epidemic begins to peak give a very rough estimate of the combination f/D, where $D = 1/v_1$ is the average interval between infection and diagnosed AIDS. For example, if a peak incidence of clinical AIDS of 2–3 per cent of the at-risk population were found each year, we could roughly estimate $f \sim 10$ per cent if D is around 3–4 years—or $f \sim 50$ per cent if D is around 15–20 years—and so on.

The long-term public health issues, however, depend more on the total fraction of the at-risk population who are likely to develop clinical AIDS, that is (for R_0 large) upon f. As discussed above, the observed levels of seropositivity suggest R_0 is unlikely to be less than around three, and it may well have a value of five or more. With $\beta c \sim 1 \, yr^{-1}$, this means the factor inside the square brackets two paragraphs above is likely to have a value of 5 years or more. But this value could be attained in two ways, which have different implications for estimates of f. On the one hand, if $v_1 \simeq v_2$, we have the estimates that D is around 5 years or more, whence observations about peak incidence of AIDS lead to a crude estimate of f. On the other hand, if $1/v_2 \gg 1/v_1$, it could be that the value of $R_0/\beta c$ is determined essentially by $1/v_2$, whence the above argument gives virtually no information about D, and thus is of no help in putting bounds on f.

These arguments can be refined into more quantitative estimates, with the help of numerical studies of the kind reported in Figs. 11.22 and 11.23(a, b). An essential ambiguity remains, however, in whether diagnosed AIDS-developers and carriers do or do not have similar durations of infectiousness; that is, whether $v_1 \simeq v_2$ or not. The analysis presented above suggests some ways of gathering information to resolve this issue.

Consider first the incidence of infection (as revealed by seropositivity) as a function of time, among classes of individuals distinguished according to levels of sexual activity. As shown in Fig. 11.31(a), if $v_1 = v_2$ there is a tendency for the more sexually active individuals to acquire infection earlier, and less active individuals later, so that the ratio of more sexually active to less sexually active individuals among those infected shifts as the epidemic progresses.

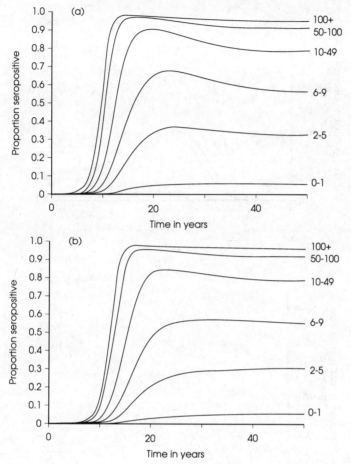

Fig. 11.31. Changes in seropositivity in six classes denoting different rates of change of sexual partners (0–1, 2–5, 6–9, 10–49, 50–99, 100+ per year) as predicted by the heterogeneous mixing model with variable incubation periods defined in eqns (11.68) to (11.72). In graph (a) the parameters v_1 and v_2 are set equal at $1/8$ yr^{-1}. In graph (b) $v_1 = 1/5$ yr^{-1} and $v_2 = 1/20$ yr^{-1}.

As seen in Fig. 11.31(b), this tendency is much more pronounced if v_1 is substantially greater than v_2 (carriers on average remain infectious significantly longer than diagnosed AIDS-developers): the more active people tend to acquire infection early on, whereas infection among the less active fraction of the population slowly builds up over time, depending primarily on the long-lived infectiousness of carriers. Systematically compiled serological data that discriminate among the levels of sexual activity of recently infected individuals, over time, should in this way be capable of shedding light on the ratio between v_1 and v_2.

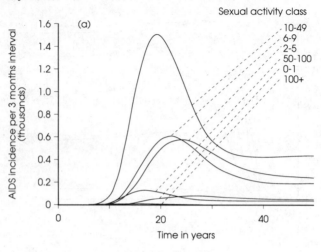

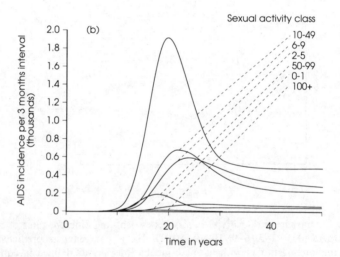

Fig. 11.32. Changes in the incidence of AIDS in sex classes denoting different rates of change of sexual partners, as defined in the legend to Fig. 11.31. In (a) the parameters v_1 and v_2 are set at $1/8 \, \text{yr}^{-1}$. In (b) $v_1 = 1/5 \, \text{yr}^{-1}$ and $v_2 = 1/20 \, \text{yr}^{-1}$.

The same general considerations apply to incidence of newly diagnosed cases of full-blown AIDS, distinguished according to levels of sexual activity in the patients, as a function of time. Here, however, the patterns are more blurred, ·by virtue of the statistical distribution of times between acquiring infection and manifesting full-blown AIDS. Figures 11.32(a) and (b) correspond to Figs. 11.31(a) and (b), illustrating the incidence of cases of diagnosed AIDS disease, among more sexually active individuals and among less active ones, as a function of time. Figure 11.32(a) is for $v_1 = v_2$ and Fig. 11.32(b) is for $v_1 = 0.2 \text{ yr}^{-1}$ and $v_2 = 0.05 \text{ yr}^{-1}$. The trends seen in Figs. 11.31(a) and (b) are again evident, although somewhat less pronounced. Again, systematic investigation of data of this kind could help determine the ratio of v_1 to v_2.

On another tack, it would be helpful to look at the incidence of diagnosed AIDS disease, as a function of time, among those individuals who were most sexually active. Most of these people are likely to have acquired infection early on, so that their distribution of incidence of disease over time gives a reasonable indication of the actual distribution of incubation times (in a way that is not possible if all data, from more active along with less active people, are combined). Such analyses could help provide an independent estimate of whether the distribution of incubation times found among those infected with HIV by blood transfusions are indeed representative of broader categories of HIV infections.

Whether AIDS will establish itself as an endemic disease in the USA and Europe depends on whether sexual habits change sufficiently to push R_0 below unity. This requires the distribution in the number of sexual partners per unit time among homosexuals to decrease to a level such that

$$c' < c/R_0. \tag{11.96}$$

Here R_0 is the initial value of the basic reproductive rate for AIDS, estimates of which we have just discussed, and c and c' are the initial and later values, respectively, of the appropriate average over the distribution in sexual habits ($c = m + \sigma^2/m = \langle i^2 \rangle / \langle i \rangle$). Downward changes in the mean clearly help. But downward changes at the high end of the distribution help disproportionately, because they have more effect on $\langle i^2 \rangle$. Alternatively, R_0 can be lowered by changes in the intrinsic transmission parameter β ('safe sex'). In either event, it is clear that the magnitude of the changes needed to drive R_0 below unity depend on how large R_0 originally was; as we have seen, this number is uncertain, but is unlikely to be less than five or so.

All the above discussion has treated AIDS as a disease of homosexuals. Needle-sharing among intravenous drug users involves the same ideas, with different values for the transmission factors β and c, but the same parameters characterizing the course of infection. For such transmission, βc can be estimated from initial doubling times, and the above discussion repeated, *mutatis mutandis*.

The same is true for heterosexual transmission, which is currently low in developed countries but high in many sub-Saharan African countries. As we have seen, simple models for purely heterosexual transmission suggest that in the earlier stages of the epidemic—before any subgroup becomes saturated with infection—the incidence of HIV infection and of AIDS cases among males and among females grows roughly exponentially at the same rate in both populations. The doubling rate (which previously was $\beta c - 1/D$) is now approximately $(\beta c \beta' c')^{1/2} - 1/D$, where D is the average duration of infectiousness. In developing countries, we would expect to find the female-to-male transmission probability, β', and probably also the male-to-female transmission probability, β, less than the transmission probability among homosexuals. We would also expect the appropriately averaged rates of acquiring new sexual partners by women and by men, c' and c, to be less than the corresponding quantity for homosexuals in large cities in the developed world in the early 1980s. As was discussed in the section on epidemiological parameters, data from recent studies in the United Kingdom suggest a factor 10 to 20 difference in the average rate at which male homosexuals and male heterosexuals acquire new partners (see Fig. 11.16). Overall, therefore, we would expect the doubling rate to be smaller—and the doubling time to be longer—for HIV infections transmitted along heterosexual chains than along homosexual ones in developed countries.

Whether or not a self-sustaining epidemic can be generated by purely heterosexual transmission in developed countries depends on the magnitude of the basic reproductive rate for such transmission; this quantity is given approximately by $R_0 = (\beta c \beta' c')^{1/2} D$. Such an epidemic is likely to take off if R_0 exceeds unity, and not otherwise. At present, uncertainty surrounds each one of the five quantities entering into this expression for R_0 (especially the female-to-male transmission probability, β'), nor are there enough data to attempt the kind of indirect inference of R_0 from population-level considerations, as we did for homosexual transmission in developed countries. We believe that reasonable estimates span a range of R_0 values from below unity to above unity.

Bearing all this in mind, our guess is that, in developed countries, HIV could well spread by purely heterosexual transmission within relatively promiscuous subgroups. The long-term possibility of a much more generally disseminated epidemic seems to us to depend crucially on whether a significant fraction of HIV infectees remain asymptomatic carriers (never developing AIDS), transmitting infection with some low probability essentially for the remainder of their sexually active lives. If this is so, then quite modest levels of promiscuity could result in HIV infections spreading slowly, over many decades, among a population who would not think of themselves as promiscuous. In our earlier language, such a long duration of infectiousness among a significant fraction of infectees corresponds to the basic reproductive rate, R_0, for heterosexually transmitted HIV being appreciably greater than unity.

This brings us to a final and important point to do with predicting AIDS cases. It might at first seem that the larger the fraction of HIV infectees who go on to develop AIDS and die, the larger the eventual number of deaths from the epidemic. This is not necessarily so. Contrast the following two possibilities, neither of which can be completely ruled out by currently available data: in Case A, 30 per cent of those infected develop AIDS, remaining infectious typically for 5 years and then dying, while the remaining 70 per cent of those infected remain asymptomatic yet infectious for 30 years; in Case B, 100 per cent of those infected develop AIDS, remaining infectious typically for 8 years and then dying. Notice immediately that the characteristic duration of infectiousness is larger in Case A ($0.3 \times 5 + 0.7 \times 30 = 22.5$ years) than in Case B (8 years); this means that the basic reproductive rate for HIV infection is almost three times greater under assumption A than under B, if the transmission probability is assumed to be the same in both cases. The total number of deaths caused by AIDS in either case depends on the fraction ever infected with HIV and on the fraction of those infected who develop AIDS. For Case A, with its substantially larger basic reproductive rate, a larger fraction of the population will acquire HIV infection, but a smaller proportion (30 per cent) of these will die. In contrast, in Case B a smaller fraction will be infected, but all who are will die. We simply cannot say whether Case A or Case B will result in a larger total number of deaths, until we have made a detailed analysis of the non-linear way in which the differences in the basic reproductive rates are likely to affect the numbers ever infected. The results of such a calculation are sensitive to the amount of variability in degrees of sexual activity; the greater this variability, the more likely that Case A will lead to more deaths than Case B, in defiance of simple intuition.

For homosexually transmitted HIV infection in developed countries, our preliminary calculations suggest that the total number of AIDS deaths increases as f (the fraction of HIV infectees going on to develop full-blown AIDS) increases up to around 50 per cent or so, but that total deaths remain roughly constant, or can even decrease, as f increases toward 100 per cent. As emphasized at the outset, current evidence cannot rule out f values as low as 20–30 per cent nor as high as 100 per cent. Given this uncertainty, it is well to recognize that projected total deaths do not simply rise as estimates of f rise, but rather that non-linearities in the transmission processes can produce counter-intuitive outcomes not easily foreseen by curve-fitting.

11.4 Summary

We begin this chapter by discussing the endemic maintenance of sexually transmitted diseases, STDs. In particular, we outline the work of Hethcote, Yorke and others on gonorrhoea in the USA, highlighting their conclusion that heterogeneity in degrees of sexual activity within the overall population is important in transmission and control. A more formal discussion is given of STDs in populations where the variability in sexual habits is described by the distribution of probabilities, $P(i)$, of having i sexual partners per unit time; the epidemiologically appropriate 'average' number of partners is seen to be roughly $c = m + \sigma^2/m$, where m is the mean and σ^2 the variance of the $P(i)$ distribution.

We then give an extensive account of the epidemic transmission of STDs, using homosexually transmitted AIDS in developed countries and hetero-sexually transmitted AIDS in developing countries as examples. We review the epidemiological and other data that are available, emphasizing both the relation between the data and information needed to predict the future course of events, and the role that mathematical models can play in this process.

12

Spatial and other kinds of heterogeneity

The main aim of this chapter is to consider how the design of immunization programmes can be affected when a population is distributed non-uniformly in space in such a way that the rates of transmission of an infectious disease are significantly higher in some places than in others.

We begin by sketching some of the background to this problem, paying attention to such scanty data as are available about the way transmission rates depend on population density. Several workers have noted that spatial or other inhomogeneities can result in the basic reproductive rate, R_0, of a microparasitic infection being in reality larger than would be estimated by treating the population as if it were homogeneously mixed. This, in turn, implies that the infection may be harder to eradicate under a uniformly applied immunization programme—a larger proportion of the population must be vaccinated—than simple estimates might suggest. We next give an explicit analysis of this phenomenon, using a simple model which has the advantage of making the basic ideas clear (but which undoubtedly overestimates the effects of spatial inhomogeneities in population density upon transmission rates). We go on to define an optimum eradication programme as that which, by treating different groups differently, achieves its aim by immunizing the smallest overall number of people. This optimum programme is seen to require *fewer* immunizations than would be estimated under the (false) assumption that the population is homogeneously mixed. The chapter concludes by outlining how these ideas about optimal versus uniform immunization programmes may be applied in other contexts, where the effects of family size or other social factors can lead to variabilities in transmission rates.

12.1 Spatial heterogeneity

12.1.1 *Dependence of transmission coefficients on population density*

Up to this point, we have been in the habit of writing a simple relationship between the force of infection, λ, and the transmission coefficient, β, as $\lambda = \beta Y$, where Y is the total number or density of infectives. Equivalently, we could write

$$\lambda = (\beta N)(Y/N). \tag{12.1}$$

Throughout this chapter, as in Chapter 11, we omit the 'bar' denoting total numbers, so that X, Y, N are the total numbers or density of susceptibles, infectives, and hosts (summed over all ages), respectively. In eqn (12.1) Y/N represents the fraction infected, or the probability that any one, randomly chosen, contact is infected, while βN represents the effective number of 'contacts' with other people times the probability that such a contact (if infected) will transmit infection. As written, the dependence of βN on the total population size or density, N, has been irrelevant, because up to this point we have consistently assumed N to be unchanging. But once N is changing over time (Chapter 13), or varying among groups (as here), we must face the question of how the transmission factor βN actually varies with N. At one extreme, it could be that a typical individual's number of contacts with others increases linearly with N, in which case the appropriate transmission factor would be just βN, with β a constant. At the other extreme, it could be that each individual has effective contact with some roughly fixed number of people, with the number determined by social and environmental factors but independent of N; in this case we would have βN roughly constant, corresponding to β itself depending on N roughly as $\beta(N) = \beta_0/N$.

Some data bearing on the dependence of the transmission factor, βN, upon population density, N, for childhood diseases are given in Fig. 12.1 (from Anderson 1982*b*). These data suggest that βN has behaviour intermediate between the extremes of depending linearly on N and not depending on N at all. The observed N-dependence can be characterized by writing $\beta N \rightarrow \beta_0 N^v$ ($1 \geqslant v \geqslant 0$), with the parameter v having small but finite values; this corresponds to

$$\beta(N) = \beta_0 N^{v-1}. \tag{12.2}$$

Further evidence for the significant—although much weaker than linear—dependence of βN on population density comes from Arita *et al.*'s (1986) study of smallpox eradication, which was discussed in Chapter 5. In Chapter 3, Fig. 3.10(b) showed that the median age of measles cases in West and Central Africa was significantly lower in urban regions than in rural ones. As discussed earlier, low ages at infection imply high forces of infection, and thus relatively high transmission rates, so that Fig. 3.10(b) can be taken as testimony that transmission rates in Africa are higher (by as much as a factor of three) in dense urban aggregations than in isolated villages. Unlike the data in Fig. 12.1, however, these smallpox and measles data do not lend themselves to a quantitative assessment of the functional dependence of $\beta(N)$ on N.

12.1.2 *Effects of variable transmission rates on immunization programmes*

Motivated by the above considerations, Murray and Cliff (1975) used stochastic simulations in pursuit of an understanding of the observed epidemiology of measles in circumstances where several distinct regions are linked relatively weakly. Mathematical models embodying such spatial heterogeneity have been explored by several authors (Hethcote 1978; Nold 1980; Post *et al.* 1983; C. C. Travis and S. M. Lenhart, private communication); most of this work is concerned with formal expressions for the conditions under which the infection can maintain itself in the population.

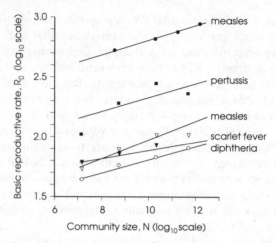

Fig. 12.1. The relationship between the logarithm of the basic reproductive rate, R_0, and community size, N, for various childhood microparasitic infections. The squares, circles, and triangles represent estimated values of R_0 based on case notification data: measles (open triangles), England and Wales 1950–5; measles (full circles), USA 1918–19; pertussis (full squares), USA 1918–19; scarlet fever (full triangles), USA 1918–19; diphtheria (open circles), USA 1918–19. The full lines denote the best fit linear models (slopes lie between 0.03 and 0.07) (from Anderson 1982*b*)..

Other authors have adopted a somewhat more intuitive approach, pointing out that the effects of spatial heterogeneity upon R_0 can sometimes be estimated as

$$R_0 = \bar{R}_0(1 + \text{var}(\beta)). \tag{12.3}$$

Here $\bar{R}_0$ is the value of the basic reproductive rate obtained by using the *average* value of the transmission parameters β, and var(β) represents the variance exhibited by β. In detail, most of the studies that lead to eqn (12.3)—or something essentially equivalent—are for schistosomiasis (Barbour 1978), malaria (Dye and Hasibeder 1986), or other parasites whose transmission cycle involves an intermediate vector (Dietz 1980); in this case, var(β) more specifically corresponds to the covariance between rates of transmission from primary to intermediate hosts and from intermediate to primary hosts. In general, however, eqn (12.3) can represent any circumstances where spatial heterogeneity leads to variability in the transmission parameter (Fine 1982; Anderson 1982*b*). Although it is acknowledged that the covariance effects could in principle be negative (for instance, patterns of human settlement could lead to patches of high vector density being associated with low host density, or dense urban aggregates could have higher standards of hygiene that effectively reduced trans- mission rates), most of the above authors have emphasized that the effects encapsulated in eqn (12.3) are likely to result in the actual value of R_0 being larger than estimated from average contact rates, $\bar{R}_0$.

Our earlier discussions, in Chapter 5, emphasized that, for a homogeneously mixed population, the critical fraction, p_c, that must be successfully immunized in order to eradicate infection is

$$p_c = 1 - x^*. \tag{12.4}$$

Here x^* is the fraction of the population who are susceptible, in the equilibrium state before any immunization. Equation (12.4), it will be remembered, itself derived from the result $p_c = 1 - (1/R_0)$ (which was derived on essentially ecological grounds), along with the relation $R_0 x^* = 1$ for a homogeneously mixed population at equilibrium.

If the population is not homogeneously mixed, it will still usually be true that $p_c = 1 - (1/R_0)$, where R_0 is the true reproductive rate of the infection (that is, the R_0 on the left-hand side of eqn (12.3)). But eqn (12.3) suggests that the actual vaue of R_0 is usually larger than that estimated from average contact rates, $\bar{R}_0$. It follows that p_c will usually be higher than estimated from eqn (12.4) using the simple average value of x^* (which is closer to $1/\bar{R}_0$ than to $1/R_0$).

In short, spatial inhomogeneities are likely to result in an infection being more difficult to eradicate (that is, requiring a larger proportion of the population to be immunized) under an uniformly applied immunization programme than simple estimates based on homogeneous mixing (eqn (12.4)) suggest. The essential reason for this is intuitively understandable: by immunizing the same fraction in all groups, we are immunizing relatively too many in small groups and relatively too few in large groups; the latter effect outweighs the former, and to eradicate the infection we simply must immunize a larger fraction than suggested by estimates that assume homogeneity.

We now proceed to give a more explicit account of these and other considerations, within the framework of a deliberately oversimplified model.

12.1.3 *A model with spatial heterogeneity*

Following Hethcote (1978), Post *et al.* (1983), and others, we consider a populaton that is subdivided spatially into n groups, with N_i individuals in the ith group. Births and deaths are assumed to balance in each group, so that all N_i are constant. In this spatially inhomogeneous situation, we assume that the force of infection in the ith group, λ_i, is a weighted sum over all infected individuals:

$$\lambda_i = \sum_{j=1}^{n} \beta_{ij} Y_j. \tag{12.5}$$

This leads to a particular case of the general formalism set out in Chapter 10, eqns (10.21)–(10.30).

In order to proceed, we must make some explicit assumption about the dependence of β_{ij} on N_j. For our illustrative calculations, we make the extreme assumption that transmission probability rises linearly with population density.

That is, we assume that, within any one patch, the parameter $\beta_{ii}(N_i)$ is simply a constant, β, so that the overall transmission factor is βN_i. Likewise the inter-group transmission probability, β_{ij}, is some constant (independent of N_j); the probability of an individual in patch i suffering an infection derived from patch j is $\beta_{ij}Y_j$ or $\beta_{ij}N_j(Y_j/N_j)$, which tends to increase as population density in patch j, N_j, increases.

This assumption is unrealistically extreme. We have already seen, in the data in Fig. 12.1, that $\beta(N)$ might more realistically be represented by eqn (12.2) as $\beta_0 N^{\nu-1}$ (and thus $\lambda \sim \beta_0 N^{\nu}(Y/N)$), with ν significantly less than unity. D. Schenzle (private communication) has suggested the alternative form

$$\beta Y = \frac{\beta_0 K Y}{N + K} = \left(\frac{\beta_0 N K}{N + K}\right)\left(\frac{Y}{N}\right). \tag{12.6}$$

Here K is some characteristic density of the host population: for densities, N, significantly below K, the chance of a susceptible becoming infected tends to rise linearly as population density increases; for N significantly above K, the transmission factor saturates to β_0, so that further increases in population density have no effect on disease transmission. Hethcote and Van Ark (1986) have advanced yet another idea, which essentially corresponds to the extreme assumption $\nu = 0$ in eqn (12.2) (opposite to our assumption that $\nu = 1$). Their assumption means that the force of infection depends only on the fraction infected, and not at all on density as such; that is, $\lambda = \beta(Y/N)$, with β a constant. Although Hethcote and Van Ark's assumption of $\nu = 0$ in eqn (12.2) is probably closer to reality than our simple assumption that $\nu = 1$ (such data as we have suggest small, but finite, ν), Schenzle's formula (12.6) or our formula (12.2) with finite $\nu < 1$ are probably more realistic than either extreme.

Having chosen to assume that the transmission parameters β_{ij} are constants, not dependent on N_j, we make the further simplifying assumption that these coefficients have one value, β, for contacts within a group, and another, smaller value, $\varepsilon\beta(\varepsilon < 1)$, for contacts between groups:

$$\beta_{ij} = \beta, \qquad \text{if } i = j, \tag{12.7a}$$

$$\beta_{ij} = \varepsilon\beta \qquad \text{if } i \neq j. \tag{12.7b}$$

We can now turn the handle on the machinery that was constructed in Chapter 10, to get some interesting results.

12.1.4 *Uniform immunization programme*

Let p_i denote the fraction immunized in group i, under some defined programme. If the fraction immunized is the same in each group, regardless of its relative size, we have $p_i = p$ for all i. The critical value of p at which eradication is just achieved, p_c, can then be estimated from eqns (10.25) and (10.26). This leads to the conclusion that p_c is given by

$$p_c = 1 - (1/\Lambda_0). \tag{12.8}$$

Here Λ_0 is the dominant eigenvalue of the $n \times n$ matrix **A** whose elements are $A_{ij} = \beta_{ij} N_j/(\mu + v)$, with β_{ij} given by eqn (12.7). It is convenient to define the quantity ρ as

$$\rho \equiv \beta N/(\mu + v). \tag{12.9}$$

This quantity ρ essentially sets the scale of the basic reproductive rate of the infection, but in this heterogeneous situation R_0 is not exactly equal to ρ (unless the homogeneous limit is recovered by putting $\varepsilon = 1$ in eqn (12.7), so that all $\beta_{ij} = \beta$).

Let f_i denote the fraction of the total population that is present in group i; that is, $N_i = f_i N$. With this notational interlude now complete, we have that Λ_0 is the dominant eigenvalue of the matrix whose elements are $A_{ij} = \rho f_j[\varepsilon + (1 - \varepsilon) \delta_{ij}]$. Here $\delta_{ij} = 1$ if $i = j$, and $\delta_{ij} = 0$ otherwise. The eigenvalues Λ of such a matrix can be seen to obey the relation (see Appendix E)

$$1 + \sum_{j=1}^{n} \frac{\rho \varepsilon f_i}{(1 - \varepsilon)\rho f_i - \Lambda} = 0. \tag{12.10}$$

In general, this will be a polynomial equation of order n for Λ, although simplifications occur if two or more values of f_j are equal.

The exact value of x^*, the overall fraction remaining susceptible (at equilibrium before any immunization), can be obtained from the pair of eqns (10.21) and (10.22), as discussed in Chapter 10. If all forces of infection, λ_j, are significantly in excess of the natural mortality rate, μ, we have for x^* the excellent approximation $x^* \simeq x^{*\prime}$, with $x^{*\prime}$ given by

$$x^{*\prime} = \frac{1}{\rho} \sum_{j=1}^{n} \frac{f_j}{\varepsilon + (1 - \varepsilon)f_j}. \tag{12.11}$$

As mentioned above, a rough estimate of the critical fraction that must be immunized to achieve eradication can be obtained from the approximation

$$\hat{p}_c = 1 - x^*. \tag{12.12}$$

Comparison of eqn (12.11) (which gives an excellent approximation to x^*) or the more exact expressions obtained from eqns (10.21) and (10.22) for x^*, with eqn (12.10) (which gives the dominant eigenvalue Λ_0 for substitution into eqn (12.8)), makes it clear that in general $x^* \neq 1/\Lambda_0$. The two quantities are equal when $\varepsilon = 1$, or when all f_i are equal ($f_i = 1/n$ for all i); in both these cases, all individuals see the same world, so that homogeneity is effectively recovered. Indeed, it can be shown generally that $x^* \geq 1/\Lambda_0$ in the above model, which is to say (May and Anderson 1984)

$$p_c \geq \hat{p}_c. \tag{12.13}$$

This is the statement whose practical implications were stressed above: under a uniformly applied immunization programme, the overall fraction that must be immunized in order to eradicate infection is larger than would be estimated by (incorrectly) assuming the population to be homogeneously mixed, and using eqn (12.12).

12.1.5 *Optimal immunization programme*

Is it sensible to apply immunization homogeneously in such an inhomogeneous situation? To answer this question, May and Anderson (1984) define the optimal immunization schedule as that which minimizes the overall fraction which must be immunized to eradicate infection. If a proportion p_i are immunized in the ith group, then the overall proportion immunized is

$$P = \sum_{i=1}^{n} p_i N_i / N = \sum_{i=1}^{n} p_i f_i. \tag{12.14}$$

Then the optimal schedule is that which minimizes P, yet eradicates infection. We denote the critical fraction immunized under this optimal scheme to be p_{opt}.

These ideas about optimal programmes should not be confused with other studies of 'optimal control', such as those by Sethi (1974) or Wickwire (1977), which ask different questions about the dynamics of changing rates of immunization within homogeneously mixed populations.

It is notationally convenient to define g_i as the fraction remaining unimmunized in the ith group:

$$q_i \equiv 1 - p_i. \tag{12.15}$$

Then our optimal task is to maximize Q, the unimmunized fraction,

$$Q = \sum_{i=1}^{n} q_i f_i, \tag{12.16}$$

subject to the constraint that the programme just achieves eradication. This critical constraint is given by eqns (10.25) and (10.26), which with β_{ij} from eqn (12.7) reduces to the requirement

$$\det \| A_{ij} \| = 0. \tag{12.17}$$

The elements of the $n \times n$ matrix $\mathbf{A}$ are given by

$$A_{ij} = \rho q_j f_j [\varepsilon + (1 - \varepsilon) \delta_{ij}] - \delta_{ij}. \tag{12.18}$$

After some matrix manipulation, along the same lines that gave eqn (12.10), eqn (12.17) can be reduced to the relationship (May and Anderson 1984; see also Appendix E)

$$1 + \sum_{j=1}^{n} \frac{\rho \varepsilon q_j f_j}{(1 - \varepsilon) \rho q_j f_j - 1} = 0. \tag{12.19}$$

The optimal schedule thus uses a set $\{q_i\}$ which maximizes the Q of eqn (12.16) subject to the constraint of eqn (12.19).

This problem in constrained optimization can be solved by standard techniques (using Lagrange multipliers, for instance). The details are set out in Appendix G, and discussed more fully in May and Anderson (1984). The solution is that the critical fraction remaining unimmunized in the ith patch is

$$q_i(=1-p_i) = \frac{1}{f_i \rho (1 - \varepsilon + n\varepsilon)}. \tag{12.20}$$

Summing over all patches, we find from eqn (12.14) that

$$p_{\text{opt}} = 1 - \frac{n}{\rho(1 - \varepsilon + n\varepsilon)}. \tag{12.21}$$

Several comments need to be made about this optimal schedule.

The first comment is a mathematical one. The basic result, eqn (12.20), is obtained under the assumption that all the q_i thus determined obey $q_i \leqslant 1$. This is obviously true if, but only if, all $f_i \geqslant 1/[\rho(1 - \varepsilon + n\varepsilon)]$. Thus eqns (12.20) and (12.21) are likely to be pertinent if $\rho \gg 1$, so long as none of the f_i are very small. In the event that the right-hand side of eqn (12.20) exceeds unity for a particular value of f_i, we put $q_i = 1$ and $p_i = 0$ in that patch (corresponding to no immunization in that patch); the constrained optimization problem is then solved for the remaining variables q_i. These complications are discussed fully by May and Anderson (1984).

The second, related comment is more biological. The optimal condition, eqn (12.20), requires that $q_i f_i$ be the same constant for all groups. That is, the same total number of individuals—not the same fraction—are to remain unimmunized in each group under the optimal schedule. In other words, a larger proportion is immunized in large groups than in small ones. This makes good sense.

It can, moreover, be shown generally that the total fraction immunized under the optimal programme (p_{opt} of eqn (12.21)) is always less than, or at worst equal to, the fraction estimated by using homogeneous mixing ($\hat{p}_c$ from eqn (12.12)). The proof that $\hat{p}_c \geqslant p_{\text{opt}}$ is given in May and Anderson (1984), and—as can be seen by comparing eqn (12.11) with eqn (12.21)—it consists essentially of demonstrating that

$$\sum_{i=1}^{n} \frac{\bar{f}}{\varepsilon + (1 - \varepsilon)\bar{f}} \geqslant \sum_{i=1}^{n} \frac{f_i}{\varepsilon + (1 - \varepsilon)f_i}. \tag{12.22}$$

Here $\bar{f} = 1/n$ is the mean value of f_i; the equality holds when all $f_i = \bar{f}$.

Thus, in summary, we have that

$$p_c \geqslant \hat{p}_c \geqslant p_{\text{opt}}, \tag{12.23}$$

within the framework of our simple model. We now briefly sketch some numerical examples, to give verisimilitude to a bald and unconvincing narrative. Then we ask how robust these conclusions may be.

12.1.6 *An explicit example: 'city and villages'*

As an illustrative example of the above ideas, suppose a fraction f of the total population lives in one big 'city', with the remaining fraction $(1 - f)$ being evenly distributed among m small 'villages' (with a fraction $(1 - f)/m$ in each village).

For any specified set of values of the parameters f, m, ε, and ρ (with ρ given by eqn (12.9)), we can now calculate the overall fraction of the population to be immunized in order to eradicate the infection: (A) under the optimal programme (the p_{opt} of eqn (12.21)); (B) according to the crude estimate based simply on x^* (the $\hat{p}_{\mathrm{c}}$ of eqn (12.12)), which only applies accurately to homogeneously mixed populations; and (C) under the uniformly applied programme (the p_{c} of eqns (12.8) and (12.10)).

Figure 12.2 illustrates the outcome of such calculations, showing the overall fractions *not* immunized (under the policies A, B, and C just defined) as

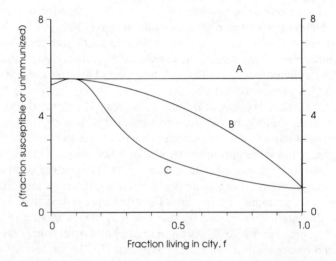

Fraction living in city, f

Fig. 12.2. Curve A shows the critical fraction not immunized (multiplied by $\rho = \beta N/(\mu + v)$), $\rho q_{\mathrm{opt}} = \rho(1 - p_{\mathrm{opt}})$, under the optimal eradication programme. Curve C shows the corresponding quantity, $\rho q_{\mathrm{c}} = \rho(1 - p_{\mathrm{c}})$, under a programme that immunizes the same fraction in every patch. Curve B shows the total fraction susceptible before immunization (multiplied by ρ), ρx^*. All quantities are shown as functions of f, the fraction of the population living in the one 'city', as distinct from the remaining fraction who are equally divided among m 'villages'. These curves are all drawn for the limit $\rho \to \infty$ (ρ being roughly proportional to the reproductive rate of the infection), in the case where $m = 10$ and $\varepsilon = 0.1$. The features of these results are as discussed in the main text. Note in particular that the optimal programme (curve A) requires fewer immunizations, and the uniform programme (curve C) more immunizations, than would be estimated (curve B) by assuming the population to be homogeneously mixed. After May and Anderson (1984).

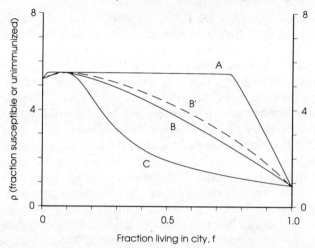

Fig. 12.3. As for Fig. 12.2, except now $\rho = 20$. Note the 'edge effects' that are manifested by curve A for the optimal eradication programme when ρ is finite. Curve A drops down to join curves B and C at the right corresponding to no immunization in villages for large f; conversely, the drop at the left corresponds to no immunization in the city for small f. For a fuller discussion see May and Anderson (1984). (The Curve B' is for x^* calculated from the exact eqns (10.21) and (10.22), instead of eqn (12.11).)

functions of f, the fraction of city dwellers, for $\varepsilon = 0.1$, m = 10, and $\rho \gg 1$. Figure 12.3 differs from Fig. 12.2 in that it exhibits the kinds of 'edge effects' which arise when ρ is finite: as $f \to 1$ the optimal policy immunizes no villagers, and as $f \to 0$ it immunizes no city people. These and other examples of a similar kind are analysed and discussed in May and Anderson (1984).

Figures 12.2 and 12.3 make plain the essential message of this chapter. For a population subdivided into groups where intra-group transmission rates are higher than inter-group ones, the optimally applied immunization coverage needed to eradicate infection (the curves A) is *lower* than would be estimated by treating the population as if it were homogeneously mixed (the curves B). This contrasts with the fact (which several public health workers have emphasized) that uniformly applied immunization coverage (the curves C) must be *higher* than estimated by assuming homogeneous mixing.

12.1.7 *More realistic models*
The assumption that transmission rates increase linearly with population density has the consequence that the differences among the critical levels of coverage under different immunization strategies—as illustrated in Figs. 12.2 and 12.3—are likely to be unrealistically high. This point has been emphasized by D. Schenzle (private communication) and Hethcote and Van Ark (1986).

If the form suggested by Schenzle is used for $\beta(N)$, eqn (12.6), then in the spatially inhomogeneous case we may replace the simple eqn (12.7) for β_{ij} with the expression $\beta_{ij} = [\beta_0 K/(K + N_j)]b_{ij}$; here $b_{ij} = 1$ if $i = j$, and $b_{ij} = \varepsilon$ otherwise. All the calculations that were carried out above can now be repeated, *mutatis mutandis*, to obtain the corresponding formulae for p_c, $\hat{p}_c$, and p_{opt}. In the limit $K \to \infty$ we obviously recover the results of the simple model of May and Anderson (1984). For smaller K values, the same qualitative results are obtained, with the main conclusion that $p_c \geqslant \hat{p}_c \geqslant p_{opt}$ remaining intact. The quantitative differences in coverage required for eradiction under different immunization strategies can, however, be a lot less than suggested by Figs. 12.2 and 12.3 if K is small enough. Indeed, in the limit $K \to 0$ (with $\beta_0 K$ finite) the transmission factor $\beta_{ij}N_j$ has no dependence at all on the population density, N_j, and so transmission rates are the same in all patches, regardless of their density; in this limit we thus have an effectively homogeneous population, and all three curves in Figs. 12.2 and 12.3 coincide ($p_c = \hat{p}_c = p_{opt}$).

Hethcote and Van Ark (1986) have adopted a somewhat different approach, based on the assumption that, in any one patch, $\beta_{jj}N_j$ is some constant which does not depend on population density N_j (although it may depend on other social variables). Revisiting May and Anderson's (1984) illustrative 'city and villages' model, these authors assume $\beta_{jj}N_j$ has one, density-independent, value (b_0 say) in the city, and another value (b_1) in each of the m villages. It is assumed that b_1 is usually somewhat smaller than b_0 (by a factor of two or so), but that b_1 has no dependence on the population size or density in the 'villages' as such. Transmission between patches is taken to be at rates intermedate between b_0 and b_1, discounted by a factor (analogous to ε above) which describes the amount of movement among patches. As in the city and villages model above, Hethcote and Van Ark use the parameter f to represent the fraction of the total population located in the single city. The kinds of calculations outlined above in eqns (12.8)–(12.23) can again be carried out under these assumptions about $\beta_{ij}(N_j)$, and again May and Anderson's essential conclusion that $p_c \geqslant \hat{p}_c \geqslant p_{opt}$ is confirmed. Again, however, Hethcote and Van Ark find that the differences among the critical coverage levels are significantly less than derived in Figs. 12.2 and 12.3 for the simplest model. (Hethcote and Van Ark's (1986) assumptions do have one curious feature, in that their transmission rates are always lower in a village than in the city, $b_0 > b_1$, even in the limit $f \to 0$ when in fact there are more people in any one 'village' than in the 'city'.)

In summary, when more complicated and more realistic models are analysed along the lines laid down by May and Anderson (1984), the difference between the critical coverage required under a uniformly applied immunization programme, p_c, and an optimal one, p_{opt}, can be substantially less than suggested by a simple model in which transmission rises linearly with population density. By the same token, however, both p_c and p_{opt} are closer to the crude estimate based on assuming homogeneous mixing, $\hat{p}_c$, in these more realistic computations.

In refining the details of the mathematical models, it sometimes seems to be forgotten that the original motivation for the work described in this chapter was a growing worry among public health workers that the effects of spatial or other heterogeneities might always require higher levels of immunization for eradication than estimated crudely from $\hat{p}_{c}$. To our minds, the pleasing thing about the more refined models discussed in this subsection is that they confirm our essential conclusion of eqn (12.23), namely that $p_{c} \geqslant \hat{p}_{c} \geqslant p_{opt}$. This means that if we determine the fraction susceptible, x^{*}, before any immunization, then the simple formula $p_{c} = 1 - x^{*}$ in general gives too *optimistic* an estimate if immunizations are carried out at random, but it gives too *pessimistic* an estimate if immunizations are delivered according to an optimal schedule. In practice, of course, all manner of realistic complications and uncertainties about parameter estimates will make any simple application of the optimal schedule difficult. But the basic conclusions— particularly that there may be some advantage to making greater efforts to immunize people in regions of higher density—seem encouraging.

12.2 Family size

In the preceding two chapters and up to this point in the present chapter, we have seen how the transmission and maintenance of infectious diseases can be influenced by heterogeneities within the population having to do with genetic constitution, number of sexual partners, or geographical circumstances. The list of such innate, cultural, and environmental heterogeneities can be extended virtually endlessly, and in each case the basic formalism developed in Chapter 10 can be applied. We content ourselves with a brief discussion of one last heterogeneity, namely that having to do with the effects of family size.

One of the best studies of the effect of family size on the epidemiology of a microparasitic infection is Black's (1959) serological study of measles in New Haven. The results are shown in Fig. 3.10(a), which gives the age-specific proportion of children from families with one or two children who show antibodies for measles, and contrasts this with the corresponding proportions of children from families with three or more children. The differences in the age-specific serological profiles are quite marked, which suggests similarly marked differences in the forces of infection between the two groups. Other studies include Becker and Angulo's (1981) demonstration that transmission rates for variola minor within households are typically much greater than between households.

For a formal discussion, the effects of family size can be treated in much the same way as we have just treated the effects of spatial heterogeneity. We could, for instance, divide the total population into n families, with one transmission rate within a family of size k and another for contacts outside the family (assumptions about birth and death rates can complicate things; the simplest assumption is that births and deaths are such as to preserve the distribution of family sizes unchanging). An alternative approach is to assume that a fraction $f(k)$ of the total population are members of families of size k ($k = 1, 2, 3, \ldots$), and then to make some specific assumption about the dependence of the force of infection, $\lambda(k)$, upon family size, k. The analysis of such models will not be given here, but it follows the lines laid down earlier in this chapter and in the two preceding ones. In general, we find the critical fraction that must be immunized under a uniformly applied programme, p_c, is greater than would be estimated by ignoring the epidemiological effects associated with family size and using $\hat{p}_c = 1 - x^*$. Conversely, the critical coverage under an optimal programme (in the sense of that requiring the least immunization) is in general below $\hat{p}_c$. That is, we again have $p_c \geqslant \hat{p}_c \geqslant p_{opt}$.

In these models, we usually assume the force of infection depends on family size, k, in a way that corresponds to β_{ij} factoring ($\beta_{ij} = g_i h_j$), as discussed in Chapter 10. The result is that the optimal strategy of immunization is what is called 'bang-bang': all individuals in families of size above k_T are immunized; no one in families of size below k_T is immunized; and the fraction of individuals immunized in families of some critical size, k_T, is adjusted to satisfy the constraint of eqns (10.25) and (10.26). This result is similar to that found for endemic STDs in Chapter 11. Such a 'bang-bang' strategy would, of course, be both unfeasible and silly in practice. These results do, however, suggest that—in so far as transmission is higher in larger families, as Fig. 3.10(a) shows—efficiencies can be realized by making somewhat more strenuous efforts to immunize members of larger families.

We conclude this section by sketching a very rough estimate of the extent to which the critical coverage under a uniformly applied immunization programme, p_c, must exceed the simple estimate $\hat{p}_c = 1 - x^*$, if the effects of family size are indeed significant.

As suggested above, we assume that a fraction $f(k)$ of the population are members of families of size k ($k = 1, 2, 3, \ldots$), and that this distribution is not changing over time. We further assume that members of families of size k experience a force of infection that depends simply on k and on the total density of infectives,

$$\lambda(k) = \beta g(k) Y. \tag{12.24}$$

If family size has no discernible epidemiological effects, then $g(k) = 1$ and eqn (12.24) becomes the familiar relation between λ and Y for a homogeneously mixed population. Finally, we assume (as usually is reasonable) that $\lambda(k) \gg \mu$ for all k, so that eqn (10.21) for x^* reduces to $x^* = \mu \sum_k f(k)/\lambda(k)$, and eqn (10.22) for $\lambda(k)$ reduces to $\lambda(k) = \mu\beta N g(k)/(\mu + v)$.

With the model thus defined, we have for x^* the excellent approximation

$$x^* = (1/\rho) \sum_k f(k)/g(k). \tag{12.25}$$

Here ρ is defined as $\rho = \beta N/(\mu + v)$. The critical fraction to be immunized under a uniformly applied programme, p_c, follows directly from eqn (10.30) of Chapter 10, which here gives

$$1 = (1 - p_c)\rho \sum_k f(k)g(k). \tag{12.26}$$

Eliminating ρ between eqns (12.25) and (12.26), we get

$$p_c = 1 - \frac{x^*}{\langle g(k) \rangle \langle 1/g(k) \rangle}. \tag{12.27}$$

Here $\langle F(k) \rangle$ denotes the average of the function $F(k)$, averaged over the distribution of k values described by $f(k)$.

If transmission does not depend on family size, we have $g(k) = 1$ and thence the standard estimate $p_c = 1 - x^*$. More generally, $g(k)$ will tend to increase with k (see Fig. 3.10(a)). If this k dependence is not too marked, we can get a rough feeling for what eqn (12.27) says, as follows. First, expand $F(k)$ (where $F = g$ or $1/g$) in Taylor series around the mean value of k, $\bar{k}$:

$$F(k) = F(\bar{k}) + (k - \bar{k})F'(\bar{k}) + \tfrac{1}{2}(k - \bar{k})^2 F''(\bar{k}) + \cdots. \tag{12.28}$$

Here $F'(\bar{k})$ denotes the first derivative of F, dF/dk, and so on. Second, we find $\langle F(k) \rangle$ by substituting eqn (12.28) into the appropriate summation to get:

$$\sum_k F(k)f(k) = F(\bar{k}) + \tfrac{1}{2}\sigma^2 F''(\bar{k}) + \cdots. \tag{12.29}$$

Here σ^2 is the variance in family size, $\sigma^2 = \langle (k - \bar{k})^2 \rangle$. For $F = g(k)$ we then have

$$\langle g(k) \rangle = g(\bar{k}) + \tfrac{1}{2}\sigma^2 g''(\bar{k}) + \cdots. \tag{12.30}$$

For $F = 1/g(k)$ the corresponding result is

$$\langle 1/g(k) \rangle = \frac{1}{g(\bar{k})} \left\{ 1 - \frac{\sigma^2}{2} \left[\frac{g''(\bar{k})}{g(\bar{k})} - 2 \left(\frac{g'(\bar{k})}{g(\bar{k})} \right)^2 \right] \right\}. \tag{12.31}$$

Putting eqns (12.30) and (12.31) together, and substituting into eqn (12.27), we end up with

$$p_c = 1 - \frac{x^*}{1 + \sigma^2 (g'(\bar{k})/g(\bar{k}))^2 + \cdots}. \tag{12.32}$$

This expression shows clearly that p_c is indeed estimated accurately by $1 - x^*$ either if the variance in family size is small (σ^2 small) or if the dependence of transmission on family size is weak ($g'(k)/g(k)$ small). For the special case where the force of infection rises linearly with family size, $g(k) \sim k$, eqn (12.32) gives the rough estimate

$$p_c \simeq 1 - \frac{x^*}{1 + (CV)^2}. \tag{12.33}$$

Here CV is the coefficient of variation for the distribution of family sizes, $CV = \sigma/\bar{k}$. We see that, for this fairly strong dependence of transmission rates on k, p_c can be significantly larger than $1 - x^*$ if the coefficient of variation in family sizes is big enough.

12.3 Summary

Variability in transmission rates for infections can arise when some hosts live in dense aggregates while others live in small or remote groups, or when some hosts are members of large families and others of small ones, or from other social or geographical heterogeneities. Under these circumstances, the critical fraction of the population that must be immunized to eradicate infection, under a uniformly applied programme, can be significantly larger than that estimated by (incorrectly) treating the population as if it were homogeneously mixed; that is, $p_c \geqslant \hat{p}_c$, where $\hat{p}_c = 1 - x^*$. But if we define an optimal eradication programme as that which—by treating different groups differently—achieves its aim by immunizing the smallest overall number in each cohort of new-borns, then this optimal programme in general requires fewer immunizations than estimated from $\hat{p}_c$; that is $\hat{p}_c \geqslant p_{opt}$. These ideas have implications for control programmes, particularly in circumstances where the epidemiological effects of spatial heterogeneity or of family size are pronounced.

13

Endemic infections in developing countries

The basic model discussed in Chapters 4, 5, and 6 contains the assumptions that the infection is not itself a cause of mortality and that the human population has zero growth, with net births exactly balancing net deaths such that the population is of constant size. Essentially all conventional mathematical models for endemic or epidemic infections of humans contain this assumption (Waltman 1974; Bailey 1975; Hoppensteadt 1975; Anderson and May 1982a). Given that the epidemiological time-scales (such as the average age at infection) are typically much shorter than the time-scales characterizing demographic change (such as population doubling time), the assumption of an unchanging host population is often a useful approximation.

In developed countries in particular, childhood infections such as measles and pertussis are more a cause of morbidity than mortality and, furthermore, net population growth rates in such regions tend to be just above or just below zero.

The situation is rather different, however, in the developing world where annual rates of population growth are invariably positive and may be as high as 2–3 per cent or more (Table 13.1). In addition, many of the common viral and bacterial infections of childhood are significant causes of mortality in the developing world, particularly when infection is linked with serious malnutrition (Morley et al. 1963; Morley 1969a,b; Aaby et al. 1983) (Fig. 13.1). For example, Walsh estimates that of the order of 900 000 deaths from measles infection occur each year in developing nations (Walsh 1983). This viral infection induces serious complications such as acute diarrhoea, encephalitis, otitis media, pneumonia, and exacerbation of protein energy malnutrition (Krugman and Katz 1981).

In this chapter we address the issues surrounding the description and analysis of microparasitic transmission in human communities where population growth rates are positive and where the infection induces mortality as well as morbidity. We start by considering simple models of transmission in a growing population, ignoring the complications introduced by case fatalities.

13.1 Transmission in growing populations

The effects of an ever increasing host population upon the incidence of a particular infection will depend upon the detailed assumptions made about the transmission and demographic processes (May and Anderson 1985). As described in Chapters 4 and 12, for a homogeneously mixing population, the rate at which new infections arise is usually assumed to be proportional to the densities of

Table 13.1 Demographic properties of human communities in various countries in the developing world (McLean and Anderson 1988*a*)

Country	Crude birth rate per 1000 per year	The reciprocal of the average birth rate (years)	Female life-expectancy at birth (years)	Population growth rate per 1000 per year
Malawi	48.5	20.6	44.2	23.4
Ecuador	41.6	24.0	61.8	31.2
Thailand	32.2	31.0	58.7	23.4
United Kingdom	12.18	78.1	76.6	1.1

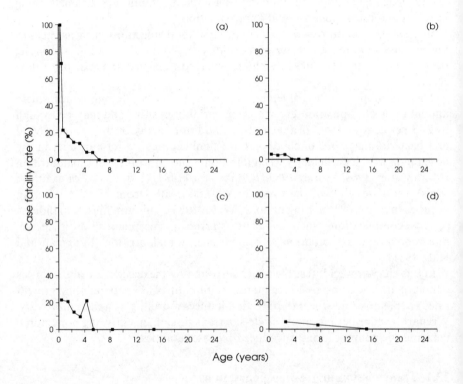

Fig. 13.1. Age-stratified case fatality rates arising from measles infection in developing countries. (a) Mortality in The Gambia over a nine-month study period following infection (Hull *et al.* 1983). (b) Study in Machakos, Kenya 1976–7 (Muller *et al.* 1977). (c) Study in Vellore, India (John *et al.* 1980). (d) Study in three Guatemalan villages 1959–63 (Gordon *et al.* 1965). Graphs adapted from McLean and Anderson (1988*a*).

susceptible hosts, X, and of infectious hosts, Y. Transmission is at the rate $\beta X Y$, where β is the transmission coefficient. A variety of assumptions may then be made about the way in which transmission is affected by the total number of people, which here is increasing over time. At one extreme, we may assume that the growing population spreads into new territory (the city boundary spreads further and further), so that the population density remains roughly constant. In this case the force of infection experienced by the average susceptible, βY, will on average be unaffected by population growth because the density of infectives remains roughly constant. At the opposite extreme, we may assume that the population growth takes place in a constrained, finite region (the city boundaries are fixed), so that the population density steadily increases. In this case the force of infection, βY, is likely to increase as the average host density, and thence the average density of infectives, increases. The realities of cities like London and New York in the eighteenth and nineteenth centuries, or of Calcutta, Lagos, and Nairobi today, lie somewhere between these two extremes. But precisely where is not clear at present.

In the case where densities do change as total populations grow, there remains the question of how transmission responds to such changes. As documented in Chapter 12, it is unlikely that transmission rates increase linearly with increases in population density. Some formulae for ways in which the force of infection, λ, may depend on total density were reviewed in Chapter 12: these include a power-law dependence, $\lambda = \beta_0 \bar{N}^v (\bar{Y}/\bar{N})$, with $v < 1$, suggested by Anderson (1982b), and the saturation equation $\lambda = [\beta_0 \bar{N}/(K + \bar{N})](\bar{Y}/\bar{N})$ suggested by Schenzle (Chapter 12).

In this chapter we consider two extreme cases. To start with we employ the assumption of the linear dependence, where net transmission is simply $\beta X Y$, to consider how a growing population influences our observation of the basic or case reproductive rate of infection R_0. We shall later consider the case where population size has no effect on transmission.

We formulate the problem along lines identical to those outlined in Chapters 4 and 5, but with the additional complication that the population is growing exponentially. For simplicity we again ignore the complications of maternally derived antibodies and the latent period. The equations of the basic model have the form

$$\frac{\partial X}{\partial a} + \frac{\partial X}{\partial t} = -(\lambda(t) + \mu(a))X(a, t), \tag{13.1}$$

$$\frac{\partial Y}{\partial a} + \frac{\partial Y}{\partial t} = \lambda(t)X(a, t) - (v + \mu(a))Y(a, t), \tag{13.2}$$

$$\frac{\partial Z}{\partial a} + \frac{\partial Z}{\partial t} = vY(a, t) - \mu(a)Z(a, t), \tag{13.3}$$

$$\frac{\partial N}{\partial a} + \frac{\partial N}{\partial t} = -\mu(a)N(a, t). \tag{13.4}$$

Here $\lambda(t)$, the force of infection at time t, is given independent of age as

$$\lambda(t) = \beta \bar{Y}(t) \tag{13.5}$$

with $\bar{Y}$ the total number of infectious individuals per unit area:

$$\bar{Y}(t) = \int_0^\infty Y(a, t)\, \mathrm{d}a. \tag{13.6}$$

The other quantities have their usual definitions: v is the recovery rate, $\mu(a)$ the age-specific mortality rate, and immunity is taken to be lifelong. These partial differential equations have as one set of boundary conditions that $Y(0, t) = Z(0, t) = 0$ and $X(0, t) = N(0, t)$, with the number per unit area in the new-born age class being

$$N(0, t) = \int_0^\infty m(a)N(a, t)\, \mathrm{d}a. \tag{13.7}$$

Here $m(a)$ is the age-specific birth rate, assumed to be independent of time. The other set of boundary conditions will consist of some arbitrarily-specified set of age profiles at time $t = 0$: $X(a, 0)$, $Y(a, 0)$, $Z(a, 0)$, $N(a, 0)$. It is well known that the total population will settle to a stable age distribution, undergoing net population growth at an overall rate r which is given in terms of the birth and death schedules, $m(a)$ and $\ell(a)$ (see Keyfitz and Flieger 1971), by the Euler equation

$$\int_0^\infty \mathrm{e}^{-ra}m(a)\ell(a)\, \mathrm{d}a = 1. \tag{13.8}$$

Here the survivorship function $\ell(a)$ is defined as

$$\ell(a) = \exp\left(-\int_0^a \mu(a)\, \mathrm{d}a\right). \tag{13.9}$$

Asymptotically we can then write

$$N(0, t) = N(0, 0)\, \mathrm{e}^{rt}. \tag{13.10}$$

The asymptotic age profile is defined as

$$N(a, t) = \ell(a)\, \mathrm{e}^{-ra} N(0, t). \tag{13.11}$$

In this new situation with a growing population, it remains possible to derive the formal solution of eqn (13.1) for the number of susceptibles:

$$X(a, t) = N(a, t)\exp\left(-\int_{t-a}^t \lambda(t')\, \mathrm{d}t'\right). \tag{13.12}$$

The difficulty here, as before, is that the force of infection, $\lambda(t)$, itself depends on Y and thence on $X(a, t)$. Some approximate but useful results can, however, be obtained by specifying the survivorship function $\ell(a)$ as either Type I or Type II (see Chapter 3).

For Type I survivorship ($\mu(a) = 0$ for $a < L$, $\mu(a) = \infty$ for $a > L$), it is possible (see May and Anderson (1985) for details) to reduce the system of equations defined by (13.1) to (13.4) to two differential equations for the force of infection $\lambda(t)$ and a quantity $\zeta(t)$ defined as

$$\zeta(t) = X(t)/N_T. \tag{13.13}$$

Here $X(t)$ is the total number of susceptibles and N_T is the threshold host density

$$N_T = v/\beta. \tag{13.14}$$

The two equations are

$$\frac{1}{\lambda}\frac{d\lambda}{dt} = v(\zeta(t) - 1), \tag{13.15}$$

$$\frac{d\zeta}{dt} = -\lambda\zeta + C\,e^{rt}. \tag{13.16}$$

The constant C is defined as

$$C = N(0, 0)/N_T. \tag{13.17}$$

Asymptotically, when the system has settled to its stable age distribution, λ and ζ have the values

$$\lambda(t) \simeq C\,e^{rt}/[1 + (r/v)], \tag{13.18}$$

$$\zeta(t) \simeq 1 + (r/v) \tag{13.19}$$

provided $rt \gg 1$ (May and Anderson 1985).

For Type II survivorship ($\mu(a) = \mu$ for all a) the equivalent equations are

$$\frac{1}{\lambda}\frac{d\lambda}{dt} = (v + \mu)(\zeta(t) - 1), \tag{13.20}$$

$$\frac{d\zeta}{dt} = -(\lambda + \mu)\zeta + C\,e^{rt}. \tag{13.21}$$

Here C and $\zeta(t)$ are again defined by eqns (13.17) and (13.13), respectively. The definition of the threshold host density in eqn (13.13) is, however, appropriately modified for Type II survivorship to replace eqn (13.14) by

$$N_T = (v + \mu)/\beta. \tag{13.22}$$

The asymptotic solutions for $rt \gg 1$ are now

$$\lambda(t) \simeq C\,e^{rt}/\zeta, \tag{13.23}$$

$$\zeta(t) \simeq r/(v + \mu). \tag{13.24}$$

13.1.1 *The basic reproductive rate R_0*

The basic reproductive rate R_0 in a growing population is a function of time t, $R_0(t)$, as a result of our assumption that net transmission is linearly proportional to the density of susceptibles times the density of infectious people. For a stably maintained endemic infection, the effective reproductive rate is unity. But this effective reproductive rate in a homogeneously mixing population is R_0 discounted by the overall fraction of the population who are susceptible, whence,

$$R_0(t) = \bar{N}(t)/\bar{X}(t). \tag{13.25}$$

In extending this familiar argument (see Chapters 5 and 6), we have explicitly made use of the fact that, for most infections, the average duration of infectiousness $(1/v)$ is very much shorter than the time-scale characterizing host population growth $(1/r)$.

Using eqn (13.25), we may estimate the value of $R_0(t)$ at any particular time t from serological studies that permit an evaluation of the total number of susceptibles, $\bar{X}(t)$, given information on total population size, $\bar{N}(t)$. It is, however, often useful to be able to make a rough assessment of R_0 from summary epidemiological quantities such as the average age at infection, A. The expressions outlined in Chapter 4 that permit estimates to be made of R_0, given A, can be extended to growing populations (May and Anderson 1985). In brief

$$R_0(t) = B\lambda(t), \tag{13.26}$$

where B is defined as

$$B = \int_0^\infty N(a, t)\mathrm{d}a/N(0, t). \tag{13.27}$$

The quantity B is the reciprocal of the average birth rate (i.e. B is the reciprocal of the number in the new-born age class, $N(0, t)$, divided by the total population at time t, $\bar{N}(t)$).

For an unchanging host population, the force of infection, λ, is related to the average age at infection, A, by the simple relation defined in eqn (4.29) (i.e. $A = 1/\lambda$), given Type I survivorship. In a growing population the simple relation of eqn (4.29) is complicated by the fact that A depends on patterns of susceptibility, which in turn involve forces of infection that typically reach out a time of order A back into the past. However, significant changes in population density usually take place on time-scales substantially longer than A, so that eqn (4.29) will remain a good approximation. This intuitive argument—the essentials of which were sketched in Chapter 4—is made more precise in May and Anderson (1985).

In brief, the expression

$$R_0 \simeq B/A \qquad (13.28)$$

remains an excellent approximation for the relationship between the basic reproductive rate R_0, the average age at infection A, and the reciprocal of the average birth rate B.

This result for a growing population differs from the standard result (eqn (4.36)) used throughout the earlier chapters, in that B replaces life expectancy L. Biologically it makes sense that the relevant demographic time-scale should, in the general case, be the reciprocal of the birth rate (i.e. the rate at which susceptibles enter the population). It is worth reiterating the example that was given in Chapter 4. Consider a country like India, where for the past 30 years or more birth rates have been around 40 per 1000 ($B = 25$ yr, from eqn (13.27)), while average life expectancy has been around $L \simeq 40$ years (and $r \simeq 0.02$ yr^{-1}). Inappropriate use of the 'zero population growth' result ($R_0 = L/A$) in this dynamic situation, instead of the appropriate formula ($R_0 = B/A$), would thus give estimates of R_0 that were too high by almost a factor of two.

13.1.2 *Changing patterns of susceptibility*

To end this section of the chapter that addresses the influence of growing populations on transmission, we briefly turn to the question of how age-specific trends in susceptibility to infection alter as a population increases in density. To examine this problem we employ the asymptotic results for temporal changes in the force of infection $\lambda(t)$ and the quantity $\zeta(t)$ (see eqn (13.13)), under the assumption of Type I survivorship. The expressions for $\lambda(t)$ and $\zeta(t)$, given in eqns (13.18) and (13.19) respectively, will be exact solutions if the initial conditions happen to be $\zeta(0) = 1 + (r/v)$ and $\lambda(0) = C/\zeta(0)$ where C is as defined in eqn (13.17)). For the purpose of providing an illustrative numerical example of the way in which age-specific patterns of susceptibility change over time we assume these initial conditions.

The number of susceptibles of age a at time t is then, from eqns (13.12) and (13.18)

$$X(a, t) = N(a, t) \exp\left(-\int_{t-a}^{t} \frac{R_0(0)\, e^{rt'}\, dt'}{B(1 + r/v)}\right). \qquad (13.29)$$

The total number of people of age a at time t is given by eqns (13.10) and (13.11):

$$N(a, t) = N(0, 0)\, e^{r(t-a)}. \qquad (13.30)$$

Figure 13.2 illustrates these expressions showing the age profiles and age-specific susceptibilities at time $t = 0$ and $t = 75$ for an infection whose basic reproductive rate is initially $R_0(0) = 4$ at $t = 0$. The human population is taken to have Type I survivorship with $L = 50$ years, and is assumed to be growing at the rate $r = 0.02$ yr^{-1}. Although the total population is increasing over time,

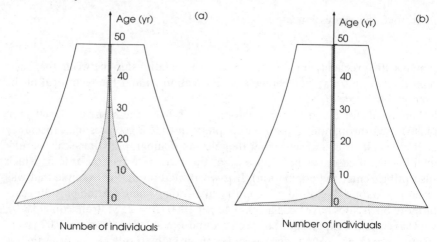

Fig. 13.2. The outer curves are the conventionally displayed age profiles—number of individuals (*x* axis) as a function of age (*y* axis)—in a population which has been and is growing at 2 per cent per annum, and where all individuals live exactly 50 years. The shaded region shows the number of individuals in the various age classes who remain susceptible to a particular infection; the remaining individuals, represented by the unshaded regions, are either infected or recovered and immune. In (a), taken to be at time $t = 0$, the basic reproductive rate of the infection is $R_0(0) = 4$. In (b), time t is equal to 75 years and the population is 4.48 times its original size; R_0 is now larger, and the average age at at infection is correspondingly lower. Adapted from May and Anderson (1985).

the two graphs in Fig. 13.2 are shown with the same baseline, because our main interest is in the fraction susceptible as a function of age and time.

   The changing patterns of susceptibility depicted in Fig. 13.2 are as we would expect. As total population size grows, infection rates increase and average ages at infection move systematically downwards.

13.2 Epidemiological patterns and demographic patterns in developing countries

So far in this chapter our discussions of transmission in growing populations have been technical in character, without much reference to empirical trends. We now turn to examine in more detail how observed patterns of infectious disease transmission differ between developed (static populations) and developing (growing populations) countries. To provide focus, we concentrate on one particular infectious disease, namely measles. First we consider the available epidemiological and demographic data and discuss the summary statistics such as the average age at infection, A, and the basic reproductive rate, R_0. We then turn to more complicated models that incorporate disease-induced mortality, positive population growth rates, a class of infants who are protected from infection by maternally derived antibodies, and a class of infecteds who are latent and not yet infectious. The model is used to assess how different vaccination programmes influence transmission of the measles virus.

The epidemiology of measles in many developing countries is somewhat similar to that of the same infection in England prior to the twentieth century. The average age at infection, for example, is typically low in urban centres, at around one to three years of age. This is to be compared with the equivalent statistics of four to six years that pertained in most industrialized countries just before the introduction of mass immunization in the mid-1960s (Morley 1968*a,b*; Anderson and May 1982*d*; Walsh 1983). High rates of transmission in developing countries are a consequence of behavioural and demographic factors. One implication of high transmission is that virtually all women of child-bearing age have experienced the infection such that most children are born with maternally derived antibodies to measles virus antigens. These protect from infection and disease for roughly three to twelve months. However, they also prevent effective immunization with current vaccines, for a similar duration (Albrecht *et al.* 1977; Halsey *et al.* 1985). These two factors, high transmission rates and the inhibitory effect of maternally derived antibodies on the efficacy of immunization, combine to cause what has to be termed the age 'window' problem which was briefly mentioned in Chapter 4 (McLean and Anderson 1988*a,b*). This issue centres on the observation that in urban centres, in contrast to similar centres in developed countries, a substantial proportion of a cohort of children will have experienced infection by the age at which maternally derived protection has waned for almost all children. The problem is illustrated schematically in Fig. 13.3.

The age 'window' problem is important in the design of mass vaccination programmes in developing countries with high intrinsic rates of transmission of the measles virus. A central question in the design of such programmes is what is the best age at which to vaccinate children so as to protect as many susceptibles as possible while minimizing the number of vaccinations that are 'wasted' on children who still possess significant titres of maternally derived antibodies specific to measles virus antigens?

The nature of this problem is dramatically underlined by the observation (K. Dietz, private communication) that if R_0 is big enough, it may be impossible to eradicate infection by a programme that immunizes only at one age, a_v say, even if we achieve 100 per cent coverage with a vaccine that is 100 per cent effective! In general, if a_v is too low then the fraction of children still protected by maternal antibodies (and therefore not having the lasting immunity evoked by immunization) is large enough to maintain endemic infection, while if a_v is too high the number of children experiencing infection at ages below a_v is enough to maintain endemic infection. If R_0 is sufficiently large, it can happen that there is no intermediate range of a_v-values for which eradication is possible.

The possibility of this happenstance can be illustrated by a simple calculation, along the lines discussed in Chapter 5. We first assume that essentially all

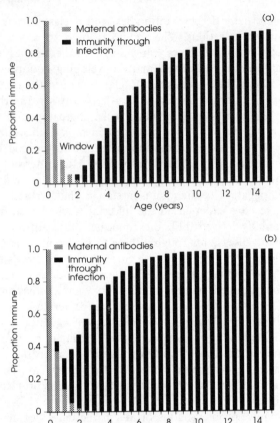

Fig. 13.3. Schematic illustration of the age 'window' problem. (a) A hypothetical serological profile that might be observed from a community in the developed world prior·to the introduction of mass vaccination. The average age at infection is about six years and there are few cases of infection in children below two years of age. This leaves an age 'window' during the second year of life when virtually all children are susceptible to infection and hence available for immunization. (b) The serological profile that might be observed in a community in a developing country. The average age at infection is two and a half years and there are many cases of infection in children below two years of age. There is no age 'window' when a high proportion of a cohort are susceptible to infection and 'susceptible' for vaccination..

offspring are born with protection from maternal antibodies, because essentially all mothers have either experienced infection at some time in their life (before the immunization programmes began), or because the mother has had antibodies evoked by immunization (following an aggressive campaign), or some mixture. If new-borns move out of the class protected by maternal antibodies at a constant rate, d, then the proportion of the population thus protected—and which is consequently unimmunizable—at age a (as discussed in Chapters 4 and 5) is

$$m(a) = e^{-da}. \tag{13.31}$$

The critical condition for eradication corresponds to the limit as the force of infection tends to zero, $\lambda \to 0$, again as discussed in Chapter 5. In this limit, all individuals are either protected by maternal antibodies, susceptible, or have acquired immunity by vaccination; the critical condition for eradication corresponds to naturally acquired infections becoming vanishingly small. Accordingly, the fraction remaining susceptible at age a, $x^*(a)$, can be seen to be:

$$x^*(a) = 1 - \exp(-da) \qquad \text{if } a < a_v, \tag{13.32}$$

$$x^*(a) = [1 - \exp(-da)] - p_c[1 - \exp(-da_v)] \qquad \text{if } a > a_v. \tag{13.33}$$

Here p_c is the proportion successfully immunized at some fixed age, a_v. Below a_v all those not protected by maternal antibodies are susceptible; above a_v this is still true, except that a proportion p_c of all those who were susceptible at age a_v are now protected. Integrating over all ages, we see the overall fraction of the population remaining susceptible is

$$x^* = \frac{d}{\mu + d} - p_c[1 - \exp(-da_v)] \exp(-\mu a_v). \tag{13.34}$$

Here we have assumed Type II mortality, at a constant rate $\mu = 1/L$; a similar expression is obtained for Type I mortality.

As explained in Chapter 5, the critical p_c value must obey the constraint that $R_0 x^* = 1$. That is to say, p_c and a_v are linked to the epidemiological and demographic parameters R_0, μ, and d through the relation

$$p_c = \frac{[d/(\mu + d)] - (1/R_0)}{[1 - \exp(-da_v)] \exp(-\mu a_v)}. \tag{13.35}$$

The best single age at which to vaccinate, a_v', is that which maximizes the denominator on the right-hand side of eqn (13.35) (thus minimizing p_c). It is a routine exercise to show that this optimum age is in fact

$$a_v' = M \ln[(L + M)/M]. \tag{13.36}$$

Here we have written the average age at which protection by maternal antibodies is lost as $M = 1/d$. Recall that L is the average life expectancy ($L = 1/\mu$), and usually $L \gg M$. Substituting from eqn (13.36) for a_v' into eqn (13.35) we see that the minimum value of the critical coverage level, p_c', is

$$p_c' = \left[1 - \frac{L + M}{L} \left(\frac{1}{R_0} \right) \right] \exp(a_v'/L). \tag{13.37}$$

But coverage levels can never exceed 100 per cent, and so eradication will not be possible under this single-age vaccination programme if the right-hand side of eqn (13.37) exceeds unity. This will happen if R_0 exceeds the value

$$R_0 > \left(\frac{L+M}{L}\right)\left[1 - \left(\frac{M}{L+M}\right)^{M/L}\right]^{-1}. \tag{13.38}$$

Given that $L \gg M$, to an excellent approximation eqn (13.38) reduces to the condition

$$R_0 > \frac{L/M}{\ln(L/M)}. \tag{13.39}$$

The same approximate value is obtained if Type I survivorship is assumed.

More accurately, we should acknowledge that under these assumptions some individuals are susceptible in later life (as can be seen from eqn (13.33)), so that not all children will be born with maternal antibody protection. This complication can be included in a self-consistent way. The corresponding calculation is more algebraically complicated than that just given, but it leads to the conclusion that eradication is not possible if R_0 exceeds a critical value given by

$$\frac{1}{R_0} = \left(\frac{1}{L+M}\right) - \left(\frac{L-M}{L}\right)\left(\frac{L(R_0-1)}{MR_0}\right)^{-M/(L-M)}. \tag{13.40}$$

This result is a more self-consistent version of eqn (13.38). In the limit $L \gg M$, however, eqn (13.40) also reduces simply to the excellent approximation given by eqn (13.39).

In brief, eradication cannot be attained with a single-age immunization scheme if R_0 exceeds the value set approximately by eqn (13.39). This critical R_0-value is illustrated, as a function of the ratio M/L, in Fig. 13.4; this figure is drawn from the exact formula, eqn (13.40).

Typically, in a developing country, L may be around 50 years and M around 0.5 years, whence $L/M \sim 100$. It follows that the above phenomenon arises only if R_0 is in excess of 20 or more, which is higher—though not a lot higher—than is commonly observed for microparasitic infections.

This illustrative calculation is based on an excessively simple model, which ignored age-dependent transmission rates, along with other kinds of relevant and realistic complications. We now go on to show how more detailed mathematical models can be used to explore problems of the design of vaccination programmes in developing countries. Successful use of such models, however, depends on accurate estimates of the variety of epidemiological and demographic parameters that control transmission of the virus. We therefore first discuss these estimates.

13.2.1 *Parameter estimates*

In a recent publication, McLean and Anderson (1988a) have reviewed the available epidemiological data relating to the transmission of measles in

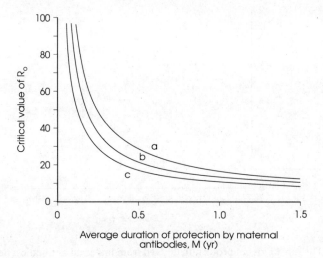

Fig. 13.4. The critical value of R_0, above which the 'window' effect makes it impossible to eradicate infection by immunization at a single age (even with 100 per cent coverage), as a function of the average duration of protection by maternal antibodies, M. This relationship is displayed for three different values of average life expectancy: (a) $L = 70$ years; (b) $L = 50$ years; and (c) $L = 35$ years.

communities with high population growth rates. Some examples of the patterns documented in this study are presented in Figs. 13.1, 13.5, 13.6, 13.7. These figures illustrate, respectively, patterns in age-stratified case fatalities, the average duration of detectable titres of maternally derived antibodies, age distribution of cases of infection, and age-stratified serological profiles for a variety of communities in different countries. The data reveal that the typical duration of maternally derived protection is similar in developed and developing countries, while the average age at infection is lower and case fatality rates higher in developing countries. An illustration of the major demographic differences between developing and developed countries is presented in Fig. 13.8.

The combination of high transmission rates and case fatalities seriously complicates the estimation of the force of infection, and of the rate at which infants lose maternally derived protection, from age-stratified data (McLean and Anderson 1988a). Most serological tests are unable to discriminate between those children with antibodies derived from their mothers and those with antibodies arising from recovery from infection. This means that an estimation technique must be employed that allows for the fact that, in certain age classes of infants and children, those found to be seropositive for antibodies specific to measles antigens include individuals with maternally derived protection and individuals with immunity derived from natural infection. In addition, the technique must also take into account the fact that the observed proportion seropositive at a given age does not represent the true proportion of that age

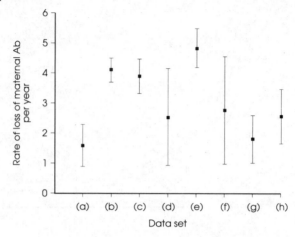

Fig. 13.5. The rate of loss of protection derived from maternal antibodies. Best estimates of the rate of decay, *d*, of maternal antibody protection assuming that the duration of protection is exponentially distributed. The results of eight surveys are recorded from Mexico, Tanzania, Kenya, India, Nigeria, New York, USA, Bulawayo, and Nigeria respectively from left to right on the horizontal azis of the graph. Data sources are given in McLean and Anderson (1988*a*).

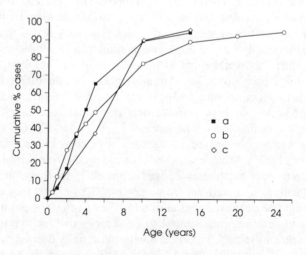

Fig. 13.6. Age-stratified case reports of measles infection in various countries (data sources given in McLean and Anderson (1988*a*). (a) Abidjan, Ivory Coast, 1972–5; (b) South West Somalia, 1978; (c) West Bengal, India, 1976–8.

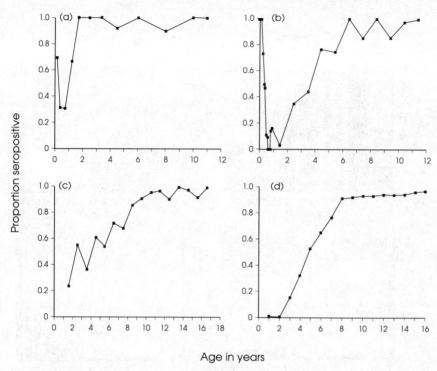

Fig. 13.7. Age-stratified horizontal surveys for the presence of antibodies to antigens of the measles virus (data sources given in McLean and Anderson (1988a)). (a) Dakar, Senegal, 1957; (b) Bangkok, Thailand, 1967; (c) Paraguay, 1971; (d) New Haven, Connecticut, USA, 1958.

cohort who have experienced infection, because a fraction of these will have died from the disease and thus will not be recorded in the serological survey. A full discussion of these problems and some suggestions for methods of parameter estimations are presented in the paper of McLean and Anderson (1988a). The major conclusion of this paper is that a very detailed set of data, concerning both the epidemiological and demographic characteristics of a given community, is required to enable accurate estimates to be obtained for the central statistics that summarize virus transmission, namely the average age at infection and the basic reproductive rate.

13.2.2 *Summary epidemiological parameters*

We showed in Chapter 4 that for populations of constant size the average age at infection, A, was simply the sum of the reciprocals of the force of infection, λ, and the rate of decay in maternally derived protection, d (eqn (4.52)). This

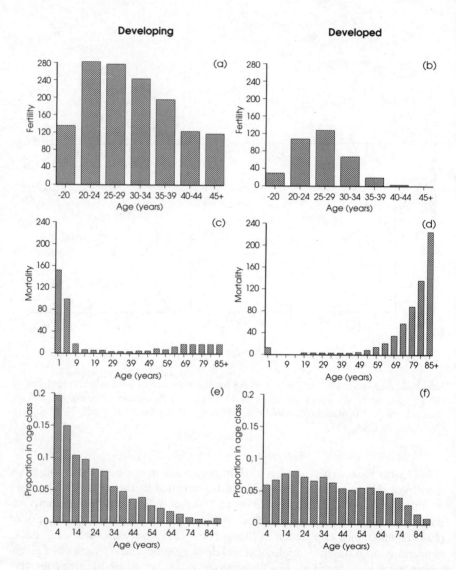

Fig. 13.8. A comparison of demographic patterns in a developing (Malawi) and a developed (United Kingdom) country (adapted from McLean and Anderson (1988*a*)). (a), (b) Age-specific fertility rates (live births per 1000 women per year) in (a) Malawi and (b) the United Kingdom. (c), (d) Age-specific death rates (deaths per 1000 per year) in (c) Malawi and (d) the United Kingdom. (e), (f) Age distribution of the population in (e) Malawi and (f) the United Kingdom. The data are from the *United Nations Demographic Yearbook*, 1982.

result can easily be extended for growing populations with a per capita growth rate r to give

$$A = 1/(r + \mu + \lambda) + 1/(r + \mu + d). \tag{13.41}$$

This result is based on the assumption that the force of infection, λ, and the death rate, μ, are constant and independent of age and that net transmission is proportional to the fraction, rather than the density or number, of infectives. It is possible to expand this result to encompass age-dependent forces of infection and mortality rates, but eqn (13.41) captures the essential interrelationships among the various epidemiological and demographic parameters. It makes clear that the average age at infection depends not only on the force of infection but also on the growth and mortality rates of the host population. This point is illustrated in Table 13.2 by a series of numerical examples in which estimates of A (and R_0) are derived (using an algorithm that takes account of age dependency in λ and μ; see McLean and Anderson (1988a)) for various values of the demographic parameters. Aside from the average age at infection, A, a further summary statistic is also recorded in Table 13.2, namely the basic reproductive rate. The relationship between R_0, B, and A (where B is the reciprocal of the average per capita birth rate defined earlier (eqn (13.28)) can be easily modified to take account of the duration of maternally derived protection M (where $M = 1/d$) such that

$$R_0 = B/(A - M). \tag{13.42}$$

As discussed in Chapter 5 (see eqn (5.2)), the magnitude of R_0 determines the critical proportion of a community that must be immunized for the eradication or interruption of virus transmission. The larger the value of R_0, the greater the value of the critical proportion to be immunized. As illustrated in Table 13.2 and by eqn (13.41), the demographic properties of a community have a central influence on the magnitude of R_0. It is informative to consider two communities with similar serological profiles (and hence similar average ages at infection prior to control) but with different birth rates. Equation (13.42)

Table 13.2 Numerical examples of the influence of demographic parameters on the estimation of the average age at infection, A, for measles in developing countries. Case fatality rates were derived from data from rural Kenya (Muller *et al.* 1977)

B (years)	r (per 1000 yr^{-1})	Case fatality rate (yr^{-1})	d (yr^{-1})	A (years)	R_0
19.1	41.9	Low	2	3.55	6.26
25.9	25.4	Low	2	3.67	8.17
34.2	11.0	Low	2	3.78	10.43

shows that the community with the greater birth rate will have the lower value for the basic reproductive rate R_0. Eradication will therefore be more easily achieved in the sense that the actual proportion that must be immunized to achieve eradication is lower. This does not imply, however, that an increase in the birth rate leads to a decrease in the critical vaccination proportion for eradication. It should be interpreted to mean that it will be easier to interrupt transmission by mass vaccination in a community with a low average age at infection because of a high birth rate than in a community with a low birth rate in which the low average age at infection is a consequence of behavioural patterns that enhance viral transmission. This example well illustrates the subtle interplay between demographic and transmission-related parameters that determine observed epidemiological patterns. Such subtleties can confound simple-minded intuitions.

13.2.3 *The impact of mass vaccination*

In the previous section we showed how a knowledge of various epidemiological and demographic parameters could facilitate the estimation of the basic reproductive rate of an infection in a growing population, and thence the critical proportion of a community that must be vaccinated to eradicate viral transmissions (eqns (13.41) and (5.2)). In practice, however, the problems of vaccination programme design in developing countries centre less on the question of what proportion to vaccinate and more on the issue of what is the best age at which to vaccinate to achieve the maximum impact on the incidences of infection related to morbidity and mortality. This arises as a consequence of the age 'window' problem discussed earlier (see Fig. 13.3) in which the combination of high transmission rates and low efficacy of vaccination in those children with measurable titres of maternally derived antibodies, creates difficulties in the choice of an age at which the majority of children are susceptible to infection (and hence susceptible to vaccination) (Hopkins *et al.* 1982; Heymann *et al.* 1983; Walsh 1983). Vaccination at too young an age 'wastes' too much vaccine on children with maternally derived protection that lowers vaccine efficacy, while vaccination at too old an age fails to have a significant impact on transmission or on morbidity and mortality in the infant and child classes.

Analytical studies of this problem are difficult, given the necessity to build models of transmission that incorporate the epidemiological complications raised by age-specific forces of infection, case fatalities, background death rates, and birth rates. An alternative and more practical option is to build a model whose complexity is dictated by the availability of epidemiological data, and then explore its properties by numerical methods. A recent paper by McLean and Anderson (1988*b*) adopts this approach to investigate different vaccination programmes in developing countries. The model consists of a set of five partial differential equations representing infants with maternally derived protection, susceptibles, latents, infectives, and immunes. The model is based upon the assumption that net transmission is proportional to the fraction of infectives

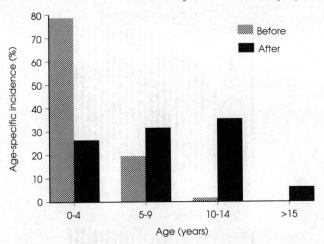

Fig. 13.9. Changes in the age distribution of cases of measles infection following introduction of mass vaccination. Data from the People's Republic of China (Yihao and Wannian 1983).

(as opposed to the number or density of infectives) and incorporates age dependency in the force of infection, in the rates of disease-induced and background mortality, and in fertility.

One motivation lying behind this study was the suggestion by Black that the age 'window' problem might be overcome by adopting a two-phase vaccination programme in which vaccination is initially targeted at very young children, and then, after a few years, switched to older age classes. The rationale behind this suggestion is that the initial phase of mass vaccination at an early age will raise the average age at infection and hence widen the age window of susceptibility in which children can be successfully immunized. Once the window is increased in width, the programme can be switched to older children, all of whom have lost their maternally derived protection. The suggestion that mass vaccination increases the average age at infection is not in doubt since theory (see Chapters 4 and 5) and observation (Fig. 13.9) support this view. However, it is not at all clear that the two-phase approach will lead to a greater reduction in morbidity and mortality in areas of high transmission than will a one-stage approach (vaccination at one age) or a two-stage (simultaneous vaccination of two age classes) programme with high coverage at the age at which susceptibility to infection is at its highest. A schematic representation of the differences between one- and two-stage programmes and two-phase programmes is depicted in Fig. 13.10.

Extensive numerical studies by McLean and Anderson (1988*b*) of model behaviour under the impact of the different programmes suggest that neither the two-phase nor the two-stage programme result in any improvement (in terms of reductions in morbidity and mortality) over a one-stage programme,

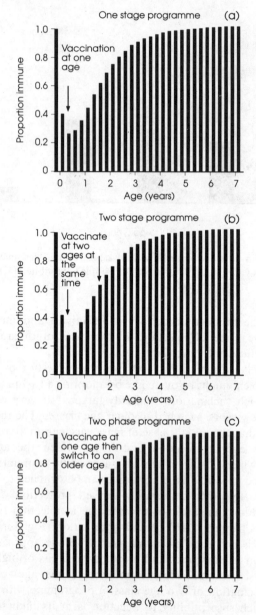

Fig. 13.10. Schematic representation of one-stage, two-stage, and two-phase vaccination programmes. One-stage programmes find an optimal age for vaccination and target all immunization effort on this age group. Two-phase programmes start by targeting one age group and then switch to targeting an older age group. Two-stage programmes target two age groups simultaneously.

targeted at nine-month-old infants, that achieved the same overall level of coverage as the more complex strategies. The explanation underlying the conclusion hinges on the influence of high intrinsic rates of transmission. With respect to the two-phase programme, for example, once immunization is shifted to the older age group the high intrinsic rate of transmission generates many cases of infection in the young unprotected infants just as it did in the pre-vaccination era. A clear picture of this chain of events is depicted in Fig. 13.11, which records the predicted impacts of a one-stage programme and two types of two-phase programmes on the age distribution of cases over a ten-year period following the introduction of mass vaccination.

The central conclusion of these numerical studies is that the greatest impact on morbidity and mortality is achieved by targeting high vaccination coverage at the age class in which susceptibility is greatest prior to the introduction of control (McLean and Anderson 1988b). The best age at which to vaccinate depends initially on the pattern of susceptibility prior to control. In areas of intense transmission this age will be between six to nine months of age while in areas of lower transmission the age will be typically around 1.5 years. This point is illustrated in Fig. 13.12 which depicts the predicted impacts of various one-stage programmes (with a 50 per cent vaccination coverage), aimed at different age groups, on mortality over a ten-year period following the introduction of control. Two examples are recorded, one depicting the predicted impact in an area of high transmission intensity and the other the predicted input in an area of low transmission intensity (McLean and Anderson 1988b).

The conclusions derived from numerical studies of models from measles transmission in developing countries are of practical significance given the recent implementation of the World Health Organization (WHO) Expanded Programme for Immunization (EPI), which aims to make measles vaccine available to all children by the middle 1990s (EPI 1986). There has been much debate in recent years over whether or not it is possible to eradicate measles in the developing world by mass vaccination (Hinman 1982) and over the economic considerations surrounding this goal (DeQuadros 1980). Central questions in this debate have been the best age at which to immunize and whether or not to recommend single- or multiple-phase/stage programmes (Black 1982; Katz 1983; Rabo and Taranger 1984).

Progress towards the resolution of these issues would be facilitated by a greater appreciation both of the need for precise epidemiological and demographic data and of the capabilities of mathematical models rapidly to explore the potential impacts of different types of vaccination programmes.

13.3 The demographic impact of AIDS

The large number of cases of acquired immunodeficiency syndrome (AIDS) now being reported to the World Health Organization (WHO) (in July 1989 149 countries reported at least one case), plus the degree to which the

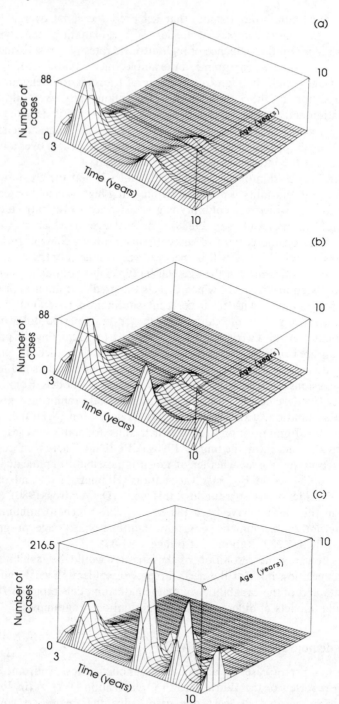

aetiological agent of the disease, the human immunodeficiency virus (HIV), has penetrated heterosexual communities in developing countries (particlarly in sub-Saharan Africa—with a range from a few per cent to more than 20 per cent of the general population infected, Fig. 13.13), has prompted governments and international agencies to give urgent consideration to the degree to which the pandemic will influence the demography and socio-economic development of large areas of the world.

Scientific assessment of this problem is complicated by our limited understanding of the epidemiology of the infection (HIV) and the disease (AIDS), as documented in Chapter 11. Uncertainties include: the fraction of those infected who will proceed to develop AIDS, and the time-scale of this progression; the likelihood of vertical transmission from infected mother to child *in utero*, during childbirth, and by breast feeding; the pathogenicities of human retroviruses other than HIV-1 (such as HIV-2) that are currently spreading in certain countries; the importance of co-factors such as genital ulcers in heterosexual transmission; the degree to which the infectiousness of infected patients changes throughout incubation of the disease; the probabilities of horizontal transmission from male to female and vice versa; and patterns of sexual behaviour in defined communities (see Chapter 11 and Anderson *et al.* 1988). The long and variable incubation period of AIDS means that epidemiological knowledge will only be accumulated slowly from long-term studies of infection and disease incidence, the rise in the former preceding that in the latter by many years. Current estimates of the mean period between HIV infection and development of AIDS, derived from transfusion-associated cases in the United States, are 8–10 years, although the mean may be lower in developing countries where people are exposed more frequently, and to a larger range of infectious agents, than in the developed world. A combination of social and political sensitivities, and the more practical difficulties in accurate diagnosis and reporting of infection and disease in poor countries, has hindered the study of the spread of infection in these parts of the world.

Quantitative data on the epidemiological processes outlined above, plus data on age-specific fertility and mortality, is essential for precise predictive work

---

Fig. 13.11. The predicted impact of a one-stage (a) and two-phase vaccination programmes (b) and (c) on the age and time distribution of cases of measles infection (adapted from McLean and Anderson (1988*b*). (a) Total cases, stratified by age, over a seven-year period following the introduction of a one-stage programme at time $t = 4$ that targets 75 per cent of 9-month-old susceptible infants. (b) Similar to (a) but representing the predicted impact of a two-phase programme. At time $t' = 4$ years a programme is introduced that targets 75 per cent of nine-month-old susceptible infants. At time $t = 6$ years the targeting is switched to the 1-year-old susceptible children at a coverage of 75 per cent. (c) Similar to (b) but representing the predicted impact of a two-phase programme in which, at $t = 6$ years, the targeting is switched to susceptible children of age 1.5 years. Note that the one-stage programme is predicted to have the greatest impact on total cases of infection.

on the demographic impact of AIDS. There is urgent need to assess the magnitude of the problem, however, to help governments and international aid agencies make long-term plans. It therefore seems sensible to study mathematical models that combine the demography of populations having positive net growth rates with the currently known epidemiological characteristics of the hetero-sexual transmission of HIV-1. In this chapter we develop simple models with the aim of obtaining a crude understanding of how AIDS deaths might affect demographic patterns, of the time-scales of such effects, and of the influence of demographic and epidemiological parameters on population sizes. Mathematical study of these deliberately simplified models is a preliminary to future numerical exploration of much more complicated and realistic models that will be possible

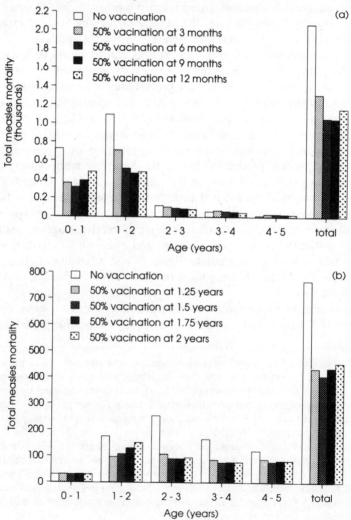

once data accumulate. The qualitative understanding that simple models can provide makes it easier to recognize what needs to be measured, together with the appropriate time-scales and parameter ranges in subsequent and more elaborate studies (Anderson and May 1988*a*).

13.3.1 *Basic model with no age structure*

We begin by considering a total population $N(t)$ at time t, subdivided into $X(t)$ susceptibles and $Y(t)$ infecteds (assumed to be infectious), all of whom develop AIDS on some characteristic long time-scale (a growing body of evidence suggests that a very high fraction of those infected will eventually develop symptoms of the disease (see Chapter 11), so in this basic model the fraction, f, of infecteds who develop AIDS is assumed to be one). For simplicity, we do not consider a separate class for AIDS, as the average incubation period, $1/(\alpha + \mu)$, appears long in relation to the life expectancy of an AIDS patient ($1/(\alpha + \mu)$ is more than nine years while life expectancy is about 1 year). In this calculation α is the disease-related death rate and deaths from all other causes occur at a constant rate μ (Type II survival, giving an exponential age distribution which is a reasonable approximation for many developing countries).

These assumptions yield the following pair of differential equation for $N(t)$ and $Y(t)$:

$$dN/dt = N[(v - \mu) - (\alpha + (1 - \varepsilon)v)(Y/N)], \tag{13.43}$$

$$dY/dt = Y[(\beta c - \mu - \alpha) - \beta c(Y/N)]. \tag{13.44}$$

We define the net birth rate of the community B as

$$B = v[N - (1 - \varepsilon)Y]. \tag{13.45}$$

Here v is the per capita birth rate (females per female, or equivalently offspring per capita for a 1:1 sex ratio) in the absence of infection; ε is the fraction of all

---

Fig. 13.12. Numerical studies of the predicted impacts of one-stage vaccination programmes targeted at different age groups of susceptible children. The groups record morbidity arising from measles infection over a ten-year period in the past vaccination era, stratified by age group (adapted from McLean and Anderson 1988*b*). (a) Prediction for an area of high transmission prior to the introduction of mass vaccination in which vaccination is targeted at a 50 per cent level of coverage of children of different ages. Five simulation studies are depicted, representing no vaccination, vaccination at 3 months of age, vaccination at 6 months of age, vaccination at 9 months of age, and vaccination at 1 year. The optimal age at which to vaccinate is predicted to be around 6–9 months of age to attain the greatest reduction in mortality. (b) Similar to (a) but recording prediction for an area of moderate transmission prior to the introduction of mass vaccination. Coverage was again set at 50 per cent and the five cases examined are: no vaccination, vaccination at 1.25 years of age, vaccination at 1.5 years of age, vaccinations at 1.75 years of age, and vaccination at 2 years of age. The optimal age at vaccination is predicted to be 1.5 years of age with respect to the overall reduction in mortality.

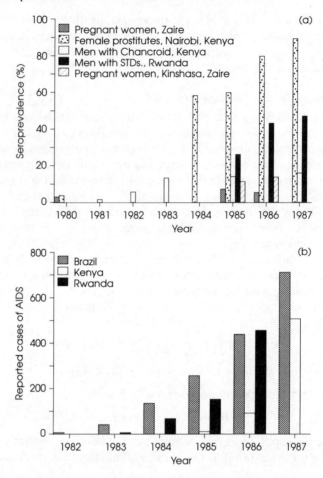

Fig. 13.13. Longitudinal changes in the proportion of people in various at-risk groups in Africa, who have antibodies in HIV antigens (serpositive) (for data sources see Anderson *et al.* 1988*a*). (b) Longitudinal trends in cases of AIDS reported to WHO in Brazil, Kenya, and Rwanda.

offspring born to infected mothers who survive, and $1 - \varepsilon$ is the fraction who acquire infection by vertical transmission and die rapidly from AIDS (effectively at birth)). The per capita rate at which adults acquire infection, λ, is assumed to be given by $\lambda = \beta c Y/N$ where β is the probability of acquiring infection from any one infected partner, c is the average rate of acquiring partners (c is not the mean number, but is the mean, m, plus the variance to mean ratio, σ^2/m, of the relevant distribution of partner-change rates), and Y/N is the probability that any one partner is infected. More generally for heterosexual transmission we should deal with two distinct populations, N_1 of males and N_2 of females, with females acquiring infection from males at a rate $\beta_1 c_1$, and vice versa for female-to-male transmission at a rate $\beta_2 c_2$. However, for simplicity we assume that $\beta_1 c_1 = \beta_2 c_2 = \beta c$ such that the two-sex model collapses to eqns (13.43) and (13.44). This appears to be a reasonable assumption, as we have shown elsewhere (May and Anderson 1987) that in the early stages of the epidemic the ratio of the number of seropositive males to seropositive females is roughly $(\beta_1 c_1 / \beta_2 c_2)^{1/2}$. Observations in a variety of African countries suggest that these rates are roughly equal.

To clarify discussion we introduce the following notation: r is defined as the growth rate of the population before the initial HIV infection, Λ as the initial exponential growth rate of the infection within the population, and θ as the extra mortality linked to infection (arising from horizontal and vertical transmission). These rates are given by

$$r = v - \mu, \quad \Lambda = \beta c - (\mu + \alpha), \quad \theta = \alpha + v(1 - \varepsilon). \tag{13.46}$$

The model defined by eqns (13.43) and (13.44) has an exact solution for $N(t)$ and for the prevalence of infection $y(t)$ $(= Y(t)/N(t))$ where

$$N(t) = N(0)\, e^{rt}[1 + (b/a)\,\Delta(e^{at} - 1)]^{-\theta/b} \tag{13.47}$$

and

$$y(t) = (\Delta\, e^{at})/[1 + (b/a)\,\Delta(e^{at} - 1)]. \tag{13.48}$$

Here $N(0)$ and $Y(0)$ (where $\Delta = Y(0)/N(0)$) are respectively the initial total population and number of infected at time $t = 0$. The parameter combinations a and b are defined as

$$a = \Lambda - r, \quad b = a + \varepsilon v. \tag{13.49}$$

The model exhibits three patterns of behaviour. The basic reproductive rate of infection, R_0, defined as the number of secondary cases of infection typically generated by one primary case in a susceptible population, is given by (see Chapter 11):

$$R_0 = \beta c/(\mu + \alpha). \tag{13.50}$$

Hence if $R_0 < 1$ (which implies $\Lambda < 0$, see eqn (13.46)) the infection cannot establish and there will be no epidemic (note that eqn (13.50) defines the control problem: sexual behaviour, c, must be changed such that $R_0 < 1$). Given the rapid spread of HIV in certain countries, of more importance are the two cases that arise when $R_0 > 1$. If $\Lambda/\beta c > r/\theta$, mortality associated with infection is so high that deaths eventually exceed births and the population begins to decline. In principle, therefore, sexually transmitted infections that also spread via vertical transmission are capable of causing the extinction of their host population.

Alternatively if $0 < \Lambda/\beta c < r/\theta$ the population will eventually settle to exponential growth, the infection being maintained within it, provided $R_0 > 1$. The critical combination of parameter values that divides the two cases is when

$$\varepsilon v = (\mu + \alpha)(\Lambda - r)/\Lambda. \tag{13.51}$$

When the right-hand side exceeds the left-hand side, extinction occurs; in the opposite case, sustained growth occurs. Note that extinction cannot occur unless $\Lambda > r$; that is, the exponential rate at which the infection initially spreads must exceed the overall population growth rate, otherwise a decreasing fraction will experience infection, even though the absolute number of infected individuals is growing. When the population continues to grow with the infection being maintained, the prevalence of infection approaches a constant value, y^* (as $t \to \infty$), where

$$y^* = (\Lambda - r)/[(\Lambda - r) + \varepsilon v]. \tag{13.52}$$

The asymptotic exponential rate at which $N(t)$ and $Y(t)$ grow, ρ (provided that the fraction infected who develop AIDS, f, is equal to 1), is

$$\rho = -(\mu + \alpha) + [\varepsilon v(\Lambda + \mu + \alpha)]/[\Lambda - r + \varepsilon v]. \tag{13.53}$$

In the case where $\rho < 0$ and population growth is eventually halted by AIDS, the period of time before the population ceases its previously exponential growth, t_c, is given by

$$t_c = \left(\frac{1}{\Lambda - r}\right) \ln\left(\frac{r[1 - \Delta(b/a)]}{\Delta[\theta - r(b/a)]}\right) \tag{13.54}$$

where Δ is the fraction infected at $t = 0$.

13.3.2 *Time-delayed recruitment*

The basic model dealt with the total population with an overall average birth rate v. In reality, however, HIV spreads predominantly among sexually active adults, and births occur from sexually mature females, so that it is more realistic to interpret $N(t)$ as the population of sexually active adults (subdivided into $X(t)$ and $Y(t)$). If τ is the average time taken to attain sexual maturity (say 15 years), the relationship between the average birth rate expressed per adult, w, and the average birth rate per member of the total population, v, is

$$v = w\,e^{-(\mu + r)\tau}. \tag{13.55}$$

Here $\exp(-\mu\tau)$ defines the proportion of new births that survive to sexual maturity at age τ with mortality rate μ; the factor $\exp(-r\tau)$ measures the sexually mature fraction of the population (assuming Type II survival). The demography and epidemiology of HIV in the adult population is now described by eqns (13.43), (13.44), and (13.45) but with the original v replaced by the v defined in eqn (13.55), and with time delays between birth and recruitment to the sexually active adult population. The time delays make these equations significantly more complicated and no exact solution is possible. However, we get the earlier results for ρ (eqn (13.53)) and for y^*, the asymptotic fraction infected (eqn (13.52)), with v now being replaced by

$$v \to w\,e^{-\mu\tau - \rho\tau}. \tag{13.56}$$

The replacement is also made in $r = v - \mu$. This again leads to eqn (13.51) being the critical condition dividing population growth ($\rho > 0$) from population decline ($\rho < 0$), with the proviso that v in eqn (13.51) is interpreted as $w \exp(-\mu\tau)$ and r is interpreted as $w \exp(-\mu\tau) - \mu$.

13.3.3 *Epidemiological parameters*

The models reveal that whether or not AIDS will change positive population growth rates to negative ones, and the time-scale of such changes, depends critically on the magnitudes of various key demographic and epidemiological parameters. The demographic parameters (birth, death, and population growth rates, v, μ, and r respectively) for a series of countries in which HIV is spreading rapidly (Kenya, Zaire, and Uganda) are recorded in Table 13.3. For comparison, data from the United Kingdom are also presented. Note the very high population growth rates in the developing countries (4 per cent per annum in Kenya). As mentioned earlier, epidemiological data are extremely limited and in certain areas we can only guess at parameter ranges. The fraction of those infected who will eventually develop AIDS, f, appears likely to be very high as long-term studies of infected homosexual men in developed countries reveal no decrease in the rate (2–7 per cent per annum) of conversion from HIV infection to AIDS. Disease progression in African heterosexuals appears to occur at similar rates, although much uncertainty remains concerning the clinical pattern of infection and disease in African patients. Roughly 30–40 per cent of infected male homosexuals appear to develop AIDS on an 8–9 year time-scale, and it seems likely that

Table 13.3 AIDS cases reported to WHO as at July 1989 and demographic parameters for a selection of countries (from World Bank and United Nations data series)

	Kenya	Zaire	Uganda	UK
Total number of AIDS cases	5949	335	6772	2296
Case rate per 100 000 population	6.8	1.1	1.5	1.0
Time period to which demographic data apply	1984–5	1984–5	1984–5	1984–5
Crude population size 1987 (millions)	22 397	31 796	16 018	55 678
Crude live birth rate per 1000 population yr^{-1}	55.1	44.8	50.3	12.9
Crude per capita birth rate yr^{-1}, v	0.0540	0.0442	0.0495	0.0129
Life expectancy at birth (years)	52.9	52.0	51.0	73.7
Crude per capita death rate yr^{-1}, μ	0.9189	0.0192	0.0196	0.0136
Population growth rate per 1000 yr^{-1}	41.4	30.3	33.5	1.5
Crude per capita growth rate yr^{-1}, r	0.0403	0.0299	0.033	0.0015
Urban population (per cent of total)	15.5	36.6	9.5	87.7
Dependency ratio (ages <15, >64)/(ages 15–64)	1.190	0.928	1.023	0.529
Child dependency age <15/(ages 15–64)	1.150	0.871	0.973	0.298
Population density (km^{-2})	38.0	13.6	68.0	230.0

most of the rest will convert to disease over a longer period (perhaps 15–20 years).

Limited studies from North America and Europe have recorded HIV infection in 30–65 per cent of babies of HIV seropositive mothers and similar studies in Nairobi, Kenya and Kinshasa, Zaire, suggest figures of 46–51 per cent (see Chapter 11). *In utero* infection appears to be the dominant mode of vertical transmission, and death rates among infected babies are very high— nearly 20 times that of children born to uninfected mothers in one study.

Data on the transmission probability, β (either from men to women or vice versa), in heterosexuals and the effective rate of partner change, c, are very limited at present for developing countries. One study suggests a value of β in the range 0.05–0.1 per partner for female to male transmission, provided co-factors (genital ulcers) are present. A rough guide to the parameter combination βc can be obtained indirectly from a knowledge of the rate of increase of the infected population (or from the doubling time of the epidemic). The limited data on trends in the rise in seropositivity in specific African countries are summarized in Table 13.4. The rate of spread is highest in urban areas in Africa, and is particularly fast in people with multiple sexual partners (Fig. 13.14), in those who have a high rate of infection with other sexually transmitted diseases (STDs) such as chancroid, and in prostitutes. For example, the doubling time, t_d, of the epidemic among prostitutes in Nairobi from 1981 to 1985 was approximately 1.0 years. In the general urban populations in Kenya, Uganda, and Zaire (as indicated by the proportion of pregnant women attending health clinics, found to be infected) the rate of spread is slower, but still alarming, doubling times ranging from 1 to 3.5 years (Table 13.4).

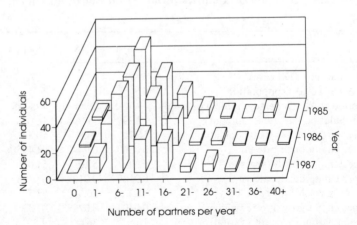

Fig. 13.14. Rates of sexual partner change recorded by interview of heterosexual males from two pastoralist Southern Nilotic groups in East Africa. The mean number of different sexual partners per year (average over three years) was 11.8 with a variance of 47.4 (from Konnings *et al.* 1989).

Table 13.4 Estimates of the rate of spread of HIV infection in various populations in developing countries (see text for details)

Location	Years	Population surveyed	Doubling time, t_d (years)	Rate of spread of infection Λ (yr^{-1})	Parameter combination, βc ($1/(\alpha + \mu) = 15$ years)	Basic reproductive rate, R_0 ($1/(\alpha + \mu) = 15$ years)
Nairobi, Kenya	1981–5	Prostitutes	1.00	0.681	0.748	11.2
Nairobi, Kenya	1982–5	Men with chancroid	1.00	0.677	0.744	11.1
Nairobi, Kenya	1981–5	Men with STDs	1.67	0.414	0.480	7.2
Nairobi, Kenya	1981–2	Women with STDs	1.00	0.686	0.753	11.3
Nairobi, Kenya	1970–86	Pregnant women	2.87	0.241	0.308	4.6
Kinshasa, Zaire	1970–86	Mothers	3.0	0.198	0.308	4.6
Kampala, Uganda	1985–7	Women—antenatal	1.12	0.619	0.686	10.3

Assuming equality of transmission from female to male and vice versa, given the observed 1:1 sex ratio in seropositivity, and an average incubation period (=average infectious period) of roughly 15 years ($1/(\alpha + \mu)$), these doubling times in the general population yield estimates of R_0 (the number of people infected by a single seropositive individual) and βc (the rate of transmission) in the respective ranges of 4–12 and 0.2–0.8. The associated estimates of the rate of increase, Λ, in the infected population, $Y(t)$, in the early stages of the epidemic in different countries/populations are recorded in Table 13.4 (range 0.2–0.8 yr^{-1}).

On the basis of these estimates we choose the following parameter ranges to explore the properties of the model with time-delays in recruitment (Section 13.3.2): $\varepsilon = 0.3$–0.7; $1/(\alpha + \mu) = 8$–20 years; $\mu = 0.019 \text{ yr}^{-1}$; $\Lambda = 0.2$–0.5 yr^{-1} (for the general urban population); $\tau = 15$ years; $v = 0.02$–0.06 yr^{-1} (where v is the birth rate per member of the population, before AIDS). Note that from Tables 13.3 and 13.4 it appears that Λ always exceeds r in value; hence the infection is predicted to have a severe effect on population growth.

13.3.4 *Population growth rates*

A wide range of parameter values, all within the bounds suggested by current empirical studies, predict asymptotically negative population growth rates even when recruitment delays are taken into account. The relationship between the asymptotic growth rate, a range of values for the rate of infection, Λ, and the fraction of babies born to infected mothers who do not acquire HIV via vertical transmission, ε, is recorded in Fig. 13.15 for various values of the incubation period. In these examples the growth rate per head of population before HIV infection, r, was assumed to be 0.04 yr^{-1} (4 per cent growth per annum) with life expectancy 52 years. As ε decreases and Λ increases the asymptotic growth rate is predicted to become negative. Concomitantly, as $\varepsilon \to 0$ and Λ rises, the asymptotic prevalence of HIV infection is predicted to rise in the adult population (age greater than 15 years) to high levels (Fig. 13.15). For plausible ranges of parameter values, HIV infection resulting in AIDS is predicted to induce the severe changes in the population size shown in Fig. 13.16(a) and (b). The critical value of the basic reproductive rate, R_0, of HIV that can bring the population growth rate, r, asymptotically to exactly zero (stationary population) for a specified value of the fraction infected who develop AIDS, f, is shown in Fig. 13.16(c).

The period t_c, denoting the time taken before the population begins to decline after invasion by HIV, is given very approximately by

$$t_c \sim [\ln(1/\Delta)]/(\Lambda - r) \tag{13.57}$$

where Δ is the fraction infected at time $t = 0$. This relationship is depicted in Fig. 13.16(d) for a range of values for the pre-HIV infection population growth rate, r (chosen to mimic developing countries—see Table 13.3), and the rate of HIV infection, Λ (see Table 13.4). Note that for low to moderate infection rates

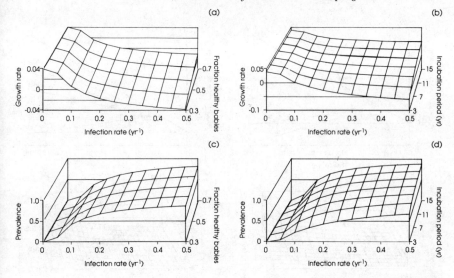

Fig. 13.15. (a), (b) The asymptotic population growth rate per head, ρ. (c), (d) The asymptotic prevalence, that is the fraction of population infected, y^*. Each graph refers to a human population infected with HIV with varying values for the epidemiological parameters Λ (rate of infection per capita per year), ε (fraction of babies born to infected mothers who do not acquire infection via vertical transmission), and $1/(\alpha + \mu)$ (average incubation period). Predictions are based on the simple delayed-recruitment model described in the main text. In (a) and (c) the duration of the incubation (=infectious) period was set at 8 years. In (b) and (d), the fraction of healthy babies born to infected mothers was set at 0.5.

(like those observed in the general population in Zaire, Uganda, and Kenya whose $\Lambda = 0.1$–0.2 yr^{-1}) the time to the onset of population decline, t_c, is predicted to be very long (20–70 years), even in countries with low growth rates ($r = 0.02$ yr^{-1}). Following onset, asymptotic rates of population decline may be dramatic (Fig. 13.15).

13.3.5 *Changes in age structure*

The simple model defined above can easily be extended to incorporate a variety of realistic refinements. These include: asymmetric probabilities of transmission from females to males, and males to females; asymmetries in the probability that a male or female partner will be infected, reflecting age dependency in the choice of partners of the opposite sex; only a fraction of those infected proceeding to develop AIDS; and, most importantly, a full age structure to reflect the demographic impact of AIDS on the age distribution of infected populations.

We consider a closed heterosexual population (no immigration or emigration) where $N_k(a, t)$ denotes the number (or density) of people of sex k ($k = 1$ denotes females and $k = 2$ denotes males) of age a at time t. Aside from the stratification

352   Microparasites

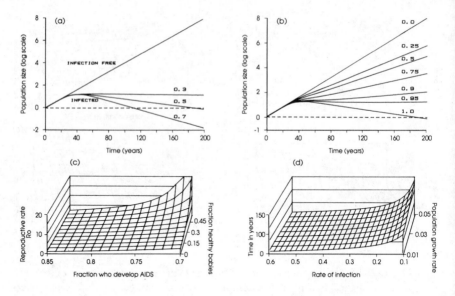

Fig. 13.16. (a) Population trajectories through time (recorded as ln $(N(t)/N(0))$, where $N(0)$ is the population size at time $t = 0$ when the infection was introduced), as predicted by the delayed-recruitment model defined in the main text, for various values of the fraction, ε, of babies born to infected mothers who do not acquire HIV infection via vertical transmission. The top line denotes 4 per cent growth in an uninfected population. The remaining trajectories, from bottom to top, denote predictions with ε set at 0.3, 0.5, and 0.7 respectively. The death rate of uninfecteds was set at $\mu = 0.019$ per capita per year (life expectancy of 52 years), the incubation period of the disease was set at 8 years ($= 1/(\alpha + \mu)$), and the time period to recruitment to the reproductively mature age class (τ) was fixed at 15 years. The rate of infection Λ was set at 0.233 per capita per year. (b) Population trajectories through time, as in (a) but varying the fraction, f, of infected adults who proceed to develop AIDS and die. The top line denotes 4 per cent population growth in an uninfected population. The remaining trajectories, from top to bottom, denote predictions with f set at 0.25, 0.5, 0.75, 0.9, 0.95, and 1 respectively. The inclusion of the fraction f into the delayed-recruitment model defined in the main text is as described in May et al. (1988a,b). Parameter values as in (a), with ε fixed at 0.5, and assuming that an equal fraction of children born to seropositive-recovered women die effectively at birth. (c) The critical value of the basic reproductive rate R_0 required to bring the growth rate of the population, r, to zero for various values of the fraction, f, who develop AIDS and the fraction of healthy babies, ε, born to infected mothers. The other epidemiological and demographic parameters are: $\Lambda = 0.4$ per capita per year, $1/(\alpha + \mu) = 10$ years; $\mu = 0.02$ yr^{-1}; $\tau = 15$ years. The top line is for $\varepsilon = 0$ and the bottom for $\varepsilon = 0.5$. (d) The period of time, t_c, predicted before an infected population ceases its previous pattern of exponential growth and begins to decline after invasion by HIV (eqn (13.57)) as a function of the rate of spread of infection, Λ, and the population growth rate, r (see Anderson et al. 1988).

by age and sex, the population is divided into four sub-populations denoting those susceptible to infection (i.e. uninfected), $X_k(a, t)$, those infected, $Y_k(a, t)$, those infecteds who recover and do not develop AIDS (assumed to be non-infectious), $Z_k(a, t)$, and those infecteds who develop AIDS, $A_k(a, t)$. For simplicity we consider that all infecteds in the $Y_k(a, t)$ class are infectious (see Anderson and May 1988*a*). Sexually mature susceptibles are assumed to acquire infection via sexual contact with an infected partner at a rate $\lambda_k(a, t)$. Newly born infants are assumed to acquire infection vertically from infected mothers. A fraction $1 - \varepsilon$ of births to infected mothers are assumed to acquire HIV infection. The model does not incorporate transmission via blood transfusions or via contaminated injecting equipment.

The model is compartmental in structure where susceptibles, on acquiring infection, move to the infected (=infectious) class $Y_k(a, t)$ at a per capita rate $\lambda_k(a, t)$ and leave at a rate $\gamma(a)$. The rate of leaving is assumed to be independent of sex but to depend on age. The average incubation (=infectious) period is therefore $1/\gamma(a)$ at age a. A fraction $1 - f$ 'recover' to join a non-infectious class $Z_k(a, t)$ while the remaining fraction f develop AIDS and join the class $A_k(a, t)$. Individuals with AIDS die at a rate α (independent of age and sex). We assume that the incubation period in those who acquire infection via sexual contact is constant and independent of age and sex (roughly 8–10 years on the basis of current evidence—see Anderson and Medley 1988). In the case of infants infected via vertical transmission we assume that the incubation period is much shorter, of the order of 2 years. We define the background mortality rate as $\mu(a)$. The system of partial differential equations, describing the changes in the number of individuals of age a at time t in each of the four compartments, is as follows:

$$\partial X_k(a, t)/\partial t + \partial X_k(a, t)/\partial a = -(\lambda_k(a, t) + \mu(a))X_k(a, t), \qquad (13.58)$$

$$\partial Y_k(a, t)/\partial t + \partial Y_k(a, t)/\partial a = \lambda_k(a, t)X_k(a, t) - (\gamma(a) + \mu(a))Y_k(a, t), (13.59)$$

$$\partial Z_k(a, t)/\partial t + \partial Z_k(a, t)/\partial a = (1 - f)\gamma(a)Y_k(a, t) - \mu(a)Z_k(a, t), \qquad (13.60)$$

$$\partial A_k(a, t)/\partial t + \partial A_k(a, t)/\partial a = f\gamma(a)Y_k(a, t) - (\alpha + \mu(a))A_k(a, t). \qquad (13.61)$$

The force, or per capita rate, of infection (via horizontal—that is, sexual—transmission) $\lambda_k(a, t)$ is defined as

$$\lambda_k(a, t) = c_k(t)\beta_{k'} \int_\tau^T \left(\rho_k(a, a', t) \frac{Y_{k'}(a', t)}{N_{k'}(a', t)} \right) da'. \qquad (13.62)$$

Here β_k and c_k are respectively the transmission probability and mean rate of acquiring new sexual partners for sex k, T and τ denote respectively the upper and lower age limits of sexual activity, k' denotes the opposite sex. The quantity $\rho_k(a, a', t)$ defines the probability that a susceptible of sex k and age a will choose a partner of age a' of the opposite sex at time t; thus defined, ρ_k involves both the intrinsic preference of individuals of age a for partners of age a' and the number of such partners that are available at time t. The variable $N_k(a, t)$ defines the total population of sex k and age a at time t.

One boundary condition for the system of eqns (13.58)–(13.62) is the requirement

$$Y_k(0, t) = \int_\tau^T m(a)(1 - \varepsilon) Y_k(a, t) \mathrm{d}a$$

and

$$X_k(0, t) = \int_\tau^T m(a)[N_k(a, t) - (1 - \varepsilon) Y_k(a, t)] \, \mathrm{d}a$$

with $m(a)$ defining the age-specific fertility rate (defined per head of population). The other boundary condition is given by specifying $X_k(a, 0)$, $Y_k(a, 0)$, and $N_k(a, 0)$ at $t = 0$.

The model is complex in structure and hence numerical methods must be employed to generate time-dependent changes in the age structure of the male and female segments of the population following the introduction of HIV-1. To start with, we consider behaviour under a series of simplifying assumptions before moving on to examine more complex (and hopefully more realistic) assumptions. We assume that $\mu(a) = \mu$ (reasonable for most developing countries), that the birth rate $m(a) = w$ for $T > a > \tau$, $m(a) = 0$ otherwise (where $\tau = 15$ years and $T = 50$ years), and that the fraction who develop AIDS, f, is equal to one. The quantity $\rho(a, a')$ is taken to have the value $N(a')/\int N(a') \, \mathrm{d}a'$, which corresponds to no age preference; if sexually active adults choose partners independent of age, then the probability of choosing a partner of age a', $\rho(a, a')$, is simply given by the fraction of the available population who are in that age class. We also assume that the fraction of children born to infected mothers that develop AIDS, $1 - \varepsilon$, survive for an average of two years from birth. In these circumstances we obtain eqn (13.53) with v defined as

$$v = \exp[-(\mu + \rho)\tau]. \tag{13.63}$$

Here v is the birth rate per adult, and ρ is the asymptotic growth rate of the population. The asymptotic prevalence of HIV infection y^* is given by

$$y^* = \left(\int_0^\infty (Y_1(a) + Y_2(a)) \, \mathrm{d}a \right) \left(\int_0^\infty (N_1(a) + N_2(a)) \, \mathrm{d}a \right)^{-1}$$

$$= (\Lambda - \rho)/\beta c. \tag{13.64}$$

Here Λ is the initial growth rate of the seroprevalence of HIV. Again for simplicity we have assumed that $\beta_1 c_1 = \beta_2 c_2 = \beta c$.

An example of the asymptotic age distribution generated by this model is presented in Fig. 13.17 which records, for comparison, the distribution in an infected and an uninfected population (Anderson *et al.* 1988; May *et al.* 1988a,b).

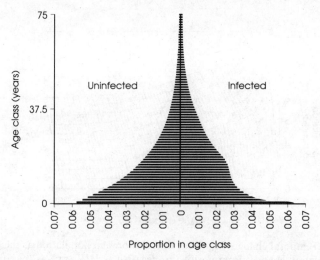

Fig. 13.17. Asymptotic age distributions (fraction in each age class) of an uninfected (left-hand side) and an infected (right-hand side) population. The growth rate, r, is 4 per cent and life expectancy, $1/\mu$, is 52 years in the absence of HIV. The incubation period was set at 15 years $(1/(\alpha + \mu))$ with the fraction of healthy babies born to infected mothers, ε, set at 0.3. The rate of infection in the early stages, Λ, was set at 0.233 yr^{-1} (Anderson *et al.* 1988).

The age profiles before and after the establishment of HIV infection are represented as the relative proportions in different age classes (as opposed to absolute numbers in the declining infected population).

An impression of the temporal evolution of the epidemic and its impact on the age structure of the population is presented in Fig. 13.18. Note how AIDS-induced mortality in infants (vertical transmission) and sexually active adults (horizontal transmission) changes the smooth exponential age distribution (at $t = 0$) to a much more complex shape. The predicted effect of AIDS upon the dependency ratio—which is taken to be the population below age 15 and that above age 64 years, divided by that aged 15 to 64 years—is not as great as might be expected (or has been widely suggested). On the one hand, the direct effects of mortality in the sexually active adult age classes due to AIDS tends to increase the ratio. On the other hand, the general depression of overall population growth rates due to adult deaths, and to the reduction in effective birth rate due to the deaths of infected babies, tends to decrease the ratio. With the caution that the dependency ratio takes no account of the extra burden that would be imposed by the care of infants and adult AIDS patients, this simple model suggests that, for some plausible ranges of parameter values, AIDS will have little effect on the dependency ratio (Anderson *et al.* 1988, 1989*b*). This result is in sharp contrast with the views of many informed discussants of this problem (Quinn *et al.* 1986; Piot *et al.* 1988).

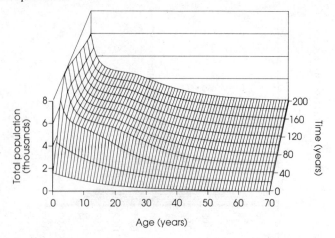

Fig. 13.18. Temporal changes in the age distribution of a population as the growth rate of the population changes from positive to negative as HIV spreads (parameter values as for right-hand side of Fig. 13.17).

Analyses based on very simple models of the major demographic and epidemiological processes yield three major conclusions. First, for plausible ranges of parameter values the disease AIDS is predicted to be capable of significantly reducing population growth rates, and even depressing them to negative values. Second, the time for these effects to become fully manifest, after the initial introduction of HIV infection, is predicted to be long, of the order of many decades. Third, whether or not AIDS will decrease or increase the dependency ratio within a given population depends critically on the values of the major demographic and epidemiological parameters prevailing in the community. For plausible parameter ranges (Tables 13.3 and 13.4) our analyses suggest little change or a small, but beneficial, change. This conclusion appears fairly insensitive to variations in the fraction of those infected, *f*, who eventually die. Similar analyses of the impact of directly transmitted infections such as smallpox and bubonic plague, that were of great historical significance as causes of human morbidity and mortality, suggest that AIDS has greater potential to depress human population growth rates significantly. This stems from the ability of HIV to transmit both horizontally via sexual contact and vertically from mother to unborn offspring, the high mortality associated with infection, and the apparently long period over which infected person are asymptomatic but infectious to their sexual partners.

Before proceeding to discuss these conclusions further we consider a series of realistic refinements to the basic age-structure model that focus on the areas in which simplifying assumptions were made to obtain the results presented in Figs. 13.17–13.19. The first concerns the assumption that the mortality and fertility rates were constant and independent of age (that is constant fertility

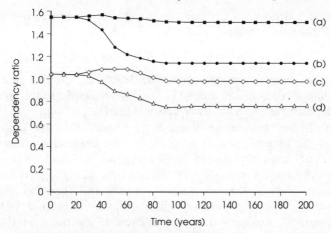

Fig. 13.19. Temporal changes in the dependency ratio ((ages < 15 and > 64)/ages 15–64) as HIV spreads. Four different numerical simulations of age-structured models are recorded. In all, $\tau = 15$ years, $\mu = 0.019$ per capita per year, $1/(\alpha + \mu) = 15$ years. The parameters r and ε are varied as follows: (a) $r = 0.04$ per capita per year, $\varepsilon = 0.7$; (b) $r = 0.04$ per capita per year, $\varepsilon = 0.3$; (c) $r = 0.02$ per capita per year, $\varepsilon = 0.7$; (d) $r = 0.02$ per capita per year, $\varepsilon = 0.3$.

over the reproductively mature age classes τ to T). The inclusion of age-specific mortality and fertility rates to mirror those typically observed in developing countries has no significant impact on the conclusions arrived at on the basis of the predictions of the simpler model. The dependency ratio again seems little affected by the epidemic. The remaining complications concern sexual behaviour and they are of sufficient importance to be considered under a separate section title.

13.3.6 *Age dependency in sexual activity and partner choice*

The model defined in eqns (13.58)–(13.62) contains a term $\rho_k(a, a', t)$ which denotes the probability that a person of sex k and age a has sexual contact with a person of the opposite sex of age a' at time t. It therefore represents a sexual partner choice or preference function (Anderson *et al.* 1989a), where choice or preference is based on age. Whether choice is based on age, sexual activity class (i.e. new partners per unit of time), or other factors, such as spatial location (i.e. urban or rural dweller), the function ρ_k is subject to a series of constraints (Jacquez *et al.* 1988; Gupta *et al.* 1989). In the case of choice, or preference, based on age these may be stated as follows:

$$1 > \rho_k(a, a', t) > 0, \tag{13.65}$$

$$\int_\tau^T \rho_k(a, a', t) \, da' = 1. \tag{13.66}$$

Here T and τ denote respectively the upper and lower age limits of sexual activity. Finally we require

$$N_1(a, t)c_1(a, t)\rho_1(a, a', t) = N_2(a', t)c_2(a', t)\rho_2(a', a, t) \qquad (13.67)$$

where $c_k(a, t)$ denotes the age- and time-dependent effective rate of sexual partner change of sex k. Equation (13.67) defines a simple 'supply and demand' rule. The partnerships made by a person of sex k and age a at time t with individuals of the opposite sex of age a' must equal those available in the age class a' of the opposite sex. It is clear that the constraints defined in eqns (13.65)–(13.67) must be satisfied at all times (all values of t). In the case of AIDS, which induces mortality in the sexually active age classes via the transmission of HIV through sexual contact, the changing demographic structure of the infected population is likely to create imbalances in the 'supply and demand' of sexual partners via differential mortality as the epidemic progresses in different strata of the population (i.e. age, sex, or sexual activity classes). In these circumstances a series of 'behavioural rules' must be defined in order that the constraints on the choice function $\rho_k(a, a', t)$ are satisfied at all times. The first of these concerns what precisely changes as the epidemic unfolds. Is it the choice or preference function, the mean rates of sexual partner change, or both? Once this has been decided it is then necessary to decide on a second set of rules which define the detail of precisely who changes behaviour. For example, if the impact of AIDS creates a change in the sex ratio of the sexually active population, say, with an excess of males, do females increase their rates of partner change to accommodate the demands of an increasing fraction of males in the population, or do males decrease their rates of pair formation in response to a constant level of activity per female but a declining fraction of females in the total population?

Similar problems apply if we consider changes in population distribution between age or sexual activity classes, as opposed to simply the two sexes. In deciding which behavioural rules to build into a model (that incorporates demographic and epidemiological processes) we require detailed information on preference functions and rates of sexual partner change, and how these alter under temporal changes in population structure resulting from AIDS-induced mortality. Such data are not available at present and hence published theoretical studies are more orientated to 'what if' questions as opposed to attempting to mirror observed behaviour.

A very simple method of ensuring that the constraints detailed in eqns (13.65)–(13.67) are satisfied for all values of t has been described by Anderson *et al.* (1989a,b). This is based on defining a set of initial conditions concerning the structure of the choice or preference function, $\rho_k(a, a', 0)$, and the mean rate of partner change, $c_k(0)$, at time $t = 0$. For simplicity we assume that the rate of partner change is independent of age a, and that both the choice functions and the mean rates of partner change for both sexes alter as the epidemic induces changes in population size and distribution between the age and sex classes.

The method assumes that the effective mean rate of sexual partner change of women depends on the number of men, and that female choice with respect to male age depends on the age distribution of men. A simple way of achieving this is to define

$$c_1(t) = k_1 N_2(t)/(N_1(t)/N_2(t)) \qquad (13.68)$$

where k_1 is an initial condition of sexual activity (at $t = 0$);

$$k_1 = c_1(0)(N_1(0) + N_2(0))/N_2(0). \qquad (13.69)$$

The age-dependent partner choice function for females is defined as

$$\rho_1(a, a', t) = (N_2(a', t)/N_2(t))(N_2(0)/N_2(a', 0))\rho_1(a, a', 0). \qquad (13.70)$$

The equivalent expressions for rate of sexual partner change of men, $c_2(t)$, and the male age-dependent partner choice function, $\rho_2(a, a', t)$, are arrived at by changing the subscripts $(1 \rightarrow 2, 2 \rightarrow 1)$ in eqns (13.69) and (13.70). The simple idea embodied in these definitions is that both the rate of sexual partner change and the choice function of either sex is dependent on the fraction of the population that is of the opposite sex (Anderson *et al.* 1989*a,b*).

The constraints and behavioural rules defined above allow us to consider the impact of different choice functions, different probabilities of transmissions between females and males and vice versa ($\beta_1 \neq \beta_2$), and age-dependent rates of sexual partner change, on the pattern of the epidemic.

We consider first differences by age in the way in which males and females choose sexual partners of the opposite sex. In many developing and developed countries males tend, on average, to form sexual partnerships with females younger than themselves. In developed countries the average difference is typically of the order of 2–3 years. However, in many developing countries a much greater difference is often observed (e.g. 5–10 years). Age- and sex-stratified data on the prevalence of HIV infection and the incidence of AIDS provide a clear indication of this trend. For example, Fig. 13.20(a) records the reported incidence of AIDS by age and sex in Uganda up to 31 July 1988, while Fig. 13.20(b) records those seropositive for HIV in Kinshasa, Zaire (1984–5) by age and sex (Quinn *et al.* 1986; Berkley *et al.* 1989). In both examples, the distributions (of cases of AIDS and HIV infection) are skewed to the younger age class of females by comparison with males. There is a 5–10 year difference between males and females in the age at which disease incidence or the prevalence of infection attains a maximum.

Heterogeneity in mixing between the different age classes has a significant influence on the predicted demographic impact of the epidemic. An illustration of this is presented in Fig. 13.21 where predicted temporal changes in total population size following the introduction of HIV-1 (at time $t = 0$) into a population of 16.6 million people (with a 3.8 per cent annual growth rate prior to the introduction) are recorded (Anderson *et al.* 1989*b*). The simulations are based on a homogeneous mixing assumption (i.e. no stratification by sexual

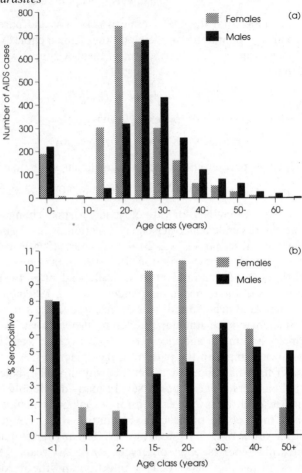

Fig. 13.20. (a) Age and sex distribution of reported cases of AIDS in Uganda up to the end of July 1988 (Berkley *et al.* 1989) and (b) of the percentage infected with HIV in Kinshasa, Zaire (1984–5) (Quinn *et al.* 1986).

activity class) but where partner choice is dependent on age. Two simulations are recorded: in one, males and females restrict their partner choice to within their own age class (restricted choice), while in the other, males, on average, choose female partners younger than themselves. Note that the latter assumption is predicted to result in HIV having a more severe demographic impact than that induced by restricted within-age-class mixing (Anderson 1989).

Models of this kind generate age and sex distributions of HIV seroprevalence and AIDS incidence similar to those observed in many sub-Saharan countries, where HIV has spread extensively in the general population (Fig. 13.22; compare with Fig. 13.20(a)). With the efficiency of vertical transmission (i.e.

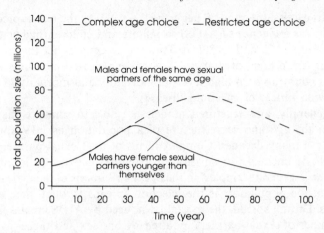

Fig. 13.21. The influence of two different assumptions concerning sexual partner choice by age on the predicted demographic impact of AIDS (see Anderson *et al.* (1989*b*) for details of simulations). At time $t = 0$, HIV was introduced into a population of size 16.6 million with a 3.8 per cent annual growth rate (in the absence of infection). The two simulations record projected changes in population size as the epidemic spreads, for a choice function $(\rho_k(a, a', t))$ in which males and females only choose sexual partners of the same age and in which males, on average, choose sexual partners younger than themselves ($\beta_1 c_1 = \beta_2 c_2$, doubling time $t_d = 1.5$ years, efficiency of vertical transmission $1 - \varepsilon = 0.5$).

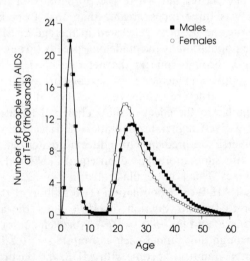

Fig. 13.22. Predicted age distribution of people with AIDS (males and females recorded separately) at $t = 90$ years after the start of the epidemic (see Anderson *et al.* 1989*b*). The major assumptions concerning transmission and mixing are as defined in the legend to Fig. 13.21 (with males having younger female partners).

perinatal transmission) set at 50 per cent ($1 - \varepsilon = 0.5$), the model predicts levels of infection (or incidence of AIDS) in infants and children higher than those observed (Figs. 13.22 and 13.20(a)). This may suggest either that the figure of 50 per cent is too high, or that AIDS is under-reported in infants and young children in countries with high levels of morbidity and mortality in the young due to a wide variety of infectious diseases.

More generally, age-structured models are able to simulate the details of changes in the age and sex structure of a population as HIV spreads over time-scales of many decades. Complex forms of the 'sexual partner choice by age matrix', or unequal transmission probabilities between males and females and vice versa, generate 'ripples' in the age distributions of the male and female segments of the population as the infection spreads through time and across age classes. During spread, the mortality induced by AIDS creates imbalances in the number of sexual partners required by one sex and those 'available' of the opposite sex. As outlined earlier, the mean rate of sexual partner change and/or the structure of the choice or preference matrix must change through time to accommodate these imbalances. This is especially apparent if the probability of transmission is higher from males to females than vice versa. Current evidence suggests there may be a two- to threefold difference in the probabilities (Johnson and Laga 1988; Anderson and Medley 1988). An illustration of the influence of unequal probabilities of transmission between the two sexes on the predicted temporal evolution of the epidemic is presented in Fig. 13.23. The projections are based on simulations in which mixing was restricted within age classes but where the probability of transmission from males to females was three times greater than that from females to males ($\beta_1 c_1 = 3\beta_2 c_2$). Note the 'ripples' generated in the age distributions of males and females in the population as the epidemic spreads through time. These are induced by changes through time in the net rate of HIV transmission as a consequence of 'supply and demand' of sexual partners in a population of changing age and sex structure (Anderson *et al.* 1989*b*).

In a manner similar to the effect of male choice of female sexual partners younger than themselves, higher probabilities of transmission from males to females than vice versa are predicted to induce a greater demographic impact when compared with simulations based on equal likelihoods of transmission between the two sexes. This point is illustrated in Fig. 13.24 which records the predicted impact of AIDS on a population (16.6 million at $t = 0$, 3.8 per cent growth rate prior to the introduction of HIV) under the assumptions that $\beta_1 c_1 = \beta_2 c_2$ (full curve) and that $\beta_1 c_1 = 3\beta_2 c_2$ (broken curve). The projections record changes through time, under each assumption, in total population size, total number infected, number of people with AIDS, and the proportion infected with HIV.

A point of particular interest revealed by numerical studies of model behaviour concerns the comparative influences of preferential choice of sexual partners by age, and unequal transmission probabilities of infection between the two sexes, on the potential demographic impact of AIDS. Figure 13.25 records temporal changes in total population size (with restricted within-age-class mixing) for four different sets of female to male and male to female transmission probabilities. In each the value of R_0 was held constant at 4.7 (with an initial doubling time, t_d, of 1.5 years) but the ratio $\beta_2 c_2/\beta_1 c_1$ was varied with values of 1, 3, 6, and 9 (reflecting an increasing bias towards more efficient transmission from males to females than vice versa). A rising bias increases the demographic impact due to the influence on net fertility of higher levels of infection amongst females by comparison with males, but the effect is less than that predicted by preferential mixing in which males, on average, choose female sexual partners younger than themselves (compare Figs. 13.21 and 13.25).

It is also of interest to note that a threefold difference in the efficiency of transmission between the two sexes is not predicted to result in very marked differences in the proportions of males and females infected in the total population (Fig. 13.26). In the case of homogeneous mixing (by age and sexual activity class) simple models predict that the ratio of the number of seropositive males to seropositive females is not unity, but is roughly $(\beta_1 c_1/\beta_2 c_2)^{1/2}$ (May and Anderson 1987). Obviously the average number of heterosexual partners of females and males, m_1 and m_2, are equal, but the effective average c_1 ($c_k = m_k + \sigma_k^2/m_k$) could significantly exceed c_2 if the variance of the distribution of acquiring new sexual partners by females (associated with the concentrated activities of female prostitutes) is greater than that of males, irrespective of the fact that transmission efficacy from males to females appears to be greater than that from females to males. The situation is made more complicated by changes through time in rates of sexual partner change, and the structure of the 'preference by age mixing matrix', as AIDS-induced mortality influences the 'supply and demand' of sexual partners of the opposite sex. This factor is largely responsible for the approximately equal proportions of males and females infected (slightly higher proportion of females infected) depicted in Fig. 13.26.

The limited quantitative data that are available on patterns of sexual partner change suggest a further modification in model structure. In both developed and developing countries rates of sexual partner change vary with age, tending (on average) to be higher in the younger, as opposed to the older, sexually active age classes (Anderson 1988b; Anderson et al. 1989a). An illustration of the predicted impact of such trends is presented in Fig. 13.27, based on the model defined by eqns (13.58)–(13.62) with the added refinement of age-dependency in the effective rates of sexual partner change (c_1 and c_2) (see Anderson et al. 1989a, 1990). Three scenarios are considered, to provide comparisons between the effects of age-dependent mixing and age-dependent rates of sexual partner change. Case 1 represents restricted (or assortative) mixing where individuals only choose sexual partners in their own age class, and where the effective rate of sexual partner change is fixed at 3.4 yr^{-1} (at $t = 0$) for all age and sex classes. Case 2 represents male preference for females of a younger age than themselves with a fixed effective rate of sexual

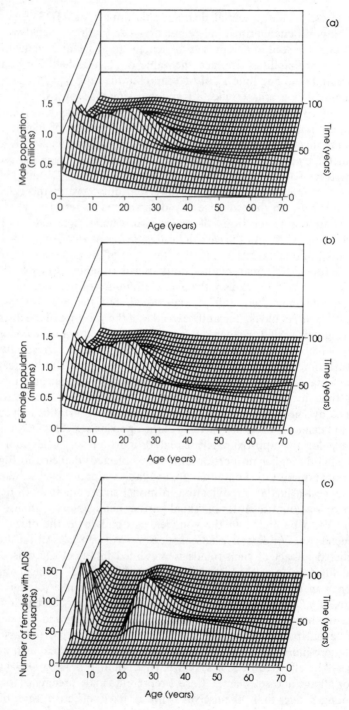

(d)

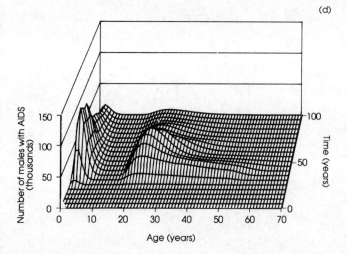

Fig. 13.23. Predicted changes in the age distribution of males (a) and females (b), along with the number of cases of AIDS among females (c) and males (d). As discussed more fully on p. 362, these figures assume that partners are chosen within age-classes, but that transmission from male-to-female is three times larger than the converse. Note the 'ripples' in age-structure and AIDS incidence as the epidemic progresses. For details see Anderson *et al.* (1989*b*).

partner change of 3.4 yr^{-1} (at $t = 0$) for all sexually active age and sex classes. Case 3 represents restricted mixing within each age class but with the effective mean rate of partner change being higher in young men and women than older individuals (but with the overall mean across all age classes fixed at 3.4 yr^{-1} at $t = 0$). The efficiency of transmission from males to females is three times that from females to males.

Figure 13.27 records predicted temporal changes in the proportion of the population infected (graph A), the total population size (graph B), and the number of people with AIDS (graph C). With the set of parameter values employed, all three cases are predicted to result in a reversal of the sign of the net population growth rate from positive to negative over a time-scale of a few decades. The least impact, over the 100-year time span of the simulations, occurs when mixing is restricted within age classes, with an effective rate of sexual partner change independent of age (case 1). A more severe impact results when older men tend, on average, to have sexual contract with women younger than themselves (case 2). The most severe impact, however, results when the effective rate of sexual partner change is highest in young men and women (case 3). The severity of the impact recorded in case 3 would be further enhanced if the assumption of restriction of within-age-class mixing was relaxed to allow men to have the greatest degree of sexual contact with women younger than themselves.

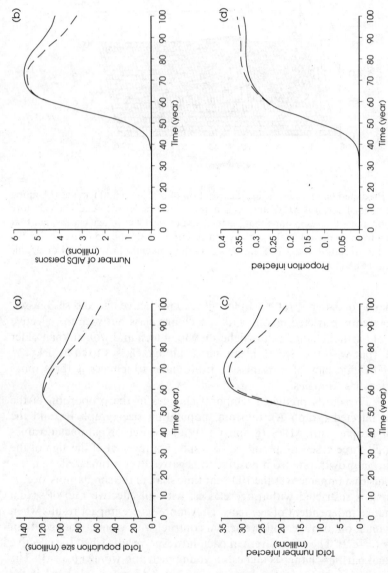

Fig. 13.24. The influence of unequal transmission probabilities from male to female and vice versa. The results from two simulations, described in Anderson *et al.* (1989*b*), are recorded in four graphs with $\beta_1 c_1 = \beta_2 c_2$ (full curve) and $\beta_1 c_1 = 3\beta_2 c_2$ (broken curve) ($t_d = 2.5$ years, $R_0 = 3.2$, $\varepsilon = 0.5$). (a) Changes in total population size; (b) changes in the number of people with AIDS: (c) changes in the total number infected; and (d) changes in the proportion infected.

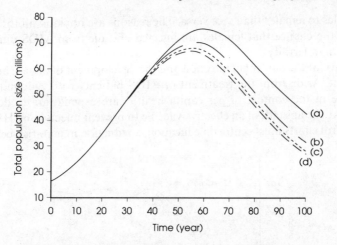

Fig. 13.25. Similar to Fig. 13.22 but recording predicted changes in total population size with the ratio of transmission efficiency of males to females divided by that from females to males ($\beta_2 c_2 / \beta_1 c_1$) set at: (a) 1, (b) 3, (c) 6, and (d) 9 (see Anderson *et al.* (1989*b*)).

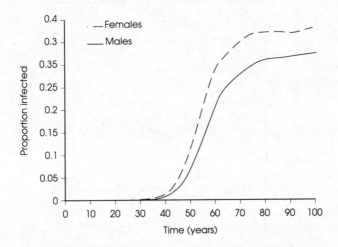

Fig. 13.26. Temporal changes in the proportion of males (full curve) and females (broken curve) infected with HIV under the assumption that $\beta_1 c_1 = 3\beta_2 c_2$ (Anderson *et al.* 1989*b*).

The depressing conclusion to emerge from these numerical studies of age-structured models of the transmission dynamics of HIV is that the likelihood of the disease AIDS inducing a severe demographic impact is much enhanced by three realistic refinements concerning sexual behaviour and the likelihood of transmission between the two sexes. These are age dependency in sexual activity (from high to low as people age), male preference for female sexual partners younger than themselves, and a higher likelihood of transmission from males to females than vice versa. The reasons are obvious; all three factors enhance the chance that females are infected and die from AIDS during their years of high fertility.

Options for the control of infection and the development of disease are limited at present. Aside from the treatment of AIDS patients with Zidovudine (very expensive in the context of per capita health care expenditure in developing countries), the absence of an effective vaccine to prevent infection by HIV means that control efforts must centre on education, a reduction in high-risk behaviours,

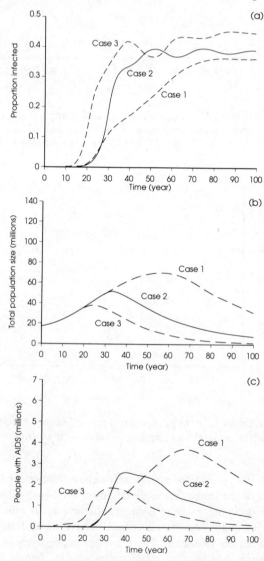

the use of condoms, and the screening of blood and blood products. Mathematical models can be used to assess the potential effectiveness of control measures, particularly in the context of their intensity and the timing of their introduction (Anderson *et al.* 1989; Rowley *et al.* 1989). An illustration of such an application is presented in Fig. 13.28 which records temporal changes in total population size (following the introduction of HIV at time $t = 0$) under the assumption that $\beta_1 c_1$ and $\beta_2 c_2$ are halved in magnitude (as a result of an increased use of condoms (influencing β_k) and/or reduction in the effective average rate of sexual partner change (c_k)) at time points 10, 20, and 30 years after the introduction of the virus. The simulations reveal that the timing of changes in behaviour has a very substantial impact on the predicted demographic impact of the disease. If control is introduced at an early stage ($t = 10$ years), the simulations suggest that over a time-scale of 100 years, AIDS will not reverse the sign of the population growth rate (in reality other factors, such as limitation of resources or a reduction in the birth rate, would act to limit population growth over this time-scale). The general conclusions to emerge from such studies are to some degree obvious, but they serve to emphasize the urgent need in many countries to develop and forcefully apply education programmes aimed at changing sexual behaviour. Models simply serve to highlight both the urgency of implementation and the non-linear benefits that accrue from early introduction, and the degree to which behaviour needs to be changed.

A striking impression of the magnitude of the AIDS problem in developing countries is provided by current serological data that indicate the degree to which HIV has spread both in high-risk groups and the general population in African countries (Figs. 13.29 and 13.30). A cursory inspection of the maps, even in the knowledge of the limited data upon which they are based, leads us to the conclusion that AIDS will cause major demographic changes in some developing countries over the next two decades. There is no doubt, however, that its effects will vary widely from one region, or one country, to the next, due to great variability in patterns of sexual behaviour. A simple illustration

---

Fig. 13.27. Numerical projections of the demographic impact of HIV and AIDS in a developing country (population size 16.6 million at $t = 0$, 3.8 per cent annual population growth rate prior to HIV introduction at $t = 0$), under different assumptions concerning both sexual partner by age and age-related changes in sexual activity (see Anderson *et al.* 1989b; Ng and Anderson 1989). (a), (b), (c) Record temporal changes in the proportion infected (a), total population size (b), and people with AIDS (c). Case 1 denotes restricted mixing where individuals only choose sexual partners in their own age class, and where the effective mean rate of sexual partner change per year is 3.4 for all sexually active age classes. Case 2 represents male preference for females younger than themselves with a fixed mean of 3.4 yr^{-1} across all sexually active age classes. Case 3 represents restricted mixing within each age class, but with the mean rate of partner change being higher in younger men and women than older individuals (but with the overall mean across all age classes fixed at 3.4 yr^{-1} at time $t = 0$) ($\beta_1 c_1 = 3\beta_2 c_2$, $t_d = 1.5$ years, $\varepsilon = 0.05$).

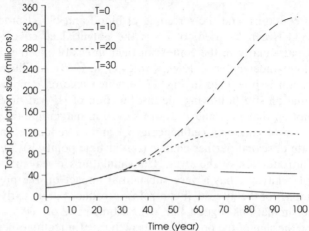

Fig. 13.28. Predicted temporal changes in total population size (16.6 million at $t = 0$, with a 3.8 per cent annual growth rate prior to the introduction of HIV at time $t = 0$) under the assumption that changes in sexual behaviour reduce the efficiency of horizontal transmission by 50 per cent at different time points from the start of the epidemic ($T = 10$, 20, and 30 years). The full curve denotes the predicted temporal pattern under the assumption of no changes in behaviour (see Anderson *et al.* 1989*b*).

of this point is provided in Fig. 13.31 which records HIV seroprevalence in urban and rural areas, and in prostitutes and pregnant women, in different African countries. In general, heterogeneity in sexual activity, whether between urban and rural areas, or between different groups in a given community, is likely to decrease the demographic impact predicted by our simple model. For any chosen values of the early doubling rate and incubation interval (Fig. 13.32),

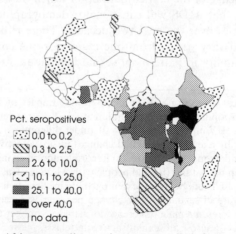

Fig. 13.29. Map of Africa recording estimates compiled from published and unpublished serological surveys of HIV seroprevalence (per cent) in high-risk urban populations (AIDS surveillance data base, United States Bureau of Census, April 1989).

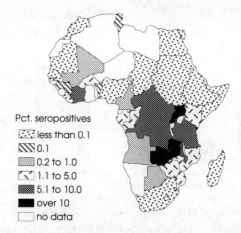

Pct. seropositives
- less than 0.1
- 0.1
- 0.2 to 1.0
- 1.1 to 5.0
- 5.1 to 10.0
- over 10
- no data

Fig. 13.30. Map of Africa recording estimates compiled from published and unpublished serological surveys of HIV seroprevalence (per cent) in the general population in urban areas (AIDS surveillance data base, United States Bureau of the Census, April 1989).

the eventual prevalence of endemic infection will be higher if all individuals are equally active sexually than if much variability exists (in which case core infection tends to be concentrated within the more active categories). Our parameter values, based on current data, may well lead to conclusions more representative of, say, Kinshasa and Nairobi than of Zaire and Kenya as a whole. But any assessment of the effects of such heterogeneities simply requires better data than that we have at present.

Simple models, such as those described here, are useful for setting the agenda for data collection to improve the accuracy of predictions. There is a clear need for the collection of much more detailed data on all the parameters discussed above, although the social, ethical, and practical problems surrounding such research are formidable. A start has been made with recent work that has begun to address some of the important complications induced by heterogeneity in rates of sexual partner change, and by complex networks of sexual and social interactions.

With these limitations in mind, we conclude by returning to two major predictions of the simple model. First, the AIDS epidemic is likely to have little impact on dependency ratios, a prediction which directly contradicts current views of this problem. From this it might be concluded that the epidemic will be less disruptive to the social organisation and economic fitness of badly afflicted countries than previously feared. We do not believe this to be the case, however, as the very high predicted mortality due to a disease which requires repeated hospitalization, perhaps over periods of a few years, and which is thought to enhance morbidity due to other infections such as tuberculosis, will be devastating to already overloaded health-care systems in poor countries.

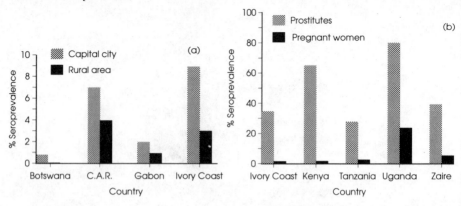

Fig. 13.31. Comparison of HIV seroprevalence in different at-risk groups in different countries. (a) Capital cities and rural areas, the general population (United States Bureau of Census, April 1989). (b) Prostitutes and pregnant women (United States Bureau of Census, April 1989).

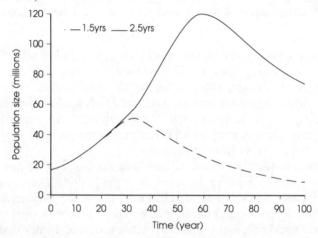

Fig. 13.32. The predicted impact of AIDS on total population size under two different assumptions concerning the doubling time, t_d, of the epidemic in its early stages (broken curve, $t_d = 1.5$ years; full curve, $t_d = 2.5$ years). Population size at time $t = 0$ was 16.6 million, and the population had an annual growth rate of 3.8 per cent prior to the introduction of HIV (Anderson *et al.* 1989*b*).

Small changes in the dependency ratio (whether plus or minus) are irrelevant under such circumstances.

The second prediction, that of a long time-period between the establishment of HIV infection and the reversal of exponential population growth, offers hope in the sense that it provides time for educational programmes to change behaviour, for the development of more effective drugs, and (we hope) for the discovery of an effective vaccine. It should be remembered, however, that the availability of cheap and effective vaccines (such as that against measles) is not always beneficial to people living in very poor countries where the cost of immunization is prohibitive to individuals and governments. For the foreseeable future the main hope for checking the spread of HIV lies in education programmes aimed at changing behaviour.

13.4 Summary

We extend the framework of our basic model to encompass host populations with positive population growth rates. The new models are used to obtain expressions relating the basic reproductive rate and the average age at infection to each other, and to various epidemiological and demographic characteristics of the infection and the host population. These expressions show clearly how demographic and epidemiological parameters combine to determine observed patterns of susceptibility and infection in developing countries. More complex models are then discussed that incorporate age dependences in case fatalities, in background mortality, and in the force of infection and choice of sexual partners. These are used to study the impacts of various vaccination programmes for the control of measles, and the potential demographic impact of AIDS in communities in the developing world.

14

Indirectly transmitted microparasites

Many important microparasitic infections of humans are indirectly transmitted from person to person by biting arthropods such as mosquitoes. A list of the major infections is presented in Table 14.1. An idea of their global significance is provided by the observation that the protozoan malarial infections on the continent of Africa alone are estimated to cause in excess of one million child deaths annually (Walsh and Warren 1979). The term 'vector transmitted' is often used to describe these infections but it should be noted that the vector is invariably a true intermediate host, in the sense that the parasite undergoes a phase of obligatory development (and often reproduction) within the arthropod.

In this chapter we consider the complications that the involvement of a second species of host introduces in the study of transmission, control, and the interpretation of observed epidemiological patterns. By way of illustration we concentrate on one particular infection, namely malaria. This is because of the disease's global significance as a cause of human mortality, its role in the early beginnings of epidemic and endemic theory, and the relative wealth of empirical information available on the biology and epidemiology of this disease. The investigation of the transmission dynamics of malaria, however, illustrates a much broader class of problems that are relevant to the study of a wide range of infections transmitted by vectors. We attempt to emphasize this point at appropriate stages in the chapter by reference to other viral and protozoan infections.

14.1 Biology and life cycle

Malaria in humans is due to infection by one of four protozoan species belonging to the genus *Plasmodium*, namely *P. falciparum*, *P. vivax*, *P. malariae*, and *P. ovale*. In some areas of the world, more than one species may be endemic in the same geographical locality, so that individuals may harbour concurrent infections of two or more species. The most pathogenic species is *P. falciparum* (falciparum malaria) which is a major cause of child mortality in many areas of the developing world. The different species have similar life histories but there are quite a number of differences in biological detail.

The infection in humans begins when sporozoites (infective stages) are injected into the blood by a female mosquito of the genus *Anopheles*; the females need blood-meals to produce their eggs. The sporozoites migrate to the liver where they enter liver cells (hepatocytes) and develop into schizonts which give rise, via asexual reproduction, to the form which invades the blood cells, the merozoites. These enter red blood cells and become first trophozoites and then

Table 14.1 Major indirectly transmitted microparasitic infections

Group	Disease	Infectious agent	Location	Intermediate host
Viruses	Yellow fever	Yellow fever virus	Africa, Central, and South America	*Aedes* spp. and *Haemagogus* spp.
	Dengue fever	Dengue fever virus	S.E. Asia, India, Pakistan, Africa, Caribbean, Pacific Islands	*Aedes* spp.
Rickettsiae	Q fever	*Coxiella burnetti*	World-wide	*Amblyomma* spp. and *Dermacentor* spp.
Protozoa	Malaria	*Plasmodium vivax*	World-wide; tropical, sub-tropical, warmer temperate	*Anopheles* spp.
	Malaria	*Plasmodium malariae*	World-wide; tropical, sub-tropical	*Anopheles* spp.
	Malaria	*Plasmodium falciparum*	World-wide; tropical, sub-tropical, warmer temperate	*Anopheles* spp.
	Trypanosomiasis	*Trypanosoma brucei*	West, East, Central Southern Africa	*Glossina* spp.
	Trypanosomiasis	*Trypanosoma congolense*	West, East, Central Africa	*Glossina* spp.
	Leishmaniasis	*Leishmania donovani*		
		L. d. donovani	Asia (including China, USSR, India), Africa	*Phlebotomus* spp.
		L. d. chagasi	Mexico, Central and South America	*Lutzomyia* spp.
	Leishmaniasis	*Leishmania mexicana*	Mexico, Central and South America, USA (Texas)	*Lutzomyia* spp.
	Leishmaniasis	*Leishmania braziliensis*	Central and South America	*Lutzomyia* spp.
	Leishmaniasis	*Leishmania tropica* and *Leishmania major*	Asia (including USSR, India), Africa, and Southern Europe	*Phlebotomus* spp.
	Leishmaniasis	*Leishmania peruviana*	Peru	*Lutzomyia* spp.
	Leishmaniasis	*Leishmania aethiopica*	East and N.E. Africa	*Phlebotomus* spp.

erythrocytic schizonts (by a phase of asexual reproduction). For each schizont, 12–24 merozoites are released to invade further blood cells. Some sporozoites may remain dormant in the liver as hypnozoites. They may later, after an interval of several months, develop into schizonts and then merozoites which enter the blood. Some merozoites develop into gametocytes and are ingested by a mosquito when it ingests human blood. Within the mosquito they develop into microgametes and macrogametes (the male and female gametes) that fuse to form a zygote (the sexual phase). This becomes a motile ookinete form which bores through the gut wall of the vector and forms an oocyst from which large numbers of sporozoites are released. These invade the salivary glands of the mosquito from which they are injected into the human host when the vector feeds (see Garnham (1966) for further details).

Bouts of fever are associated with the rupture of the schizonts, which event occurs approximately every 48 hours with *P. falciparum*, *P. vivax*, and *P. ovale* and every 72 hours with *P. malariae*. The liver and spleen are grossly enlarged in infected individuals and haemolytic anaemia may be severe.

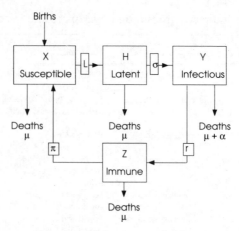

Fig. 14.1. Diagrammatic flow chart illustrating transitions between classes of the human population. The human population is divided into susceptibles (X), latent individuals (H), infectious individuals (Y) and immune individuals (Z). Rate parameters determine the flow of individuals between these classes: the per capita transmission rate L, the natural death rate μ, the disease-induced death rate α, the recovery rate γ, the rate at which individuals become infectious σ, and the rate of loss of immunity π.

The foregoing description is in broad qualitative terms and quantitative details vary from one species of the parasite to another and between different people and different species of vector. Mathematical studies of malaria transmission are conventionally based on the employment of the classical microparasite compartmental models (the prevalence framework) discussed in earlier chapters. A diagrammatic flow-chart of the principal population compartments based on such a framework is illustrated in Fig. 14.1. The basic malaria model described in a later section is based on this simple, idealized structure.

However, it should be noted that for protozoan parasites in particular, this framework ignores two important complications; these complications are less relevant for vector-transmitted viruses (the arboviruses). The first concerns the course of infection within an individual patient. In the case of malaria, for example, it is possible to obtain quantitative measures not just of prevalence (presence or absence of infection) but also of the intensity of infection (based, for example, on the proportion or number of infected red blood cells per sample). Furthermore, infection does not necessarily imply infectiousness since a patient may harbour many liver and blood cell stages of the parasites but no gametocytes (the stage infective to the vector). In other words, a more relevant quantitative measure of infectiousness is provided by counts of gametocytes per unit blood sample. In the epidemiological literature concerned with malaria, the proportion of the population with detectable levels of gametocytes in their blood stream is often defined as the 'gametocyte rate' of the population (Macdonald 1957). This is a misuse of the term 'rate' since prevalence is a 'standing crop' measure and not a rate. Similar criticisms apply to the use of the term 'trophozoite rate' (proportion of the population with infected red blood cells), and the overall 'parasite rate' (the proportion of the population with any evidence of infection).

The second problem concerns the nature of acquired immunity to malarial infection. Immunity appears to depend on both the duration and the intensity of past exposure to infection. Unlike many vector-transmitted viral infections (e.g. yellow fever virus), recovery from a primary infection with malaria does not imply fully protective immunity against reinfection. Parasite population growth may be slower, and the clearance of parasites from the blood more rapid, in second or subsequent infections but individuals may still be infectious to mosquitoes (i.e. gametocytes are often produced in second or subsequent infections). The mechanisms of immunity to malaria are not fully understood at present. Antibody and cell-mediated responses are important in limiting parasite population growth within individuals, but evidence of repeated infections in the same individuals in endemic areas argues that such mechanisms may only provide partial protection against parasite invasion (Molineaux and Gramiccia 1980). However, it is becoming increasingly apparent that genetic heterogeneity in parasite populations, both within an individual (antigenic variation within a clone) and within the community as a whole (parasite strain variation), may be an important determinant of the apparent absence of fully protective immunity following recovery from a primary infection (Forsyth *et al.* 1988). In short, the preceding discussion implies that the framework portrayed in Fig. 14.1, which embodies a class of 'immune' individuals, is an oversimplification of the true complexities of acquired immunity to certain vector-transmitted infections such as malaria. In later sections, however, this simple framework provides a useful point of departure for the development of more complex models.

14.2 Epidemiological patterns

Before turning to the development of a simple model to describe the basic features of malarial transmission, in this section we summarize the type of information available for estimating parameters and for testing the predictions of models.

14.2.1 *Infection in humans*
We consider empirical information on infection within the human host under four general headings. This is followed by parallel considerations of such factors for the intermediate hosts.

14.2.1.1 *Latent and infectious periods*　The latent period for malaria is defined as the time from initial infection to the appearance of gametocytes in the blood. This period may depend on the duration of past exposure to infection (as a

Table 14.2 Latent periods of infectiousness for vector-transmitted protozoan and viral infections

Infectious agent	Latent period (days)	Duration of infectiousness	Reference
Plasmodium ovale	10–14	~2 months	Molineaux and Gramiccia (1980)
Plasmodium malariae	15–16	~4 months	Molineaux and Gramiccia (1980)
Plasmodium falciparum	9–10	~9.5 months	Molineaux and Gramiccia (1980)
Yellow fever virus	6	Short (4 days)	Anderson (1981a)
Trypanosoma brucei	10–14	Long (years?)	Anderson (1981a)

consequence of the build-up of acquired immunity). Average values for three species of human malaria are listed in Table 14.2. For comparison, the latent periods for other vector-transmitted viral and protozoan infections are also presented in this table. Note that the latent periods for malaria are relatively long in comparison with the viral infections such as yellow fever.

Periods of infectiousness are more difficult to determine (Table 14.2). In the case of malaria, infectiousness is defined as the presence of gametocytes in the blood. Their abundance (the degree of infectiousness, see Table 14.2) and the duration of their presence (the infectious period) depend both on the age of a given infection within an individual (the production of gametocytes varies during the course of a single infection) and the individual's past experience of malaria. For example, rates of recovery from infection with *P. ovale*, *P. malariae*, and *P. falciparum* appear to increase with age in endemic areas (Fig. 14.2) (Molineaux and Gramiccia 1980). Recovery is usually defined as the clearance of the parasite from the blood of a patient and it is not necessarily synonymous with the rate of clearance of gametocytes. However, the two are positively associated, with the latter being slightly more rapid than the former (Macdonald 1950).

In gaining an understanding of the duration of infectiousness, the most easily obtained information is that concerning the rate of clearance of parasites from the blood following a single response. The best series of observations on this subject is that collected by Earle *et al.* (1939) who studied a group of Puerto Ricans infected with *P. falciparum* who remained untreated over a period of 60 weeks. The data are presented in Fig. 14.3 and an analysis gives an expected duration of infection of roughly 200–300 days. A collection of estimates of infectious periods, some based on recovery rates, are presented in Table 14.2. Again note that the periods are much longer for protozoan infections than for vector-transmitted viruses.

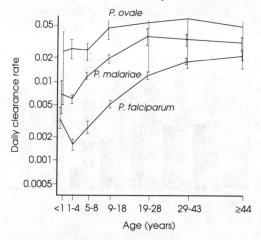

Fig. 14.2. Daily recovery rate from patent parasitaemia (clearance rate) for three species of *Plasmodium*, by age of the human host (from Moiineaux and Gramiccia 1980).

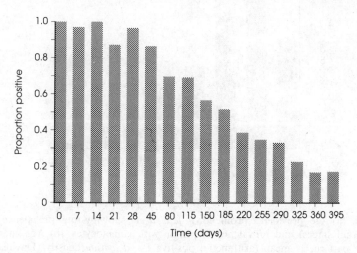

Fig. 14.3. The proportion of subjects remaining positive at succeeding intervals of time after a single infection with *P. falciparum* (Earle *et al.* 1939).

14.2.1.2 *Changes in prevalence and intensity with age*   Observed patterns of change with age in the prevalence and average intensity (defined as some measure of the degree of red blood cell invasion) of malarial infection aredisplayed in Fig. 14.4. In areas of endemic *P. falciparum* infection, they characteristically rise steeply in early childhood to attain some maximum value (depending on the intensity of transmission, but often approaching 100 per cent prevalence) in the 5–10-year-olds and then decline steadily with increasing age. The rate of increase in early childhood, the maximum prevalence attained, and the rate of

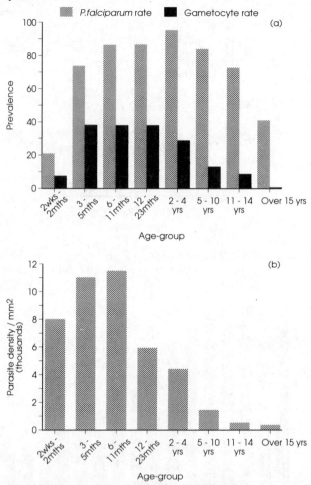

Fig. 14.4. (a) Age–prevalence profile for *P. falciparum*, showing total prevalence (sexual and asexual stages) and prevalence of people with gametocytes. (b) Age-intensity of infection pattern, as mean (arithmetic) positive *P. falciparum* density (Davidson and Draper 1953).

decline in the adult age groups from the maximum value are all positively associated with the intensity of transmission (Fig. 14.5). This association, with respect to the rate of decline in the teenage and adult age classes, is presumably a consequence of the dependence of the degree of acquired immunity on the duration and intensity of past exposure. In areas of high transmission where intensive studies have taken place, the decline in prevalence in older age classes is directly attributable to acquired immunity, because exposure to anophelene bites does not decrease with age (Carnevale *et al.* 1978) and mortality directly due to malaria is limited to the very young (Molineaux and Gramiccia 1980).

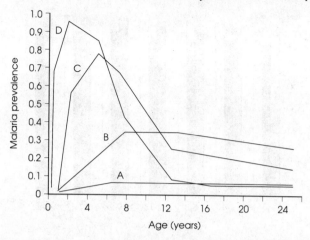

Fig. 14.5. Prevalence of acute malaria infection versus age in years, in stable indigenous populations, for differing levels of endemicity: A, low endemicity; B, moderate endemicity; C, high endemicity; D, hyperendemicity (from Boyd 1949*a*).

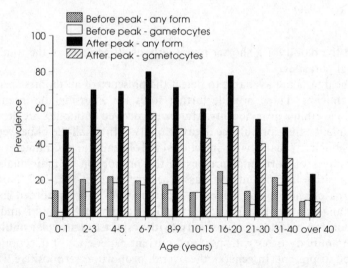

Fig. 14.6. Prevalence of gametocytes (*P. falciparum*) before and after the peak of malaria in Sundatar, Indonesia, according to age group (from Schuffner 1938).

Changes in the prevalence of people with gametocytes (infectious individuals) with respect to age (horizontal surveys) broadly reflect the patterns observed for the prevalence of infections, except that the proportions positive tend to be much lower (often by a factor 0.5 or less; see Earle (1939), Macdonald (1951)) (Fig. 14.6). Gametocytes appear an appreciable time after the first development of parasitaemia in non-immune subjects (James *et al.* 1932) and are subsequently

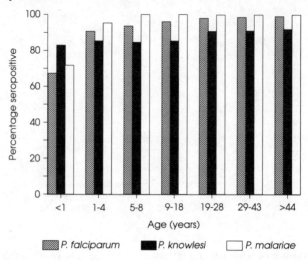

Fig. 14.7. Prevalence of antibodies to *P. falciparum*, *P. knowlesi*, and *P. malariae* according to age, determined by indirect haemagglutination antibody test (Molineaux and Gramiccia 1980).

present in the blood for a shorter time (perhaps 40 per cent of the total) than are asexual parasites.

Serological tests are available to detect the presence of antibodies specific to malarial antigens. These provide further tools for assessing the intensity of transmission within a given locality. Maternally derived antibodies are detectable in young infants; their prevalence decays rapidly with a half-life of between 3–6 months (similar to many viral infections) (Molineaux and Gramiccia 1980). Some examples of horizontal profiles of the proportion of individuals serologically positive in different age classes are recorded in Fig. 14.7. Note that the patterns of change are markedly different from those recorded for age-related changes in the prevalence of infection (compare Figs. 14.5 and 14.7). The relationship between seropositivity (with respect to particular antibodies) and mean antibody titres with past and current experience of infection is not understood at present. In general, the overall proportion seropositive within a community is positively associated with the intensity of transmission. Short-term reductions in the level of transmission (a few years) have little impact on the proportion seropositive in different age classes (Molineaux and Gramiccia 1980). However, long periods of no exposure to infection tend to result in lowered antibody titres within individuals and a reduction in the proportion seropositive within groups of people. This observation supports the notion that repeated exposure to infection is necessary to maintain a degree of acquired immunity. Longitudinal serological studies of infants in areas of endemic malaria reveal that maternally derived antibodies appear to provide little

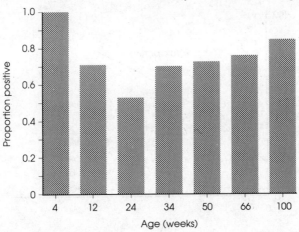

Fig. 14.8. Proportion of infants positive for malaria antibodies, by age, determined by a precipitin test (Molineaux and Gramiccia 1980).

protection against rapid infection in infancy (Fig. 14.8). Studies of the relationship between antibody titres and the prevalence of infection in different age classes have produced consistent patterns for a variety of different malarial species. In general, within areas of moderate to high transmission, the association is positive in young children and then becomes negative in older children and adults. The changeover point is often around 5 years of age. This pattern is further evidence of the significance of acquired immunity in reducing prevalence in the older age groups.

14.2.1.3 *Rates of infection and reinfection* The calculation of rates (or forces) of infection is made complicated in the case of malaria by the uncertain relationship between serology and past-plus-current experience of infection, and the build-up of acquired immunity within an exposed community. With respect to the prevalence of infection, the rate of increase over the first few years of a child's life (before immunity restricts parasite establishment) provides good data on the 'pristine' force of infection (the λ of microparasite models). Some examples of the estimation of the rate of infection in children with various species of *Plasmodium* are presented in Fig. 14.9. The data employed in these studies were collected by horizontal studies. Longitudinal observations on cohorts of children provide similar information. Provided the infection is endemic and stable within a community, estimates of the rate of infection (rate of increase in prevalence with age or time) provide a means of estimating the basic reproductive rate of the parasite. This aspect will be discussed in more detail in the section dealing with models. Horizontal or longitudinal serological surveys in young infants and children similarly provide information on the rate or force of infection. This interpretation, however, needs care due to the

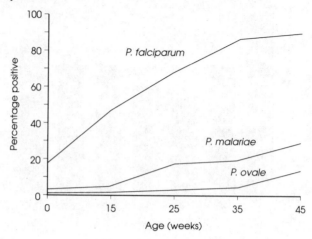

Fig. 14.9. Observed cumulative prevalence of *P. falciparum*, *P. malariae*, and *P. ovale*, by age of infants followed after birth at 10-weekly intervals (Molineaux and Gramiccia 1980).

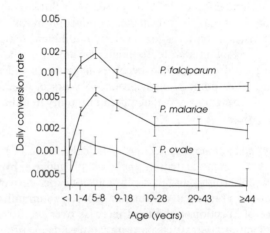

Fig. 14.10. Daily incidence rate of patent parasitaemia (i.e. conversion rate) for three species of parasite, by age (Molineaux and Gramiccia 1980).

complications introduced by maternally derived antibodies (particularly in areas of intense transmission where the percentage seropositive rises rapidly with age) (Fig. 14.8).

Longitudinal studies over a broad range of age classes enable us to assess the dependence of infection on host age. The so-called 'conversion rates' (the rate at which individuals change from parasite negative to parasite positive; see Bekessy *et al.* 1976) appear to alter with age (Fig. 14.10), although the factors involved are not clearly understood. They probably include age-related changes in exposure to mosquito bites (although this factor is not thought to be the most important) and a relative change in the proportion of 'conversions' that are new infections versus relapses of old infections. It is thought that the rate of relapses decreases with age as acquired immunity builds up beyond the ages of 5–10 years (Molineaux and Gramiccia 1980).

Studies of rates of conversion in individual patients also help us gain an understanding of within-age-class heterogeneity in exposure or susceptibility to infection. Most interestingly, the best study of this problem—which was concerned with the transmission of *P. falciparum*, *P. malariae*, and *P. ovale* in northern Nigeria (the Garki district)—showed that within any given age class there is for any particular parasite an excess (over that predicted on the basis of random exposure to infection) of persons persistently positive and of persons persistently negative (Molineaux and Gramiccia 1980). Furthermore, an analysis of the frequency of mixed-species infections revealed an excess of multiple infections over that predicted on the basis of chance alone. In short, both observations suggest a degree of predisposition to single and mixed malarial infections in individual patients. The reasons for this are not understood at present, but they could involve explanations based on human behaviour relative to mosquito biting habits, spatial factors (e.g. where an individual's house is relative to mosquito breeding or resting sites), or immunocompetence (perhaps genetically based).

14.2.1.4 *Morbidity and mortality* Malaria, particularly falciparum malaria, is a major cause of morbidity and mortality throughout many regions of the world. Mortality is invariably greatest in young infants and children and declines dramatically amongst those who survive beyond the age of 4–5 years in areas of endemic infection (Fig. 14.11). Morbidity is normally estimated by reference to spleen measurements (Christophers 1924; Macdonald 1926). In endemic areas there is a clear association between the degree of spleen enlargement and both the presence or absence of infection and the intensity of infection (Fig. 14.12). At present insufficient data are available for case complication rates (morbidity and mortality) per case of infection in a naive person (no prior experience of infection) stratified by age across child and adult age-classes.

14.2.2 *Vector biology and malarial infection*

Over the past 50 years much research effort has been devoted to the study of the ecology and population dynamics of the *Anopheles* vectors of human malaria (see Garrett-Jones 1964; Gillies and Wilkes 1965). The quantitative character of much of this work is in part a consequence of the emphasis placed by Macdonald (1957), in his simple models of the dynamics of malaria, on the detailed entomological factors involved in transmission. Further impetus was provided by the necessity to monitor the impact of control programmes based on the widespread use of insecticides (DDT in the early days of control).

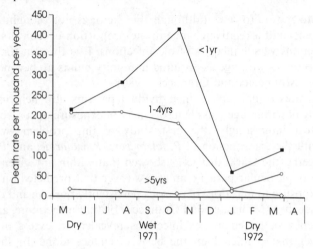

Fig. 14.11. Seasonal variation in the mortality rate, of the human host, by age (Molineaux and Gramiccia 1980).

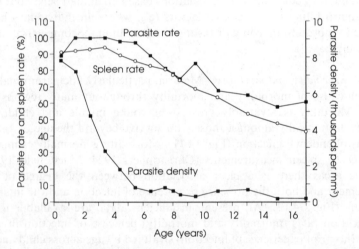

Fig. 14.12. Malaria survey in hyperendemic area of Tanzania. The parasite rate is the percentage of an age group with blood samples positive for malaria. The spleen rate is the percentage of an age group with enlarged spleens. The parasite density is the number of parasites per cubic millimetre (in thousands) in those blood samples which were positive for parasites (Christophers 1949).

Today, with the intense interest in the development of vaccines and the application of new molecular and biochemical techniques to the study of acquired immunity in humans, the research emphasis has changed from entomology to infections in humans. For completeness, however, we present in this section a brief review of the entomological data that are pertinent to an understanding of transmission. We consider this empirical information under a series of headings.

14.2.2.1 *Latent periods* The time period between infection and the beginning of infectiousness (sporozoites appearing in the salivary glands of the mosquito) varies greatly depending on extrinsic (e.g. temperature) and intrinsic (e.g. the species of mosquito) factors. A summary of the average latent periods for a range of vector transmitted infections is given in Table 14.3. In the case of *P. vivax* and *P. falciparum*, for example, the latent period depends critically on the prevailing temperature (Fig. 14.13) (Wenyon 1921; Jancso 1921; King 1929; Kligler and Mer 1937; Stratman-Thomas 1940; Knowles and Basu 1943; Siddons 1944; Boyd 1949a, b). However, over a very large range of the equatorial region of Africa temperatures show no great diurnal or seasonal fluctuations. With temperatures in the range of 25–27 °C, the latent periods for *P. falciparum* and *P. vivax* are approximately 12 days and 9 days respectively.

14.2.2.2 *Vector mortality* Arthropod vectors of microparasites have, in general, short life expectancies relative to the human host. As illustrated in Table 14.4, they range from a few days to a few months. Many factors influence survival including climatic, density-dependent, and age-related processes. For the anophelene vectors of malaria, a large number of studies have focused on the estimation

Table 14.3 Latent periods in which the vector is infected but not infectious

Parasite	Vector	Temp. (°C)	Incubation period (days)	Reference
Plasmodium falciparum	*Anopheles gambiae*	24	11	Baker (1966)
Schistosoma mansoni	*Biomphalaria glabrata*	24	35	Stirewalt (1954)
Onchocerca volvulus	*Simulium damnosum*	20	14	Blacklock (1929)
Dirofilaria immitis	*Aedes trivittatus*	22.5	16	Christensen and Hollander (1978)
Trypanosoma brucei	*Glossina morsitans*		15–35	Schmidt and Roberts (1977)
Wuchereria bancrofti	*Anopheles funestus*	20	13–15	Krafsur and Garrett-Jones (1977)
Yellow fever virus	*Aedes aegypti*		10–12	Burnet and White (1972)
SLE virus	*Culex p. pipiens*		7–19	Chamberlain *et al.* (1959)
Dengue virus	*Aedes aegypti*		7–10	Smith (1976)
Loa loa	*Chrysops dimidiatus*		10–12	Muller (1975)

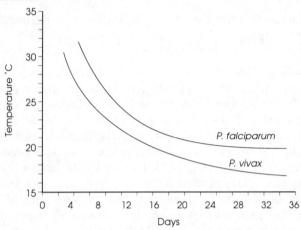

Fig. 14.13. The duration of sporogenic development (latent period) of malaria parasites in the mosquito host (*Anopheles* spp.) in relation to environmental temperature (°C) (Macdonald 1957).

Table 14.4 Expected life spans of arthropod vectors in natural environments and the laboratory

Vector	Expected life span (days)	Reference
Anopheles funestus	5.6 (field)	Krafsur and Garrett-Jones (1977)
Anopheles funestus	5.89 (field)	Gillies and Wilkes (1963)
Anopheles funestus	10.2 (field)	Garrett-Jones and Grab (1964)
Anopheles gambiae	11.26 (field)	Gillies and Wilkes (1965)
Anopheles gambiae	15.4 (field)	Garrett-Jones and Shidrawi (1969)
Anopheles gambiae	8.0 (field)	Garrett-Jones and Grab (1964)
Anopheles nili	5.8 (field)	Garrett-Jones and Grab (1964)
Anopheles coustani	8.5 (field)	Garrett-Jones and Grab (1964)
Aedes trivittatus	25 (lab.)	Christensen (1978)
Ornithonyssus bacoti	28 (lab.)	Williams and Kershaw (1961)
Glossina p. palpalis	127 (lab.)	Mulligan (1970)
Glossina morsitans	72 (lab.)	Buxton (1955)
Glossina morsitans	28–32 (field)	Jackson (1948)

of mortality rates under field and experimental conditions (for reviews see Boyd (1949a), Macdonald (1952), Brun (1973), and Garrett-Jones and Shidrawi (1969)). This body of data reveals that the life expectancy of mosquitoes under field conditions is often very short (a few days to a few weeks) and of not dissimilar magnitude to the latent period of infection. We might therefore expect the proportion of infectious mosquitoes to be low in natural populations. Infection, in most cases, is thought not to reduce life expectancy significantly below that of uninfected hosts.

14.2.2.3 *The prevalence and intensity of vector infection* In the context of malaria the prevalence of infection is conventionally referred to as the 'sporozoite rate' (defined as the proportion of the mosquito population with sporozoites in their salivary glands). Virtually without exception the prevalence of infection within vector populations is very low, irrespective of the type of disease agent or species of vector (Table 14.5). In general this is a direct consequence of the short life expectancies of vector species relative to the duration of infection in the human host and the latent period of infection in the vector. This point is well illustrated by a simple example. Suppose the mosquito population is of constant density with a stable age distribution and life expectancy of $1/\mu$ (where μ is the constant age-independent death rate). If the population is exposed to a constant rate of infection, λ, (independent of mosquito age) and the parasite has a latent period of τ time units, then the proportion of infectious vectors in the total population, p, is simply

$$p = \left(\frac{\lambda}{\lambda + \mu}\right) \exp(-\mu\tau). \tag{14.1a}$$

For high infection rates, $\lambda \gg \mu$, eqn (14.1) reduces to

$$p \simeq \exp(-\mu\tau). \tag{14.1b}$$

Table 14.5 Prevalence of infection in vector (intermediate host) populations

Vector	Parasite	Study area	Prevalence (per cent)	Reference
Anopheles gambiae	Plasmodium falciparum	Ethiopia	1.87	Krafsur and Garrett-Jones (1977)
Anopheles funestus	Plasmodium falciparum	Ethiopia	1.23	Krafsur and Garrett-Jones (1977)
Simulium damnosum	Onchocerca volvulus	West Africa	2.8	Holstein (1953)
Simulium damnosum	Onchocerca volvulus	Guatemala	5.0	Strong (1937)
Aedes trivittatus	Dirofilaria immitis	North America	1.0	Christensen (1978)
Biomphalaria glabrata	Schistosoma mansoni	St Lucia	1.3	Jordan (1977)
Bulinus nasutus productus	Schistosoma haematobium	Tanzania	3.1	Webbe (1962)
Oncomelania quadrasi	Schistosoma japonicum	Philippines	4.7	Pesigan et al. (1958)
Anopheles funestus	Wuchereria bancrofti	Tanzania	7.6	Krafsur and Garrett-Jones (1977)
Culex pipiens fatigans	Wuchereria bancrofti	Sri Lanka	6.9	Samarawickrema and Laurence (1978)
Glossina swynnertoni	Trypanosoma brucei	Tanzania	0.24	Duke (1923)
Glossina pallidipes	Trypanosoma brucei	Uganda	0.09	Molvo et al. (1971)
Glossina swynnertoni	Trypanosoma congolense and Trypanosoma vivax	Tanzania	15.5	Molvo et al. (1971)
Glossina swynnertoni	Trypanosoma vivax	Tanzania	25.9	Rogers and Boreham (1973)
Glossina morsitans	Trypanosoma vivax	Nigeria	61.8	Riordan (1977)
Rhodnius pictipes	Trypanosoma cruzi	Brazil	30.0	Lainson et al. (1979)

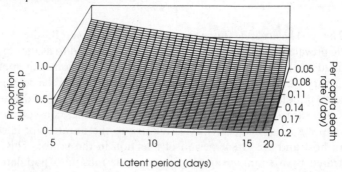

Fig. 14.14. The relationship between the proportion of infectious vectors in the total population as a function of the per capita death rate of the vector, μ, and the latent period of the parasite, τ (see eqn (14.1)).

Alternatively, eqn (14.1b) can be expressed as $p = q^\tau$ where q represents the probability of surviving one unit of time (see Macdonald 1957). If vector life expectancy, $1/\mu$, is of the same order or less than the latent period, τ, then the value of p is small (Fig. 14.14). For many vector-transmitted infections $1/\mu$ and τ are of similar magnitudes and hence we may expect the prevalence of infectious vectors to be low.

More generally, vector densities are rarely constant in size (they often exhibit marked seasonal changes in abundance) and the prevalence of infection is often related to human density, to the anthropophilic index (the proportion of blood meals taken from humans), and to the prevalence of infection in the human community. For malaria, there appears to be a positive association between the proportion of mosquitoes positive for sporozoites and the proportion of people positive for gametocytes (Fig. 14.15) (Macdonald 1952).

For protozoan parasites it is sometimes possible to score the intensity of infection and its distribution within the vector population. An example is presented in Fig. 14.16, which shows the frequency distribution of malarial oocysts in a sample of mosquitoes. This distribution is highly aggregated in form and the negative binomial probability model provides a good empirical description. The reasons for such observed heterogeneity are not fully understood at present, although genetic susceptibility to infection is undoubtedly of importance. For example, Ward (1963) in a series of laboratory selection experiments showed that the frequency distribution of oocysts of *P. gallinaceum* in anophelenes could be changed from an aggregated pattern to a random-underdispersed pattern by progressively selecting from resistant strains of the vector over many generations of laboratory inbreeding (Fig. 14.17).

14.2.2.4 *Human-biting rates*   The rate at which vectors feed on humans per unit of time is of obvious importance to the transmission of vector-borne

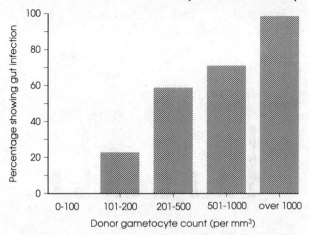

Fig. 14.15. Proportion of *Anopheles stephensi* acquiring infection, as a function of the gametocyte count of subjects infected with *P. falciparum* on which the insect hosts were fed (Knowles and Basu 1943).

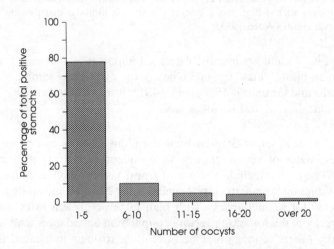

Fig. 14.16. Frequency distribution of oocysts in positive stomachs of wild-caught *Anopheles gambiae* and *Anopheles funestus* (from Muirhead-Thomson 1954).

infections. With respect to malaria this epidemiological parameter is termed the human-biting rate. Methods of data collection include the use of human volunteers to act as baits for defined units of time (the number of bites and the biting mosquitoes are recorded and collected over this interval (see WHO 1975; Molineaux and Gramiccia 1980), and the identification of blood meals (i.e. whether the meal is from humans or other mammalian species) by immuno-logical tests (to calculate the anthropophilic rate). For the malarial vectors,

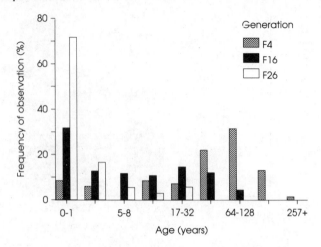

Fig. 14.17. Selection of a strain of *Aedes aegypti* resistent to infection by *Plasmodium gallinaceum*. The figure shows frequency distributions of malarial oocysts in hosts infected after varying intervals of selection. As the duration of selection progressed from generation 4 (F4) to generation 26 (F26) the distribution changed from an essentially unimodal form with a high mean oocyst count to a bimodal distribution with a low mean oocyst count (Ward 1963).

biting habits at night are usually of greatest importance in disease transmission and human-biting rates are often based on night-time sampling schedules (Molineaux and Gramiccia 1980) (Fig. 14.18). Biting habits, however, often vary on a regular diurnal and seasonal basis.

14.2.2.5 *Vector density*   Standardized sampling schemes can be employed to record estimates of vector density, independent of records of human-biting activity. These may include the use of traps, visual searches of insect resting sites, or sampling for aquatic larval stages of, for example, mosquitoes. As might be expected for animal species with high intrinsic growth rates (true for the vast majority of microparasite vectors), population abundances tend to fluctuate over many orders of magnitude and are often strongly influenced by climatic factors (Fig. 14.19).

14.3 Basic model for malaria

The earliest attempt to provide a quantitative understanding of the dynamics of malaria transmission was that of Ross (1911, 1915, 1916, 1917). The focus of his original work was malaria, but he extended this to develop a rather general theory of disease transmission which he termed '*a priori* pathometry'. Essentially, the models consisted of a few differential equations to describe changes in the densities of susceptible and infected people, and—in the case of

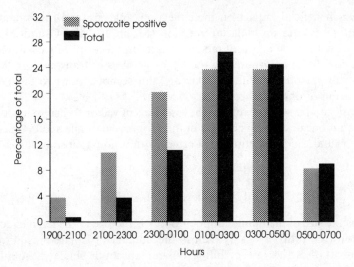

Fig. 14.18. Distribution by hour of the night of the sporozoite-positive bites, as a percentage of the total bites by *Anopheles gambiae* (from Molineaux and Gramiccia 1980).

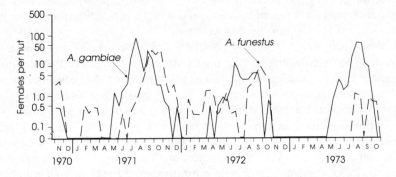

Fig. 14.19. Indoor resting densities of *Anopheles gambiae* and *Anopheles funestus*, estimated from pyrethrum spray collections in Kwaru, Northern Nigeria (Molineaux and Gramiccia 1980).

malaria—susceptible and infected mosquitoes. The analyses in Ross (1911) were extended by Lotka (1923). Then, in the early 1950s, an epidemiologist, George Macdonald, added a layer of biological realism to these early models by his careful attention to interpretation and estimation of parameters (Macdonald 1957). The value of mathematical studies to the design of malarial control programmes and the interpretation of observed epidemiological trends has been a topic of considerable controversy (Martini 1921; Moshkovskii 1950; Macdonald 1957; Bruce-Chwatt and Glanville 1973). Today, however, there is no doubt that the work of Macdonald in particular (based on Ross' early models) has had a very beneficial impact on the collection, analysis, and interpretation of epidemiological data on malarial infection (Molineaux and Gramiccia 1980).

We start with the simplest of models (based on the work of Ross (1911) and Macdonald (1957)) incorporating the major features of transmission. We then progressively introduce additional factors and complications to facilitate the interpretation of observed trends (see Aron and May 1982).

The basic model, which captures the essentials of vector transmission, consists of two equations describing changes in the proportion of infected ($=$ infectious) humans, y, and the proportion of infected ($=$ infectious) mosquitoes, $\hat{y}$.

$$\mathrm{d}y/\mathrm{d}t = (ab\hat{N}/N)\hat{y}(1 - y) - \gamma y, \tag{14.2}$$

$$\mathrm{d}\hat{y}/\mathrm{d}t = acy(1 - \hat{y}) - \mu\hat{y}. \tag{14.3}$$

Here N is the size of the human population, $\hat{N}$ is the size of the female mosquito population (the ratio $m = \hat{N}/N$ defines the number of female mosquitoes per human host), a is the rate of biting on humans by a single mosquito ('the human-biting rate' defined as the number of bites per unit of time), b is the proportion of infectious bites on humans that produces a patent infection, γ is the per capita rate of human recovery from infection ($1/\gamma$ is the average duration of infection) c is the proportion of bites by susceptible mosquitoes on infected people that produce a patent infection, and μ is the per capita rate of mosquito mortality ($1/\mu$ is mosquito life expectancy).

In this simple model, the total population of both humans and mosquitoes is assumed to be constant, so that the dynamical variables are the proportion infected in each population (y and $\hat{y}$). The first equation (14.2) describes changes in the proportion of infected humans. New infections are acquired at a rate that depends on the number of mosquito bites per person per unit time, $a\hat{N}/N$, on the probabilities that the biting mosquito is infected, $\hat{y}$, and that a bitten human is uninfected, $1 - y$, and on the chance that an uninfected person thus bitten will actually develop a patent infection. The ratio $\hat{N}/N$ arises as a direct consequence of the fact that female mosquitoes only take a fixed number of blood meals per unit of time. Thus the net rate of transmission is held to an upper limit, irrespective of the absolute densities of mosquitoes and people, by the biting rate times the number of female mosquitoes per person. This term embodies the actual difference between vector and direct transmission (see Anderson and May 1979b; Anderson 1981a). Infections are lost by infected people returning to the uninfected class at a net recovery rate γy. In this simple model it is assumed that recovered individuals have no immunity to reinfection (this assumption will be altered in a later section). Human recovery is assumed to occur at a much faster rate than human mortality (see Table 14.2) such that the rate of mortality is of negligible importance in the loss of infected people (here again this assumption is relaxed at a later stage).

The second equation, eqn (14.3), describes changes in the proportion of mosquitoes infected. The gain term depends on the number of bites per mosquito per unit of time a, on the probabilities that the biting mosquito is uninfected, $1 - \hat{y}$, and that the bitten human is infected, y, and on the chance that an uninfected mosquito acquires infection from biting an infectious person, c. The loss term arises from the death of infected mosquitoes, $\mu\hat{y}$ (mosquitoes do not appear to recover from malarial infection).

This model is, of course, highly simplified and its presentation is solely to illustrate the properties arising from vector transmissions. The major omissions, which are discussed in later sections, include the tendency of people to acquire immunity, the absence of parasite-induced mortality in humans and mosquitoes, and the absence of a class of infected but not yet infectious hosts in both the human and mosquito population (i.e. the inclusion of a latent period).

The basic reproductive rate in this simple vector transmission model is defined as follows

$$R_0 = ma^2bc/\mu\gamma. \tag{14.4}$$

(Note that in the literature on malaria R_0 is conventionally called z_0). An heuristic derivation is as follows. Take a single primary case with a recovery rate of γ; the average time spent in an infectious state is $1/\gamma$. During this time, the average number of mosquito bites received from m susceptible mosquitoes each with a biting rate a is am/γ; of these bites a proportion c are actually infectious, which gives a total of amc/γ mosquitoes infected by the primary human case. Each of these mosquitoes survives for an average time $1/\mu$ and makes a total of ab/μ infectious bites. The total number of secondary cases is thus $(ab/\mu)(amc/\gamma)$. Note that a enters twice in the numerator of eqn (14.4) since the mosquito biting rate controls transmission from humans to mosquitoes *and* mosquitoes to humans.

Equation (14.4) is usually derived algebraically by analysis of the stability properties of the differential equations (14.2) and (14.3) (Lotka 1923; Macdonald 1957; Dietz 1975; Anderson and May 1979*b*). A more transparent and more generalizable derivation can, however, be obtained by a geometrical 'phase-plane' analysis of the dynamical behaviour of the model (Aron and May 1982). Here, as illustrated in Fig. 14.20, the horizontal axis corresponds to the dynamical variable y, the proportion of people infected, and the vertical axis to the dynamical variable $\hat{y}$, the proportion of infected mosquitoes. In this figure, the variable $\hat{y}$ is unchanging along the isocline labelled by $d\hat{y}/dt = 0$; for a given value of y, $\hat{y}$ is increasing below this isocline and decreasing above it. Similarly, the variable y is unchanging along the isocline labelled $dy/dt = 0$; for given $\hat{y}$, y increases to the left of the isocline and decreases to the right of it. In the four domains of the y–$\hat{y}$ plane thus defined by the isoclines in Fig. 14.20(a), the dynamical trajectories of this system will move in the general direction indicated by the arrows. The intersection of the two isoclines represents the equilibrium state, to which all trajectories will tend in Fig. 14.20(a). The basic topological requirement for the two isoclines to intersect at positive values of y and $\hat{y}$ is that the initial slope of the $\hat{y}$ isocline (namely, ac/μ) exceed that of the y isocline

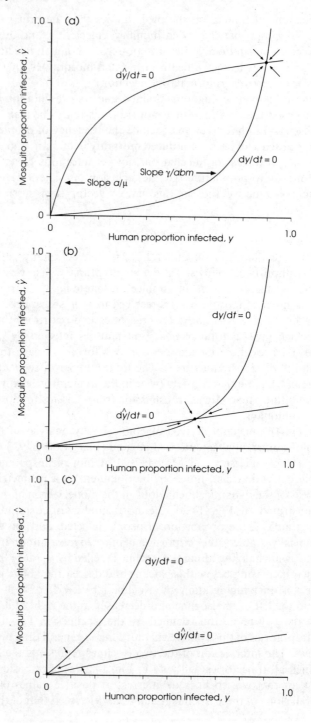

(namely, γ/abm). This gives eqn (14.4). Explicitly, the equilibrium proportion of infected humans (the prevalence of infection) is

$$y^* = (R_0 - 1)/[R_0 + (ac/\mu)]. \tag{14.5}$$

The corresponding equilibrium prevalence for mosquitoes is

$$\hat{y}^* = \left(\frac{R_0 - 1}{R_0}\right)\left(\frac{ac/\mu}{1 + ac/\mu}\right). \tag{14.6}$$

The initial slope of the $\hat{y}$ isocline, ac/μ, represents the average number of bites on human hosts made by a mosquito in its lifetime, that lead to mosquito infection. If this number is relatively large, the $\hat{y}$ isocline will rise steeply and the equilibrium point is likely to lie toward the top right-hand corner of the y–$\hat{y}$ plane in a relatively 'deep valley' in this dynamical landscape (Fig. 14.20(a)). In these circumstances small changes in mosquito density, m, or the biting rate, a, will have little effect on the equilibrium prevalence of infection in humans. This corresponds to what is called 'stable endemic malaria'. However, if ac/μ is relatively small, the $\hat{y}$ isocline will have the shallow form depicted in Fig. 14.20(b), and the equilibrium point is likely to lie in a 'shallow elongated canyon' (Aron and May 1982). In this case, small changes in mosquito density or the biting rate are more likely to result in substantial changes in the proportion of humans infected. This is the essence of Macdonald's (1957) conclusion that ac/μ is an index of stability; in areas where mosquito vectors bite humans relatively often and have relatively long life spans, this index is high and malaria tends to be endemic (Macdonald's 'stable malaria'); conversely, where mosquitoes bite on humans less often and have shorter life spans, the index is low and malaria tends to be subject to epidemic outbreaks (Macdonald's 'unstable malaria').

If the initial slope of the $\hat{y}$ isocline is less than that of the y isocline, we necessarily have $R_0 < 1$ and the infection cannot persist, being below the transmission threshold $R_0 = 1$ (Fig. 14.20(c)).

Fig. 14.20. The 'phase-plane' of the dynamical variables, y (proportion of humans infected), and $\hat{y}$ (proportion of mosquitoes infected); each point in the plane corresponds to a particular pair of values $y, \hat{y}$. The variable $\hat{y}$ is unchanging along the isocline $d\hat{y}/dt = 0$. The intersection of the two isoclines, if it exists, represents the equilibrium point of the system, and elsewhere trajectories move in the directions indicated by the arrows. In (a) the initial slope a/μ of the $\hat{y}$ isocline significantly exceeds the initial slope γ/abm of the y isocline, and the equilibrium point rests in a relatively deep valley, corresponding to Macdonald's 'stable' malaria. In (b), the initial slope a/μ is relatively small, but still exceeds γ/abm, and the equilibrium point exists, but now in a relatively shallow canyon, corresponding to Macdonald's 'unstable' malaria. In (c), the initial slope a/μ is less than γ/abm, so that the isoclines do not cross; all trajectories are directed towards the origin and the disease cannot maintain itself. (The figure follows Macdonald in putting $c = 1$.)

Table 14.6 Macdonald's stability index (ac/μ) for several regions where malaria is indigenous

Anopheles spp.	Location/time period	Stability index	Reference
A. punctulatus	Maprik, New Guinea (1957–8)	2.9	Peters and Standfast (1960)
A. balabacensis	Khmer (1960)	4.9	Slooff and Verdrager (1972)
A. minimus	Bangladesh (1966–7)	4.4	Khan and Talibi (1972)
A. gambiae	Kankiya, Nigeria (1967)	3.4	Garrett-Jones and Shidrawi (1969)
A. gambiae	Garki, Nigeria (1972)	3.9	Molineaux et al. (1979)
A. gambiae	Khashm, El Girba, Sudan (1967)	0.47	Zahar (1974)

Table 14.6 summarizes information about Macdonald's 'stability index', ac/μ, for several regions in which malaria is indigenous. The available data are rarely precise enough to permit a good estimate of both μ and a, so that the values of a/μ presented in Table 14.6 are very rough approximations (see Aron and May 1982). Often μ is inferred from age-structured data, which is permissible only if dealing with a vector population with a stable age distribution. In general, Aron and May (1982) found that sufficient information for even a rough estimate of ac/μ was available only for regions where malaria was, in Macdonald's classification, 'stable'. It is therefore not surprising that all ac/μ values in Table 14.6 are relatively large, corresponding to 'stable malaria'.

The table specifically excludes data from regions where intervention with insecticides (DDT) has occurred, because there are now additional complications in the interpretation of mosquito life-history parameters. One such complication arises from inhomogeneities in the effects of insecticides, which are usually applied to the interior surfaces of houses and are more effective against mosquitoes that rest indoors after taking a blood meal. If insecticides do not affect all mosquitoes equally, measurements of the biting rate and longevity may be severely distorted (Molineaux et al. 1979). For example, suppose after spraying there are two mosquito populations of roughly equal size: those that rest outdoors and are consequently unaffected by the spraying and those that rest indoors and suffer high mortality. For illustration $a_1 = 0.25$ bites per day and $\mu_1 = 0.05$ per day for the exophilic mosquitoes, and $a_2 = 0.5$ and $\mu_2 = 0.5$ for the endophilic ones. The correct way to calculate the index, a/μ, is to take the appropriate arithmetical average of the separate indices: $\frac{1}{2}(a_1/\mu_1 + a_2/\mu_2) = 3.0$. But if the endophilic and exophilic categories are not properly distinguished, then a/μ is likely to be estimated using average values of a and μ: $[\frac{1}{2}(a_1 + a_2)]/[\frac{1}{2}(\mu_1 + \mu_2)] = 1.4$. Molineaux et al. (1979) have analysed the consequences of this aggregation phenomenon in considerable detail. They emphasize that aggregating the groups will always underestimate the vectorial capacity of the mosquito population and hence the basic reproductive rate R_0. An excellent review of the methodology involved in the interpretation of epidemiologically relevant aspects of mosquito vector populations is by Garrett-Jones and Shidrawi (1969).

Although the basic model gives a good overview of the dynamics of malarial infection, particularly the basic factors that underlie 'stable' and 'unstable' malaria, many of its predictions are strikingly different from reality. In particular, it is clear from Fig. 14.20 that highly endemic areas ($y \to 1.0$, ac/μ relatively large) will show a high proportion of mosquitoes infected. It follows from eqn (14.6) that $\hat{y} \simeq 1$ when R_0 and ac/μ are significantly greater than zero. However, as shown in Table 14.5, the sporozoite rate in mosquitoes (the prevalence of sporozoite infection) is typically a few per cent even in areas of high prevalence within the human community.

14.4 Beyond the basic model for malaria

14.4.1 *Latent periods*

An obvious modification to the basic model is the incorporation of latent periods during which infected hosts are infected but not yet infectious (see Tables 14.2 and 14.3). We denote these periods as τ_1 and τ_2 in the human and mosquito hosts respectively. Further, we represent mortality in the human population as occurring at a rate μ_1, and that in the mosquito population as occurring at a rate μ_2 (i.e. the μ in eqns (14.3)–(14.6) is replaced by μ_2). The proportion of infected but not yet infectious hosts are defined as $h(t)$ and $\hat{h}(t)$ for man and mosquitoes respectively. The variables $y(t)$ and $\hat{y}(t)$ now denote infectious hosts. The model is of the form

$$dh(t)/dt = abm\hat{y}(t)(1 - y(t)) - \mu_1 h(t) - abm\hat{y}(t - \tau_1)(1 - y(t - \tau_1)), \quad (14.7)$$

$$dy(t)/dt = abm\hat{y}(t - \tau_1)(1 - y(1 - \tau_1)) - \mu_1 y(t) - \gamma y(t), \quad (14.8)$$

$$d\hat{h}(t)/dt = acy(t)(1 - \hat{y}(t)) - \mu_2 \hat{h}(t) - acy(t - \tau_2)(1 - \hat{y}(t - \tau_2)), \quad (14.9)$$

$$d\hat{y}(t)/dt = acy(t - \tau_2)(1 - \hat{y}(t - \tau_2)) - \mu_2 \hat{y}(t). \quad (14.10)$$

It is here assumed that latent and infectious hosts have identical mortality rates.

The equilibrium solution is found by putting $dy/dt = d\hat{y}/dt = dh/dt = d\hat{h}/dt = 0$, and solving the ensuing set of algebraic equations. The basic reproductive rate of malarial infection is now

$$R_0 = \left(\frac{ma^2 cb}{\gamma \mu_2}\right) \exp(-\mu_1 \tau_1 - \mu_2 \tau_2). \quad (14.11)$$

Here b is now the proportion of bites by sporozoite-bearing mosquitoes that result in infection and c is the proportion of bites by susceptible mosquitoes on gametocyte-bearing people that result in mosquito infection. The introduction of latent periods diminishes the value of R_0 compared with that derived from the basic model (eqn (14.4)) by a factor $\exp[-(\mu_1\tau_1 + \mu_2\tau_2)]$. The importance is therefore very much dependent on the magnitudes of the death rates μ_1 and μ_2 and the latent periods τ_1 and τ_2. In humans the death rate is normally very small on a scale relevant to the latent periods (i.e. $1/\mu_1 \simeq 40$–50 years, $\tau_1 \simeq 0.5$–1 year) such that the term $\exp(-\mu_1\tau_1)$ is essentially unity. This is not the case, however, for the mosquito population. Vector life expectancy $(1/\mu_2)$ is often shorter than the latent period (τ_2) such that the factor $\exp(-\mu_2\tau_2)$ is significantly less than unity in value (see Table 14.3). Under the assumption that $\mu_1 \to 0$, the equilibrium prevalence of sporozoite-infected mosquitoes becomes

$$\hat{y}^* = \left(\frac{R_0 - 1}{R_0}\right)\left(\frac{ac/\mu_2}{1 + ac/\mu_2}\right)\exp(-\mu_2\tau_2) \qquad (14.12)$$

where R_0 is as defined in eqn (14.11) with $\mu_1 = 0$. In other words the prevalence of infection in humans, y^*, can approach unity but the prevalence of sporozoite-infected mosquitoes, $\hat{y}^*$, cannot exceed $\exp(-\mu_2\tau_2)$. Mosquito prevalence can be a few per cent even when R_0 and ac/μ_2 are significantly greater than unity.

This relatively simple refinement, which goes a long way to making the model more realistic, has been discussed by Macdonald (1957). Macdonald drew from eqn (14.11) the important qualitative conclusion that killing adult mosquitoes is more effective than killing larvae. The larval survivorship enters into R_0 (eqn (14.11)) linearly, via the absolute mosquito density $\hat{N}/N$. In contrast, the adult mosquito survivorship enters in a highly non-linear way via the factor $\exp(-\mu_2\tau_2)/\mu_2^2$ (allowing for the latent period and effects on absolute density) (Aron and May 1982). Reduction of larval recruitment by a factor of two would only halve the basic reproductive rate R_0, but a doubling of the adult mortality rate (doubling μ_2) would produce an exponentially severe decrease in R_0. The change in emphasis in control measures directed against the mosquito vectors of malaria, largely as a consequence of Macdonald's insights, is described by Harrison (1978).

14.4.2   *Variable mosquito density*

Macdonald (1957) used the simple model to make broad geographical comparisons between the 'stable' malaria of Africa and the unstable malaria of parts of India. On a smaller scale, the basic model suggests that areas of high transmission will be less sensitive to fluctuation in mosquito population density than areas of low transmission, with respect to observed changes in prevalence within human communities. In Sri Lanka, before control by DDT, there was considerable local variation in the endemicity of malaria. Figures 14.21(a) and 14.21(b) are hospital records of monthly malaria cases, over several years, from two different localities. Although Fig. 14.21(a), for the region of greater transmission, shows variability and marked decline following control measures

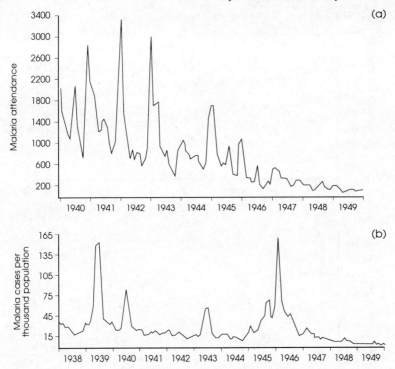

Fig. 14.21. (a) Monthly malaria attendance at the civil hospital in Anurodhapura in the endemic zone of Sri Lanka (Rayendran and Jayewickreme 1951*b*). (b) Monthly malaria attendance per 1000 population in the upper catchments of the Deduru Oya and Matia Oya basins in the epidemic zone of Sri Lanka (Rayendran and Jayewickreme 1951*a*).

after World War II, it nevertheless has a steady seasonal pattern from year to year. The region of lesser transmission, illustrated in Fig. 14.21(b), is prone to severe outbreaks which subside (Rayendran and Jayewickreme 1951*a, b*).

The basic model of eqns (14.2) and (14.3) demonstrates this pattern nicely if the total mosquito population, $\hat{N}$, varies seasonally with an amplitude that fluctuates randomly from year to year (Aron and May 1982). Figure 14.22 shows the dynamical behaviour of such a system when the transmission rate is very high (average value of $R_0 \gg 1$) and when the transmission rate is just above the threshold (R_0 slightly above unity in value). In both cases, the systems are subject to the same kind of (multiplicatively random) fluctuations, but the latter is much more affected than the former. Areas of low transmission are also more sensitive to sudden non-seasonal drops in the mosquito density, as happened when the plain of Philippi in Macedonia had a big drop in malaria following a dry year, while the neighbouring plain of Chrysopulis (where malaria transmission was more endemic) was scarcely affected (Boyd 1949*b*).

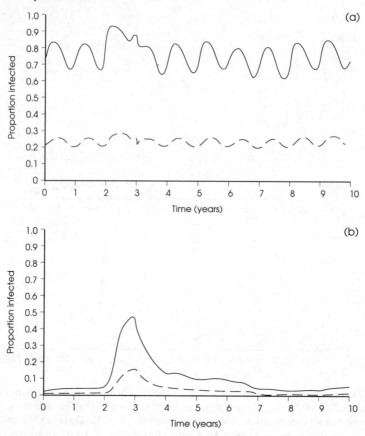

Fig. 14.22. (a) Proportion of infected humans (full curve) and mosquitoes (broken curve) versus time from simulation of basic model with a large reproductive rate R_0 and variable mosquito density $M(t)$. Explicitly, $M(t) = A[B + \varepsilon \sin(2\pi t)]$ where t is measured in years. Here, $B = 50$, $\varepsilon = 20$, and A is a random sequence which fluctuates around unity during the first half of the year (upper half of sine wave), but is otherwise equal to unity. The parameters used in the simulation are $a = 20\ \mathrm{yr}^{-1}$, $\mu = 50\ \mathrm{yr}^{-1}$, $\gamma = 4\ \mathrm{yr}^{-1}$, $N = 20$, $b = 1$. When $M = B$, $R_0 = 5$. (b) Same as for (a) but with small reproductive rate R_0. Here, $B = 10.5$ and $\varepsilon = 1$, and A, a, μ, γ, N, and b are the same as for (a). When $M = B$, $R_0 = 1.05$. (From Aron and May 1982.).

Regular changes in mosquito population abundance caused by seasonality also helps explain other patterns in the overall dynamics of malaria. It is obvious that a rise in the mosquito population can lead to a malaria epidemic among the human population, but less obvious when the maximum prevalence in mosquitoes should occur relative to that in humans. Peters and Standfast (1960) note an inverse relationship, over the year, between mosquito abundance and the sporozoite rate (prevalence in mosquitoes). More detailed studies show that the peak of mosquito density occurs either before (Boyd 1949*b*) or during (Christophers 1949) the peak of human malaria cases, but that the maximum prevalence among mosquitoes follows both the peak in prevalence within humans and the peak of mosquito abundance.

There has been some confusion in the epidemiological literature concerning the mechanisms that underly these observations (see Boyd 1949*b*; Peters and Standfast 1960). Our view of the sequences of events is that, at first, mosquito density rises due to the seasonal increase in the number of emerging adults. As the total density rises, the density of infected mosquitoes also rises, followed by a peak in human cases. The rise in prevalence among mosquitoes occurs after the peak in human cases, not just from latent period delays, but because by then fewer mosquitoes are emerging into the population to swell the ranks of the uninfected vectors, thus causing the proportion infected to increase.

Exactly these patterns can be produced by the basic model of eqns (14.2) and (14.3). For the dynamics of the mosquito population, $\hat{N}$, we write

$$d\hat{N}/dt = E(t) - \mu_2\hat{N}. \tag{14.13}$$

Here μ_2 is as defined earlier, and $E(t)$ is the rate of emergence. We take $E(t)$ to vary sinusoidally over the year; the mosquito density will then also be sinusoidal, with a lag of about the mean lifetime of a mosquito (Aron and May 1982). Note that it is assumed that the variation in mosquito density arises from the periodicity in the rate of adult emergence; the mortality rate may also vary but we believe seasonality in emergence is of greater importance. Equation (14.2) for the proportion of humans infected is as before. Equation (14.3), for the proportion of mosquitoes infected, was originally derived under the assumption that the total number of mosquitoes was constant. Under our new assumptions it becomes

$$d\hat{y}/dt = acy(1 - \hat{y}) - [\mu_2 + (d\hat{N}/dt)/\hat{N}]\hat{y}. \tag{14.14}$$

The steady annual cycles to which the solutions of this system of eqns (14.2), (14.13), and (14.14) tend are illustrated in Fig. 14.23. Figure 14.23(a) shows first the peak for the mosquito density, $\hat{N}(t)$, then the peak for the total number of infected mosquitoes, $\hat{y}(t)\hat{N}(t)$, and finally (as the total population is declining) the peak for the proportion infected, $\hat{y}(t)$. Figures 14.23(b), (c), and (d) show that the peak for human prevalence, $y(t)$, follows the maximum both for total density, $\hat{N}(t)$, and for the number of infected mosquitoes, $\hat{y}(t)\hat{N}(t)$, but precedes the maximum for the mosquito prevalence, $\hat{y}(t)$. This basic model does not incorporate latent periods, the inclusion of which would accentuate the lags. Latency is clearly important in determining the exact timing of the peaks (Dietz *et al.* 1974), but the relative timing during the transmission season is simply a consequence of the seasonal growth dynamics of the mosquito population.

In summary, the basic model can—with a few refinements—account for the main patterns exhibited within the mosquito population. We now turn to the more important problems presented by infection within the human community,

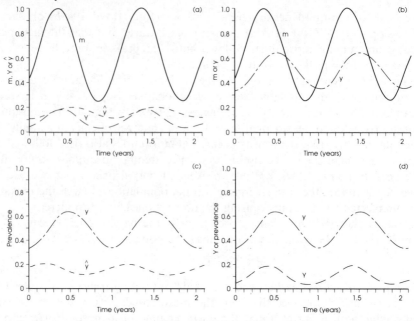

Fig. 14.23. (a) The absolute number of mosquitoes per host, m ($m = \hat{N}/N$), number of infected mosquitoes, Y ($Y = \hat{y}\hat{N}$), and the proportion of mosquitoes infected, $\hat{y}$, are shown as functions of time. These curves are obtained from the basic dynamical model defined by eqns (14.2), (14.13), and (14.14). The rate of emergence is taken to vary sinusoidally, with a 1-year period. The parameters used in these simulations are $a = 20 \text{ yr}^{-1}$, $\mu_2 = 50 \text{ yr}^{-1}$, $\gamma = 4 \text{ yr}^{-1}$, $b = 1$, $N = 20$, and $m(t) = 25 + [15 \sin(2\pi t)]$ (so that $m_{\max} = 40$). The total number, m, and the total number of infected mosquitoes Y are plotted as proportions of $m_{\max}$; the prevalence $\hat{y}$ is by definition a fraction $0 < \hat{y} < 1$, and the time is plotted in years (from Aron and May 1982). (b) The total mosquito population, m, and the proportion of humans infected, y, are plotted as functions of time, with units as for (a). (c) The prevalence of malaria among mosquitoes, $\hat{y}$, and humans, y, as function of time, with units as for (a). (d) The absolute number of infected mosquitoes, Y, and the human prevalence of malaria, y, are shown as functions of time, with units as for (a).

to investigate how various details about the biology of the infection between the malarial parasites and humans can be incorporated.

14.4.3 *Multiple infections in humans*

We have so far assumed that an infected person is not subject to further infection. There is evidence to suggest that this is not the case and that at any one time a given individual may harbour more than one infective inoculation of parasites via multiple infectious bites (Cohen 1973a; Molineaux and Gramiccia 1980). This problem is often referred to as superinfection, and it has been considered by a variety of researchers (Macdonald 1957; Bailey 1975; Fine 1975;

Aron and May 1982). Superinfection may arise as a consequence of concurrent infections with different species of malaria, or from different genetic strains, or from different inocula of the same strain.

There are several models for superinfection, forming a continuum of descriptions for the effect of a subsequent infection when one is present already. One extreme is the original Ross model, already discussed, in which secondary infections are lost (i.e. superinfection is ignored). The other extreme is Macdonald's (1950, 1957) model, in which successive infections are effectively 'stacked', waiting to express themselves when the previous infection is over. An intermediate version is the model introduced by Dietz (described in Bailey 1975, pp. 317–22) in which infections arrive and run their course totally independently of each other. (Macdonald's version was intended to correspond to the situation described by Dietz, but there was a mathematical misunderstanding; see Fine (1975).)

These various assumptions may be compactly written by replacing eqn (14.2) with the more general form

$$\mathrm{d}y/\mathrm{d}t = \lambda(1 - y) - py. \tag{14.15}$$

Here λ is the force of infection (the parameter referred to as h or 'happenings' in the paper of Ross (1911)), and is defined, in the notation of the basic model (eqns (14.2) and (14.3)), as

$$\lambda = (ab\hat{N}/N)\hat{y}. \tag{14.16}$$

The quantity p is the rate of recovery to the uninfected state, and is defined variously as

$$\text{Ross:} \quad p = \gamma, \tag{14.17}$$

$$\text{Dietz:} \quad p = \lambda/[\exp(\lambda/\gamma) - 1], \tag{14.18}$$

$$\text{Macdonald:} \quad p = \gamma - \lambda \quad (\gamma > \lambda), \tag{14.19}$$

$$p = 0 \quad (\gamma < \lambda).$$

As before γ is the rate of recovery from a single infection.

Contrary to what is sometimes implied in Macdonald's work, the different assumptions about the nature of superinfection make for quantitative, rather than qualitative, differences in the overall dynamic behaviour. This is clearly seen by returning to the phase-plane analysis of Fig. 14.20, and replacing the y isocline (along which $\mathrm{d}y/\mathrm{d}t = 0$) of the original Ross model by the corresponding y isocline generated by the Dietz and Macdonald formulae (eqns (14.18) and (14.19) respectively). This is done in Fig. 14.24. There is no difference between the models at low prevalence levels, so that the basic reproductive rate, R_0, is the same for all three, and all have the same criterion for the maintenance of infection (i.e. there are no differences at low transmission intensities, where superinfection is rare). On the other hand, the equilibrium values of the

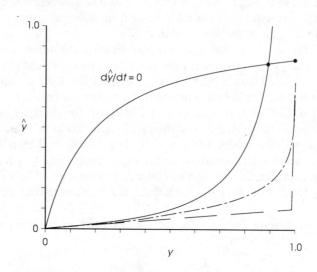

Fig. 14.24. The phase-plane of the dynamical variables y and $\hat{y}$ is shown as in Fig. 14.20. The $\hat{y}$ isocline, along which the proportion of mosquitoes infected is unchanging, is as before. The y isocline, along which the proportion of humans infected is unchanging, is calculated under various assumptions about the nature of superinfection: the full curve, as before, assumes no superinfection (Ross model); the broken curve assumes 'stacked' infections (Macdonald model); the dot-dashed curve corresponds to the Dietz model. At lower prevalence levels the three models are essentially the same, and the qualitative dynamics are essentially similar; the detailed locations of the equilibrium points are different for the three models. (From Aron and May 1982.)

proportions of humans and of mosquitoes infected, y^* and $\hat{y}^*$, do depend on how superinfection is defined. As one moves from the original Ross model, to that of Dietz, to that of Macdonald, both y^* and $\hat{y}^*$ increase somewhat. Thus the details, but not the overall stability properties, are affected by the inclusion of superinfection.

To proceed further in our refinements, with the aim of understanding observed patterns in human communities, we need to consider the question of acquired immunity. First, however, by way of introducing the problem we turn to the treatment of age structure within the human population.

14.4.4 *Age structure*

The basic model of Ross can be easily extended to encompass age structure within the human community. To do this we consider population densities, as opposed to proportions, and define $Y(a, t)$ as the number of infected people of age a at time t. The model is now of the form

$$\partial Y(a, t)/\partial t + \partial Y(a, t)/\partial a = (ab\hat{Y}(t)/N)(N(a) - Y(a, t)) - (\gamma + \mu_1)Y(a, t),$$

$$(14.20)$$

$$d\hat{Y}(t)/dt = (ac\bar{Y}(t)/N)(\hat{N} - \hat{Y}(t)) - \mu_2\hat{Y}(t).$$ $$(14.21)$$

Here $\hat{Y}(t)$ defines the density of infected mosquitoes, $N(a)$ denotes the density of humans of age a, and N and $\hat{N}$ the total densities of humans and mosquitoes respectively (both assumed to be constant). Human and mosquito mortality are represented by the rates μ_1 and μ_2 as in eqns (14.7) and (14.8). The term $\bar{Y}(t)$ denotes the total density of infected people weighted by the proportional representation of each age class in the community

$$\bar{Y}(t) = \left(\int_0^\infty Y(a, t) \exp(-\mu_1 a) \, da\right)\left(\int_0^\infty \exp(-\mu_1 a) \, da\right)^{-1}. \quad (14.22)$$

It is here assumed that human mortality is constant and independent of age (Type II survivorship). Thus the total density of humans N is given by $N(0)L$ where $N(0)$ is the cohort size at birth (assumed constant) and L is human life expectancy ($L = 1/\mu_1$).

At equilibrium ($\partial Y(a, t)/\partial t = d\hat{Y}/dt = 0$), eqn (14.20) becomes

$$dy^*/da = \lambda(1 - y^*(a)) - (\gamma + \mu_1)y^*(a). \quad (14.23)$$

Here $y^*(a)$ denotes the equilibrium proportion of infected people of age a. The force of infection, λ, is defined as

$$\lambda = (ab\hat{N}/N)\hat{y}^* \quad (14.24)$$

where $\hat{y}^*$ is the equilibrium proportion of infected mosquitoes. The solution of eqn (14.23) is

$$y^*(a) = [\lambda/(\lambda + \gamma + \mu_1)]\{1 - \exp[-(\lambda + \gamma + \mu_1)a]\}, \quad (14.25)$$

given that $y(0) = 0$ (i.e. infants are uninfected at birth). The simple model therefore predicts that the prevalence of infection within the human community rises monotonically with age to a plateau, $\lambda/(\lambda + \gamma + \mu_1)$, in the older individuals. This pattern, however, differs markedly from those observed in human communities with endemic malaria infection (Fig. 14.5). Observed trends are normally convex in form; the prevalence rises rapidly with age in the young infants and children, attains a peak, and declines in the older children to reach a low level in adults. It is clear that the basic model must be modified to encompass some description of the acquisition of immunity to infection. Before turning to this problem, however, it is worth considering the parameter λ, the force of infection, in a bit more detail.

A good estimate of the pristine force of infection can be obtained from the rate of increase of prevalence with age in young children, before acquired

Table 14.7 Estimates of force of infection

Age group	Location	Daily force of infection	Reference
Infants	Nyanza Province, Kenya	0.0084	Pull and Grab (1974)
0–4 years	Maputo, Mozambique	0.001–0.0075[a]	Schapira *et al.* (1990)
5–14 years	Maputo, Mozambique	0.001–0.013[a]	
Infants	Garki, Nigeria	0.0015–0.0323[a]	Bekessy *et al.* (1976)
1–4 years	Garki, Nigeria	0.007–0.0220[a]	
5+ years	Garki, Nigeria	0.0171–0.0233[a]	
0–14 years	Gambela, West Ethiopia	0.0064–0.0255[a]	Krafsur and Armstrong
15+ years	Gambela, West Ethiopia	0.0037–0.0151[a]	(1977)

[a] Range from dry to wet season.

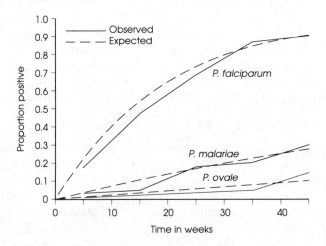

Fig. 14.25. The fit of eqn (14.25) in the main text to the data recorded in Fig. 14.9 for (a) *P. falciparum*, (b) *P. malariae*, and (c) *P. ovale*. The estimated forces of infection (λ) are (a) $\lambda = 2.7 \text{ yr}^{-1}$, (b) $\lambda = 0.37 \text{ yr}^{-1}$, (c) $\lambda = 0.126 \text{ yr}^{-1}$ (for $\gamma = 1 \text{ yr}^{-1}$, $\mu = 0$). The average ages at first infection for the three parasites are approximately (a) 0.37, (b) 2.67, and (c) 7.91 (years).

immunity complicates the interpretation of observed trends. A variety of epidemiological studies have focused on the rate of increase of prevalence over the first few years of life in children born within areas of endemic infection (e.g. Macdonald 1950; Molineaux and Gramiccia 1980). Table 14.7 reveals various estimates of λ that are derived from a wide variety of data sets. Examples of fitting the model defined by eqn (14.25) to certain records of change in prevalence with age in children are displayed in Fig. 14.25. In many instances the model provides a good description of observed trends in children between the ages of 0 and 2 years.

In areas of stable endemic malaria we can express the basic reproductive rate R_0 in terms of the parameter λ, the equilibrium prevalence of sporozoite-infected mosquitoes (the sporozoite rate), $\hat{y}^*$, and certain other parameters via the use of eqns (14.4) and (14.24):

$$R_0 = \lambda ac/\mu_2\gamma\hat{y}^*. \qquad (14.26)$$

To estimate the value of R_0 for a given area, we therefore require a number of separate bits of epidemiological data. The parameters λ and $\hat{y}^*$ may be reliably estimated from data on changes in prevalence with age in humans (as indicated in Fig. 14.25) and by sampling mosquitoes to measure the sporozoite rate (note, however, that this may vary on a seasonal basis; see Fig. 14.23). The remaining parameters, however, are more difficult to determine (i.e. the biting rate, a, the probability that a bite on an infectious person results in a patent infection in the mosquito, c, and mosquito life expectancy, μ_2). As noted in Fig. 14.22, the probability c depends on the density of gametocytes within an individual patient. However, by way of a numerical example suppose $c = 0.5$, $a/\mu_2 = 5$, $\hat{y}^* = 0.05$, $\lambda = 0.005$ day^{-1}, and $\gamma = 0.005$ day^{-1}. The substitution of these values in eqn (14.26) yields an R_0 value of 50. Some crude estimates of R_0 for different localities and times are recorded in Table 14.8. Note that the

Table 14.8 Estimates of the basic reproductive rate, R_0, of *Plasmodium* spp.

Infectious agent	Location/time period	R_0	Reference
P. falciparum	Northern Nigeria (1970s)	~80	Molineaux and Gramiccia (1980)
P. malariae	Northern Nigeria (1970s)	~16	Molineaux and Gramiccia (1980)

values for areas of stable endemic infection (particularly in Africa) are somewhat higher than those typically estimated for directly transmitted viral infections such as measles (see Table 4.1). This observation is in part corroborated by the observation that the average age at which a child typically first acquires malarial infection in an endemic area is normally much lower (i.e. 2–6 months) than that recorded for viral infections such as measles (i.e. 1–3 years, see Chapter 13). However, it must be remembered that—in contrast to what one might believe from reading some descriptions of the derivation of R_0 for malaria— many uncertainties surround the estimating of the parameters, a, c, and μ_2 in any given locality. The values presented in Table 14.8 are no more than rough approximations.

14.4.5 *Acquired immunity*
Models for the transmission dynamics of malaria have only recently begun to take account of the phenomenon of acquired immunity, despite it obvious relevance as a determinant of observed age-related changes in the prevalence of

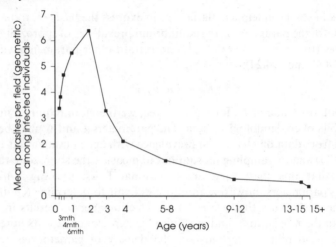

Fig. 14.26. The mean number of parasites per microscope field, according to the age of the human host (from Putnam 1931).

infection. This is in part a consequence of the early focus in malaria models on the vector components of transmission, deriving from the initial aim of global eradication of malaria based on the application of DDT (see Macdonald 1957; Bruce-Chwatt and Glanville 1973; Yekutiel 1980). The failure of this campaign owing to the problems of resistance to insecticide, along with recent advances in immunology and molecular biology, has shifted the focus of research to the mechanisms of immunity in man. Recent work, for example, on the immunogenicity of various sporozoite, merozoite, and gametocyte antigens, plus the use of recombinant DNA technology in the expression of the genes that encode for particular antigens within bacteria, has raised the hope that vaccines to protect against malarial infection will be developed in the coming few years (Zavala *et al.* 1985).

In this subsection we turn to the question of whether enough is understood about immunity to malaria to formulate sensible models for the impact of herd immunity on transmission within a community. The standard characterization of the epidemiology of malaria is, as discussed earlier, based on age–prevalence curves, which show the proportion of each age group whose blood slides contain infected cells. In endemic areas, the prevalence peaks at a very early age and then declines slowly (Fig. 14.5); at the same time the number of infected cells and gametocytes found in those slides positive for parasites decreases relatively quickly with age (Fig. 14.26). Unfortunately, however, the measurement of such patterns does not provide sufficient information with which to unravel the various components of acquired immunity and their dependence on the intensity of transmission. Observed curves can be fitted by a wide variety of models that contain very different assumptions (Dietz *et al.* 1974; Elderkin

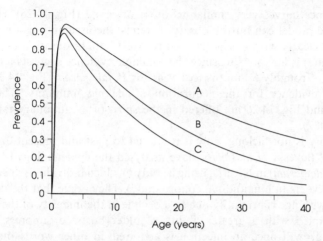

Fig. 14.27. Prevalence of infection versus age according to eqn (14.30), derived from the simple model with lifelong immunity. A single infection rate λ is used with three different recovery rates, γ: $\lambda = 20\ \text{yr}^{-1}$; and A, $\gamma = 0.03\ \text{yr}^{-1}$; B, $\gamma = 0.05\ \text{yr}^{-1}$; C, $\gamma = 0.07\ \text{yr}^{-1}$.

et al. 1977; Aron and May 1982; Aron 1983). However, with this caveat in mind, we start with the simplest possible assumption, namely, that on recovery from first exposure an individual acquires sterile immunity for life (in line with the assumption made in the simple compartmental models for directly transmitted microparasites discussed in earlier chapters).

The age-structured model defined in eqns (14.20)–(14.21) can be simply modified to incorporate an immune class of individuals as follows. We consider the system at equilibrium and define $x^*(a)$, $y^*(a)$, and $z^*(a)$ as the proportion of susceptible, infected, and immune individuals of age a, respectively. The rates of change of these variables, with respect to age, may be expressed as

$$dx/da = -(\lambda + \mu_1)x, \tag{14.27}$$

$$dy/da = \lambda x - (\gamma + \mu_1)y, \tag{14.28}$$

$$dz/da = \gamma y - \mu_1 z. \tag{14.29}$$

The term λ, the force of infection, is as defined in eqn (14.24), γ denotes the recovery rate (where recovery takes an individual into the immune class), and μ_1 represents the rate of human mortality (note that no account is taken of disease-induced mortality). The initial condition is $x(0) = 1$, and it follows that $x(a) + y(a) + z(a) = \exp(-\mu_1 a)$ for all ages a. This set of equations can be integrated to obtain an explicit description of the experiences of a cohort as it ages

$$y(a) = \{\exp[-(\gamma + \mu_1)a] - \exp[-(\lambda + \mu_1)a]\}[\lambda/(\lambda - \gamma)]. \tag{14.30}$$

In Fig. 14.27 we choose $\lambda = 2\ \text{yr}^{-1}$ and γ between 0.07 and 0.03 yr^{-1} (corresponding to mean durations of infection of 15–30 years), to obtain age–prevalence curves very similar to those observed (Fig. 14.26). However, although the model can mirror observed trends, the assumptions on which it is based are clearly wrong. The inferred recovery rate (a duration of infection of 15–30 years) is far too slow since the available evidence suggests a duration of infection of roughly 6 months to 1 year for *P. falciparum* (Fig. 14.3), nor is there good evidence for the acquisition of lifelong immunity. The above discussion and Fig. 14.26 are offered in the spirit of a cautionary tale (Aron and May 1982).

If immunity is not lifelong, how is it related to past and present experience of infection? Bekessy *et al.* (1976) have analysed the epidemiology of malaria (mostly *P. falciparum*) in Nigeria, using a study in which individuals are followed over several years (a longitudinal cohort study). They argue that the decline in prevalence with age is primarily due to a decline in the intensity of the parasite burden, coupled with a greater ability of older hosts to suppress parasite population growth once an infection is acquired; in other words the rate of parasite replication within the host is inversely related to the host's accumulated past experience of infection. A marked seasonal pattern in parasitaemia continued even for the adults, indicating that they are still susceptible. Dietz *et al.* (1974) have incorporated those ideas into a model of the epidemiology of malaria. In it, there are two classes of individuals: one class has a slow recovery rate from malaria; the other has a fast recovery rate, and infections only have a 70 per cent chance of being detected (owing to the low densities of parasites in the fast recovery class). Both classes are repeatedly exposed, become infected, and recover, remaining within their own class except for a fixed rate of transition from the relatively susceptible class (low recovery) to the relatively immune class (fast recovery). This model is illustrated schematically in Fig. 14.28. The model gave a good fit to data collected in an extensive study of malaria in northern Nigeria (see Molineaux and Gramiccia 1980), but parameter estimation was based to a large extent on the patterns which the model was intended to reflect. The major deficiency in the model of Dietz *et al.* (1974), however, is its failure to account for the loss of immunity that is known to occur when transmission is significantly reduced. For villages in the same Nigerian study used by Dietz *et al.* (1974), Cornille-Brögger *et al.* (1978) showed that two transmission seasons with massive intervention in the form of drug administration and insecticide spraying were followed, in the next season in which no control was attempted, by a higher than usual prevalence of malaria. Figure 14.29 illustrates the results of these studies, showing the relative rise in prevalence in 1974 for those over 10 years old (younger individuals still received drugs to prevent serious morbidity and mortality). In subsequent years, following the cessation of control, the prevalence of infection within adults settled back to the levels recorded in a set of comparison villages (in which no control was attempted). Although the loss of immunity amongst adults was small and easily recovered in this particular field study, the phenomenon is clearly an important feature of the transmission biology of malaria.

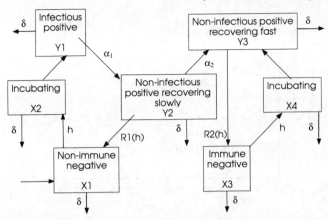

Fig. 14.28. States and transitions of the Dietz model (Dietz *et al.* 1974). Humans are born into the non-immune negative state X1; i.e. passive immunity is ignored. Non-immune negatives are innoculated at a rate h and move to the incubating class X2, remaining for a fixed incubation of N days. After this they become positive and infectious, in class Y1. Infectivity is lost at a rate α_1, while persons move to a positive but non-infectious state Y2. From here a person may either recover from infection and return to the non-immune negative state X1, at a rate $R1(h)$, or become an 'immune positive' at a constant rate α_2. The actual recovery rate $R1(h)$ is a function of a constant, r_1, which is the basic recovery rate of non-immunes, and of h, the effective inoculation rate: as inoculation rate increases the recovery rate decreases, i.e. superinfection prevents recovery and an increasing proportion of Y2 move to Y3. The 'immune positives' in Y3 recover from infection at a rate $R2(h)$, which is a function of r_2, the basic recovery rate of immunes, and of h; r_2 is larger than r_1: immunes tend to recover faster than non-immunes, but superinfection again reduces the recovery rate. If an immune positive (Y3) recovers from infection he or she becomes an immune negative (X3). Immune negatives are successfully inoculated at the same rate (h) as the non-immune negatives, and incubate the infection for the same period of N days (X4) after which they are 'immune positives' (Y3). δ denotes the death rate from each class (from Molineaux and Gramiccia 1980).

Pringle and Avery-Jones (1966) have demonstrated similar effects in African children. The children received antimalarial drugs for a few weeks, and were then taken off the drugs; they then had higher parasitaemias than at the start of the study. In short, it seems that continued exposure to infection helps maintain immunity.

Recently, Aron and May (1982) and Aron (1983) have described a simple way to incorporate this mechanism. Suppose there are three classes of individuals: susceptibles, infecteds, and immunes. Assume that immunity lasts for some fixed period of time, τ, in the absence of re-exposure, but that if a person is further exposed before τ units have elapsed, immunity is sustained and another interval of duration τ without infection is required before immunity is lost. If infection occurs at a per capita rate λ (as a Poisson process), the average

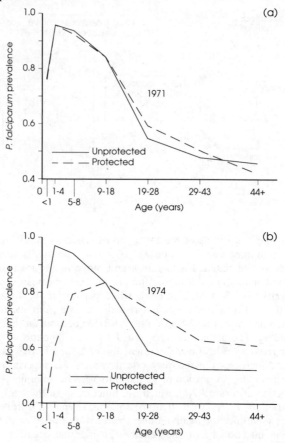

Fig. 14.29. (a) Prevalence of infection versus age in years in an endemic area in 1971 before intervention. There is no difference as yet between the two villages (full and broken curves). In 1972 and 1973 there was massive intervention in the form of drug administration and anti-mosquito spraying in one of the groups, which was subsequently halted for adults in 1974. (b) Prevalence of infection versus age in years in 1974. The adults in the once-protected group (broken curve) show significantly higher prevalences than in the comparative villages (full curve) (from Cornille-Brögger *et al.* 1978).

time spent in the immune state, $T(\lambda, \tau)$, can be calculated as a function of λ (see Aron (1983)):

$$T(\lambda, \tau) = [\exp(\lambda \tau) - 1]/\lambda. \tag{14.31}$$

Hence the average per capita rate of loss of immunity, $v(\lambda, \tau)$, as a function of λ and τ, is simply

$$v(\lambda, \tau) = 1/T(\lambda, \tau). \tag{14.32}$$

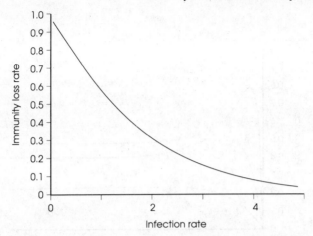

Fig. 14.30. This figures shows the rate of loss of immunity, $v(\lambda, \tau)$, as a function of infection rate, λ, for eqn (14.32). In this model, repeated infection helps maintain immunity. The 'immune interval', τ, is taken to be 1 year.

An illustration of the relationship between v and λ as predicted by eqn (14.32) is depicted in Fig. 14.30.

This simple description of immunity as a function of exposure can now be incorporated into the equilibrium age–prevalence model defined in eqns (14.27)–(14.29):

$$dx/da = v(\lambda, \tau)z - (\lambda + \mu_1)x, \tag{14.33}$$

$$dy/da = \lambda x - (\gamma + \mu_1)y, \tag{14.34}$$

$$dz/da = \gamma y - (v(\lambda, \tau) + \mu_1)z. \tag{14.35}$$

The only difference is that now immunity is not permanent. As before, this linear set of differential equations can be integrated to construct age–prevalence curves given the initial condition $x(0) = 1$ (all uninfected at birth).

The patterns predicted by this simple model are illuminating. First, if v is held to be a predetermined constant such that the average duration of immunity is $1/v$, then complex changes in prevalence with age can arise as shown in Fig. 14.31. However, note that the shapes of these curves bear little similarity to those actually observed (Fig. 14.5). If we now employ the function defined in eqns (14.31) and (14.32), where loss of immunity is a function of the rate of exposure to infection, λ, then a different picture emerges as illustrated in Fig. 14.32. The patterns are much closer to those observed for parameter values that are chosen to accord with observations on recovery rates and the duration of immunity.

Although this model represents an advance on the simpler models discussed in the earlier sections, it is still a very crude description of the true complexities

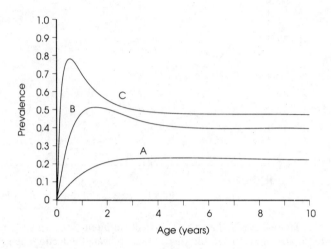

Fig. 14.31. Age structure curves for malaria calculated from the model defined by eqns (14.33)–(14.35), assuming both the intrinsic recovery rate, γ, and the rate of loss of immunity, $v(\lambda, \tau)$, are constants, independent of the transmission rate, λ (specifically $\gamma = 0.5 \text{ yr}^{-1}$, $v(\lambda, \tau) = 0.5 \text{ yr}^{-1}$) and $\lambda = 0.2 \text{ yr}^{-1}$ (A), 1 yr^{-1} (B), and 5 yr^{-1} (C).

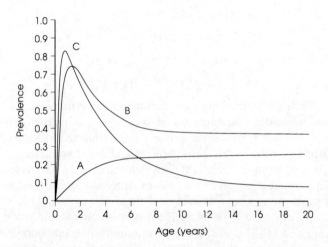

Fig. 14.32. As for Fig. 14.31 except here the rate of loss of immunity $v(\lambda, \tau)$ depends on the transmission rate, λ, as described by eqns (14.31) and (14.32). Specifically, the figure is for $\gamma = 0.25 \text{ yr}^{-1}$ and $\tau = 1.3$ year; the three curves are for the different transmission rates; A, $\lambda = 0.1 \text{ yr}^{-1}$; B, $\lambda = 2 \text{ yr}^{-1}$; C, $\lambda = 4 \text{ yr}^{-1}$.

of immunity to malarial infection. In particular, the classification into three discrete categories—susceptible, infected, and immune—is a poor reflection of the observation that populations of malarial parasites can exist at various densities within individual people. In many respects, the transmission dynamics of malaria depends on the quantitative distribution of parasite abundance within the human community, rather than on mere presence or absence of infection. A related complication arises in the determination of prevalence from blood slides, especially at lower parasite densities, because 'false' negatives become common (Miller 1958; Molineaux and Gramiccia 1980; Aron 1982). This problem can affect the reliability of estimates of infection and recovery rates.

All detailed descriptions of the acquisition and loss of immunity, whether in hospital or in the natural environment, indicate that the phenomenon is gradual. In the studies of Crica *et al.* (1934), in which *P. vivax* infections were administered therapeutically to a group of patients, there was a steady decline in the manifestation of clinical symptoms from the first inoculation to the fifth and last (which induced no clinically measurable symptoms). The gradual acquisition and loss of immunity has been demonstrated in laboratory rodent hosts. For example, Zuckerman (1974) showed that serum from immune rats (used to protect non-immune animals) became more and more effective as the number of infections given to the immune donor rats increased. Furthermore, Sergent and Poncet (1956) have shown loss of immunity in rats to be gradual; the longer the interval to a subsequent infection, the greater was the proportion of rats producing parasitaemias and the greater was the intensity of the parasitaemias.

These observations combine to suggest that an accurate mathematical description will need to abandon the compartmental, or prevalence-based, structure of conventional microparasite models and move toward a more detailed description of the growth and decay of parasite abundance within individuals. This latter approach is conventionally restricted to the description of the transmission dynamics of macroparasites, but many protozoan infections—such as malaria, trypanosomiasis, and leishmaniasis—fall in the buffer zone between the extremes presented by viral infections, where a compartmental framework is a good description of observed events, and helminth parasites, where notice must be taken of parasite abundance within the host.

An earlier attempt to model the malarial parasite population within an individual host and the acquisition of immunity is that of Elderkin *et al.* (1977). The dynamical variables in this model are the population of asexual stages in the human host, the population of gametocyte sexual stages in the blood, and the level of resistance (immunity) of the host. We make no attempt to discuss this model in detail, but simply note that it can generate convex changes in the parasite density within the host as people age. A somewhat simpler approach is to consider a single variable, $M(a)$, denoting the mean number of malarial parasites (asexual and sexual stages) in a person of age a. Suppose that new

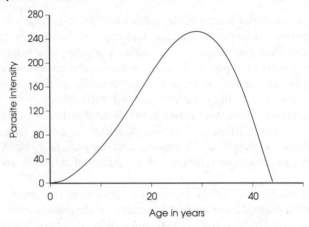

Fig. 14.33. Numerical solution of eqn (14.38) with parameter values $\Lambda = 0.1$, $b = 1.0$, d and $\delta = 0.0003$ (arbitrary time units).

parasites arrive at a per capita rate Λ (via inoculation by the mosquito vector) and that the population within the host has per capita birth and death rates b and d respectively. Further assume that immunity acts to increase the death rate, $d(\bar{M}(a))$, of the parasite (as seems likely from experimental studies) in a manner linearly dependent on the accumulated sum of the hosts' past experience of infection $\bar{M}(a)$; that is,

$$\bar{M}(a) = \int_0^a M(\alpha)\, d\alpha \tag{14.36}$$

and

$$d(\bar{M}(a)) = d + \delta\bar{M}(a). \tag{14.37}$$

Here d is the death rate in naive hosts and δ measures the severity of the acquired immunological response. We may therefore represent changes in $M(a)$ with respect to age by the simple differential equation

$$dM(a)/da = \Lambda + M(a)[b - d(\bar{M}(a))]. \tag{14.38}$$

As illustrated in Fig. 14.33, this model, with an appropriate choice of parameter values, can generate convex patterns of change in the mean parasite density with host age that are reminiscent of those observed in endemic areas (see Fig. 14.26). A further discussion of this type of model of acquired immunity is developed in Chapter 18 in the context of macroparasites.

In short, this example further illustrates the point that a variety of models for acquired immunity, each containing different assumptions, can generate patterns similar to those observed in areas of endemic infection. It is impossible at present to discriminate among these models with respect to their biological accuracy, since the detailed mechanisms of human immune responses to malaria are not well understood.

Further complications arise if we consider the significance of genetic heterogeneity within both the human and mosquito hosts and within the parasite population. It is well understood that different people exhibit different innate susceptibilities to malaria infection and different abilities to acquire immunity. This is sometimes mediated by factors other than genetic background, such as nutritional status (Scrimshaw *et al.* 1968). However, laboratory studies with rodent malaria models demonstrate well the importance of genetic background as a determinant of innate resistance and the development of specific immunity (Cox 1982). With respect to humans, the sickle cell genetic trait is known to confer a degree of innate resistance with heterozygous individuals (Allison 1964). More broadly, Armstrong (1978) demonstrated that two tribes living adjacently in Ethiopia had significantly different susceptibilities to *P. vivax*. Even within a community, genetic background undoubtedly influences the effectiveness of an individual's immune response to invasion by malarial parasites. The complexity of the issue is further compounded by variation among strains within the parasite population. Recent evidence suggests that *P. falciparum* populations exhibit considerable antigenic variation even within a defined locality (Forsyth *et al.* 1988).

Little is understood about these factors at present, yet they are likely to be of some importance to the development and community-wide use of potential malarial vaccines. The ideal vaccine will probably have to incorporate antigens from different parasite developmental stages and different strains. However, the major problem may concern genetic variability in immunocompetence within the human community. An effective vaccine must be able to convert 'low responders' (the genetically less immunocompetent individuals who suffer most from mortality and morbidity) into 'high responders'.

14.5 Control

The problems outlined above lead us to the issue of community-wide control. Past attempts have been based on chemotherapy and vector control. The successes and failures are well documented in the literature and we do not intend to go into any detail concerning these methods (see Molineaux and Gramiccia 1980). The problems of insecticide and drug resistance are acute at present in many regions of the world and this has added an increased urgency to research on the development of malaria vaccines (Ballou *et al.* 1987).

What can simple theory tell us about the use of vaccines (or other control measures) for the community-wide control of malaria? It is our view that mathematical models of the kind reviewed in this chapter—in which the characterization of acquired immunity is admittedly phenomenological· and imperfect—do provide some useful insights. These fall under four general headings.

14.5.1 *Reduction in transmission intensity*

Ideally, control measures should aim to reduce the value of the effective reproductive rate of the parasite, R, below unity. This is irrespective of whether intervention is based on the application of insecticides, the use of antimalarial drugs, mass vaccination, or some combination of these methods. In practice, however, this objective is rarely achieved. Intervention normally results in a reduced transmission efficiency but with the parasite persisting at some lower overall abundance.

In terms of the simple model defined in eqns (14.33)–(14.35), which incorporates a crude description of acquired immunity, a reduction in transmission implies a lowering in the magnitude of the force of infection, λ. On the assumption that acquired immunity plays an important role, a reduction in λ will sometimes result in a decreased prevalence of infection in the younger age classes but an increased abundance of the parasite in the adult groups. Reduced transmission implies less experience of infection in childhood and hence lower immunity to infection as these children move into the adult classes. Prior to control, those that survive childhood will have built up strong acquired immunity due to the intensity of their exposure. The problem is illustrated in Fig. 14.34, where the pattern of age-related change in prevalence, $y^*(a)$, predicted by eqns (14.33)–(14.35) is shown for various values of λ (moving from a high value representing the pre-control situation to a lower value depicting the results of increased intervention). Note that we discussed an empirical example of this phenomenon in an earlier section (see Fig. 14.29).

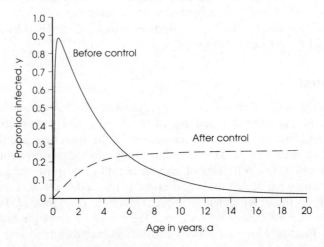

Fig. 14.34. An illustration of the impact of control (a reduction in the force of infection) on the age–prevalence profile of malaria as predicted by eqns (14.33)–(14.35) (parameter values, $\tau = 1.3$ years, $\mu = 0$, $\gamma = 0.25$ yr^{-1}). Prior to control $\lambda = 4$ yr^{-1}, and after $\lambda = 0.1$ yr^{-1}.

This problem—whereby control measures can have a perverse outcome—is one we have encountered in earlier chapters where, in the context of mass vaccination against directly transmitted viral infections, it was predicted (and observed) that reduced transmission tends to shift the age distribution of the incidence of infection and increase the average age at first exposure (Chapter 5). In the case of malaria, whether or not this phenomenon is of practical significance depends on the manner in which the risk of mortality and serious morbidity due to infection changes with age. Fortunately (or unfortunately in the pre-control situation), these risks appear to be greatest in infants and young children. Thus even low to moderate reductions in transmission, whether induced by insecticide application or mass vaccination, will tend to reduce the overall incidence of disease in endemic areas. It is still important, however, to recognize the fact that control measures can act to increase the prevalence and intensity of malarial infections in adult age classes over the levels pertaining prior to control.

14.5.2 *Eradication by mass vaccination*
The criterion for eradication by mass vaccination, when and if vaccines become available, remains as defined in Chapter 5 in the context of directly transmitted viral infections. With respect to malaria, the crude estimation procedures outlined earlier suggest that the value of the basic reproductive rate, R_0, is typically much higher in endemic areas than is normally the case for many important childhood viral and bacterial infections (Table 14.8). This implies that the level of vaccination coverage required to eradicate malaria in hyper-endemic regions will be very high. To take a simple numerical example, if the value of R_0 is 50 (Table 14.8), then eqn (5.2) indicates that eradication requires approximately 98 per cent of each cohort of children to be effectively immunized soon after birth with a vaccine that gives lifelong protection. In practice, therefore, the goal of eradication is likely to prove extremely difficult to attain. This point is not well appreciated by those who believe that the advent of malarial vaccines heralds the demise of malarial parasites world-wide. A bleaker view is that vaccines will certainly be of benefit to the Western traveller to tropical regions, but may have less impact on the inhabitants of these regions. It is important to remember in this context that the development of cheap, safe, and effective vaccines is only a first step (albeit an essential one) in the community-wide control of an infection. Economic and motivational issues are at least as important as technological ones. For example, a cheap, effective, and safe vaccine for measles has been available since the late 1960s and yet the infection remains one of the major causes of child mortality in the world today (Anderson and May 1985c).

14.5.3 *What age to vaccinate?*
The principles involved in this issue are identical to those discussed in Chapter 13. The central issue is that the maximum impact on transmission is achieved

by immunizing as young as is practically possible, taking into account the rate of decay of maternally derived protection and the rate at which children acquire infection prior to intervention. For malaria, maternal antibodies do not appear to provide significant protection to infection. Hence, in principle, vaccination can take place almost immediately after birth. However, weighed against this advantage (by comparison with viral infections such as measles) are the disquieting observations that in endemic areas the average age at first infection is often as low as 3–6 months of age and that morbidity and mortality are most severe in young infants and children. Thus the 'age window' in which vaccines can be administered to best advantage is very small. But, as indicated earlier, low to moderate levels of vaccination at the start of an immunization programme will tend to widen the 'age window' (by lowering the net rate of transmission) provided vaccine is administered well before the average age at first infection pertaining before intervention.

14.5.4 *Reinfection following cessation of control*

A further consequence of high basic reproductive rates, in addition to the requirements of high levels of vaccine coverage for eradication and a narrow age window in which to administer the vaccine, is that the rate of return to the pre-control prevalence of infection will be extremely rapid following a cessation of intervention measures (irrespective of whether they involve insecticides, chemotherapy, or vaccines). The experience gained in past malaria control campaigns clearly supports this prediction. For example, results from the 'Garki' project in northern Nigeria, reported by Molineaux and Gramiccia (1980), show that the prevalence of infection in a series of study villages rapidly returned to its pre-control state (as recorded in 1971) following insecticide spraying and drug administration over a period from April 1972 to October 1973. The resurgence of malaria was monitored in 1974 and 1975; the observed patterns are recorded in Fig. 14.35.

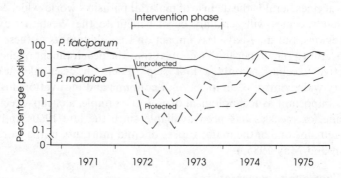

Fig. 14.35. Prevalence of *P. falciparum* and *P. malariae* in an unprotected population and a population protected in 1972–3 by drug administration and antimosquito spraying (Molineaux and Gramiccia 1980).

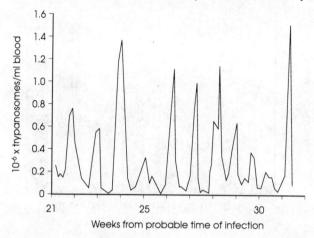

Fig. 14.36. Fluctuation of parasitaemia in a case of human trypanosomiasis (*Trypanosoma gambiense*) (Ross and Thomson 1910).

14.6 Other indirectly transmitted infections

Although much of this chapter has been devoted to malaria, the principles outlined apply equally well to many other important viral and protozoan infections that are transmitted by vectors. In this section we outline a few points of epidemiological interest with respect to these other diseases.

14.6.1 *African trypanosomiasis*

The trypanosome protozoa in Africa cause a number of important diseases in humans. The most notorious is *Trypanosoma brucei gambiense* which is the cause of African sleeping sickness. The parasite is transmitted by tsetse flies of the genus *Glossina*. Control has proved to be very difficult: effective non-toxic drugs are unavailable at present, and vector management is ineffective because of the presence of animal reservoirs of the parasite, the wide distribution of the flies, and the underground habitat of their pupal stages. Parasite populations in humans undergo cycles of 'antigenic variation'. During the course of infection the number of trypanosomes in blood and lymphatic fluids fluctuates in a characteristic oscillatory fashion (Fig. 14.36). Each decline in parasitaemia is a result of antibody-mediated destruction of trypanosomes having a particular surface antigen. The subsequent growth of the population in the next 'epidemic' cycle within the host is due to the emergence of a different antigen type of the parasite (Vickerman 1978; Hoare 1972; Cross 1978). It appears that each parasite is able to express somewhere in the order of 100 different variable surface antigens (called VATs, variable antigen types). This has frustrated all attempts to develop effective vaccines. Antigenic variation within the host is

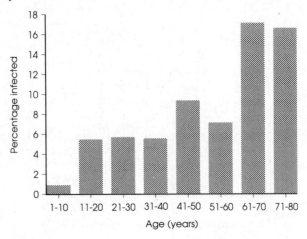

Fig. 14.37. Age–prevalence pattern for human sleeping sickness cases (diagnosed parasitologically) from the Timbo area of Central Nyanza, Kenya (Rogers 1988).

clearly an effective strategy to enhance the parasite's ability to persist, both within an individual host and within the community as a whole.

The principal differences between the transmission dynamics of African trypanosomes and malaria may be summarized as follows:

1. As a result of antigenic variation (the evasion of the host's immunological attack) trypanosome infections tend to be persistent in character such that following a single inoculation an infected person may harbour parasites for many years.

2. In endemic areas, the basic reproductive rate of the parasite appears to be much lower than that typically estimated for *P. falciparum*. As illustrated in Fig. 14.37, the prevalence of trypanosome infection usually rises slowly with host age.

3. Certain species of trypanosomes, such as *T. brucei gambiense*, are a significant cause of mortality. Deaths due to infection, however, more typically occur after childhood since the disease is progressive in character.

4. Reservoirs of infection exist in animal species other than humans, in areas of endemic human infection. In the case of *T. brucei gambiense* these reservoirs are typically pigs and dogs while for *T. brucei rhodesiense* they are often various species of antelopes and wild dogs (Hoare 1972). Reservoirs often play an important role in maintaining transmission in human communities where the 'within human' transmission component of R_0 is less than unity in value (Rogers 1988; Mulligan *et al.* 1988).

5. The insect vector has a much lower reproductive rate and longer life

expectancy than the mosquito intermediate hosts of malaria. In current ecological jargon, tsetse flies lie to the *K*-selected end of the life history spectrum among insects (Rogers 1988).

Most of the factors mentioned above create problems in the design of effective control programmes. The only methods currently available are those of vector control by insecticide application, and environmental management to destroy the habitats both of the vector and of the mammalian species that act as reservoir hosts. No detailed study of the transmission dynamics of African trypanosomes has been completed as yet. It is clearly an area that demands greater attention, given the global significance of these parasites as causes of mortality and morbidity (Walsh and Warren 1979; Molineaux 1985).

14.6.2 *Leishmaniasis*

Leishmania species are obligate intracellular protozoan parasites in the mammalian host that are transmitted by the bites of infected sand flies. They are, in a broad sense, the trypanosomes of the New World. Transmission to humans is usually from other infected mammalian species that act as reservoirs of infection. Depending on the species of the parasite, infection can result in cutaneous, mucocutaneous (espundia), or visceral (kala azar) disease. Non-toxic chemotherapeutic agents and vaccines are unavailable at present and vector control can be very difficult due to the behavioural habits of sand flies. In many of its principal features the epidemiology of *Leishmania* species is similar to that of the trypanosome parasites. The infection is persistent in character although the latent period may be long for infections such as *L. donovani* (3–6 months) in contrast to trypanosome infections. If an individual recovers strong immunity is acquired and endemic as opposed to epidemic patterns are more commonly observed within communities. The vector is relatively long-lived and has a low reproductive rate in comparison with species such as mosquitoes. In some cases reservoir hosts facilitate disease persistence within human populations. This class of infections has not received much attention with respect to the quantitative study of transmission dynamics.

14.6.3 *Arboviruses*

Arthropod-borne viruses form an important group of infectious diseases of humans. Roughly 400 arthropod-borne viruses of vertebrates are currently recognized, and about 20 per cent of these are known to infect humans. In contrast to the protozoan vector-borne infections, most viral diseases are of very short duration and if a person recovers long-lasting or lifelong immunity is usually acquired. The two most important groups of viruses are those that cause yellow fever and those that induce dengue fever.

14.6.3.1 *Yellow fever* This infection is caused by viruses that are transmitted by the mosquito *Aedes aegypti*. Two forms are distinguished on the basis of

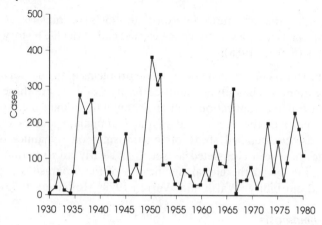

Fig. 14.38. Annual incidence of reported cases of yellow fever in South America (Warren and Mahmoud 1984).

transmission: urban yellow fever in which the virus is spread from person to person by *A. aegypti* strains that breed in urban habitats; and jungle or sylvan yellow fever which is transmitted by forest-dwelling strains of the mosquito between non-human primates and thence to, and sometimes between, people. In past history, yellow fever was one of the great epidemic scourges of humankind until the development and deployment of an effective vaccine in the twentieth century. However, yellow fever persists today in tropical areas of the Americas and Africa although it has not as yet appeared in Asia or the Pacific region (Theiler and Smith 1973).

The epidemiology of yellow fever is markedly different from that described for malaria and other vector-borne protozoas. First, the infection is typically epidemic in character such that the incidence of disease in a defined locality tends to fluctuate greatly from year to year (Fig. 14.38). Second, the latent and infectious periods in humans tend to be short (of the order of a few days; see Table 14.2) while those in the mosquito vector are not dissimilar from protozoan infections such as malaria (Table 14.3). Third, on recovery an individual tends to acquire long-lasting (if not lifelong) immunity to reinfection. Fourth and finally, transmission within human communities may be maintained, in the presence of a high degree of herd immunity, either by reservoir hosts (other primates) or vertical transmission of the virus within mosquito populations.

In light of these observations it is clear that, at least in the case of urban yellow fever, a simple compartmental model should capture the main features of transmission. If we ignore age structure for simplicity, the appropriate set of equations to describe changes in the proportions of infected mosquitoes, $\hat{y}$, and humans, y, and immune people, z, are very similar to those presented in earlier sections for malaria (see eqns (14.2) and (14.3)). Using the same notation as

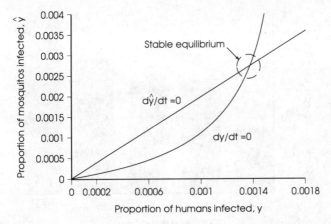

Fig. 14.39. Phase plane of the proportion of infectious mosquitoes, $\hat{y}$, and the proportion of infected humans, y, showing the isoclines $d\hat{y}/dt = 0$ and $dy/dt = 0$ for eqns (14.39)–(14.41). In the case of yellow fever it is assumed that immunity is lifelong. Parameter values $ab\hat{N}/N = 0.1$, $1/\mu_1 = 30$ years, $1/\mu_2 = 10$ days, $1/\gamma = 20$ days, and $ac = 0.2$.

that described for the basic malaria model, an appropriate model is of the form

$$dy/dt = (ab\hat{N}/N)\hat{y}(1 - y - z) - (\gamma + \mu_1)y, \tag{14.39}$$

$$dz/dt = \gamma y - \mu_1 z, \tag{14.40}$$

$$d\hat{y}/dt = acy(1 - \hat{y}) - \mu_2 \hat{y}. \tag{14.41}$$

Here μ_1 and μ_2 denote the death rates within human and mosquito populations respectively (note that disease-induced mortality in people is ignored). The properties of this model are broadly similar to those outlined for the basic malaria model. For example, the basic reproductive rate R_0 is as defined in eqn (14.4) with γ replaced by $\gamma + \mu_1$. However, there is one important difference induced by the presence of an immune class. This is best illustrated by a geometrical 'phase-plane' analysis of the dynamical behaviour of eqns (14.39)–(14.41). We consider dynamical changes in three dimensions created by the variables y, z, and $\hat{y}$ by reference to the isoclines obtained by setting $dy/dt = dz/dt = d\hat{y}/dt = 0$. An example is illustrated in Fig. 14.39 for the situation $R_0 > 1$. A stable equilibrium exists, but the dynamical trajectories to this state may be oscillating in character. In other words, the system has a propensity to exhibit weakly damped oscillations as a direct consequence of the inclusion of an immune class. The properties of the system are very similar to those described earlier (see Chapter 6) for directly transmitted viral and bacterial infections. The phase and amplitude of the epidemic cycles will be dependent on the magnitude of R_0 and the generation time of the virus (the sum of the latent plus infectious periods in both hosts). The model can be easily extended to include age structure as illustrated earlier in eqns (14.20) and (14.21), and by

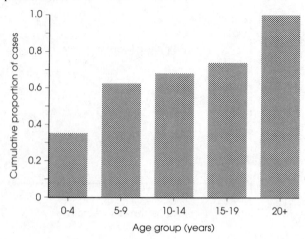

Fig. 14.40. Cumulative proportion by age of individuals who experienced infection by the yellow fever virus in Ghana from 1977–80. Data based on case reports of infection (Agadzi *et al.* 1984).

the equilibrium age distribution model defined in eqns (14.27)–(14.29). This latter set of equations is directly applicable to the study of yellow fever.

The above discussion prompts the question of why yellow fever incidence fluctuates so erratically in endemic areas when infections such as measles tend to exhibit more regular oscillatory patterns. The reason is unclear at present, but a variety of observations provide some clues. First, in endemic urban areas, where vaccination is (or was) low, the proportion seropositive for antibodies to the yellow fever virus tends to rise steadily with age, to approach a plateau in older age classes (Fig. 14.40). This is not dissimilar to measles, although the rate of rise with age is slower for yellow fever (which has a lower R_0 and larger average age at first infection, A). These age–seropositivity curves suggest that either many people acquire inapparent infections (with a mild and short-duration fever) or that case reporting is highly inaccurate. Both are likely to be true, and the former is backed by a body of clinical evidence (Monath 1985).

In rural areas, the erratic patterns of incidence in humans are more easily explained. Human density may often be too low to maintain R_0 above unity in the absence of non-human primate reservoirs and vertical transmission in the mosquito population. Epidemics in human communities will therefore occur at infrequent intervals when herd susceptibility rises to a sufficient level to trigger an outbreak of infections transmitted solely among humans.

14.6.3.2 *Dengue fever*   Dengue viruses are vector-transmitted, single-stranded, enveloped RNA viruses of the genus *Togaviridae*. They are transmitted by various species of day-biting *Aedes* mosquitoes (principally *A. aegypti*) and

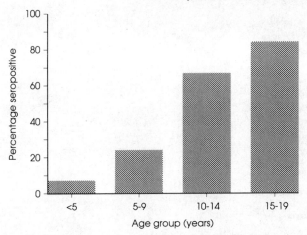

Fig. 14.41. Prevalence of dengue virus antibodies detected by immunoglobulin G enzyme-linked immunosorbent assay in children in Tahiti (April–June 1987) (Chunque *et al.* 1989).

may, in certain areas, also infect non-human primates. As for yellow fever, dengue viruses are transmitted in two basic patterns, either urban or sylvan. They can produce a spectrum of diseases in humans ranging from undifferentiated fever, dengue fever syndrome to dengue haemorrhagic fever. There appear to be four major antigenic types of the virus (labelled types 1 to 4), although evidence exists for extensive genetic heterogeneity within the group.

The epidemiology of dengue virus infection is broadly similar to that described for yellow fever. In brief, latent and infectious periods in humans are of short duration (a few days), immunity or recovery is long lasting, patterns of disease tend to be epidemic in character, non-human primates enhance population persistence, and inapparent infections in humans are common. Serological surveys in areas of endemic infection often reveal high levels of seropositivity in children and young adults, indicating that the virus can have a significant transmission potential (R_0 large) in certain areas (Fig. 14.41). The transmission dynamics of these viruses have been little studied but the model outlined for yellow fever would seem to be appropriate. At present, control is based on reductions in vector abundance. Vaccines are under development. However, an effective vaccine must be able to protect against infection by all four of the major strains of the virus since they often occur together within human communities (Halstead 1984).

Part II

Macroparasites

15

Biology of host–macroparasite associations

15.1 Introduction

Many important diseases of humans, particularly in tropical and subtropical regions, arise from infection by macroparasites or metazoan (multicellular) organisms. The major parasites belong to the helminth and arthropod groups. and include flukes (the trematodes), tapeworms (the cestodes), nematodes, lice, fleas, and ticks. These organisms tend to have much longer generation times than microparasites; they often possess complex life cycles involving two or more obligatory host species, and direct multiplication within the definitive or final host (i.e. humans) is either absent or occurs at a low rate. Sexual reproduction often occurs in the human host, but this process entails the production of transmission stages, such as eggs or larvae, which leave the host to complete further development and maturation. Direct asexual reproduction may occur in intermediate hosts such as in the life cycle of the digenetic flukes (e.g. the schistosome parasites).

Macroparasites infect very large numbers of people throughout the world and present a major medical problem, especially in tropical and subtropical countries (Table 15.1). The diseases caused are diverse and human immune responses against the different parasites vary considerably. The responses to metazoan organisms, however, do share a number of common features. Their larger size, in comparison to microparasites, entails the existence of more antigens, both in number and kind. For the parasites with complicated life histories involving many developmental stages, some of these antigens may be specific to a particular stage of development (Maizels *et al.* 1983). Macroparasitic infections are generally chronic in form and they are more a cause of morbidity than mortality. This is in part a consequence of the inability of humans, in the majority of instances, to develop fully protective immunity to reinfection following first exposure to parasite invasion. Macroparasitic infections therefore tend to be *persistent* in character; in endemic areas, people usually harbour parasites for the majority of their lives as a consequence of repeated reinfection.

Among the consequences of chronic or persistent infection are the presence of circulating antigens, persistent antigenic stimulation, and the formation of immune complexes (Butterworth *et al.* 1982). Levels of immunoglobulins are typically raised by many macroparasitic infections, such as IgE in helminth infection. Splenomegaly is often pronounced and there is evidence that parasite antigens can act to induce the mitosis of lymphocytes (the major effector cells of the vertebrate immune system) (Roitt 1988). In addition to the immune

Table 15.1 The major helminth (=macro-parasite) infections of humans (see Muller 1975)

Intestinal nematodes	*Ascaris lumbricoides*
	Trichuris trichiura
	Ancylostoma duodenale
	Necator americanus
	Enterobius vermicularis
Flukes	*Schistosoma mansoni*
	Schistosoma haematobium
	Schistosoma japonicum
	Opisthorcis sinensis
	Fasciola hepatica
	Paragonimus westermani
Filarial nematodes	*Onchocerca volvulus*
	Wuchereria bancrofti
	Loa loa
	Brugia malayi
	Dracunculus medinensis
Tapeworms	*Echinococcus granulosus*
	Taenia saginata
	Taenia solium

responses directed against the parasite, immunosuppression and immunopatho-logical effects are observed. As a consequence of their antigenic complexity and complicated developmental cycles within the human host, no single immunological effector mechanism acts in isolation; there are always several. Macroparasites have therefore evolved many different ways of evading the host's defences to ensure persistence, both within an individual host and within the population.

In this, and the following chapters, our focus is primarily directed towards the major helminth infections of man. These include the intestinal nematode infections (*Ascaris lumbricoides*—the roundworm, *Necator americanus* and *Ancylostoma duodenale*—the hookworms, *Trichuris trichiura*—the whipworm, and *Enterobius vermicularis*—the pinworm), the schistosome blood flukes (*Schistosoma mansoni*, *S. haematobium*, *S. japonicum*, and *S. intercalatum*), the filarial nematodes (*Onchocerca volvulus*, *Wuchereria bancrofti*, *Brugia malayi*, and *Dracunculus medinensis*), and intestinal or encysted tapeworm infections (*Hymenolepsis nana*, *Taenia saginata*, and *Echinococcus granulosus*) (see Muller 1975). Their life cycles are sometimes direct (e.g. the intestinal nematodes and *Hymenolepsis nana*) where transmission between hosts is achieved by means of eggs or larvae which pass into the external environment via the host's faeces.

The faecal–oral route of horizontal transmission is very effective in poor communities in developing countries with low standards of hygiene and sanitation. Indirect transmission may be via molluscan intermediate hosts, as in the case of the schistosome flukes, or via biting arthropods, as in the case of the filarial worms. Humans are usually the definitive host (the host in which the parasite attains reproductive maturity). Once the parasite has gained entry to the definitive host, a sequence of developmental changes normally occurs (often involving complex migratory patterns within the body of the host) before the organism arrives at its preferred site and attains reproductive maturity. A time-delay therefore exists between entry to the definitive host and the point when the parasite begins the production of eggs or larvae for transmission to other hosts. This delay may be just a few days in length or it may stretch for many weeks, depending on the species of parasite.

The principal population processes involved in the life cycles of three of the most important helminth parasites of man (e.g. *Ascaris lumbricoides*, *Schistosoma mansoni*, and *Onchocerca volvulus*) are portrayed diagrammatically in Figs. 15.1–15.3.

15.2 Population processes

15.2.1 *The basic reproductive rate, R_0*

The transmission potential of a parasite with a complex life cycle that involves many distinct developmental stages and, concomitantly, many population-determining rate processes (i.e. birth, death, and infection rates), is best described by reference to the basic reproductive rate, R_0, of the organism. This

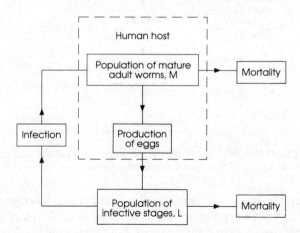

Fig. 15.1. Diagrammatic flow chart of the principal population and rate processes involved in the life cycles of directly transmitted intestinal helminths of humans.

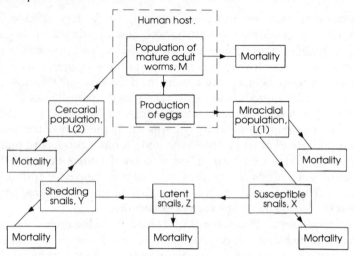

Fig. 15.2. Diagrammatic flow chart of the principal population and rate processes involved in the life cycle of schistosome parasites of humans.

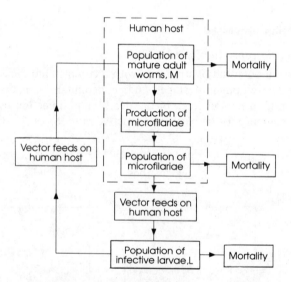

Fig. 15.3. Diagrammatic flow chart of the principal population and rate processes involved in the life cycles of the filarial nematodes of humans.

parameter, in the case of macroparasites, defines the average number of offspring (or female offspring in the case of a dioecius species) produced throughout the reproductive life span of a mature parasite that themselves survive to reproductive maturity in the absence of density-dependent constraints on population growth (see Anderson 1982*b*; Anderson and May 1979*b*,

1985b,d). As discussed earlier, R_0 is directly equivalent to Fisher's definition of net reproductive rate for free-living species (see Fisher 1930). The value of R_0 is determined by the many rate processes that control the flow of a parasite through its life cycle. The manner in which these birth, death, and infection rates interact with the density of the host (or hosts for an indirect cycle) to determine the value of R_0 is described in detail in subsequent chapters that deal with mathematical models. For a given species of parasite the value of R_0 will vary from one human community to another depending on the prevailing densities of hosts, and climatic, social, and environmental conditions. Its magnitude may therefore alter on a regular seasonal basis.

By definition, a parasite population will fail to establish within a host community unless the magnitude of R_0 exceeds unity. However, as for microparasites, once established the effective reproductive rate R of the parasite under steady-state or equilibrium conditions will tend to unity in value. Note that R_0 is defined per generation time (the average time from birth to the attainment of reproductive maturity) of the parasite.

15.2.2 *Parasite mortality and average life spans*

The average duration of stay in any one developmental state within a macroparasite's life cycle varies greatly, both between species and between developmental stages. However, for the major helminth species some generalities emerge. The human host typically has a life span an order of magnitude or more in excess of any of the parasitic or free-living stages of the disease agent (Table 15.2). Certain of the filarial nematodes are thought to be an exception to this trend since life expectancy of adult worms in humans is often quoted as 10 years or more (Dietz 1982*a*). However, obvious practical problems surround the estimation of mortality rates of endoparasites of humans, and the conventional wisdom for this group of parasites may be false (Anderson and May 1985*b*). The free-living stages of helminths, or the developmental stages within insect or molluscan intermediate hosts, have life spans much shorter than those of the sexually mature parasites in humans (Table 15.2). A good illustration of these trends is provided by the blood fluke *Schistosoma mansoni*. The adult parasite in humans is thought to have an expected life span of 3–5 years, the infected molluscan intermediate host typically has a life span of the order of a few weeks, while the free-living aquatic stages responsible for transmission from man to snail (the miracidia) and from snail to man (the cercaria) have average life spans of a few hours.

In this context, it is important to note that the epidemiological and parasitological literatures often contain conflicting reports concerning parasite life expectancies, as a consequence of the failure to distinguish between maximum life span and average life expectancy. The former quantity is, of course, much greater than the latter, For example, *S. mansoni*'s maximum life span may be 10 to 20 years while life expectancy is estimated to be between 3

Table 15.2 (a) Parasite life expectancies in the human host (see Anderson and May (1979*b*, 1985*b,c*) and Anderson (1981) for source references)

Parasite	Life expectancy (years)[a]
Enterobius vermicularis	<1
Trichuris trichiura	1–2
Ascaris lumbricoides	1–2
Necator americanus	2–3
Ancylostoma duodenale	2–3
Schistosoma mansoni	3–5
Schistosoma haematobium	3–5
Wuchereria bancrofti	3–5
Onchecerca volvulus	8–10

[a] Rough approximation due to the practical difficulties inherent in estimation.

Table 15.2(b) Parasite life expectancies in the intermediate host

Parasite	Host	Life expectancy (days)[b]
Schistosoma mansoni	*Biomphalaria glabrata*	7–42
Schistosoma haematobium	*Bulinus globosus*	14–28
Schistosoma japonicum	*Oncomelania hupensis*	28–42
Wuchereria bancrofti	*Anopheles funestus*	5–10
Onchocerca vulvulus	*Simulium damnosum*	14–28

[b] Life expectancy highly dependent on prevailing environmental conditions.

Table 15.2(c) Parasitic life expectancies of free-living infective stages

Parasite	Life cycle stage	Life expectancy[b]
Schistosoma mansoni	Miracidia	4–16 hours
Schistosoma mansoni	Cercaria	8–20 hours
Ascaris lumbricoides	Egg	28–84 days
Necator americanus	Infective larvae	3–10 days
Ancylostoma duodenale	Infective larvae	3–10 days
Tricuris trichiura	Egg	10–30 days
Enterobius vermicularis	Egg	14–56 days

[b] Life expectancy highly dependent on prevailing environmental conditions.

and 5 years (Anderson 1987). A further complication arises from the use of prevalence data (the proportion or percentage of hosts infected) as opposed to intensity data (an indirect measure of parasite burden per host) in the estimation of life expectancy. For groups of infected people who ceased to be exposed to reinfection, the decay in average intensity of infection through time is much more rapid than the decay in prevalence (this issue is discussed more fully in the sections on macroparasite models).

The relative time-scales on which the dynamics of host and parasite populations operate are largely determined by the expected life spans of the human host and the various developmental stages of the parasite. The empirical observations on the differences in such life expectancies in the case of helminth parasites enable significant simplifications to be made in the construction of mathematical models to mimic their transmission dynamics (see Anderson and May 1982c). The dynamical changes in the population of mature adult parasites in man can be examined under the assumption that the human population is approximately constant in size on a time-scale appropriate to changes in parasite abundance. Furthermore, it is reasonable to assume, in most cases, that the populations of free-living infective stages or infected intermediate hosts are essentially at equilibrium, due to the rapidity with which changes in these populations occur compared with those in mature adult parasite populations. This observation is of particular relevance for the study of intestinal nematodes, schistosome flukes, and the filarial worms. As such, it is often appropriate to study the population dynamics of these species by reference to a mathematical model based on a single equation to describe changes in the average adult parasite burden within the human community. From an epidemiological standpoint, this is most convenient since it is the parasite in man which is of prime interest as the cause of disease and morbidity. In most instances, the severity of disease symptoms is likely to be directly related to the parasite burden harboured by an individual.

Simple estimates of life expectancy hide many biological complications. A few of these deserve mention. The study of patterns of parasite mortality in humans is difficult for practical and ethical reasons, and hence our knowledge of their relationships with other variables, such as parasite age, host nutritional status, host genetic background, or the host's past experience of infection, is largely derived from experimental work with laboratory rodent models and their associated helminth parasites. Most organisms, whether parasitic or free-living, exhibit age-dependent survival (see Hutchinson 1978). Helminth parasites of mammals are no exception. As illustrated in Fig. 15.4, survival following infection is often biphasic, where at first a substantial proportion of the initial inoculum fail to establish and thereafter the mortality rate increases with the age of the parasite. The pattern of this curve, for a given species of helminth, is often dependent on the genetic background of the host and on its nutritional status. Poor nutritional status of the host may increase (as in the case of intestinal infections in mice) or decrease (as in the case of *S. mansoni*

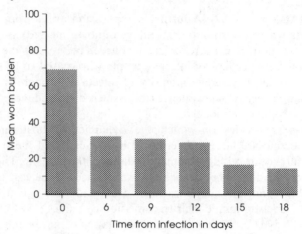

Fig. 15.4. The survival of *Schistosoma mansoni* in CBA/Ca mice infected with 70 cercaria on day 0. The graph records the decay in worm burden (mean in ten mice) through time (parasite life expectancy = 12 days).

in mice) parasite survival (Fig. 15.5). The outcome appears to depend on the balance between the indirect impact of low nutritional status on the host's immunological defences, versus its direct impact on parasite nutrition and growth.

In addition to the above complications, the pattern of parasite survival in a well nourished host often depends on the host's prior experience of infection.

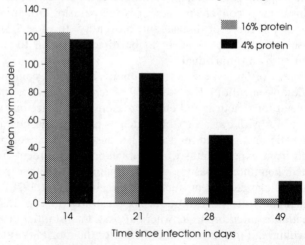

Fig. 15.5. The survival of *Trichuris muris* in 4-week-old (at day 0) CBZ/Ca mice given 650 larvae on day 0 (from Michael and Bundy 1989). The graph records parasite survival (mean burden) in mice fed on either a low (4 per cent) or a high (16 per cent) protein diet, at various times post-infection.

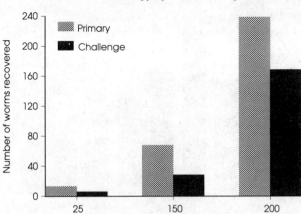

Fig. 15.6. The impact of past experience of infection on the number of *Heligmosomoides polygyrus* (nematode) that survive for 14 days post infection in mice (from Maema 1986). Different batches of mice were exposed to 25, 150, and 200 infected larvae on day 0. The histogram plots the number of worms surviving 14 days post-infection, at the three infection levels, in naive mice (primary infection) and in mice who had been immunised with a dose of 150 larvae (parasites subsequently cleared with an anthelminthic).

Parasite survival in challenge infections following a primary exposure is often curtailed as a consequence of acquired immunity (Fig. 15.6). Unfortunately, little is understood about these complications for the major helminths of man. At present we can only assume that they are of relevance by analogy with laboratory research with rodent models (Slater and Keymer 1986; Slater 1988).

With respect to free-living infective stages, or the survival of larval parasites in intermediate hosts (invariably poikilotherms), environmental factors such as temperature or humidity are important determinants of mortality rates (Fig. 15.7). Seasonal changes in temperature, for example, can induce substantial changes in the life expectancies of free-living infective stages, such as the L_3 infective larvae of hookworms or the miracidia or cercaria of schistosomes. These may result in seasonal fluctuations in the magnitude of the basic reproductive rate, R_0.

15.2.3 *Rates of infection*

For parasitic species, transmission between hosts is essentially equivalent to a birth process since it places the parasite in a location where reproduction (either sexual or asexual) can take place. Transmission rates are therefore of central importance to an understanding of the population dynamics and epidemiology of infectious disease agents.

One of the principal determinants of the net rate of infection of the human host is its relationship with the density (or densities in the case of indirectly

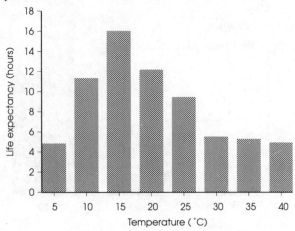

Fig. 15.7. The relationship between the life expectancy (in hours) of the miracidia of *Schistosoma mansoni* and water temperature (°C) (from Anderson *et al.* 1982).

transmitted species) of hosts and the density of infective stages (or intermediate hosts). A variety of experimental studies (employing laboratory models) suggest that the net rate of infection is directly proportional to the density of the host times the density of infective stages (Fig. 15.8). In other words, where infection is achieved via exposure to free-living infective stages, the relationship between the number of parasites that establish within a single host, and the density of infective stages to which the host is exposed, is linear in form. Ultimately, of course, saturation must occur since the physical size of the host (or the organs or tissues that are the preferred site of infection) will eventually limit the rate of establishment. In natural habitats, however, such considerations are unimportant in most instances. The linear relationship (Fig. 15.8) appears to hold for directly transmitted parasites and for those that are indirectly transmitted between hosts by free-living infective stages. The slope of the linear relationship is determined by many factors including the species of host and parasite, host genetic background, host nutritional status, the host's past experience of infection, and various climatic factors, such as temperature or humidity, that influence the 'infectivity' of the transmission stages.

In the case of indirectly transmitted parasites that utilize a biting vector, such as the filarial worms, the relationship between the net transmission rate and the densities of human and vectors is somewhat more complex. As in the case of malaria (see Chapter 14), the net gain of parasites is related to the ratio of vector density divided by human density, since the vector can only take a fixed number of bites per unit of time (in other words a saturation effect). The principal determinant of the rate of transmission is thus the 'human-biting rate' of the vector. This is to be contrasted with the case of schistosome parasites, where transmission from man to snail and snail to man is achieved via a

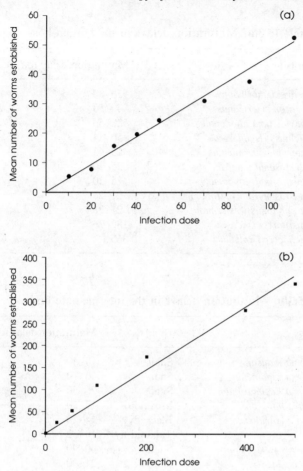

Fig. 15.8. (a) Number of *Schistosoma mansoni* worms recovered 6 weeks post-infection from naive mice (CBA/Ca) exposed to a single infection of varying intensity (0–110 cercariae). Full line is the best-fit linear model, $y = ax$, where $a = 0.4711$ (after Crombie and Anderson 1985). (b) Number of *Heligmosomoides polygyrus* worms recovered 14 days after the exposure of naive mice (CBA/Ca) to varying doses of infective larvae (50–500). Full line is the best-fit linear model, $y = ax$, where $a = 0.721$ (Maema 1986).

short-lived free-living infective stage. In this circumstance, the net gain of parasites in the human population is proportional to the density of humans times the density of snails. These issues are described in more detail in the subsequent sections on mathematical models

15.2.4 *Maturation delays*

For most helminth parasites, a not insignificant time delay occurs between the time of entry to the host and the time when the parasite attains reproductive

Table 15.3(a) Maturation delays in the human host

Parasite	Maturation delay (days)
Ascaris lumbricoides	50–80
Necator americanus	40–50
Ancylostoma duodenale	28–50
Trichuris trichiura	50–84
Enterobius vermiculus	15–43
Schistosoma mansoni	25–30
Schistosoma japonicum	25–30
Schistosoma haematobium	21–28
Paragonimus westermani	21–28
Opisthorcis sinensis	182–365
Onchocerca volvulus	365+

Table 15.3(b) Maturation delays in the intermediate host

Parasite	Host	Maturation delay (days)[a]
Schistosoma mansoni	Snail	18–40
Schistosoma japonicum	Snail	30–70
Schistosoma haematobium	Snail	20–50
Wuchereria bancrofti	Mosquito	13–20
Onchocerca volvulus	Black fly	14–20
Loa loa	Tabanid fly	10–12
Paragonimus westermani	Snail	60–90
Opisthorcis sinensis	Snail	21–30
Opisthorcis sinensis	Fish	20–30

[a] Dependent on climate conditions.

maturity. In the case of the human host, this maturation delay (often termed the latent period) is usually much less than the typical life expectancy of the parasite (Table 15.3). These delays are therefore of limited significance to the overall transmission dynamics of the parasite in humans. It is possible that the lengths of these delays are to some extent influenced by the host's past experience of infection (as suggested by evidence from laboratory work on rodents) but quantitative data for human infections are not available at present (Befus 1975). With respect to the intermediate hosts of the schistosome flukes and filarial worms, the maturation delay may be relatively long compared with the life expectancy of the infected host (Table 15.3). For example, in the case of *S. mansoni*, the delay from the point of infection of a snail by a miracidium to the time when cercariae are first released from the snail is of the order of 4–5 weeks. In most natural habitats, the snail host *Biomphalaria glabrata* has a very limited life expectancy, in the range of 4–8 weeks (Anderson and May 1979a). Thus, in these circumstances, the maturation delay has a very important effect on the density of 'infectious' vectors within the habitat. Short life expectancy combined with long maturation delays can result in a very low 'standing crop' of infectious intermediate hosts, irrespective of the intensity of transmission from human to invertebrate host (May 1977a; Barbour 1978; Anderson and May 1979a).

More generally, in the case of poikilothermic hosts, the maturation delay or latent period will be influenced by environmental variables such as temperature. High temperatures usually induce rapid parasite development, and vice versa (Fig. 15.9).

15.2.5 Parasite reproduction

Most macroparasites exhibit very high rates of egg production within the human host. Table 15.4 documents estimates of these rates for the major helminth infections of man. As for free-living species (see Southwood 1981), the rate of reproduction for the major helminth species is closely correlated with size (e.g. length or weight) (Fig. 15.10). High productivity of transmission stages offset the low probability that any one infective stage gains entry to a new host.

Many factors can influence the rate of parasite reproduction in humans. These include parasite age, host nutritional status, and past experience of infection. Egg or larval production by helminths is invariably age related; the rate, as a function of age, is usually convex in form where the peak per capita fecundity occurs somewhere between the point of reproductive maturation and the average life expectancy of the adult worm (Fig. 15.11). Low nutritional status of the host may act to decrease or increase parasite fecundity, depending

Table 15.4 Rates of egg production by mature parasites in the human host

Parasite	Rate of egg production (per female per day)
Schistosoma mansoni	100–300
Schistosoma japonicum	100–300
Schistosoma haematobium	500–3000
Diphyllobothrium latum	1 000 000
Necator americanus	3000–6000
Ancylostoma duodenale	10 000–20 000
Ascaris lumbricoides	200 000
Trichuris trichiura	50–84

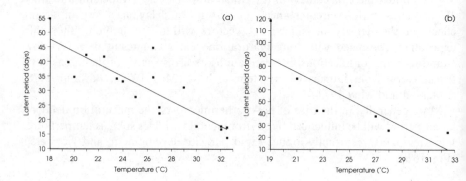

Fig. 15.9. The dependence on water temperature of the latent period, τ, of schistosome species in their intermediate snail hosts (from Anderson and May 1979*b*). (a) Latent period of *Schistosoma mansoni* in *Biomphalaria glabrata* and *Biomphalaria pfeifferi*. (b) Latent period of *Schistosoma haematobium* in *Bulinus globosus*. Full lines are best-fit linear models.

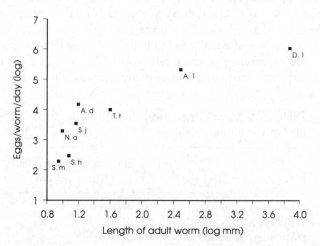

Fig. 15.10. The relationship (on a log–log scale) between the average length of mature female parasites in the human host and the daily per capita rate of egg production. The labels denote estimates for a range of species: S.m. = *Schistosoma mansoni*, S.h. = *Schistosoma haematobium*, S.j. = *Schistosoma japonicum*, N.a. = *Necator americanus*, A.d. = *Ancylostoma duodenale*, T.t. = *Trihuris trichiuria*, A.l. = *Ascaris lumbricoides*, D.l. = *Diphyllobothrium latum*.

on the species of host and parasite and the niche occupied by the parasite within the host. For the blood flukes, poor nutrition tends to decrease fecundity, while for the intestinal worms, the converse situation arises (Fig. 15.12). Past experience of infection is thought to influence parasite fecundity, particularly in the case of the filarial worms, but quantitative data for human infection are limited at present. In the case of the intestinal nematodes of man, average per capita fecundity appears to be independent of past experience of infection (as measured by host age in areas of endemic infection) (Fig. 15.13).

For indirectly transmitted species, where a phase of asexual reproduction occurs in a poikilothermic invertebrate host species (e.g. for the schistosome parasites), the production of transmission stages is influenced by a wide variety of factors such as temperature, host nutritional status, and host age and size. Cercarial production by *Biomphalaria glabrata* infected with *S. mansoni*, for example, is decreased by poor nutritional status of the host, rises with water temperature, and is positively correlated with molluscan size (and thus with age) (Anderson and May 1979a).

One of the most important factors determining the production of transmission stages by adult helminth parasites is the sexual habits or behaviour of the species. Most of the major helminth parasites of man are dioecius and many are thought to be polygamous. This latter factor is of particular importance to parasitic species, owing to their isolation within individual hosts. On gaining entry to a host, an individual parasite cannot leave to seek an alternative habitat if the current one contains no member of the opposite sex. Polygamy implies that a single male is potentially able to fertilize a number of different females

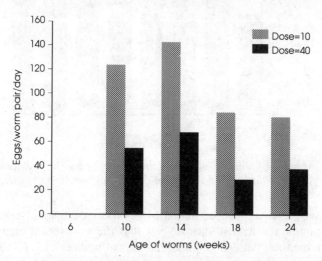

Fig. 15.11. Age-dependent fecundity in *Schistosoma mansoni* infection in laboratory mice (CBA/Ca). The pattern of egg production (recorded as a mean eggs per worm per pair per day in faeces) is recorded for mice given single infection dose of either 10 or 40 cerariae (Sithithaworn 1986).

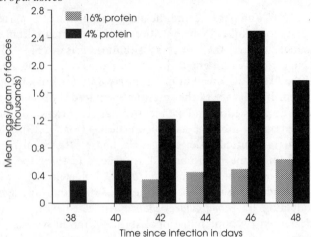

Fig. 15.12. Fecundity of *Trichuris muris* in 4-week-old (at day 0) CBA/Ca mice given 650 larvae on day 0 (from Michael 1989). The graph records eggs per gram of faeces (mean) in mice fed on either a low (4 per cent) or a high (16 per cent) protein diet, at various times post infection.

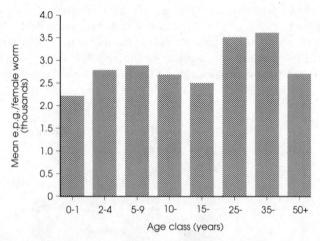

Fig. 15.13. Mean egg production (eggs per gram of faeces, e.p.g.) by *Ascaris lumbricoides*, per female worm, as a function of the age of the human host (from Elkins *et al* 1986).

or, conversely, a female can be mated by a variety of different males. Within human communities, field studies suggest that the sex ratio of male to female parasites in the total parasite population tends to be close to 1:1. However, the overall frequency distribution of male and female parasites per host may vary widely from the overall ratio within individual people. Aggregated distributions of parasite numbers per person are clearly advantageous with respect to maximizing the probability that a female worm finds a partner of the opposite sex.

An exception to the general trend for polygamy is thought to be the schistosome flukes, where pairs of males and females appear to live '*in copulo*' throughout their adult lives. Here again, however, there is the need to find a partner of the opposite sex on initial entry to the host. Certain tapeworm species, such as *Hymenolepis nana*, are hermaphroditic, although exchange of gametes between different worms will occur in multiple infections. Hermaphroditism is clearly advantageous for a parasite species, particularly when parasite abundance is low.

More broadly, knowledge of the reproductive biology of the major helminth species is limited at present. It is widely assumed that the intestinal and filarial nematodes are polygamous but quantitative data are unavailable. Furthermore, it is not known for any of the human helminths how frequently a female worm needs to be mated to maintain fertile egg production throughout her life span. These factors are of obvious important to an understanding of transmission dynamics.

15.2.6 *Density-dependent population processes*

Rates of adult parasite survival, fecundity, and maturation are often inversely associated with the density of parasites within an individual host (see Anderson and May 1978; May and Anderson 1978; Keymer 1982). In the parasitological literature such patterns are often referred to as the 'crowding effect' (Read 1950; Kennedy 1975) while in the ecological literature they are more generally referred to as density-dependent processes (Begon and Mortimer 1981). These patterns may arise either as a consequence of limitation of resources in the habitat within the host (such as space, nutrients, etc.) or as a result of host responses (immunological or non-specific) where the severity of the response rises faster than linearly with increases in parasite burden (Anderson 1978b).

Owing to practical and ethical problems, quantitative data on density dependence for human helminths are hard to come by. In the case of the intestinal worms, however, drug expulsion techniques can be employed to assess the relationship between egg output in the faeces of the host and female worm burden (Cross *et al.* 1982; Schad and Anderson 1985; Anderson and May 1985b; Elkins *et al.* 1986). In most instances per capita fecundity appears to decline as worm burden rises (Fig. 15.14). Sex ratios, on the other hand, appear to be independent of worm burden (Anderson and Schad 1985; Elkins *et al.* 1986). By analogy with laboratory studies of helminth infections of rodents, it is likely that worm establishment, survival, and maturation in humans are also dependent on parasite burden (Fig. 15.15). However, at present no data are available on these aspects (Anderson and May 1985b).

Density-dependent processes are of central importance as regulatory constraints on parasite population growth, not only within individual hosts but also within the human community as a whole. Their net severity will be dependent on the statistical distribution of worm numbers per host (Anderson and May 1978; May and Anderson 1978; Anderson 1979). Within human

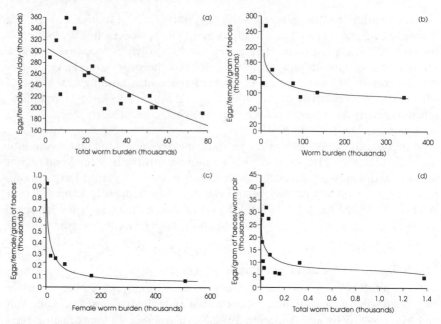

Fig. 15.14. Examples of density-dependent fecundity in intestinal nematodes. (a) *Ascaris lumbricoides*—a study of 20 patients in Malaysia (Sinniah *et al.* 1983). The full line is the best-fit exponential model; $y = a \, exp(-bx)$, $a = 3.07 \times 10^5$, $b = 0.00767$. (b) Mixed hookworm infections (*Necator americanus* and *Ancylostoma duodenale*) in India (Schad and Anderson 1985). The full curve is the best-fit power function, $y = ax^b$, $a = 287.4$, $b = -0.210$. (c) *Trichuris trichiura* in Jamaica and St Lucia (Bundy *et al.* 1985a). The full curve is the best-fit power function, $y = ax^b$, $a = 202$, $b = -0.58$. (d) *Schistosoma mansoni* autopsy data collected by Cheever (1968) (see Medley and Anderson 1985). The full curve is the best-fit power function, $y = ax^b$, $a = 45.48$, $b = -0.2887$.

communities, density-dependent parasite fecundity by itself will be sufficient to regulate the population growth of the total parasite population.

In indirect life cycles, density-dependent mechanisms are also of significance within intermediate hosts. In the case of the schistosome flukes, cercarial output by infected snails appears to be independent of the number of miracidia that have penetrated the host (Anderson 1978b; Anderson and May 1979b, 1985b). This is an extreme form of regulation, since the rate of production of transmission stages is essentially independent of parasite recruitment. A different situation arises for filarial worm infection of arthropod vectors. In this case, vector survival appears to be inversely related to larval nematode burden (Fig. 15.16). Parasite-induced host mortality, when the rate of mortality is dependent on burden, is a further form of density dependence.

More generally, in complex life cycles a variety of density-dependent mechanisms act to constrain the flow of parasites between hosts. However, we only need a single such constraint to regulate population growth over the complete cycle.

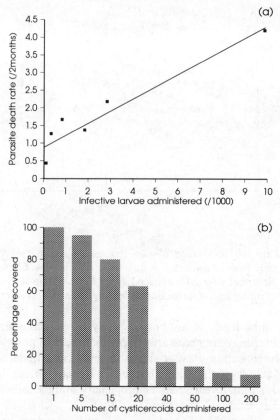

Fig. 15.15. Density-dependent parasite mortality and establishment. (a) The death rate of the dog hookworm *Ancylostoma caninum* (per 2-month period) as a function of the number of larvae administered to the dog host (data from Krupp 1962). The full line is the best-fit linear model, $y = a + bx$, where $a = 0.891$ and $b = 0.34 \times 10^{-3}$. (b) The influence of the number of cysticeroids of the tapeworm *Hymenoepis nana* administered to the rat host on the percentage of worms recovered (data from Hesselberg and Andreassen 1975).

15.2.7 *Acquired immunity*

In the epidemiological literature concerned with macroparasitic infections of humans no single topic has aroused more controversy than the question of the relevance of acquired immunity to observed parasite distributions and abundances (Bradley 1972; Warren 1973). The issue is complex and hinges on the interpretation and relevance of observations from a variety of different sources. There is little doubt that helminth parasites are able to elicit immunological responses, because antibody and cellular responses to specific parasite antigens (surface and excretory) are observed (Wakelin 1984; Pritchard *et al.* 1989). These responses may be measured using a variety of conventional immunological

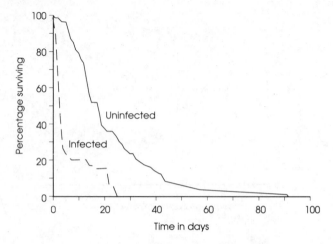

Fig. 15.16. Showing the percentage of two batches of mosquitoes (*Aedes aegypti*) surviving days after feeding on either a dog infected with *Dirofilaria immitis* or an uninfected dog. Note that survival is reduced in the batch fed on the infected dog as a direct result of acquiring microfilariae during feeding (from Kershaw *et al.* 1953).

tests that determine levels of antibody activity or cellular sensitization. The responses, however may not necessarily imply that the host possesses any degree of immunity to reinfection. Past attempts to relate, in a quantitative manner, immunological activity with parasite burdens in human patients have produced poor correlations and reveal great heterogeneity among individuals. It may therefore be that many of the responses that are elicited by infection are irrelevant to parasite establishment, survival, and reproduction. Antibody or cellular activity may represent responses to antigens that are not critical to parasite survival or to the functional integrity of antigens. Some of the surface and excreted antigens of the parasite may have evolved to distract the attention of the host immunological attack away from those that control the vital functions of the infectious agent. Protective immunity can only be measured by parameters that reflect parasite establishment, survival, and reproduction. In order to understand the relationship between protection and immune effector mechanisms, it is necessary to turn to experimental manipulations of laboratory host–parasite systems. There are, in the immunological literature, many papers describing immunological responses to macroparasites, and many describing the expression of resistance in terms of parasite abundance within a host. However, in relatively few have the two phenomena been clearly interrelated. In addition to this problem is the growing realization that the genetic background of the host is of major significance as a determinant of resistance to a specific parasite (Wakelin and Blackwell 1988).

With these problems in mind, it is possible to draw some very tentative general conclusions about acquired immunity to helminth infection. Laboratory studies clearly show that mammalian hosts are able to develop protective immunity to infection following initial exposure (Wakelin 1984). Acquired immunity acts to decrease parasite establishment and/or survival and/or reproduction and/or maturation. The degree of protection appears, in certain cases, to depend on the accumulated sum of past experience of infection, but the duration of 'immunological memory' of such experiences seems to be short relative to the life span of the host. Protection is therefore partial and short-lived. This is in marked contrast to mammalian responses to microparasites, such as viruses, where protection is often complete and memory is very long-lived. By analogy with such laboratory-derived information, it would seem highly probable that acquired immunity to macroparasites is of some significance in human communities within areas of endemic infection. The degree of protection of an individual, however, is likely to be linked to genetic background and nutritional status. In the context of parasite transmission, a degree of herd immunity may be built up in areas where transmission intensity is moderate to intense, such that the adult age classes are more resistant to infection than are the infant and child age classes (Anderson and May 1985*d*). A firm link between specific effector mechanisms and protective immunity to helminth infection in humans, however, remains to be established (Butterworth *et al.* 1984, 1985).

15.3 Epidemiological patterns

Before turning to the development and analysis of mathematical models of helminth transmission, we briefly consider the epidemiological data which are available to test predictions and to refine model structure. What can be measured concerning the distribution and abundance of endoparasites within human communities? The options are clearly limited by practical and ethical considerations but a variety of approaches are possible. Most measures are indirect because of the endoparasitic mode of life. They involve the assessment of parasite burden within individal patients via measures of helminth egg abundance in the faeces or urine (as in the case of the intestinal nematodes and tapeworms, and the schistosome flukes), or via sampling host tissue to record the abundance of larval parasites ('skin snip' tests for the density of larval filarial worms) (Muller 1975). The association between the rate of production of transmission stages and the adult worm burden, however, is made complicated by density-dependent fecundity and by single-worm or single-sex infections (i.e. no transmission stages are produced by unfertilized females or by male-only infections) (Anderson and Schad 1985). Direct measurement is sometimes possible for intestinal tract infections, by means of drug administration to expel worms in the faeces for collection and counting. In recent years, this method has become more widely used; it has helped to provide detailed quantitative data on worm abundance and distribution, on the age, sex, and size structure of parasite populations, and on the relationship between fecundity and worm burden (Cross *et al.* 1982; Thein-Hliang 1985; Anderson and Medley 1985; Bundy *et al.* 1985*a*; Anderson and Schad 1985; Schad and Anderson 1985; Elkins *et al.* 1986).

The two most widely used statistics in the epidemiological study of macroparasites are the prevalence of infection (the proportion or percentage of hosts infected in the sample) and the intensity of infection (a record of worm abundance measured via direct or indirect methods). With respect to the latter quantity, average values and variance around the mean can be calculated for different strata of the population, according to age, sex, or social groups. Changes in prevalence or average intensity of infection are commonly recorded by cross-sectional sampling schemes (where membership of a section is based on age, sex, or social status) either horizontally (at one point in time across different sections of the same population) or longitudinally (through time and across the different sections). Horizontal or longitudinal changes in prevalence and intensity of infection with host age are of particular value in the study of transmission dynamics, because age often reflects duration of exposure to infection in areas of endemic parasitism (Anderson and May 1985*b*). Incidence defines the rate of appearance of new cases of infection and it can be quantified via changes in prevalence with age or through time.

Field studies of reinfection following chemotherapy are also of great value in the study of helminth population dynamics. Rates of reinfection in people of differing ages (with different past experiences of infection) can help to shed light on the relevance of acquired immunity, provide information on immune effector mechanisms to parasite invasion, help to assess age-dependent changes in exposure to infection, and facilitate the measurement of the basic reproductive rate, R_0 (Croll *et al.* 1982; Anderson 1980; Anderson and May 1982*c*, 1985*b*).

Recent advances in immunology and molecular biology have created new techniques for the assessment of parasite distributions and abundances in human communities (Haswell-Elkins *et al.* 1989). Serological surveys for the presence or absence of antibodies specific to parasite antigens in individual patients can provide information on present and past experience of infection. Monoclonal or polyclonal antibody production methods can greatly enhance the specificity of serological tests. Unfortunately, however, due to uncertainties concerning the duration of antibody production following exposure to macroparasitic antigens, seronegativity cannot be interpreted to mean no past exposure to the parasite. More sophisticated techniques, such as DNA probes or the polymerase chain reaction (PCR), offer great potential in future epidemiological research. They potentially enable a precise assessment to be made of the presence or absence of live parasites within the patient.

15.3.1 *Distribution of parasite numbers per person*
The epidemiological measures of prevalence and average intensity of infection are summary statistics of the frequency or probability distribution of parasite numbers per host. The form of these distributions is of great significance both

to the population dynamics of the parasite and to the prevalence of symptoms of disease within human communities (morbidity is, in general, positively correlated with parasite burden). For helminth parasites, the distributions are invariably highly aggregated or contagious in form such that most individuals harbour few parasites and a few individuals harbour the majority of the parasite population. In statistical terms this implies that the variance in parasite load per person is much greater in value than the mean or average burden (for a random (Poisson) distribution the mean is equal to the variance).

Observed patterns are well described empirically by the negative binomial distribution model (Fig. 15.17). This distribution is characterized by two parameters: the mean, m, and a parameter, k, which varies inversely with the degree of parasite aggregation ($k \to 0$ as the total parasite population is concentrated on fewer and fewer people, while $k \to \infty$ as the distribution becomes more random in character) (see Bliss and Fisher 1953). The probability of observing i parasites per person, $p(i)$, for the negative binomial model is defined as

$$p(i) = \frac{(k + i - 1)!}{i!(k - 1)!} (1 + m/k)^{-k-i}(m/k)^i. \qquad (15.1)$$

The prevalence of infection (the proportion infected), P, is simply

$$P = 1 - (1 + m/k)^{-k}. \qquad (15.2)$$

A method for fitting this distribution to empirical observations is described by Bliss and Fisher (1953). The technique involves a maximum-likelihood procedure for the estimation of the value of the aggregation parameter k. Goodness of fit is assessed in the usual manner employing the χ^2 test. As k becomes large (in practical terms $k > 5$ or so), eqn (15.1) converges to the Poisson series,

$$p(i) \to m^i \exp(-m)/i!. \qquad (15.3)$$

Most observed distributions of helminths within human communities are remarkable for their high degrees of aggregation. Values of the aggregation parameter k typically lie in the range 0.1–1.0 (small values indicating severe contagion) (Table 15.5). It is not uncommon, in these circumstances, for more than 80 per cent of the total parasite population to be harboured by less than 20 per cent of the human community. As such, severe morbidity due to helminth infection is often restricted to a small fraction of 'wormy people'.

Parasite aggregation may arise as a consequence of a wide variety of factors either acting alone or concomitantly (see Boswell and Patil 1970; Anderson and Gordon 1982). These include heterogeneity in exposure to infection (due to social, environmental, or behavioural factors, or to aggregation in the spatial distribution of infective stages or infected intermediate hosts), differences in susceptibility to infection (due to genetic or nutritional factors, or to varying past experiences of infection), or to variability in parasite survival within

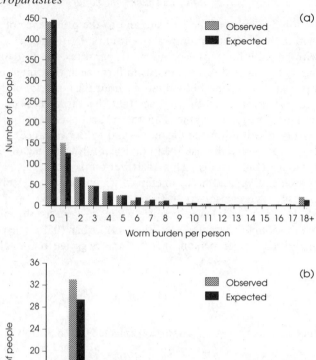

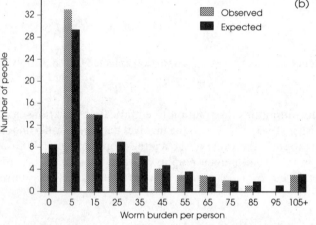

Fig. 15.17. Examples of the frequency distribution of parasite numbers per person. (a) *Ascaris lumbricoides* in Korea (Seo 1980). (Negative binomial fit, mean, $m = 2.18$ worms per person, variance, $\sigma^2 = 5.05$, $k = 0.319$.) (b) *Ancylostoma duodenale* in India (Schad and Anderson 1985). (Negative binomial fit, mean $m = 24.54$ worms per person, $k = 0.618$.)

different individuals (due to genetic, immunological, or nutritional factors). Which factors are of major importance as determinants of observed patterns is difficult to ascertain in the absence of information in addition to the frequency distribution. It is futile to try to reach conclusions about the mechanisms underlying a particular pattern simply by comparison of its goodness of fit to an empirical model such as the negative binomial distribution. This probability model, for example, can be generated by a wide variety of distinct population

Table 15.5 Degree of parasite aggregation in the human or intermediate host population, as measured inversely by the negative binomial parameter, *k* (see Anderson and May (1985*c*) for source references)

Parasite	Geographical location	Host	*k*
Ascaris lumbricoides	Iran	Man	0.2 –0.9
	Burma	Man	0.3 –0.9
	Korea	Man	0.3 –0.55
	India	Man	
	Bangladesh	Man	0.2 –0.5
	Japan	Man	0.2 –0.5
Necator americanus	India	Man	0.03–0.6
	Taiwan	Man	0.05–0.4
Trichuris trichura	Jamaica	Man	0.2 –0.3
	St Lucia	Man	0.2 –0.4
Enterobius vermicularis	Korea	Man	0.3 –0.4
Schistosoma mansoni	Brazil	Man	0.03–0.5
Wuchereria bancrofti	Surinam and Samoa	Man	0.6 –0.7
Wuchereria bancrofti		*Culex* spp. and *Anopheles* spp.	0.2 –1.7
Onchocera spp.		*Simulium dmonosum*	0.04–0.07

processes, including the compounding of a series of Poisson variates with different means or the generalization of two different distributions (see Pielou 1969). The observation that the negative binomial model is a good description of recorded patterns in human communities should therefore simply be regarded as a convenience, in the sense of giving a useful two-parameter distribution model to describe observed trends. Its goodness of fit to data can never, by itself, suffice to 'explain' the pattern of parasite abundance.

In quantifying the degree of parasite contagion within a human community great care should be exercised in the design and stratification of the sampling programme. Suppose, for example, that the parasite was randomly distributed within an age class of people but that the mean worm burden per class increased rapidly with age (often the case in practice). If our observed distribution was formed from individuals drawn from a variety of different age classes, we would arrive at the conclusion that the parasites were aggregated within the human community (because the compounding of a series of Poisson distributions with different means gives an aggregated distribution with variance greater than the mean). This is, of course, a correct conclusion, but it hides the important fact that the parasites are randomly distributed within an age class (i.e. equal susceptibility/exposure to infection at a given age). Similar problems can arise from the failure to take account of sex, social status, and various other factors. In practice it is difficult to acquire data on worm distributions within human communities and it is only recently that drug expulsion techniques have been used extensively to investigate such patterns for the intestinal nematodes (Fig. 15.17; Seo *et al.* 1979; Croll *et al.* 1982; Schad and Anderson 1985; Bundy *et al.* 1986; Haswell-Elkins *et al.* 1987*b*). For the indirectly transmitted helminths, data are very limited except in the case of *S. mansoni* where an autopsy study by Cheever (1968) produced confirmation on worm distributions. Rarely, however, have the sampling programmes allowed a detailed comparison of parasite aggregation among age or sex classes. Such data as are available suggest that the degree of aggregation (as measured by the negative binomial parameter k) is reasonably constant across age classes but with a slight tendency to decrease with host age (Table 15.6). More research is required in this area.

A further practical implication of parasite aggregation concerns the relationship between the prevalence of infection and the mean parasite burden (eqn (15.2)). For small k, fairly large changes in the mean, m, only induce relatively small changes in the prevalence P (Fig. 15.18). This observation has important implications for monitoring the effects of control programmes. Often such monitoring is based on changes in prevalence but, as indicated in Fig. 15.18, this approach may falsely lead one to the conclusion that control has had little impact; there will often be large changes in mean worm load but small changes in prevalence (Anderson and Medley 1985; Anderson and May 1985*b,d*).

Aggregation within the host community has important implications for the population biology and epidemiology of the parasite. First, it enhances the likelihood of an individual parasite finding a mate of the opposite sex. It therefore enhances the net reproductive rate of the total parasite population. Second, it increases the net regulatory impact of density-dependent constraints on parasite establishment, survival, and reproduction. Third, it results in severe symptoms of disease being focused on a relatively small fraction of the total population. Finally, it has important implications for the design of control programmes; these will discussed in later chapters.

15.3.2 *Predisposition to heavy or light infection*

Are those individuals in the tail of the probability distribution of worm numbers per person predisposed to this state, not by chance, but by social, behavioural, genetic, or nutritional factors? This intriguing question has only recently been addressed via the use of drug treatment and the monitoring of patterns of reinfection in individual patients (see Schad and Anderson 1985; Bundy *et al.* 1985*b*; Bensted-Smith *et al.* 1989; Elkins *et al.* 1987*b*). For those studies that have been completed (for *Ascaris*, *Enterobius*, *Trichuris*, hookworms, and *S. mansoni*), the answer appears to be yes (Table 15.7). Many statistical problems surround the analyses of such data, however, and caution is required until more information becomes available. Here again, sampling design and stratification are of great importance since worm burdens change with the age and sex of patients. The analyses must therefore be based on records of worm abundance, before chemotherapy and after an interval of reinfection, that are standardized

Table 15.6 Variation in the negative binomial parameter, *k*, by host age group (data from Elkins *et
al.* (1986), Haswell-Elkins *et al.* (1987*b*), Anderson
1980))

Parasite	Age classes (years)	*k*
Ascaris lumbricoides	<2	0.772
	2–4	0.851
	5–9	0.403
	10–14	1.731
	15–24	0.906
Enterobius vermicularis	0–4	0.169
	5–9	0.182
	10–14	0.325
	20–29	0.313
	30–45	0.285
	40+	0.246
Necator americanus	1	0.04
	2	0.07
	3	0.13
	4	0.20
	5	0.24
	6	0.34
	7	0.50
	8	0.60
	9	0.75
	10	0.60
	11	0.60

according to the age and the sex of the patient (Bensted-Smith *et al.* 1989).
Aside from reinfection studies, a further source of evidence for predisposition to
heavy or light infection is provided by longitudinal observations on individual
patients who do not receive chemotherapy. From a study in India of hookworm
infection in patients observed over a 16-month period (faecal samples were
taken at 2-month intervals), it was observed that those with low faecal egg
counts at the beginning of the period of observation remained low, while those
who has high faecal egg counts remained high (Fig. 15.19) (Nawalinski *et al.*
1978). Care is needed in the interpretation of these observations, however, since
complications are introduced by the relatively long life span of adult hookworms
(see Table 15.2).

A further question that arises from the study of worm loads in individual
patients is that of multispecies predisposition. For example, are those individuals
who are predisposed to heavy *Ascaris* infection also predisposed on average to

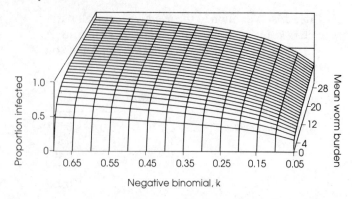

Fig. 15.18. The relationship between the proportion infected, *P*, the mean worm burden, *m*, and the aggregation parameter, *k*, for the negative binomial probability distribution of worm numbers per person.

Table 15.7 Studies of predisposition to heavy infection by helminth parasites

Parasite	Location	Evidence for predisposition	Reference
Ascaris lumbricoides	India	Yes	Haswell-Elkins *et al.* 1987*a*)
	Burma	Yes	Thein-Hliant (1989)
Enterobius vermicularis	India	Yes	Haswell-Elkins *et al.* (1987*a*)
Necator americanus	India	Yes	Schad and Anderson (1985)
Ancylostoma duodenale	India	Yes	Schad and Anderson (1985)
Trichuris trichiura	St Lucia	Yes	Bundy (1988)
Schistosoma mansoni	Kenya	Yes	Bensted-Smith *et al.* (1989)

harbour high burdens of other intestinal nematode species such as *Trichuris* and *Enterobius* and hookworms? A recent study has addressed this question and produced a positive result (Haswell-Elkins *et al.* 1987*a*). Wormy persons, at least for intestinal infections, therefore appear to be predisposed to infections with several species.

The causes of predispositions are as yet unclear but it appears likely that a variety of factors are involved, including behavioural, social, genetic, and nutritional processes. Past work has stressed the relevance of behavioural and social factors (see Schad *et al.* 1984). Laboratory studies on rodent–helminth models argue, however, that genetic and nutritional factors are probably of great significance (Wakelin 1984; Anderson 1986). It is possible that parasite aggregation reflects heterogeneity in immunocompetence to resist parasite invasion or to eliminate established worms. This may be mediated by the genetic background of the host and/or nutritional status. In general, however, it seems

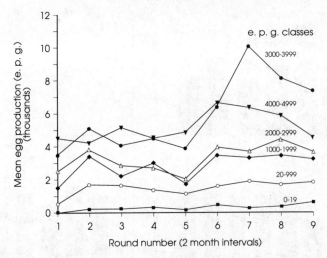

Fig. 15.19. Changes through time (by survey rounds two months apart) in the mean egg output (eggs per gram, e.p.g.) of different groups of people infected with hookworm (*Necator americanus* and *Ancylostoma duodenale*). Individuals were classified into groups on the basis of their egg counts at round 1 and at subsequent rounds were held in the classification made in the first survey (round 1). The study was conducted in a rural community north of Calcutta, India (Schad and Anderson 1985). Individuals were males and remained untreated with anthelminthics throughout the study.

likely that observed patterns result from the combined effects of behavioural factors and acquired immunity. Work in progress on the epidemiology of *S. mansoni* should help to improve our understanding of the relative importance of each factor (Butterworth *et al.* 1984, 1985, 1988; Sturrock *et al.* 1987).

15.3.3 *Age–prevalence and age–intensity profiles*

Since the major helminths of man do not reproduce within the human host to directly increase adult worm abundance, population growth in an individual is simply controlled by immigration (infection) and parasite mortality. In the simplest case in which the immigration and death rates are constant and unaffected by factors such as host age or parasite density, the average burden of adult parasites will grow monotonically as people age to reach a plateau where the immigration rate is exactly balanced by the net death rate. We might therefore expect observed age–prevalence or age–average intensity profiles to reflect some of the basic properties of an immigration–death process. Many data are available to test this hypothesis since the epidemiological literature contains a vast number of surveys of the change in helminth prevalence and average intensity (measured directly or indirectly) with host age (see Anderson and May 1985b). The majority of studies are horizontal in nature owing to the long period of study required to monitor longitudinal changes in a cohort of people over their average life span.

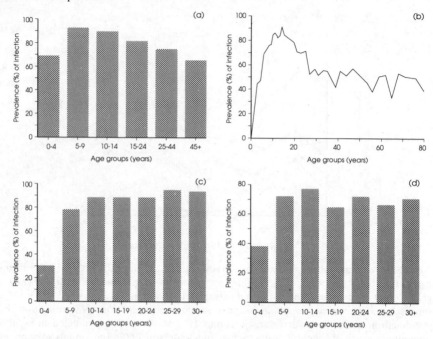

Fig. 15.20. Changes with age in the prevalence (per cent) of infection with helminth parasites in human communities. (a) *Ascaris lumbricoides* in Burma (Thein-Hliang 1989). (b) *Schistosoma haematobium* in Tanzania (Bradley and McCullough 1973). (c) Hookworm (mixed *Necator americanus* and *Ancylostoma duodenale*) in Thailand (Unhanand *et al.* 1980). (d) *Trichuris trichiura* in Thailand (Unhanand *et al.* 1980).

As illustrated in Fig. 15.20, changes in prevalence with age are often in broad agreement with the notion that worm abundance is simply controlled by constant rates of parasite input and loss. In certain instances, particularly noticeable among the intestinal nematodes, prevalence increases monotonically with age to a plateau in a manner entirely consistent with these simple ideas concerning parasite gain and loss. In other instances, however, as illustrated by the patterns recorded for schistosome flukes and filarial worms, prevalence declines after the attainment of a maximum value as people move into the older age classes. Patterns of convexity of change with age are much more apparent in profiles of average intensity of infection (Fig. 15.21). This is the case for both the intestinal nematodes and the indirectly transmitted species.

Convex patterns in intensity of infection may arise either as a result of age-related changes in exposure to infection (due to behavioural factors) and/or increased resistance to infection (where resistance may influence establishment and/or worm survival) in older individuals with considerable past experience of infection. Where parasite infection is a cause of mortality as well as morbidity, convex patterns may be due to age-dependent host mortality where the death

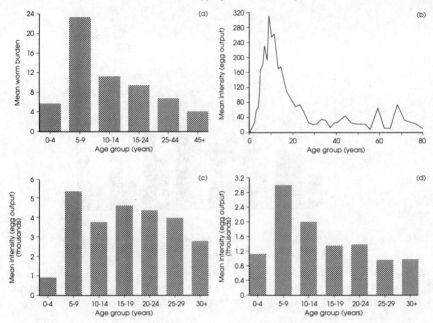

Fig. 15.21. Changes with age in the mean intensity (eggs per gram of faeces or worm burden) of infection with helminths in human communities. (a) *Ascaris lumbricoides* in Burma (Thein-Hliang 1989). (b) *Schistosoma haematobium* in Tanzania (Bradley and McCullough 1973). (c) Hookworms in Thailand (Unhanand *et al.* 1980). (d) *Trichuris trichiura* in Thailand (Unhanand *et al.* 1980).

rate is dependent on past or current experience of infection. With respect to convexity in prevalence with age, an additional factor may be of importance: a decay in prevalence within the older age groups could arise, independent of any change in the average worm load, if the degree of parasite aggregation increases with age (see Fig. 15.18). In general, therefore, convexity may arise from ecological or immunological processes, or a combination of both.

The distribution of parasite abundance among different age classes is clearly non-uniform when the average intensity follows a convex pattern. Peak intensities occur in the child or teenage segments of human communities. However, this peak is in part related to worm life expectancy. It tends to be in the child age classes (5–10-year-olds) for intestinal worms (less so for hookworm than *Ascaris* and *Trichuris*), the teenage classes of schistosome flukes, and the young adult groups for filarial worms (see Fig. 15.21). In many instances, a very large percentage of the total parasite population is harboured by the children, partly as a consequence of convexity in age–intensity changes but also as a consequence of the demography of the human population (largely children with relatively few older people in communities in developing countries with high birth rates and poor survival) (Fig. 15.22).

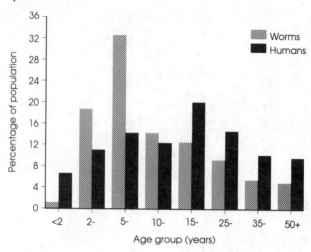

Fig. 15.22. Study of the epidemiology of *Ascaris lumbricoides* in India (from Elkins *et al.* 1986). Graph records the percentages of the total parasite population, and the human population, in different age classes of the human community.

One of the most striking features of changes in intensity with age in areas of endemic infection is the rapidity with which parasite burdens rise with age. The rate of increase reflects a variety of factors, not least of which is the transmission potential (or the magnitude of the basic reproductive rate, R_0) of the parasite. One component of this potential is the life expectancy of the adult parasite (see Table 15.2). In broad terms, the rate of increase of intensity with age in the child age classes is inversely correlated with worm life expectancy. The rate tends to be high for the short-lived intestinal nematodes, moderate for the schistosome flukes, and low for the filarial worms. Since age is equivalent to time, this rate can be used to derive estimates of the 'force of infection' (the per capita rate at which individuals acquire parasites). In turn, the force of infection, combined with a knowledge of worm life expectancy, provides information on the basic reproductive rate, R_0. The use of horizontal profiles as opposed to longitudinal data is only appropriate in areas where the parasite population has remained relatively unperturbed (no control or major cultural or environmental changes). In other words, the system must be at its stable endemic state to yield reliable estimates of R_0. Furthermore, estimates should be based on the rise in intensity in the young age classes before density-dependent constraints on parasite abundance complicate the interpretation.

Finally, it is important to note that patterns of change in prevalence and intensity with age can vary greatly according to factors such as sex, social status, and religion (Fig. 15.23). Such complications should be taken into account, both in considering the overall transmission dynamics of helminths within human communities and in the design of control programmes.

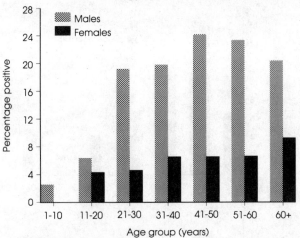

Fig. 15.23. Age and sex distribution of skin sensitivity test for *Schistosoma japonicum* among Cambodian refugees at a holding centre in Prachinburni Province, Thailand (Keittivuti *et al.* 1983). The histograms record the percentage of each age and sex group with positive skin tests (indicating presence, or past experience, of infection with *Schistosoma japonicum*).

15.3.4 *Reinfection following chemotherapeutic treatment*

A remarkable feature of the ecology of helminths in human populations is the stability of their populations in response to perturbations induced by either community-based chemotherapy programmes or transient environmental changes. Following depression, population abundance tends to return (in a monotonic manner) to the pre-control or pre-perturbation level. The rapidity with which worm burdens recover varies according to the species of parasite. It tends to be fast for the short-lived intestinal helminths and slower for the more long-lived schistosome flukes, as discussed in Chapter 16.

Rates of reinfection provide very useful data with which to estimate the value of the basic reproductive rate, R_0 (Croll *et al.* 1982). They also provide information on age-related changes in the rate of acquisition/establishment of parasites and, as discussed earlier, on the issue of predisposition to heavy or light infection. A number of recent field studies have examined parasite acquisition in relation to age, following chemotherapy (Elkins *et al.* 1986; Bundy *et al.* 1988*a*; Sturrock *et al.* 1987). Interestingly, the research suggests that net parasite acquisition is related to age, tending to be greatest in children and to decline in the older age groups (Fig. 15.24). However, the number of worms acquired over an interval of reinfection (usually 1 year), represented as a fraction of the pretreatment worm load, tends to be independent of host age (Fig. 15.24). These patterns could arise either as a consequence of age-related changes in exposure to infection, or as a result of acquired immunity (in the older age groups), or due to some combination of both mechanisms.

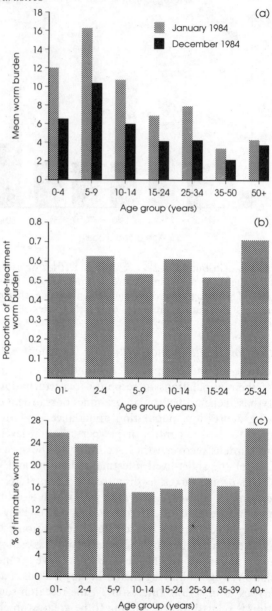

Fig. 15.24. Rate of reinfection by *Ascaris lumbricoides* following chemotherapy (over an 11-month interval) in Pulicat, India (data from Elkins *et al.* 1986). (a) The mean worm burden in various age classes in January 1984 and December 1984. (b) The data, by age group, as a proportion of the pre-treatment worm burden reacquired over the 11-month reinfection period. (c) The percentage of immature worms in the mean worm loads in December 1984 after 11 months' exposure to infection.

16

The basic model: statics

16.1 Historical background

The origins of mathematical studies of the population dynamics of host–helminth parasite systems lie in the literature concerned with theoretical ecology. In 1934 Kostitzin published a seminal paper which described a deterministic model of the flow of hosts among a series of classes denoting different infection statuses, defined by the number of parasites harboured (Kostitzin 1934). The model consisted of an infinite series of differential equations and contained many rate parameters denoting host and parasite reproduction and survival. His formulation took account both of the influence of these rate parameters on the distribution of parasite numbers per host and, concomitantly, of the effect of this distribution on the dynamical properties of the interactions of the two species. The major contribution of this work was the recognition that the classical epidemic models, which treated the host population as consisting of a few discrete classes (such as susceptibles, infected, and immunes), were inappropriate descriptions of associations in which the pathology induced by infection, the fecundity and mortality of the host and parasite, and the host responses generated by infection, all typically depend on the number or burden of parasites harboured by an individual host.

Subsequent to Kostitzin's work, interest in mathematical models of macroparasites was not rekindled until the early 1960s. The stimulus for further developments was provided by parasites of medical and veterinary significance, in particular the human schistosome flukes and the gastrointestinal nematodes of sheep and cattle (Hairston 1965a; Macdonald 1965; Tallis and Leyton 1966; Leyton 1968). The ecologist, Hairston, first aroused interest in the population biology of schistosome parasites by his attempts to employ life-table or actuarial methods to study their transmission within human communities (Hairston 1962, 1965a). He focused attention on the numerous population processes, inherent in the two-host life cycle, which contribute to the overall reproductive success of the parasite. This introduced the idea that the numerical magnitudes of the many transmission, mortality, and reproductive rates could be combined in a single composite measure of parasite transmission success. Today we refer to this measure as the basic reproductive rate, R_0.

Hairston also introduced a further technique, the use of Muench's so-called *catalytic models* to estimate rates of helminth transmission within human or intermediate host populations, from observations recording the changes in parasite prevalence with host age (Muench 1959). The term *catalytic models* derives from their origins in chemistry where they were used to study kinetic reactions involving enzymes. Prior to Hairston's work they had been employed in the study of viral and bacterial infections. They are in essence a simplification of the equilibrium microparasitic model which describes the decay in susceptibles with host age (see Chapter 4). As applied to helminth infections they are only appropriate in the estimation of forces of infection within snail intermediate host populations where infection status is based on the division of the population into susceptible and infected classes (due to the parasites' direct sexual reproduction within the host) (Hairston 1965*b*; Anderson and May 1978*b*; Anderson and Crombie 1984, 1985).

In the mid-1960's, an epidemiologist, George Macdonald, celebrated for his important work in extending the early mathematical studies of Ross (1915) and Lotka (1923) on the dynamics of human malarial infections, was also thinking along similar lines to Hairston. In 1965 Macdonald published an important paper on the dynamics of schistosome parasites within human and snail populations in which he described a simple mathematical model (Macdonald 1965). The formal details of Macdonald's model are vague in the original publication, but this does not detract from the originality of his approach. The important advance made by Macdonald was his recognition of the importance of mating success of dioecius helminths to the transmission dynamics of the parasite. Along similar lines to Hairston's work, he also argued that combinations of parameter values determined transmission success from man to snail and from snail to man.

Shortly after the publication of Macdonald's paper, Tallis and Leyton (1966) and Leyton (1968) described stochastic formulations to mimic the dynamics of dioecious helminth populations within their definitive hosts. The stimulus for their study lay in the economic importance of gastrointestinal nematode infection to the production of sheep and cattle livestock. These authors, who were unaware of Macdonald's work, provided a layer of formalism to the treatment of mating probabilities and, more importantly, demonstrated that aggregated distributions of parasite numbers per host could be generated by heterogeneity in exposure to infection within the host population.

The papers of Hairston (1962, 1965*a*), Macdonald (1965), Tallis and Leyton (1966), and Leyton (1968) stimulated a steady flow of interest in models of helminth transmission dynamics during the 1970s. Most of the published work was concerned with schistosome parasites (see Nasell and Hirsch 1972*a,b*; Lewis 1975*a,b*; Nasell 1976*a,b*, 1977; May 1977*a*; Cohen 1977; Fine and Lehman 1977; Barbour 1978; Goddard 1978; Bradley and May 1978; and Anderson and May 1979*b*), but some work had been initiated in the field of ecology with the focus on the impact of helminths on host population growth and regulation (see Crofton 1971*a,b*; Anderson 1974, 1978*b*, 1979; May 1977*b*; Anderson and May 1978, 1979*b*). In the 1980s, research interest accelerated, and models have been developed (both deterministic and stochastic) for intestinal nematode and filarial worm infection (Anderson 1980, 1981*b*, 1982*c*; Anderson and May 1982*c*,

1985*b*; Dietz 1982*a*). The main themes of this research and its applications in the study of helminth epidemiology and control are developed in the following sections and chapters.

16.2 Basic models

To start, we consider the simplest possible framework to describe changes with respect to time, t, in the number of adult parasites, $M(t)$, in a single host. Initially we ignore the age structure of the host population and examine what happens when the host is constantly exposed to infection at a rate Λ, and the adult parasite dies at a constant per capita rate, μ_1. The resultant model is a simple immigration–death process

$$dM(t)/dt = \Lambda - \mu_1 M(t), \tag{16.1}$$

with solution

$$M(t) = M^*[1 - \exp(-\mu_1 t)]. \tag{16.2}$$

It is assumed that the host is uninfected at time $t = 0$ ($M(0) = 0$). The worm burden rises montonically as time goes on, to attain a globally stable equilibrium, M^*, where the rate of infection Λ is exactly balanced by the net death rate of the parasite

$$M^* = \Lambda/\mu_1. \tag{16.3}$$

The equilibrium level is simply the rate of infection Λ times the life expectancy of the parasite $1/\mu_1$. The time taken to attain an abundance which is a fraction f of the equilibrium (starting at zero), t_f, is

$$t_f = -\ln(1 - f)/\mu_1. \tag{16.4}$$

This result is revealing; it shows that, for the simple model, the rate of approach to the equilibrium worm burden depends simply on the life expectancy of the parasite, $1/\mu_1$, and is independent of the rate of infection. The magnitude of the equilibrium, M^*, of course depends on the intensity of transmission, Λ. These principles, although derived from the very simplest model, apply to varying degrees for the most complex models developed in subsequent sections.

The equivalent stochastic formulation for eqn (16.1) predicts that the distribution of worms within a population of hosts at time t is Poisson in form with mean and variance $M(t)$ (as defined in eqn (16.2)) (Anderson 1974). In reality of course the distribution is not random but aggregated in form. This can arise if the value of Λ is itself a random variable within the population of hosts, such that exposure to infection is heterogeneous.

16.2.1 *Direct life cycle macroparasites*

The immigration–death process is of course too simple to describe the dynamics of a parasite with a complex life cycle. In reality the rate of infection, Λ, will depend on a variety of factors such as host density, the density of infective stages in the habitat, and the total size of the population of reproductively mature adult parasites in the host populaton. To capture this dependence we need to formulate a model which describes how parasites flow through a complete developmental cycle. We begin with direct life cycle parasites, such as the intestinal nematodes, which produce eggs (or larvae) in the human host that pass to the exterior to form a pool of free-living infective stages. Such a life cycle is portrayed diagrammatically in Fig. 15.1.

The life cycles of all directly transmitted nematodes are basically of similar structure, involving two principal populations: the sexually mature parasites in man and the free-living infective stages. The latter may be mobile larvae as in the hookworm life cycle or resistant eggs as in the case of *Ascaris lumbricoides*. A sensible beginning in the study of their transmission dynamics is to formulate two equations to describe the rates of changes with respect to time, t, in the mean number of sexually mature worms, $M(t)$, in a human community of density (or size) N and the number of infective larvae in the habitat, $L(t)$ (Anderson 1980, 1982a; Croll *et al.* 1982; Anderson and May 1985b). At this stage we ignore the complications introduced by the age structure of the human community and acquired immunity to infection.

The equation for the number of mature parasites, $M(t)$, must contain one gain and two loss terms. The gain term, which represents parasite recruitment to the sexually mature population, may be expressed as $\beta L(t - \tau_1)d_1$. Here β is a transmission coefficient representing the rate of contact between humans and infective stages times the probability that any one contact results in parasite establishment. The term $L(t - \tau_1)$ denotes the density of infective stages at time $t - \tau_1$. After gaining entry to the host, it is assumed that a period τ_1 elapses before the parasite develops to reproductive maturity. We use the parameter d_1 to denote the proportion of infective stages gaining entry to the host which survive to reach sexual maturity. The two loss terms represent parasite mortalities due to natural causes or host-induced effects (non-specific or immunological attack), and human mortality (since the death of the host leads to the death of the parasites contained within). If the human host's per capita death rate is μ, where $1/\mu$ denotes life expectancy, and if $p(i)$ is the probability that a host contains i worms, then the net rate of loss of parasites due to host deaths is $\mu \sum ip(i)$; this assumes that the worms do not affect the mortality rates of their hosts. Similarly, the net rate of loss due to natural or induced parasite mortality may be expressed as $\sum \mu_1(i)ip(i)$ where the term $\mu_1(i)$ represents the per capita parasite mortality rate as a function of worm burden, i. Laboratory studies of nematode infections within rats, mice, and dogs indicate that worm mortality is sometimes density dependent (see Krupp 1962; Anderson 1982c; Keymer 1982). However, the relevance of these observations to human infection is as yet unclear owing to the practical difficulties inherent in measurement.

The equation for $L(t)$, the density of infective stages at time t, also consists of one gain and two loss terms. The net output of transmission stages by the total parasite population may be roughly estimated as $s\phi N \sum i\lambda(i)p(i)$, where s represents the proportion of female worms in the population (in the case of dioecius species we usually assume $s = \frac{1}{2}$), ϕ denotes the probability that a female worm is mated (and hence able to produce fertile eggs), and $\lambda(i)$ denotes the per capita rate of egg production by female worms, expressed as a function of parasite density, i, within a host. To be exact, however, it is necessary to acknowledge the aggregated distributions of worms seen in nature, and to compute the messier quantity $\sum \sum j\lambda(n)p(n)\pi(j; n)$, where $\pi(j; n)$ is the probability for a host to contain j mated female worms, given that a total of n worms (male and female) are present. For clumped distributions of worms, this messier expression does not simply factor into $s\phi\langle i\lambda\rangle$, although—as we shall see below—the differences between the exact expression and the more intuitively accessible approximation are not usually significant in practice; these details are pursued more fully in Appendix F. In any event, it is clear that the expression for the net output of transmission stages depends both on the distribution of worms among hosts and the sexual habits of the worms (May 1977a). Table 16.1 defines the form of ϕ for various assumptions concerning the distribution of the $p(i)$ terms (i.e. Poisson or negative binomial) and the sexual habits of the worm. Notice the mating probability, ϕ, saturates to unity when mean worm burdens are high, but that ϕ can be significantly less than unity if worm burdens

Table 16.1 The mating probability function (after May 1977a)

Sexual habits and parasite distribution	Mating function
Hemaphroditic, self-fertilization possible	$\phi = 1$
Dioecious, worms monogamous (a) Random distribution of parasites	$\phi(M) = 1 - \dfrac{e^{-M}}{2\pi} \displaystyle\int_0^{2\pi} (1 - \cos\theta)\, e^{-M\cos\theta}\, d\theta$
(b) Negative binomial distribution of parasites	$\phi(M, k) = 1 - \dfrac{(1-\gamma)^{1+k}}{2\pi} \displaystyle\int_0^{2\pi} \dfrac{1 - \cos\theta}{(1 + \gamma\cos\theta)^{1+k}}\, d\theta$ where $\gamma = M/(M + k)$
Dioecious, worms polygamous (a) Random distribution of parasites	$\phi(M) = 1 - e^{-M/2}$
(b) Negative binomial distribution of parasites	$\phi(M, k) = 1 - (1 + M/2k)^{-(1+k)}$

are on average low (although even here ϕ can be close to unity if the distribution is sufficiently clumped).

As discussed in the previous chapter, helminth fecundity, $\lambda(i)$, often appears to be inversely related to total worm burden, i (see Fig. 15.14). Of the total output of transmission stages, only a proportion d_2 will survive the average time period τ_2 required to develop to the infective state. A simple estimate of net recruitment to the population of infective stages at time t is thus $sd_2\phi N \sum \lambda(i)ip(i, t - \tau_2)$. A rough guide to the lengths of the maturation delays, τ_1 and τ_2, and to the life expectancies of the infective stages and mature worms for the major intestinal nematodes of man is presented in Table 16.2. The two loss terms represent deaths due to natural mortalities in the free-living environment, at a per capita rate μ_2, and losses due to the pick-up of infective larvae by hosts (i.e. transmission) at a net rate βNL; under essentially all conditions met in the field, losses due to larval mortality will be much greater than those due to pick-up by humans.

These assumptions can be expressed in two coupled non-linear differential equations for changes in $M(t)$ and $L(t)$ with respect to time as follows:

$$dM/dt = \beta L(t - \tau_1)d_1 - \mu \sum ip(i) - \sum \mu_1(i)ip(i), \qquad (16.5)$$

$$dL/dt = sd_2\phi N \sum \lambda(i)ip(i, t - \tau_2) - \mu_2 L - \beta NL. \qquad (16.6)$$

The model is deterministic in structure, but it contains probability elements (the term ϕ and the $p(i)$s). To proceed with the investigation of its behaviour, it is helpful to make a phenomenological assumption concerning the distribution of parasite numbers per host. In practice, this distribution will itself be determined by the rate processes that control parasite and host abundance. However, a useful simplification is achieved by assuming, in line with observation (see Fig. 15.17), that the parasites are distributed in a negative binomial manner with clumping parameter k (assumed constant and independent of time or parasite density) and mean $M(t)$. This assumption of a negative binomial distribution was discussed more fully in the preceding chapter, along with the biological character of the distribution in relation to its formal, mathematical properties (eqns (15.1)–(15.3)).

This procedure is only a crude approximation to the more exact approach arising from the development of fully stochastic models (see Nasell and Hirsch 1973; Barbour 1978), but such models are somewhat intractable to analytical investigation owing to the many non-linearities that are inherent in biological problems. Our phenomenological assumption about the way in which worms are distributed among hosts generates greater flexibility without too much loss of detail, and facilitates the biological interpretation of properties of the model.

16.2.2 *Basic reproductive rate for macroparasites*

For microparasites, we saw that the basic reproductive rate—the number of secondary infections produced, on average, by each primary infection in the

Table 16.2 Maturation delays and life expectancies of intestinal nematodes of humans (see Anderson and May 1985b)

Parasite	Delay from infection of the human host to production of eggs (days)	Delay from release of eggs to development of stage infective to the human host (days)	Life expectancy of mature parasite, $1/\mu_1$ (years)	Life expectancy of infective stage, $1/\mu_2$ (days)
Ascaris lumbricoides	50–80	10–30	1–2	28–84
Necator americanus	40–50	3–6	2–4	3–10
Ancylostoma duodenale	28–50	3–6	2–4	3–10
Trichuris trichiura	50–84	11–80	1–2	10–30
Enterobius vermicularis	15–43	0.2–0.4	0.1–0.2	14–56

absence of density-dependent constraints—was an important characteristic of a particular infectious agent, of relevance both to the natural dynamics of transmission and to the design of control programmes. For macroparasites, the analogous quantity, R_0, may be defined as the average number of (female) offspring per adult (female) worm that survive to reproduction in the absence of density-dependent constraints.

It is instructive to derive an explicit formula for R_0 from eqns (16.5) and (16.6), and this we now do. We shall then discuss the kinds of density-dependent processes that ultimately limit mean worm burdens, and outline ideas about thresholds and 'breakpoints' in host–macroparasite systems.

As a deliberately oversimplified introduction, we neglect the effects that worm density within a host may have on per capita worm fecundity and mortality, assuming the constant rates λ and μ_1 respectively. We also assume, in this preliminary discussion, that the probability of mating success is unity, $\phi = 1$. The pairs of eqns (16.5) and (16.6) for the dynamics of adult worm and free-living larval stages, respectively, then become

$$dM(t)/dt = d_1\beta L(t - \tau_1) - (\mu + \mu_1)M(t), \qquad (16.7)$$

$$dL(t)/dt = sd_2\lambda NM(t - \tau_2) - (\mu_2 + \beta N)L(t). \qquad (16.8)$$

It can be shown that this pair of equations will lead to ever increasing values of $M(t)$ and $L(t)$ if $R_0 > 1$, where R_0 is defined as

$$R_0 = (s\lambda\beta Nd_1d_2)/[(\mu + \mu_1)(\mu_2 + \beta N)]. \qquad (16.9)$$

Conversely, if $R_0 < 1$ both $M(t)$ and $L(t)$ tend asymptotically to zero; the parasite population cannot maintain itself. The unbounded increase in $M(t)$ and $L(t)$ for $R_0 > 1$ is, of course, the result of our neglecting all density-dependent processes. But the *intrinsic* reproductive rate, R_0, is defined as that pertaining in the absence of density-dependent constraints, and so the above analysis is appropriate.

A major simplification can usually be made by noting the considerable differences in time-scales—set by life expectancies—between mature adult worms and infective larval stages. For the examples in Table 15.3, the life span of adult worms is an order of magnitude or more greater than the typical life spans of the infective stages (with the isolated exception of *Enterobius vermicularis*). Under these circumstances, we can focus on the dynamics of the adult worms, $M(t)$, assuming that the dynamics of the infective stages move on a much faster time-scale so as to be effectively adjusted to its equilibrium value (which, from eqn (16.8) with $dL/dt = 0$, is $L(t) = sd_2\lambda NM(t - \tau_2)/(\mu_2 + \beta N)$). The consequent differential equation for the single variable $M(t)$ is

$$dM(t)/dt = (\mu + \mu_1)[R_0M(t - \tau_1 - \tau_2) - M(t)]. \qquad (16.10)$$

Here R_0 is as defined above, in eqn (16.9). It is clear that this system will undergo exponential growth if $R_0 > 1$, and that $M(t)$ will decline toward zero otherwise. More precisely, $M(t)$ will asymptotically grow as $\exp \Lambda t$, with the growth rate Λ given implicitly by

$$\Lambda = (\mu + \mu_1)[R_0 \exp(-\Lambda(\tau_1 + \tau_2)) - 1]. \tag{16.11}$$

The maturation delays, τ_1 and τ_2, are in general short in comparison with the life expectancies of the mature worms in humans; that is $(\mu + \mu_1)(\tau_1 + \tau_2)$ is typically significantly less than unity. If this is the case, we may to an excellent approximation simply put $\tau_1 = \tau_2 = 0$. This approximation will be made throughout the remainder of this chapter. One consequence is that eqn (16.11) for the growth rate of the worm populations in the absence of density-dependent constraints reduces to

$$\Lambda = (\mu + \mu_1)(R_0 - 1). \tag{16.12}$$

This is formally analogous to eqn (2.3) for the growth of epidemics of microparasitic infections in their early stages, before the pool of susceptibles undergoes substantial depletion. The time lags, τ_1 and τ_2, have the effect of reducing the growth rate Λ below the value given by eqn (16.12), but it remains true that macroparasites will establish themselves if and only if $R_0 > 1$, with R_0 given by eqn (16.9).

The definition of R_0, eqn (16.9), is notationally complicated, but it says something simple. The basic reproductive rate of the parasite depends on the net rate of producing transmission stages, λ, on the life expectancy of adult worms, $1/(\mu + \mu_1)$, and of infective larvae, $1/(\mu_2 + \beta N)$, and on the probability that infective stages will indeed find hosts (which depends both on transmission efficiency, β, and on the host density, N). The threshold or persistence criterion $R_0 > 1$ can, from eqn (16.9), be reformulated as a condition that the population of human hosts exceed a threshold density, $N > N_T$, with N_T given by

$$N_T = \frac{\mu_2(\mu + \mu_1)/\beta}{s\lambda d_1 d_2 - (\mu + \mu_1)}. \tag{16.13}$$

For most macroparasitic organisms this threshold host density is quite low, owing to high rates of egg production (λ very large) and low rates of mortality for adult parasites ($\mu + \mu_1$ small in relation to λ). This is in marked contrast to many microparasitic infections, such as measles and other common viral infections, where threshold population sizes are large (see Chapter 4).

Confirmation of the ability of directly transmitted helminths to persist in low-density human communities is provided by observations on the types of infectious disease agents that persist endemically in primitive hunter–gatherer societies in areas such as the Amazon basin (Tyrell 1980). Intestinal helminth infections appear to have been common, while directly transmitted viruses, such as measles and influenza, appear to have been absent prior to contact with white missionaries and the encroachment of civilization into the rain forest habitats of the tribes.

16.2.3 *Density-dependent factors and the dynamics of macroparasitic infections*

Density-dependent processes acting on parasite establishment, survival, and/or fecundity will, of course, eventually constrain the growth of macroparasitic populations, and prevent the exponential 'runaway' found in the simple models above.

Empirical evidence for intestinal nematodes suggests that the decline in per capita fecundity with increasing total worm burden may be approximated by the exponential relationship (see Fig. 15.15).

$$\lambda(i) = \lambda_0 \exp[-\gamma(i - 1)]. \tag{16.14}$$

Here λ_0 is the intrinsic fecundity in the absence of density-dependent effects, and γ is a parameter characterizing the severity of such density-dependent constraints. Other, more general, functional forms for $\lambda(i)$ can of course be fitted to specific data for specific systems. Less information is available about the dependence of worm mortality upon worm load, $\mu_1(i)$, for infections in human hosts. We therefore retain the assumption that μ_1 is a constant (independent of worm burden, i), and let it be density-dependent constraints on egg output that ultimately limit worm burdens in our model systems. The essential nature of the analysis would, however, be the same if density dependence were alternatively introduced into $\mu_1(i)$, or into some combination of $\lambda(i)$ and $\mu_1(i)$. In detailed applications, the models should be constructed on the basis of carefully gathered data about these processes; unfortunately, such data are lacking for most helminth infections of humans.

If we use eqn (16.14) for $\lambda(i)$ in eqn (16.6), and assume a negative binomial distribution of worms among hosts, the simple factor λ in eqn (16.8) for $L(t)$ or in the 'collapsed' eqn (16.10) for $M(t)$ is replaced by

$$\lambda \to \lambda_0(1 + M(1 - z)/k)^{-(k+1)}. \tag{16.15}$$

Here $z \equiv \exp(-\gamma)$ measures the strength of the density-dependent effects, k is the usual clumping parameter of the negative binomial distribution, and M is the mean worm burden.

We continue to assume that developmental times (τ_1 and τ_2) and larval life expectancies are all short compared with the life expectancies of adult worms, so that we focus on the dynamical behaviour of adult worm burdens, $M(t)$. We also continue to assume that mating probabilities are unity, $\phi = 1$, although this assumption will be relaxed in the next section. Using eqn (16.15) for λ in eqn (16.10) for $M(t)$, and also putting $\tau_1 = \tau_2 = 0$, we thus have the density-dependent relationship

$$dM(t)/dt = (\mu + \mu_1)(R_0 f(M(t); z, k) - 1)M(t). \tag{16.16}$$

Here R_0 is as defined above, eqn (16.9), with λ replaced by λ_0. The function

$f(M)$ comes from the density dependence in egg output, eqn (16.15), and is

$$f(M) = (1 + M(1 - z)/k)^{-(k+1)}. \tag{16.17}$$

Notice that $f(M)$ decreases monotonically as M increases, with $f(0) = 1$.

This equation for $M(t)$ has simple dynamical behaviour. If $R_0 < 1$, $M(t)$ tends to zero and the parasite population cannot maintain itself. If, however, the parasite's basic reproductive rate is above unity, $R_0 > 1$, the system settles to a stable equilibrium value of the mean worm burden, M^*, given by

$$R_0 f(M^*) = 1. \tag{16.18}$$

That is

$$M^* = k(R_0^{1/(k+1)} - 1)/(1 - z). \tag{16.19}$$

Equation (16.19) describes how—under the above assumptions—the equilibrium worm burden, M^*, depends on the basic reproductive rate of the parasite, R_0, the degree of parasite aggregation, k, and the severity of the density-dependent constraints on worm fecundity, z. For a fixed value of the transmission parameter R_0, M^* decreases as the degree of worm clumping (measured inversely by k) increases. For fixed k and z, on the other hand, M^* increases monotonically with increasing R_0; the dependence of M^* on R_0 is most pronounced when k is small (high aggregation).

Recall that, for a negative binomial distribution of worms among hosts, the prevalence of infection, P^*, is related to M^* by

$$P^* = 1 - (1 + M^*/k)^{-k}. \tag{16.20}$$

Thus P^* tends to asymptote to unity for mean worm burdens M^* significantly in excess of unity. As shown in Fig. 16.1, higher aggregation (smaller k) results in smaller P^* for a given value of M^*.

Equation (16.19) can be employed to obtain rough estimates of the magnitude of R_0 given that we have available from field studies information on the average worm burden within the community, M^*, the severity of density-dependent constraints on fecundity, z or γ, and the degree of parasite clumping within the host population, k. The method is obviously crude; it assumes that the parasite population is at a stable equilibrium, that population regulation is due simply to density dependence of fecundity (i.e. no acquired immunity in the older age classes, or density-dependent establishment or survival) and that complications introduced by the age structure of the human community are taken into account in the estimation of M^*. Despite these cautions, however, such rough estimates of R_0 do provide a means of crudely assessing transmission potential. Table 16.3 lists some estimates of R_0 for intestinal helminth infections, calculated by this model. Note that the values of R_0 are low by comparison with many microparasitic infections (see Table 4.1). In many of these examples, estimates of M^*, k, and γ were obtained from field studies in which antihelminthic

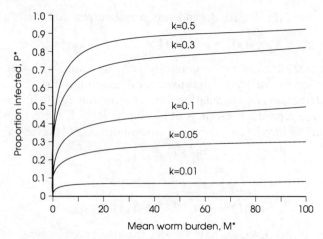

Fig. 16.1. The relationship between the prevalence of infection, P^*, the mean worm burden, M^*, and the negative binomial aggregation parameter k (eqn (16.20)). Note that for high degrees of aggregation (k small) large changes in the value of M^* may only induce small changes in the value of P^*.

Table 16.3 Estimates of the basic reproductive rate R_0 for different species of helminths in different geographical locations (see Anderson and May 1985*b*)

Parasite	R_0	Location
Ascaris lumbricoides	4–5	Iran
	1–3	Burma
	1–2	Bangladesh
Necator americanus	2–3	India
Trichuris trichiura	4–6	Jamaica
Schistosoma haematobium	2–3	Egypt
Schistosoma japonicum	1–4	Philippines
Onchocerca volvulus	50	Cameroon
	9–74	Ivory Coast

treatment was employed to count worm burdens expelled from individual patients.

16.2.4 *Mating probabilities and 'breakpoints'*
Up to this point we have been assuming that all female worms are indeed mated. This is not necessarily so, particularly at low average worm densities when a

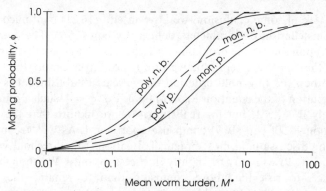

Fig. 16.2. The dependence of the probability that a female worm is mated, ϕ, on the average worm burden, M^*, for various assumptions concerning parasite distribution within the host population and the sexual habits of the parasite (see Table 16.1). Poly. n. b. denotes polygamous parasites distributed in a negative binomial pattern; poly. p. denotes polygamous worms randomly distributed (Poisson); mon. n. b. denotes monogamous worms distributed in a negative binomial pattern; and mon. p. denotes monogamous worms distributed in a random pattern (after May 1977*a*) (see also Anderson 1982).

given host may harbour no male worms. As mentioned earlier, Table 16.1 catalogues formulae for the mating probability, $\phi(M)$, under various assumptions about the distributions of male and female worms among hosts, and about the mating habits of the worms. Are, for instance, male and female worms distributed separately or together (with any one worm being male or female with probability 0.5), and are they monogamous or promiscuous? The functional form of ϕ obviously depends on these details. This dependence is illustrated graphically in Fig. 16.2 (abstracted from May (1977*a*)).

When these complications, associated with the macroparasites having a sexual stage in the definitive host, are included, eqn (16.16) takes the more general form

$$dM(t)/dt = (\mu + \mu_1)(R_0 \mathscr{F}(M) - 1)M(t). \qquad (16.21)$$

Here we have, as above, assumed that other time-scales are short compared with the life expectancy of adult worms ($\tau_1 = \tau_2 = 0$; $dL/dt = 0$), and that the only significant density-dependent constraints operate on egg output. The new features, upon which the discussion in this section is focused, have to do with the possibility that mating probabilities are significantly less than unity at low worm burdens. This effect is incorporated in the function $\mathscr{F}(M)$, which differs from the density-dependent function $f(M)$ of eqn (16.17) in that it includes the effect of worm mating. $\mathscr{F}(M)$ is calculated along the lines indicated in Appendix H. In general, $\mathscr{F}(M)$ will tend to behave as $\phi(M)$ at low values of M (when density-dependent effects are not significant) and as $f(M)$ at high M values (when mating probabilities tend to unity).

At the risk of some confusion, we have in eqn (16.21) continued to use R_0 for the constellation of parameters defined by eqn (16.9). The complications attendant upon the mating probability ϕ (which is always less than unity) mean, however, that the basic reproductive rate is no longer simply the 'R_0' of eqn (16.9). Rather, the threshold criterion for parasite establishment is that there exists a solution of the equation $R_0 \mathcal{F}(M) = 1$. For $\phi = 1$, such a solution exists if and only if $R_0 > 1$, but for realistic $\phi(M)$ we require that the parameter combination R_0 of eqn (16.9) compensate for $\phi < 1$. As will become plain in the ensuing discussion, in most practical situations this threshold value of the 'R_0' of eqn (16.9) will only be slightly in excess of unity. We thought it better, on balance, to risk the above confusion than to rename the parameter combination of eqn (16.9) at this point.

Clearly, the mating probability $\phi(M)$ will tend to zero as $M \to 0$, because at low enough mean worm densities one is unlikely to find hosts with two or more worms of either sex ('low enough' may, of course, be very low if aggregation is very pronounced; see Fig. 16.2). Conversely, at very high values of M, ϕ will asymptote to unity. The result is that, for $R_0 > 1$, there can be two alternative stable equilibrium solutions of eqn (16.21): one at $M = 0$ and one close to the 'endemic equilibrium', M^*, given by eqn (16.18) (provided M^* is large enough that $\phi(M^*) \simeq 1$). These two stable equilibria will be separated by an unstable equilibrium solution of the equation $R_0 \mathcal{F}(M) = 1$, which epidemiologists have called the 'breakpoint' and which we denote by M_B. Initial values of M less than M_B—or fluctuations in mean worm burdens below M_B—produce dynamical trajectories in which $M \to 0$ and the parasites are extinguished; initial values of M lying above the breakpoint value result in the system tending to settle to the endemic mean worm burden M^*.

As a specific example, suppose male and female worms are distributed jointly in a negative binomial pattern, and that they are polygamous (as most intestinal nematodes of humans probably are). Further assume that all females are mated if at least one male is present. If $\lambda(i)$ has the exponential dependence on total worm density given by eqn (16.14), the function $\mathcal{F}(M)$ is then (see Appendix H)

$$\mathcal{F}(M) = f(M) \left[1 - \left(\frac{1 + M(2 - z)/2k}{1 + M(1 - z)/k} \right)^{-k-1} \right]. \tag{16.22}$$

Here $f(M)$ is the density-dependent function defined earlier in eqn (16.17), while the factor in square brackets represents an effective value, ϕ', for the mating probability in this particular context. Notice that if density-dependent effects on egg output are weak, so that $z \to 1$, we have $\phi' \simeq 1 - (1 + M/2k)^{-k-1}$ which is exactly the mating probability, ϕ, for promiscuous worms, as given in Table 16.1.

Figure 16.3 shows the equilibrium solutions, M, of eqn (16.21) with $\mathcal{F}(M)$ given by eqn (16.22), as a function of R_0, for various values of k. In all cases, there is a threshold value of R_0 below which the parasites cannot persist ($M = 0$

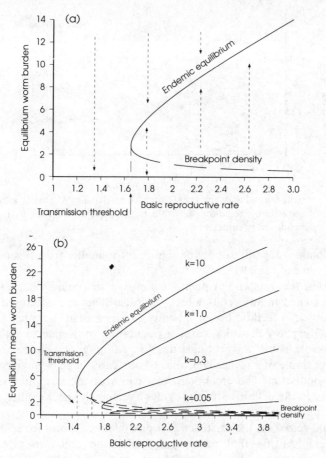

Fig. 16.3. (a) Equilibrium solutions for the mean worm burden, M, of eqn (16.21) with $\mathscr{F}(M)$ given by eqn (16.22) as a function of the basic reproductive rate, R_0. Parameter values, $k = 1.0$, $\gamma = 0.96$. (b) Similar to (a) but recording the dependence of the equilibrium solutions for M on the degree of parasite aggregation within the host population (measured inversely by the negative binomial parameter k).

is the only stationary point). Above the threshold value of R_0, there are two alternative stable states, $M = 0$ and the endemic equilibrium $M = M^*$, divided by the unstable 'breakpoint' or watershed value. Fig. 16.3(b), however, also makes it clear that the breakpoint phenomenon is most pronounced where there is little or no worm clumping (k large); for high aggregation (k small), the breakpoint worm burden, M_B, tends to be very low. This point is driven home in Fig. 16.4, which shows the maximum value of the breakpoint worm density, $M_B(\text{max})$, as a function of the degree of parasite aggregation within the host population, for various values of the density-dependence parameter, z. This maximum value of M_B is attained at the transmission threshold, and—as Fig.

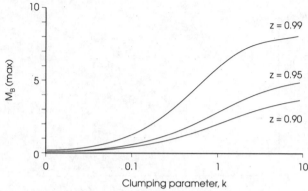

Fig. 16.4. The maximum value of the breakpoint worm density, $M_B(\text{max})$, as a function of the degree of parasite aggregation, k, within the host population for various values of the density-dependence parameter. z.

16.3 makes plain—M_B will usually be significantly smaller than this maximum value (itself typically small).

In essentials, this breakpoint phenomenon is what ecologists call the Allee effect. As discussed in any ecology text, the Allee effect is conjectured to arise when lack of social facilitation, or inability to find a mate, or other processes operating at very low densities, cause a population to decline to extinction if depressed below some low enough density. Although much discussed, no convincing example of an Allee effect has to our knowledge been given for any vertebrate population. The breakpoint that can arise for macroparasites with a sexual stage in the definitive host provides a seemingly more explicit example of the Allee phenomenon.

Macdonald seized on the existence of a possible breakpoint for schistosome infections, emphasizing that permanent eradication could in principle be achieved if average worm burdens could once be pushed below the breakpoint level. As Macdonald emphasized, in the absence of a breakpoint, eradication of a parasite requires some kind of intervention that permanently alters R_0, to hold it below threshold. But if a breakpoint exists, one can eradicate a parasite even though R_0 remains *above* threshold, by a one-time depression of mean worm burdens below the breakpoint so that the system settles to the alternative stable state, $M \to 0$. This is clearly an exciting possibility. It in effect uses the worms' sex life against them.

In his illustrative calculations, Macdonald assumed that the worms were distributed independently randomly (a Poisson distribution, $k \to \infty$), and that they were strictly monogamous. As Fig. 16.3 makes plain, the breakpoint phenomenon is much less marked—breakpoint worm burdens are much lower—when there is significant aggregation (small k), as is always the case in practice. The breakpoint is also at significantly lower worm densities if the worms are promiscuous rather than monogamous. These realistic modifications to Macdonald's work by Bradley and May (1978) and May (1977*a*) led them to conclude that the breakpoint phenomenon was not likely to be of much use in practical programmes of control. We return to this point, with some numerical estimates, at the end of this section.

Macdonald's analysis was specifically for schistosomes. These macroparasites possess an intermediate host (snails), so that the equations are different in detail from those for direct life cycles that we have used. For one thing, the density-dependent process that ultimately limited worm burdens in Macdonald's models was the assumption that snail vectors could only experience one infection (tantamount, indeed, to a kind of density dependence on egg output). These details notwithstanding, the essentials of Macdonald's studies are as outlined above, as are those of systems with other kinds of density-dependent constraints but where alternative stable states can arise by virtue of the parasite's mating system in the definitive host.

These ideas about the dependence of mating probabilities on parasite density can be tested against some empirical evidence for intestinal nematodes (Anderson 1980, 1982c). Certain such nematodes, such as *Ascaris lumbricoides*, produce infertile eggs when not mated, and these pass out in the faeces and can be distinguished from fertilized eggs. Thus, counts can be made of both the proportion of unfertilized eggs passed by a given person and the proportion of people releasing unfertilized eggs. In Japan, where a particularly successful control programme was mounted after World War II to control *Ascaris*, the proportion of faecal samples with unfertilized *Ascaris* eggs increased steadily as control measures reduced the abundance of the parasite (Yokogawa 1985). Similar patterns have been recorded in Korea as shown in Fig. 16.5.

The relationship between the prevalence of infection (the egg–parasite rate

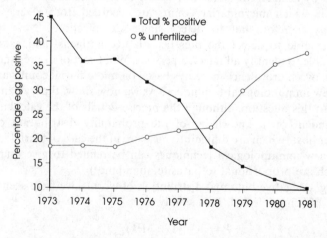

Fig. 16.5. Changing patterns in the proportion of a population in Korea infected with *Ascaris* (full squares) and the proportion passing unfertilized eggs only (open circles), during a period (1969–81) of parasite control by mass chemotherapy (Seo *et al.* 1983).

for faecal samples) and the proportion of people discharging unfertilized eggs among the infecteds can be deduced on theoretical grounds as follows. Define y as the proportion of those hosts with at least one female worm (i.e. the fraction of hosts passing eggs), and x as the proportion of those hosts with at least one female who have no male worms (i.e. the fraction of hosts either passing eggs that are unfertilized, or no eggs at all if egg production requires fertilization). Then, asuming a 1:1 male to female sex ratio, the relationship between x and y can be defined for various distribution patterns. For example, if the male and female worms are distributed independently randomly (Poisson), then

$$y = 1 - x. \tag{16.23}$$

In practice, *Ascaris* will be distributed in a contagious manner. In this event, if we assume that males and females are distributed together following a negative binomial pattern, then (May 1977a)

$$x = \{1 - y - [2(1 - y)^{-1/k} - 1]^{-k}\}/y, \tag{16.24}$$

where k is the usual aggregation parameter. Figure 16.6 shows the relationship between x and y for various values of the parameter k, along with a set of empirical observations from Komiya *et al.* (1962) for *Ascaris* infection in Japan. The model provides an adequate description of the observed trend for x to decline as y increases, with a k value of approximately 0.05–0.1.

The presence of unfertilized worms can also have an important influence on the interpretation of epidemiological data acquired by new biochemical, immunological, and molecular techniques. In the case of the filarial worms, for example, females do not produce microfilariae unless they have been successfully inseminated by a male. Measures of parasite abundance based on 'skin snip' techniques in which microfilariae counts are recorded from a series of skin samples may therefore fail to detect single-sex infections. New methods, however, are able to detect the presence of 'live antigens' and as such are potentially able to identify all infected persons. What sort of discrepancy might we expect between prevalence measures based on microfilarial counts and those based on new immunological techniques? As we now show, theory can provide an answer to this question, although the precise details of the calculations are again dependent on a knowledge of the probability distribution of worm numbers per host (which are difficult to measure in the case of filarial infections unless the new immunological techniques can be refined to give quantitative scores which are proportional to parasite abundance).

Assuming a negative binomial distribution of worms, we have seen that the probability of being infected, P, is simply

$$P = 1 - (1 + M/k)^{-k}. \tag{16.25}$$

The probability, P_T, of harbouring at least one pair of male and female worms (so that transmission stages are produced within the host), given that the males

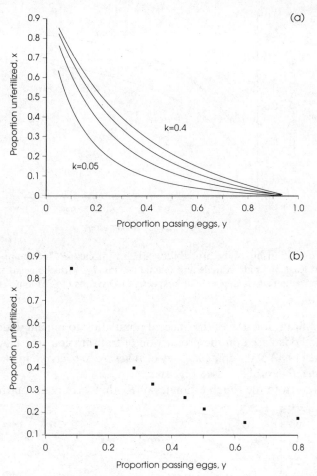

Fig. 16.6. (a) The relationship between the proportion of hosts with at least one female worm who have *no* male worms, x, and the proportion of hosts with at least one female worm (the fraction passing eggs), y, defined by eqn (16.24) for various values of the negative binomial aggregation parameter, k ($k = 0.05$, 0.1, 0.2, 0.4). (b) Empirical observations on the relationship between x and y from Japan during an intensive control programme aimed at the eradication of *Ascaris* (data from Komiya *et al.* (1962)).

and females are distributed together (not independently), is (May 1977*a*)

$$P_T = 1 - 2(1 + M/2k)^{-k} + (1 + M/k)^{-k}. \tag{16.26}$$

The magnitude of the difference between P and P_T is dependent on the degree of worm clumping (measured inversely by k), but it may be as much as 30 per cent or more for moderate mean worm burdens (say around 10) if the value of k is less than unity (see Fig. 16.7). Thus for high degrees of worm aggregation, which are the rule rather than the exception in human communities, we might

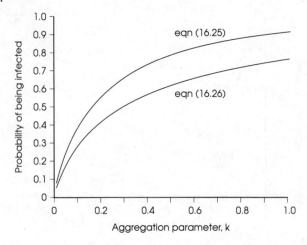

Fig. 16.7. The relationship of the probability of being infected, P, and the probability of harbouring at least one pair of male and female worms, P_T, with the negative binomial aggregation parameter k as determined, respectively, by eqns (16.25) and (16.26).

expect a significant fraction of the infected population to remain undetected by sampling methods based on the production of transmission stages. A study by Forsyth *et al.* (1990) of the epidemiology of *Wuchereria bancrofti* in New Guinea well illustrates this problem (see Fig. 16.8).

We now return to the rough estimates of R_0 that were made on the basis of

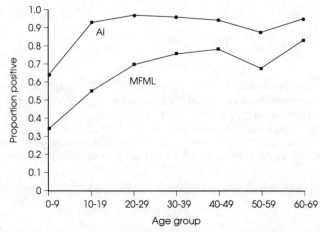

Fig. 16.8. A comparison of measurements of microfilarial density (MFML) and serum levels of *Wuchereria bancrofti* phosphorycholine containing antigen (AI) in individuals as an indirect measure of the presence of adult worms. A fraction of the infected population remain undetected when microfilarial density is assessed via blood analysis (from Forsyth *et al.* 1990).

eqn (16.19) at the end of the previous Section 16.2.3. These estimates, which are summarized in Table 16.3, can be used to make some very rough assessments of the magnitude of the breakpoint value of the mean worm burden (see Fig. 16.4). Thus, for example, a study by Croll *et al.* (1982) of the epidemiology of *Ascaris* in Iran produced the following estimates of the parameters: $M^* \simeq 22$, $k = 0.5 \pm 0.8$, $R_0 \simeq 4-5$, $\mu + \mu_1 \simeq 1 \text{ yr}^{-1}$. Used in conjunction with eqn (16.22), these estimates produce the guesstimate that the breakpoint density is around 0.1–0.3 worms per person. In other words, the unstable equilibrium values lies very close to zero. Similar calculations for other intestinal helminths such as *Trichuris* and hookworm species produce similar results. These low values are a direct consequence of high levels of parasite aggregation, where 80 per cent or more of the total worm population is harboured by 20 per cent or less of the host community (Anderson 1982*a,b*).

These rough assessments provide a retrospective justification of the approximation $\phi \to 1$ that was employed earlier in this chapter. The high degrees of parasite clumping typically found in human communities (with k in the range 0.1–0.5) imply that most worms will be mated, unless mean worm burdens are unusually low, as they may be in the later stages of a successful control programme.

The models in this section have been oriented towards exploring the dynamics of nematode infections with direct life cycles, but it is important to note that many of their properties are of relevance to the study of species with more complex life cycles. This is a consequence of the short life expectancies of most vectors and intermediate hosts relative to the life spans of adult worms in humans (see Table 15.2). Sensible discussion of the dynamics can therefore usually be based on single equations describing changes in the average worm load within the final host population. These issues are discussed in more detail in Chapter 20.

16.3 The control of transmission and morbidity

Simple models can help to further our understanding of how best to control parasite transmission and morbidity, not just within the individual patient, but within the community as a whole. In practice, the control of helminth parasites currently involves a variety of approaches including chemotherapy, improved sanitation, hygiene and education, and reduction in vector or intermediate host density. Vaccines to protect humans against infection by helminths are unavailable at present. However, the recent and rapid progress in molecular, biochemical, and immunological parasitology suggests that they may become so in the coming decade (Johnson *et al.* 1989). In this section we consider two aspects of control. The first of these concerns transmission and morbidity control by chemotherapeutic agents, applied either randomly or selectively, within a population. The second centres on the following question—given that vaccines will be developed, what properties should they possess in order to maximize their control impact at the population level?

16.3.1 *Chemotherapy*

Safe and effective drugs are now available (or will become so in the near future) for all of the major helminth infections of man. These include broad-spectrum antihelminthics such as mebendazole and albendazole for the treatment of intestinal nematode infections, the drug pyrantel pamoate for the treatment of *Ascaris*, the new drug praziquantel for the control of schistosomes, and the novel and recent use of ivermectin to treat filarial infections.

We examine both random and selective application of chemotherapeutic agents within the community. Both forms of treatment act to raise the net death rate of the parasite over the level pertaining prior to control. If a drug is administered randomly within a population by treating a proportion g of the community per unit of time, and if the drug has an efficacy h (the average proportion of the adult worm burden killed by a single or short course of treatment), the resulting increase in the per capita death rate of adult worms, c, is given by (see Anderson 1980)

$$c = -\ln(1 - gh). \tag{16.27}$$

By subtracting the additional net death rate due to treatment, cM, from the right-hand side of eqn (16.21), the average worm burden, M^*, at the new equilibrium established by the control programme is

$$M^* = k(\{R_0/[1 - A \ln(1 - gh)]\}^{1/(k+1)} - 1)/(1 - z), \tag{16.28}$$

where A denotes the life expectancy of the adult worm in the absence of treatment ($A = 1/(\mu + \mu_1)$). To eradicate the parasite, the value of the effective reproductive rate R (the basic reproductive rate R_0, modified by the action of chemotherapy) must be reduced below unity. To achieve this, the proportion of the population treated at random (independent of worm load) per unit of time must exceed a critical value g_c where

$$g_c = \{1 - \exp[(1 - R_0)/A]\}/h. \tag{16.29}$$

To take the specific example of the study of Croll *et al.* (1982) on *Ascaris* in an agricultural village in Iran, where R_0 and A were estimated as 3 and 1 year, respectively, eqn (16.29) predicts that a drug of 95 per cent efficacy ($h = 0.95$) would have to be administered to greater than 91 per cent of the population each year to eradicate the infection. If the value of R_0 was as high as 5 (with the same A and h values), then treatment at yearly intervals would not suffice to interrupt transmission. On a monthly drug administration schedule, an R_0 value of 5 would require the treatment of 28 per cent of the population at each round of chemotherapy. The predicted relationship (based on eqn (16.29)) between the critical value g_c and various values of R_0 and A is displayed graphically in Fig. 16.9. It is interesting to note that the critical value g_c can be substantially less for long-lived parasites than for short-lived species. This prediction argues that the effective control of schistosome and filarial

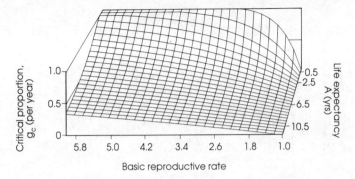

Fig. 16.9. The relationship of the critical proportion of the population that must be treated per year with an antihelminthic, g_c, and the basic reproductive rate of the parasite, R_0, plus the life expectancy of the parasite, A, as defined by eqn (16.29). Drug efficiency was set at 95 per cent ($h = 0.95$).

infections by mass drug application will be somewhat easier than for the short-lived intestinal nematodes such as *Ascaris*, *Trichuris*, and hookworms (see Table 15.2).

More generally, it is also important to note that long-term community-wide control of infection is dependent not simply on the magnitude of R_0 and A but also on the stability properties of the parasite population. In principle, if treatment lowers the average worm burden below the breakpoint (see Fig. 16.3), the population will move to extinction. However, we saw earlier that calculations based on simple theory indicate that the breakpoint is typically close to zero worms per person, owing to high levels of parasite aggregation within human communities. In practice, therefore, treatment must be continued at a rate above the critical value g_c for a period in excess of the maximum life span of the longest-lived developmental stage in the parasite's life cycle (the adult worm). Thus in the case of the long-lived filarial worms, low levels of treatment may substantially reduce the average worm burden (see Fig. 16.9), but treatment would have to be maintained over many years to achieve eradication. This result is not encouraging and argues that eradication by mass chemotherapy may not be a practical objective, given the complication of the movement of infected people from other communities into a control area.

On a more technical level, our simple model of the manner in which mass chemotherapy acts to suppress average worm burdens illustrates a theme that has emerged in earlier sections. If the parasites are highly aggregated within the human community, substantive changes in average worm load may have only a limited impact on the prevalence of infection. As illustrated in Fig. 16.10, the equilibrium worm burden, M^*, decays approximately exponentially as the intensity of treatment, g, increases. The prevalence, however, remains relatively high until the proportion treated approaches the critical value g_c.

A different approach to that of eradication by mass treatment is to aim for

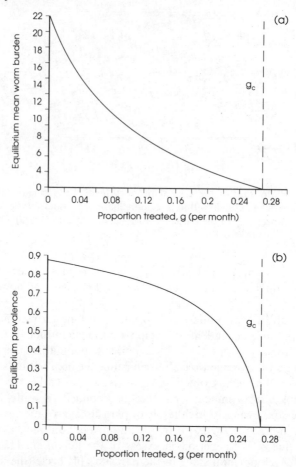

Fig. 16.10. The relationship between the equilibrium worm burden, M^* (graph (a)), and the equilibrium prevalence of infection, P^* (graph (b)), and the proportion of the population treated with antihelminthics per month, g. Parameter values: $h = 0.9$, $R_0 = 4.3$, $A = 1$ year, $k = 0.57$, $z = 0.96$. The broken vertical lines denote the value of the critical proportion g_c (see eqn (16.29)).

disease (as opposed to parasite) control. Infection with helminth parasites is not synonymous with symptoms of disease. The degree of morbidity is usually positively correlated with the burden of worms harboured by an individual (Walsh and Warren 1979; Warren 1979; Davis *et al.* 1979). If clinical symptoms of disease within communities are known typically to be absent below some characteristic intensity of infection, say m, then a sensible aim for control would be to reduce M^* (the average worm burden prior to control) below m. To reduce $M^* < m$, the critical proportion to be treated, g_c, is (for small k)

$$g_c = \{1 - \exp[(1 - R_0)(1 - m/M^*)/A(1 + (R_0 - 1)m/M^*)]\}/h. \quad (16.30)$$

The application of this approach is of course dependent on a knowledge of the value of m. In practice it may well be that because of severe parasite aggregation, m may be rather low. However, this approach would seem to be worth pursuing in the case of certain helminth species where large numbers of surveys have been carried out such that some crude estimate of the relationship between $M*$ (estimated by indirect methods such as faecal egg counts) and the incidence of disease is available (e.g. APCO 1980, 1983).

A more sophisticated approach to that outlined above is selectively to treat the most heavily infected people within the community. This approach to control was originally suggested by Smillie (1924) in the context of hookworm infections. More recently, Warren has rekindled interest in this topic (Warren and Mahmoud 1976; Warren *et al.* 1978; Mahmoud and Warren 1980; Warren 1981). There are obvious advantages attached to selective treatment in terms of cost; fewer drug treatments are required when compared with mass or blanket chemotherapy. There are benefits too if the drug induces significant side effects (such as stomach pains or nausea) or if there are worries concerning the impact of repeated mass treatment on the rate of evolution of drug-resistant strains of the parasite. However, there are certain disadvantages as well, such as the extra cost involved in identifying the most heavily infected individuals in a community prior to treatment. It has been argued that this factor alone induces cost penalties that far outweigh the advantages occurring from the reduction in the number of drug treatments required. 'Wormy people' would have to be identified by faecal egg counts, urine egg counts, skin snip larval counts, blood larval counts, or by noting the presence or absence of clinical symptoms of disease. All these procedures are time consuming, and they require trained personnel.

Two recent observations, however, argue for a reappraisal of the relative merits of selective versus mass treatment. The first of these concerns the acquisition of a substantial body of quantitative data (often via drug-induced worm expulsion techniques) on the degree to which helminths are aggregated in their distributions within human communities (see APCO 1980, 1983; Croll *et al.* 1982; Thein-Hliang 1985; Bundy *et al.* 1985a; Elkins *et al.* 1986). Almost invariably, irrespective of the species of helminth, a very substantial fraction of the total worm population is harboured by a small fraction of the human population. The second issue concerns the question of predisposition to heavy (or light) infection. It is only recently that firm statistical evidence has emerged to suggest that those few heavily infected individuals in the tail of the frequency distribution of worm numbers per person are, on average, predisposed to this state, not by chance but by some combination of social, behavioural, genetic, and nutritional factors (Anderson and Medley 1985; Thein-Hliang 1985; Schad and Anderson 1985; Elkins *et al.* 1986; Bundy *et al.* 1985a; Bensted-Smith *et al.* 1989). This evidence argues that once the heavily infected individuals in a community are identified at the start of a control programme, treatment could sensibly be focused on them at subsequent rounds of treatment without resurveying the community to assess the distribution of infection. Single, as opposed to repeated, identification clearly helps to reduce the costs involved in a selective treatment programme.

Theoretical predictions based on simple models can help to sharpen the debate on this topic. Suppose the probability that an individual receives treatment is defined as $g(i)$ such that the value of this function changes from low to high as worm burden i increases. If $p(i)$ is the probability that an individual harbours i worms and M^* is the precontrol average worm burden, then the average number of worms killed in a short interval of time, ΔM, following selective treatment with a drug of efficacy h is simply

$$\Delta M = h \sum_i ip(i)g(i). \tag{16.31}$$

In previous work (Anderson and May 1982c) we chose an arbitrary function to define $g(i)$:

$$g(i) = f[1 - (1 - \alpha) e^{-i/I}]. \tag{16.32}$$

Here the constants f and α (both <1) define the upper and lower bounds on $g(i)$, respectively. The parameter I characterizes the worm burden above which treatment is more likely. A continuous function for $g(i)$ is more realistic than, say, a step function, because in practice there is always considerable uncertainty about the worm burden harboured by any given individual. The total proportion of the population treated, $\bar{g}$, is

$$\bar{g} = \sum_i g(i)p(i). \tag{16.33}$$

Thus, given the definition of $g(i)$ in eqn (16.32), the average number of worms killed, ΔM, becomes

$$\Delta M = hf\left(\sum_i ip(i) - (1 - \alpha) \sum_i ip(i)z^i \right), \tag{16.34}$$

where $z = \exp(-1/I)$.

Suppose that the parasites are distributed in a negative binomial manner with clumping parameter k. The probability generating function, $\pi(z)$, for this distribution is

$$\pi(z) = [1 + M^*(1 - z)/k]^{-k} = \sum_i p(i)z^i. \tag{16.35}$$

Then eqn (16.34) becomes

$$\Delta M = hfM^*\{1 - z(1 - \alpha)[1 + M^*(1 - z)/k]^{-(k+1)}\}. \tag{16.36}$$

In the limits $I \to \infty$ and $I \to 0$, denoting extreme selectivity and no selectivity, respectively, we have

$$\Delta M \stackrel{I \to \infty}{=} hf\alpha M^*, \tag{16.37}$$

$$\Delta M \stackrel{I \to 0}{=} hfM^*. \tag{16.38}$$

The average proportion treated, $\bar{g}$, under the negative binomial assumption is

$$\bar{g} = f\{1 - (1 - \alpha)[1 + (1 - z)M^*/k]^{-k}\}. \tag{16.39}$$

The quantity of greatest practical relevance is the average proportion of the mean worm burden M^* killed by a single application of selective treatment within the population, $\Delta M/M^*$. Now

$$\Delta M/M^* = \bar{g}h(G(I, M^*, k)/H(I, M^*, k)), \tag{16.40}$$

where

$$G(I, M^*, k) = 1 - z(1 - \alpha)[1 + (1 - z)M^*/k]^{-(k+1)}, \tag{16.41}$$

and

$$H(I, M^*, k) = 1 - (1 - \alpha)[1 + (1 - z)M^*/k]^{-k}. \tag{16.42}$$

Similar manipulations can be performed to calculate the proportional reduction in the prevalence of infection, $\Delta P/P^*$, and the average egg output rate by individuals within the population, $\Delta E/E^*$ (where P^* and E^* are the equilibrium precontrol prevalence and average egg output rate; see Anderson and May (1982c)).

An illustration of the impact of a single application of selective treatment on $\Delta M/M^*$ (as predicted by eqn (16.40) is presented in Fig. 16.11 for various assumptions concerning the degree of parasite clumping, k, the total proportion treated, $\bar{g}$, and the degree of selectivity, I. The principal conclusion to emerge from such analyses is that selective treatment is highly beneficial in comparison to random treatment provided that the worms are highly aggregated within the human community. For example, if the selectivity index is set at 40 (with $\alpha = 0$, $f = 1$, $h = 0.95$, $M^* = 40$) a 50 per cent reduction in average worm burden is achieved by treating 8 per cent of the population when the parasites are highly clumped ($k = 0.5$). If the worms were randomly distributed ($=$ Poisson), a 50 per cent reduction can only be achieved by treating 50 per cent of the community. There is little benefit to be gained from being too selective (I large). This is fortunate given the practical difficulties involved in distinguishing via indirect methods such as faecal egg counts between individuals who harbour, say, 50 or 75 worms.

On theoretical grounds selective treatment appears highly beneficial for the control of human helminths. In practical terms, however, the need to identify those predisposed to heavy infection at the start of a control programme may

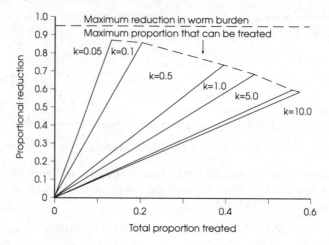

Fig. 16.11. The impact of a single application of selective treatment with an antihelminthic on $\Delta M/M^*$, as predicted by eqn (16.40), for various assumptions concerning the degree of parasite aggregation, k, and the total proportion treated. The relationship is plotted for six values of k with $z = 0.96$, $h = 0.95$, $\alpha = 0$, $M^* = 22$, $f = 1.0$ (see Anderson and May 1982c). The maximum reduction in worm burden is set by the value of h (i.e. 0.95), while the value of g (see eqn (16.39)) sets the maximum proportion that can be treated for a given set of parameter assignments.

negate the superficial cost advantage with respect to the number of drug treatments administered within the community. The relative importance of these two cost factors can only be assessed in defined localities by carefully designed field trials. Work of this kind remains to be done.

A slightly cruder approach to selectivity is that based on targeting treatment not to heavily infected individuals, but to groups of people who harbour significant fractions of the community's total worm burden. One such approach is to base targeting on the age of an individual, given the observation that average worm burdens are often highest in the child or teenage segments of human communities in developing countries (see Fig. 15.21). In practical terms these age groups are often accessible *en masse* through their attendance at schools. This approach, plus further aspects of control relating to temporal changes in parasite abundance following control intervention, will be discussed in subsequent sections dealing with age structure and the dynamic aspects of macroparasite models, respectively.

16.3.2 *Vaccination*

If vaccines are developed to combat infection by macroparasites (as seems likely in the coming decades), what can theory tell us about the level of herd immunity needed to interrupt transmission and about the ideal properties for the vaccine to make this task as simple as possible? The principles involved are identical to those outlined in earlier chapters for microparasitic infections. The task essentially revolves around the reduction of the parasite's effective reproductive rate, R, below unity. In contrast to the vaccines effective against many of the common viral infections (e.g. measles), it seems likely that macroparasitic vaccines will only provide protection against infection for a limited period of time (i.e. not lifelong protection following a single or short course of immunizations). This assumption rests on the observation that humans are unable to develop fully protective immunity under conditions of natural exposure. This observation may be pessimistic, because it may be possible to genetically engineer parasite antigens which induce stronger protection than that elicited by natural infection. However, in either case we can define the magnitude of the problem. For a vaccine which has efficacy h (defined as the proportion of people immunized that have full protection against infection) and creates immunity for an average period of v years, the proportion p that must be immunized per unit of time to interrupt transmission ($R < 1$) should satisfy

$$p > [1 - (1/R_0)]/vh. \tag{16.43}$$

For example, if a vaccine provides lifelong protection (with efficacy $h = 1$) against infection by a helminth with an R_0 value of 3 (appropriate for hookworm and *Ascaris* in areas of endemic infection; see Table 16.3), eqn (16.43) suggests that it would be necessary to protect 67 per cent of each cohort of children, soon after birth, to reduce the value of the effective reproductive rate to below unity. The relationship between the critical value of p (to reduce $R < 1$) and the basic reproductive rate, R_0, for vaccines which provide protection for varying lengths of time is illustrated graphically in Fig. 16.12.

One factor of particular importance in the implementation of vaccination programmes concerns the age at which the vaccine should be administered. In areas of endemic helminth infection, children on average acquire infection in

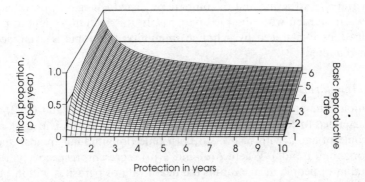

Fig. 16.12. The dependence of the critical proportion of a community that must be vaccinated per unit of time, p, and the magnitudes of R_0 and the duration of protection, v (years), provided by the vaccine (eqn (16.43)). Vaccine efficiency was set at 100 per cent ($h = 1$).

their first few years of life. As discussed earlier for microparasitic infections, if eradication is the aim of control (as opposed to morbidity control), the average age of immunization must be less than the average age at first infection (see Chapter 5).

The relative merits of immunizaton (when and if vaccines become available) versus chemotherapy will ultimately depend on cost factors, since both forms of control will probably have to be administered repeatedly to the individuals at risk (certainly so for antihelminthics, but less so for vaccines, since little is understood at present concerning the possibilities of artificially creating immunity to macroparasitic infection). The general conclusions outlined above also apply to the use of devices for the slow release of chemotherapeutic agents, which provide protection against infection for a defined period of time. Technology of this kind is not available for the treatment of human helminth infections at present, but it has been developed for the treatment of gastrointestinal nematode infections of cattle (Jones 1981).

Finally, the above analysis assumes that vaccines will provide full protection against infection. This may not necessarily be true; they may simply act to decrease parasite establishment, survival, and fecundity below the levels pertaining in unvaccinated individuals. These issues will be discussed in the chapter on acquired immunity.

16.4 Age-structured host populations

The models described in the preceding sections of this chapter do not take into account the age structure of the human community. This is an important omission since, as noted in Chapter 15 (see Figs. 15.20 and 15.21), the prevalence and intensity of infection often exhibit characteristic patterns of change with age. We now build on the insights gained from the simple models to incorporate age structure and to compare predicted changes in prevalence and mean worm burden with observed patterns. In this section we ignore possible complications introduced by acquired immunity; this topic is examined in a separate chapter.

16.4.1 *Immigration–death model*

The simple immigration–death model defined in eqns (16.1) and (16.2) can be easily extended to consider changes in the mean worm burden, $M(a, t)$, at time t in people of age a with respect to both time (longitudinal trends) and host age (horizontal trends). Where $\Lambda(a)$ and $\mu_1(a)$ represent, respectively, the rate of infection of people at age a and the death rate of parasites within hosts of age a, the appropriate partial differential equation is

$$\partial M(a, t)/\partial t + \partial M(a, t)/\partial a = \Lambda(a) - \mu_1(a)M(a, t). \qquad (16.44)$$

With the boundary and initial conditions of $M(0, t) = 0$ and $M(a, 0) = M(a)$

(where $M(0) = 0$), the solution of eqn (16.44) is, for $t > a$

$$M(a, t) = \int_0^a \Lambda(s) \exp\left(- \int_s^a \mu_1(\alpha) \, d\alpha \right) ds,$$ (16.45a)

and for $t < a$

$$M(a, t) = \int_0^t \Lambda(s) \exp\left(- \int_s^t \mu_1(\alpha) \, ds \right) ds$$

$$+ M(a - t) \exp\left(- \int_{a-t}^t \mu_1(s) \, ds \right).$$ (16.45b)

If the rate of infection and adult parasite mortality are constant and independent of host age (Λ and μ_1, respectively), eqns (16.45) simplify to

$$M(a, t) = (\Lambda/\mu_1)[1 - \exp(-\mu_1 a)],$$ (16.46a)

$$M(a, t) = (\Lambda/\mu_1)[1 - \exp(-\mu_1 t)] + M(a - t) \exp(-\mu_1 t).$$ (16.46b)

The equilibrium age distribution ($\partial M(a, t)/\partial t = 0$) is simply

$$M^*(a) = (\Lambda/\mu_1)[1 - \exp(-\mu_1 a)].$$ (16.47)

The mean worm burden therefore rises monotonically with age to a plateau at Λ/μ_1. The overall equilibrium mean worm burden, $\bar{M}^*$, in the total population of people is the integral, over all age classes, of the mean worm burden at age a, weighted by the proportion of the human community in that age class. If we define $\ell(a)$ as the probability that an individual person survives to age a, then

$$\bar{M}^* = \int_0^\infty M^*(a)\ell(a) \, da.$$ (16.48)

With Type I human survivorship, with life expectancy L, this becomes

$$\bar{M}^* = \left(\frac{\Lambda}{\mu_1} \right) L \left(1 - \frac{[1 - \exp(-\mu_1 L)]}{\mu_1 L} \right).$$ (16.49)

Alternatively, when survivorship is Type II with death rate μ,

$$\bar{M}^* = \Lambda/[\mu(\mu_1 + \mu)].$$ (16.50)

More generally, since parasite life expectancy is typically much less than that of the human host ($\mu \ll \mu_1$), then eqns (16.49) and (16.50) simplify to

$$\bar{M}^* \to \Lambda/(\mu_1 \mu).$$ (16.51)

This model provides an introduction to the incorporation of host age structure, but its structure is too simple to describe the details of parasite transmission. Most importantly, the magnitude of the infection term, Λ, will itself depend on the overall mean worm burden, $\bar{M}$.

16.4.2 *Direct life cycle macroparasites*

The simple immigration–death model can be generalized (see Anderson and May 1982c, 1985b) to take account of the dependence of the rate of host infection, Λ, on the production of transmission stages by the mature worms, as follows:

$$\partial M(a, t)/\partial t + \partial M(a, t)/\partial a = \Lambda(a, t) - f_3(M, k)M(a, t). \qquad (16.52)$$

Here the transmission or infection function, $\Lambda(a, t)$, is defined as

$$\Lambda(a, t) = f_1(a, M, k)\left(\int_0^\infty \ell(a)M(a, t)f_2(M, k)\, da\right)\left(\int_0^\infty \ell(a)\, da\right)^{-1}. \qquad (16.53)$$

The functions f_1, f_2, and f_3 represent, respectively: the collapsed details of parasite survival, reproduction, and transmission via the segments of the life cycle not involving the mature worms in man; density-dependent constraints on adult parasite fecundity; and survival of adult parasites within the host. As for the models without age structure, we assume that the distribution of parasites within the host community is well described empirically by the negative binomial probability model. We also assume that the degree of worm contagion (as measured inversely by k) is independent of host age (see Table 15.6 for empirical evidence in support of this assumption).

The net output of transmission stages into the environment is represented in eqn (16.53) by the term

$$\left(\int_0^\infty \ell(a)M(a, t)f_2(M, k)\, da\right)\left(\int_o^\infty \ell(a)\, da\right)^{-1},$$

where $\ell(a)$ denotes, as before, the probability that a person survives to age a. It is assumed that the human community is of constant size with a stable age distribution. The net output term simply represents the contribution for each age class of people weighted by their proportional representation within the total community. The rate of infection, $\Lambda(a, t)$, is therefore the net rate of production of transmission stages times the probability, $f_1(a, M, k)$, that an individual infective stage successfully invades a host and develops to join the reproductively mature worms ($M(a, t)$). The function f_1 is defined as dependent on host age, a, parasite burden, M, and parasite aggregation, k, to mirror assumptions of density-dependent parasite establishment in humans and age-specific rates of human contact with transmission stages.

With the exception of possible complications introduced by acquired immunity, the model defined in eqn (16.52) is a fairly general statement of the dynamics of helminth transmission within human communities. In order to examine its dynamical properties, however, it is helpful to consider an example in which we are able to specify particular functions for f_1, f_2, and f_3. We consider the directly transmitted intestinal nematodes and assume that the only density-dependent constraint on parasite population growth acts on adult worm fecundity through the function f_2; the functions f_1 and f_3 are taken to be independent of M and k. This assumption is based on the empirical observations displayed in Fig. 15.14 which show that per capita worm fecundity often decays exponentially as worm burden rises. The additional assumptions that f_1 and f_3 are constant and independent of worm load are made partly for convenience and partly because no quantitative information is available for human infection to suggest otherwise.

Given an exponential decay in fecundity with increased worm load and a negative binomial distribution of parasite numbers per host, the function f_2 takes the form

$$f_2(M, k) = [1 + (1 - z)M/k]^{-(k+1)} \tag{16.54}$$

where $z = \exp(-\gamma)$ and the constant γ as before denotes the severity of density dependence (see eqn (16.14)). If host contact with infective stages is taken to be independent of age, then eqn (16.53) simplifies to

$$\Lambda(t) = (R_0 \mu_1/L) \int_0^\infty \ell(a)M(a, t)[1 + (1 - z)M(a, t)/k]^{-(k+1)} \, \mathrm{d}a. \tag{16.55}$$

Here, L denotes human life expectancy ($L = \int_0^\infty \ell(a)\,\mathrm{d}a$), and R_0 is the basic reproductive rate of the parasite.

At equilibrium ($\partial M(a, t)/\partial t = 0$), the age distribution of average worm burdens, $M^*(a)$, is again given by

$$\mathrm{d}M^*(a)/\mathrm{d}a = \bar{\Lambda} - \mu_1 M^*(a). \tag{16.56}$$

Here, $\bar{\Lambda}$ is as defined in eqn (16.55) where $\Lambda(t)$ is replaced by $\bar{\Lambda}$ and $M(a, t)$ is replaced by $M^*(a)$. The solution of eqn (16.56) is as defined in eqn (16.47) with Λ replaced by $\bar{\Lambda}$. The equilibrium prevalence of infection, $P^*(a)$, is simply defined as

$$P^*(a) = 1 - (1 + M^*(a)/k)^{-k}. \tag{16.57}$$

This model can be fitted to observed data that record changes in $M^*(a)$ and $P^*(a)$ with age, such that estimates of $\bar{\Lambda}$ (the equilibrium rate of infection) can be obtained, given a knowledge of the magnitude of adult worm life expectancy, $1/\mu_1$, and the clumping parameter, k.

An example of this approach is displayed in Fig. 16.13, which employs epidemiological data of *Ascaris* infection in a series of rural villages in Iran (see Croll *et al.* 1982). Note that the predictions of this simple model accurately reflect the observed trends (mean worm burden rises monotonically with age to a plateau of approximately 22 worms per person, $\bar{\Lambda}/\mu$). In this specific example, the mean worm burden $M^*(a)$ in the majority of age classes (all but the very young children) is essentially equal to the mean worm burden within

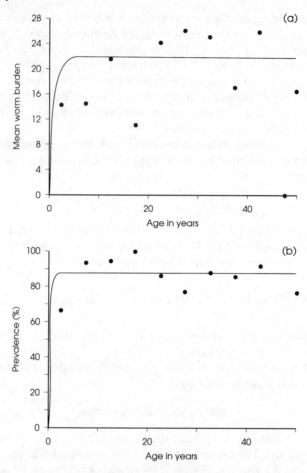

Fig. 16.13. (a) Observed age-related changes in the mean worm burden and (b) the prevalence of infection are compared with the predictions (full curves) of eqns (16.56) and (16.57). The data are from a study of the epidemiology of *Ascaris* in Iran by Croll *et al.* (1982). Parameter values: $M^* = 22$, $k = 0.57$, $z = 0.96$, $A = 1$, $R_0 = 4.3$.

the total community, $\bar{M}^*$. Thus a good estimate of $\bar{\Lambda}$ is given from eqn (16.55) as

$$\bar{\Lambda} \simeq R_0 \bar{M}^* \mu_1 [1 + (1 - z)\bar{M}^*/k]^{-(k+1)}. \tag{16.58}$$

The value of R_0 may therefore be derived from (16.58) given estimates of $\bar{\Lambda}$, μ_1, $\bar{M}^*$, z, and k. For the study in question, the values were crudely estimated as $\bar{\Lambda} = 22$, $\mu_1 = 1$, $\bar{M}^* = 22$, $k = 0.57$, $z = 0.96$; this gives an R_0 value of between 4 and 5 (Croll *et al.* 1982). This method of estimation, however, is very crude and fails to apply more generally, since monotonic changes in mean worm burden with age when the plateau Λ/μ_1 is attained very rapidly are rarely recorded in horizontal surveys of helminth abundance within human communities (see, for example, Figs. 15.20 and 15.21).

More generally, we can express eqn (16.55) at equilibrium as

$$1 = \frac{R_0}{L} \int_0^\infty \ell(a)[1 - \exp(-\mu_1 a)]$$

$$\times \left[1 + (1 - z)\left(\frac{\bar{\Lambda}}{\mu_1 k}\right)[1 - \exp(-\mu_1 a)] \right]^{-(k+1)} da, \quad (16.59)$$

since $M^*(a) = (\bar{\Lambda}/\mu_1)[1 - \exp(-\mu_1 a)]$ (see eqn (16.53). Given knowledge of $\bar{\Lambda}$ from observed changes in $M^*(a)$ with age, and independent estimates of z, μ_1, k, and $\ell(a)$ (from drug-induced worm expulsion studies and demographic data), eqn ((16.59) can be evaluated numerically to produce an estimate of R_0. The life expectancies of most human helminths are much shorter than those of their host ($L \gg 1/\mu_1$); hence, a useful approximation to eqn ((16.59) is given by taking the limit $\exp(-\mu_1 a) \to 0$:

$$R_0 \simeq [1 + (1 - z)\bar{\Lambda}/(\mu_1 k)]^{(k+1)}. \quad (16.60)$$

A slightly better approximation can be obtained via series expansion of the terms within the integral of eqn (16.59) and the omission of higher-order terms. This yields

$$R_0 \simeq (1 + B)^{k+1}\left[1 + \left(\frac{1 - kB}{1 + B}\right)\frac{1}{\mu_1 L} \right] \quad (16.61)$$

where $B = \bar{\Lambda}(1 - z)/(\mu_1 k)$. These approximations provide reliable estimates of R_0 provided parasite life expectancy is in the range of 1 to 5 years and parasite aggregation is moderate to severe. Both assumptions are usually satisfied for helminth infections of humans. A further potential problem with the model concerns the assumption that the distribution of parasites in the total community is negatively binomial in form. The precise distribution is probably fixed from a mixture of negative binomials (one for each age class) as a result of differing rates of host mortality within each age class (see Dietz 1982a). The use of a common aggregation parameter, however, is a good approximation provided that parasitic life expectancy is short in relation to that of humans, as it is for the intestinal nematodes and schistosomes flukes; the assumption is less good for the filarial worms.

Observed patterns of change in the average intensity of infection with age are commonly convex in form, where peak parasite abundance is attained in the child or teenage sections of the community (Fig. 15.21). Convexity may arise due to a variety of factors either acting alone or in combination. The two most important factors are thought to be age-related changes in contact with infective stages and the build-up of acquired immunity in older age classes due to long experience of infection (Warren 1973; Anderson and May 1985b;

Anderson 1986). The topic of acquired immunity is examined in a later chapter; in this section we briefly consider age-dependent exposure.

Equation (16.56) can be simply modified to incorporate the rate of infection as a function of age, $\bar{\Lambda}(a)$. The general solution of the modified model is

$$M^*(a) = \exp(-\mu_1 a) \int_0^a \bar{\Lambda}(s) \exp(-\mu_1 s) \, ds, \qquad (16.62)$$

given the initial condition $M^*(0) = 0$. The pattern of change in average worm burden with age will of course depend on the precise functional form of $\bar{\Lambda}(a)$. Model predictions for a series of different assumptions concerning the dependency of the infection rate on age are displayed in Fig. 16.14. In practice, however, it is very difficult (particularly in the case of the intestinal nematode infections of humans) to obtain estimates of the age dependency of $\bar{\Lambda}$, independent from observed changes in mean worm burden with age. It would require detailed quantitative scores, stratified according to age, of the behavioural habits that are relevant to contact with infective stages. Such information is not available at present for the directly transmitted helminths, although work in progress on the relationship between *Trichuris* infections and soil ingestion by children may provide some quantitative information (Bundy *et al.* 1985b; Bundy, 1988).

In the absence of independent information, if we assume that worm life expectancy is constant and independent of age, and that acquired immunity is negligible, rough estimates of $\bar{\Lambda}$ can be obtained from the solution of eqn (16.56) given observations on mean worm burden at ages a and $a + \Delta a$ ($M(a)$ and $M(a + \Delta a)$), where Δa is a smallish interval of age relative to the life expectancy of the parasite, $1/\mu_1$. More precisely,

$$\bar{\Lambda}(a \to (a + \Delta a)) = \frac{\mu_1(M^*(a + \Delta a) - M^*(a))}{\exp(-\mu_1 a)[1 - \exp(-\mu_1 \Delta a)]}. \qquad (16.63)$$

A practical illustration of this approach is presented in Fig. 16.15.

We are left with a practical dilemma. It is relatively easy to formulate models that incorporate age dependence in contact with infection, but in practice it is extremely difficult to compare prediction with observation due to the lack of data on this dependence. We will return to this issue in the following chapter which deals with temporal dynamics.

16.6 Some formal elaborations

For completeness, we briefly mention some formal approaches to the development of age-structured models of helminth transmission. These approaches are of limited interest in an epidemiological context, since their mathematical abstractness limits practical application.

A perceived shortcoming of the models developed in earlier sections of this

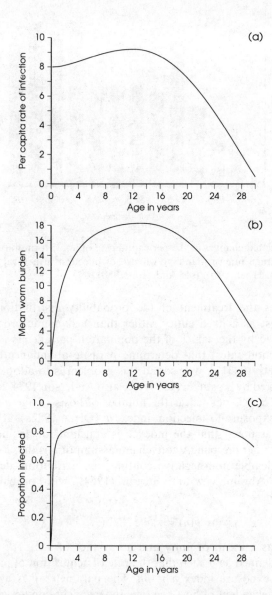

Fig. 16.14. The influence of age-related changes in the per capita rate of infection, Λ, on age-specific trends in the mean worm burden, $M^*(a)$, and the prevalence of infection, $P^*(a)$, as predicted by eqns (16.56) and (16.57). An arbitrary form of $\Lambda(a)$ was chosen and is plotted in (a). This choice generated the age-related changes in $M^*(a)$ and $P^*(a)$ recorded, respectively, in (b) and (c).

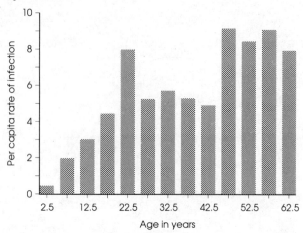

Fig. 16.15. Age-related changes in the per capita rate of hookworm infection estimated from data on average intensity and prevalence of infection in a rural community in Taiwan (data from Hsieh 1970) (see Anderson 1980).

chapter concerns the treatment of the probability distribution of parasite numbers per host as a fixed entity rather than a dynamic process in which pattern is dictated by the values of the population parameters (such as birth, death, and infection rates) that determine parasite abundance (Dietz 1982a; Hadeler and Dietz 1983). A way round this problem is to adopt an approach originally suggested by Kostitzin (1934) (see also Anderson 1974, 1980) in which a variable $n(a, i, h, t)$ is defined as the number of hosts of age a with parasite burden i and exposure-to-infection index h (Dietz 1982a) at time t. For simplicity, it is assumed that the index h is constant for an individual host throughout his or her lifespan. A convenient assumption is that h has a gamma distribution (a flexible non-negative continuous distribution, defined by two parameters; see Abramowitz and Stegun (1964)) with probability density function $g(h)$, where

$$g(h) = s^s h^s \, \mathrm{e}^{-sh} / \Gamma(s). \tag{16.64}$$

This function has a mean of unity and a variance of s^{-1}. The coefficient of transmission is defined as β such that the rate of acquisition of parasites by an individual with exposure index h is βh. The parameter β is assumed to be constant and independent of host age (age-independent contact with infection) and total parasite abundance (a constant force of infection such that changes in parasite density do not influence transmission success). As before, parasites have a constant per capita natural mortality rate μ_1, while the human host has an age-dependent death rate $\mu(a)$ and a parasite-induced death rate αi where α is a constant of proportionality (see Anderson and May 1978; May and Anderson 1978). At equilibrium ($\partial n(a, i, h, t)/\partial t = 0$), changes in $n^*(a, i, h)$ with respect to host age can be expressed as an infinite series of differential equations:

$$dn^*(a, i, h)/da = -[\beta h + \mu(a) + \mu_1 i + \alpha i]n^*(a, i, h)$$
$$+ \beta h n^*(a, i - 1, h) + \mu_1(i + 1)n^*(a, i + 1, h). \quad (16.65)$$

Via the introduction of the probability generating function (p.g.f.)

$$\pi(a, z, h) = \sum_i n^*(a, i, h)z^i, \quad (16.66)$$

the system of equations can be reduced to one partial differential equation with the solution (in terms of the p.g.f.),

$$\pi(a, z, h) = Ng(h)\exp\left(-\int_0^a b(\tau)\,d\tau - \alpha\int_0^a m^*(\tau, h)\,d\tau + m^*(a, h)(z - 1)\right).$$

$$(16.67)$$

The mean number of parasites, $m^*(a, h)$, in people of age a and exposure index h is given by

$$m^*(a, h) = [\beta h/(\alpha + \mu_1)]\{1 - \exp[-(\alpha + \mu_1)a]\}. \quad (16.68)$$

The initial and boundary conditions required to obtain these solutions are $n(0, 0, h) = Ng(h)$ where N is the total host population size (a constant at equilibrium) and $n(0, i, h) = 0$ for $i > 0$ (hosts uninfected at birth). Note that in the case where $\alpha = 0$ (no parasite-induced host death) and h adopts the same value for all individuals in the population (homogeneous exposure to infection), eqn (16.65) is identical to our earlier model (eqn (16.56) with $\bar\Lambda = \beta h$).

Not surprisingly, the distribution of parasite numbers in hosts of age a with exposure index h is Poisson (random) in form, with mean $m^*(a, h)$, as defined in eqn (16.68). The distribution of parasites in all hosts of age a (irrespective of exposure index) is negative binomial in form (with p.g.f. $G(z, a)$) due to the compounding of the separate Poisson distributions for each exposure index class whose means are distributed in a gamma form. The mean of this distribution, $M^*(a)$, is

$$M^*(a) = m^*(a, 1)/[1 + (\alpha/s)\int_0^\infty m^*(\tau, 1)\,d\tau]. \quad (16.69)$$

The average number of parasites in any one individual rises monotonically as he or she ages, to approach the plateau $\beta h/(\alpha + \mu)$. However, provided $\alpha > 0$ (i.e. the parasite is a cause of host mortality), the average number of parasites in all people of age a rises to a maximum value as a increases, but then declines to approach zero as a becomes larger. The age at which $M^*(a)$ is at a maximum depends on the magnitude of the parasite-induced death rate α. The convexity of $M^*(a)$ with age a is a direct consequence of the relatively early death of highly exposed individuals such that the average exposure index—and therefore the average parasite load—declines above a certain age (Dietz 1982*a*).

The probability generating function for the number of parasites in the total host population, $H(z)$, is a mixture of negative binomial distributions (one for each age class with p.g.f. $G(z, a)$):

$$H(z) = \left(\int_0^\infty Q(a)G(z, a)\, da \right)\left(\int_0^\infty Q(a)\, da \right)^{-1} \qquad (16.70)$$

Here, $Q(a)$ is defined as

$$Q(a) = \exp\left(-\int_0^a \mu(\tau)\, d\tau \right)\left[1 + \frac{\beta\alpha}{s(\alpha + \mu_1)}\left(a - \frac{1 - \exp[-a(\alpha + \mu_1)]}{\alpha + \mu_1} \right) \right].$$

$$(16.71)$$

The general, and somewhat obvious, conclusion to emerge from this sort of approach is that heterogeneity in exposure to infection generates heterogeneity in the distribution of parasite numbers per host within an age class.

These aggregated distributions (negative binomial in form for the specific example considered by Dietz (1982a)) differ from one age group to the next such that the overall distribution in the total community is formed from a mixture of contagious distributions. Provided that the life expectancy of the parasite, $1/\mu_1$, is short in relation to that of the human host (which is invariably the case), the mixture itself is, to a good approximation, negative binomial in form. In practical terms, therefore, it would be difficult to distinguish between the mixture pattern and a single negative binomial distribution unless a very large number of observations were available.

Aside from the virtue of simplicity, the phenomenological assumption of our earlier models, that the distribution is fixed and negative binomial in form, appears to be an excellent approximation to the predictions of much more elaborate and cumbersome models. Furthermore, it should be noted that these more formal approaches (Dietz 1982a; Hadeler and Dietz 1983) are based on the unrealistic assumption that the rate of exposure to infection is independent of the total parasite population size.

The basic model: dynamics

The preceding chapter focused on equilibrium results and (where possible) compared prediction with observations on the assumption that the parasite population under study was at its stable endemic state within a host community of constant size and stable age distribution. These assumptions can be relaxed in order to consider what happens when the parasite population is perturbed from its steady state by control intervention or environmental change. We examine four topics of practical interest, namely, the decay in parasite abundance following the cessation of transmission, reinfection following drug treatment, the dynamic consequences of repeated mass chemotherapy, and temporal changes induced by targeted or selective chemotherapy.

17.1 The decay in parasite load following a cessation in transmission

It sometimes happens that groups of infected individuals are no longer exposed to reinfection either as a result of their emigration to localities where transmission is not possible or as a result of effective control measures in their own community. Under such circumstances, observations through time on the decay in the prevalence and the average intensity of infection in a sample of people who do not receive chemotherapeutic treatment provides valuable information on the population biology of the parasites. In particular it facilitates the estimation of helminth life expectancies.

The simple models outlined in Chapter 16 enable predictions to be made concerning the manner in which prevalence and intensity will decay through time (Anderson and May 1985b). In the simplest case, where the death rate of the adult parasite is constant and independent of age, μ_1, the change in the mean worm burden, $M(t)$, in a sample of people is simply

$$M(t) = M(0) \exp(-\mu_1 t). \tag{17.1}$$

Here $M(0)$ is the initial average worm burden at time $t = 0$. Assuming that the parasites are distributed in a negative binomial pattern, then the prevalence of infection at time t, $P(t)$, is

$$P(t) = 1 - \{1 + [M(0) \exp(-\mu_1 t)]/k\}^{-k}. \tag{17.2}$$

For high degrees of parasite aggregation (small k, which is usually the case in practice) the average worm burden $M(t)$ decays much more rapidly than the prevalence $P(t)$ (Fig. 17.1). The initial decline in the prevalence is relatively slow and depends in a complicated way on the average worm burden and the degree of parasite clumping in the sample of hosts. Once the time elapsed since

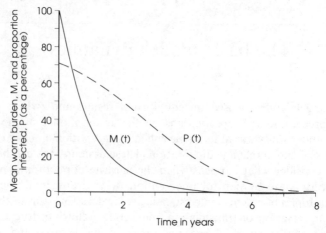

Fig. 17.1. The decay in the mean worm burden, $M(t)$, and the prevalence of infection (as a proportion), $P(t)$, through time following a cessation in transmission of exposure to infection as defined by eqns (17.1) and (17.2). Parameter values: $\mu = 1.0 \, \mathrm{yr}^{-1}$, $M(0) = 100$, $k = 0.3$.

cessation from exposure to infection is long compared with the expected life span of the parasite ($t \gg 1/\mu_1$), most hosts harbour either one or no worms. In these circumstances eqn (17.2) reduces to

$$P(t \gg 1/\mu_1) \simeq M(0) \exp(-\mu_1 t). \tag{17.3}$$

Equivalently, this relation has the form

$$\ln P \simeq \text{constant} - t\mu_1. \tag{17.4}$$

An example of the comparison of the predictions of this simple model with data concerning infection with the filarial nematode *Wuchereria bancrofti*, in a sample of people who emigrated to a country free from infection, is presented in Fig. 17.2. Equation (17.2) has three unknowns, namely $M(0)$, μ_1, and k. Non-linear statistical procedures can be used to estimate these parameters given records of the decay in $P(t)$ over many time intervals past cessation of reinfection (Anderson and May 1985b). A plot of $\ln P(t)$ against t tends towards a straight-line relationship for large values of t; the slope of this line gives a direct estimate of the rate of mortality of the parasite, μ_1, and hence its life expectancy, $1/\mu_1$. Figure 17.2 shows two phases in decay in $\ln P(t)$: an initial slow and complicated decline followed by a phase of linear decay. Webber (1975) noted this pattern in this particular data set, but the explanation he offers is unnecessarily involved. The agreement between model prediction and observation is encouraging given the crudity of the assumption embodied in eqn (17.2).

An example of the differential rates of decay in prevalence, $P(t)$, and intensity,

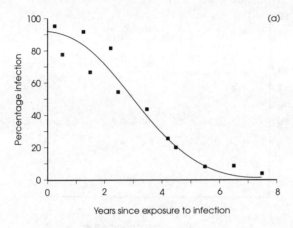

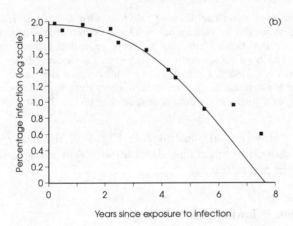

Fig. 17.2. (a) The decay in the prevalence of *Wuchereria bancrofti* infection within a sample of people no longer exposed to infection. The full squares are observed values (data from Webber 1975) and the full curve is the prediction of the model defined by eqn (17.2). Parameter values were estimated by a non-linear least-squares technique: $k = 0.61$, $\mu = 1.1 \, \mathrm{yr}^{-1}$, $M(0) = 39.2$. (b) Identical to (a) except the vertical axis is presented on a logarithmic scale (see Anderson and May 1985*b*).

$M(t)$, is provided by the control programme to prevent the transmission of *Onchocera volvulus* in western and central Africa (WHO 1985). In large areas, repeated insecticide application has substantially suppressed the abundance of the simuliid vectors of the filarial parasite and has, in certain areas, resulted in a cessation in transmission to humans (as verified by the absence of cases of infection in young children born after the initiation of the control programme). *Onchocera volvulus* appears to have a long life expectancy in man (roughly 8–12 years), and hence prevalence and intensity have decayed slowly since interruption

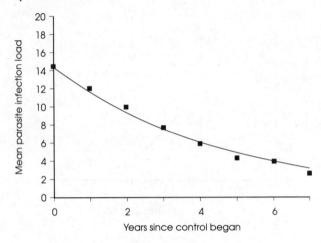

Fig. 17.3. The decay in the mean level of infection with *Onchocera volvulus* (mean microfilarial load as judged by skin snips) in human communities in the Kowlpeolgo region of north-eastern Benin, following a severe reduction (almost cessation) of transmission induced by a vector control programme (larviciding) (data from WHO (1985)). The points are observed values and the full curve is the best-fit exponential model. The mean life expectancy of a reproductively mature worm is estimated to be between 4 and 5 years with a maximum life expectancy of 11–12 years.

of transmission. However, as illustrated in Fig. 17.3, the decay in average intensity (as measured by microfilarial densities in skin snips) is much more rapid than that in prevalence.

17.2 Reinfection following chemotherapy

The pattern of reinfection by helminths following chemotherapeutic treatment provides much information about a parasite's transmission dynamics. As mentioned earlier, such patterns in individual patients provide evidence with which to test the hypothesis of predisposition to heavy or light infection. In samples of patients, change in prevalence and average intensity (measured directly via drug-induced worm expulsion or indirectly via the production of transmission stages) through time post-treatment provides a means for estimating the magnitude of the basic reproductive rate, R_0, as well as facilitating the comparison between the predictions of simple models and observed trends.

One of the more remarkable features of the population biology of helminth species is the rapidity with which the average intensity of infection returns to its pre-control level following depression by chemotherapeutic intervention. A series of examples are portrayed in Fig. 17.4. This observed stability—the return invariably appears to be monotonic in form with no 'overshoot' of the pre-control equilibrium—is in accord with the predictions of our simple models.

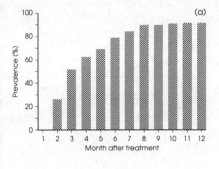

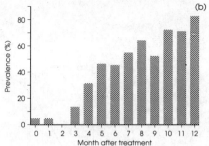

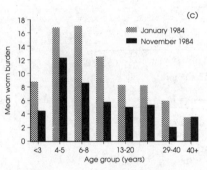

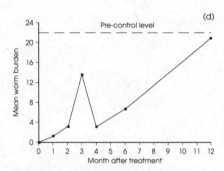

Fig. 17.4. Examples of the rapidity with which levels of infection return to their pre-control levels following a single round of mass treatment. Four examples are recorded, each of which refers to a study of the chemotherapeutic treatment of intestinal nematode infections in developing countries. (a) The rise in the prevalence of infection with *Trichuris trichuria* in a community in Malaysia (Cabrera 1980). (b) The rise in the prevalence of infection with *Ascaris lumbricoides* in a community in Burma (Thein-Hliang 1985). (c) Mean burdens of *Ascaris lumbricoides* pre-treatment (January 1984) and 11 months post-treatment (November 1984) in a village community in southern India (Elkins *et al.* 1986). (d) The rise in the mean burden of *Ascaris lumbricoides* in a rural community in Iran (Croll *et al.* 1982).

This stability is induced by the density-dependent constraints on parasite fecundity (or, alternatively, parasite survival or establishment) concomitant with the aggregation of parasite distribution within the human community which serves to enhance the net force of such regulatory mechanisms. These points are well illustrated by numerical studies of the simple non-age-structured model of changes in mean worm burden with time, $M(t)$, defined in eqn (16.21). A series of temporal realizations are displayed in Fig. 17.5 where the equilibrium mean worm burden, M^*, is depressed, via chemotherapeutic treatment, by 90 per cent. The predicted pattern of reinfection following this depression is recorded for various values of the degree of parasite aggregation, k, of parasite life expectancy, $1/\mu_1$, and of the severity of density-dependent constraints on fecundity, z. It is assumed that the worms are dioecious and polygamous, and are distributed in a negative binomial pattern. Of particular interest is the

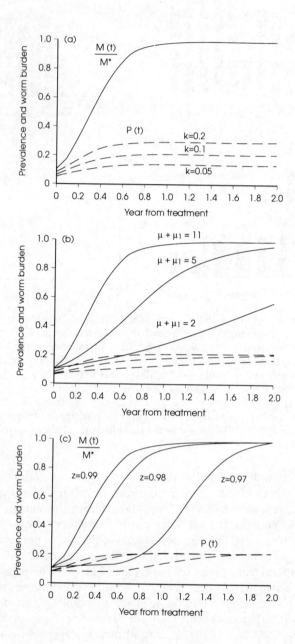

prediction that worm life expectancy (which is related to the magnitude of R_0) has a marked impact on the rate of return to the pre-control level. It is slow for long-lived species, and vice versa. This is in good agreement with observed trends. The time to return to the pre-control average intensity is often one year or less for *Ascaris* and *Trichuris* (expected life spans of one year or less), two to four years for hookworms (expected life span 2–3 years), and five years or more for schistosomes (expected life span 3–5 years). Examples of these rates of return are displayed in Fig. 17.4. It is also interesting to note that theory and observation are in good agreement with respect to relative changes in prevalence and intensity following control intervention. The prevalence, $P(t)$, rises more rapidly after treatment ceases than does the average intensity, $M(t)$ (Fig. 17.5).

These conclusions also emerge from a study of the dynamic properties of the more complicated age-structured model defined by eqn (16.44). A numerical projection of the predicted changes in $M(a, t)$ and $P(a, t)$ with age and time, following a defined drug intervention programme (across all age classes), is displayed in Fig. 17.6 (based on eqn (16.44) with the assumption that density dependence acts solely on fecundity). Age structure within the host population (in the absence of acquired immunity) does not affect the general conclusion that helminth populations are very stable to perturbation as a consequence of density-dependent constraints on population growth or reproduction within individual people combined with high degrees of aggregation in the frequency distributions of parasite numbers per person.

For indirect life cycles, of course, such density-dependent checks may act within the intermediate host (i.e. snail or arthropod). These issues are discussed in Chapter 20, but broadly speaking the general conclusion remains the same for both directly and indirectly transmitted macroparasites.

Patterns of reinfection also present an opportunity to acquire rough estimates of the magnitude of the basic reproductive rate, R_0, for a given parasite in a

---

Fig. 17.5. Temporal realizations of changes in the mean worm burden $M(t)$ (expressed as a fraction of its equilibrium value M^*) following a 90 per cent reduction induced by chemotherapy (applied independent of worm load), as predicted by eqn (16.21). In (a) the value of the negative binomial parameter k is varied (0.05, 0.1, and 0.2) and the full curve records changes in the value of $M(t)/M^*$ through time. Note that varying k does not influence the rate of return to the pre-control equilibrium value. The broken curves denote changes in the proportion infected for each value of k ($R_0 = 2$, $z = 0.99$, $\mu + \mu_1 = 11$). In (b) the value of the mortality rate term, $\mu + \mu_1$, is varied (2, 5, and 11; all yr^{-1}). The full and broken curves are as described for (a) ($R_0 = 2$, $k = 0.1$, $z = 0.99$). In (c) the magnitude of the parameter, z, that inversely records the severity of density-dependent constraints on fecundity is varied (0.99, 0.98, and 0.97). The full and broken curves are as described for (a). Note that the magnitude of z influences the shape of the pattern of return of the mean worm burden to its pre-control level ($R_0 = 2$, $k = 0.1$, $\mu + \mu_1 = 11$).

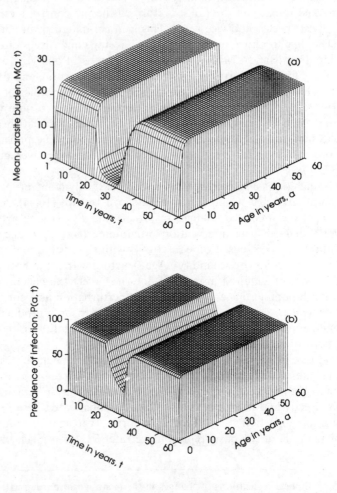

Fig. 17.6. Three-dimensional graphs generated by the numerical solution of eqn (16.44) which represents time- and age-dependent changes in the intensity (a) and prevalence (b) of infection. The simulations mirror the dynamics of *Ascaris lumbricoides* in a human community. For the first 20 years the helminth infection is at its endemic equilibrium (M^* set at 22 worms per host). In year 20 chemotherapy is applied randomly in the community on a continual basis where 20 per cent of the population is treated per month with a drug of 95 per cent efficiency. After 10 years treatment is stopped and the parasite population returns to its pre-control equilibrium. The human survivorship function was chosen to mimic typical patterns in the developing world (life expectancy of 50 years). Parameter values, $R_0 = 4.3$, $k = 0.57$, $z = 0.96$, $\mu = 1\,\mathrm{yr}^{-1}$ (from Anderson and May 1982c).

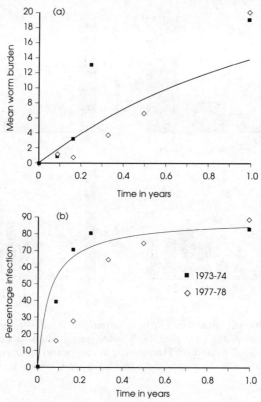

Fig. 17.7. The change in the mean worm burden of *Ascaris lumbricoides* (a) and the prevalence of infection (b) through time in samples of 111 (squares) and 110 (diamonds) people after treatment with a chemotherapeutic agent in a rural community in Iran (data from Croll *et al.* 1982). The squares represent data collected in the period 1973–4 and the diamonds represent data collected in 1977–8. The full curves represent predictions of eqn (16.21) for the rate of reinfection following treatment as denoted by mean worm burden and prevalence. Parameter values: $R_0 = 4.3$, $M^* = 22$, $k = 0.57$, $z = 0.96$, $\mu = 1\,\mathrm{yr}^{-1}$.

specific community. In the case of intestinal nematodes, for example, it is often possible, via drug-induced worm expulsion studies, to acquire data on the magnitudes of the clumping parameter, k, and the severity of constraints on fecundity, z. With a knowledge of the life expectancy of the parasite, μ_1, the model defined in eqn (16.21) can be solved numerically, and by trial and error a value of R_0 can be arrived at which maximizes the agreement between prediction and observation. An example of this approach is presented in Fig. 17.7 for a study of reinfection by *Ascaris* in a series of Iranian villages following drug treatment (Croll *et al.* 1982). Some further examples of reinfection are recorded in Fig. 17.8 for *Ascaris*, *Trichuris*, and hookworm infections. This

516   *Macroparasites*

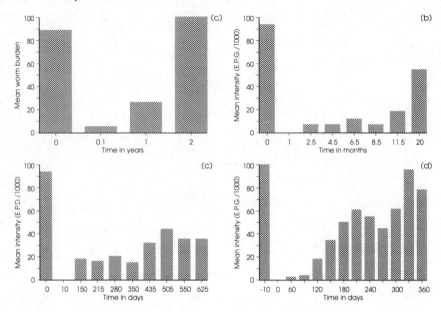

Fig. 17.8. Examples of reinfection with intestinal nematodes in groups of people following chemotherapeutic treatment. (a) Hookworm in adults and children in North America (Sweet 1925). (b) and (c) Hookworm in adults and children in India (Schad and Anderson 1985). (d) *Ascaris lumbricoides* in 'wormy' children in Burma (Thein-Hliang 1989).

method of deriving estimates of R_0 is clearly crude and is dependent on the many simplifying assumptions incorporated in the model defined in eqn (16.21). However, despite its crudity, it is the best method available at present.

Reinfection studies also provide information on rates of reacquisition of parasites in different age classes of the human population. As discussed earlier, one explanation of convex patterns of change in average intensity of infection with age is that contact with infective stages is age dependent. A number of epidemiological studies have recorded rates of reinfection following treatment in samples of patients stratified according to their age (Elkins *et al.* 1986, 1988; Bundy *et al.* 1988a; Bensted-Smith *et al.* 1989; Butterworth *et al.* 1985). Data from one such study involving reinfection by *Ascaris* over a 12-month period following treatment are displayed in Fig. 15.24. Mean worm burdens after 1 year of re-exposure to infection clearly vary with age (in a convex pattern), but when these burdens are expressed as a proportion of the pre-control worm load, it is apparent that the proportional rate of reacquisition is essentially constant and independent of the age of the host. The interpretation of the factors underlying this observation is not clear cut, since age dependency and/or acquired immunity could explain the pattern. In the absence of independent data (on, for example, immunological activity or the rate of exposure to infection in the different age classes), it is not possible to discriminate between these two alternative explanations (Anderson 1986).

17.3 Repeated mass chemotherapy—long-term control

The rapidity with which average worm burdens return to their pre-control levels following a single chemotherapeutic intervention in a community argues that effective long-term control will require both extensive coverage and repeated application (APCO 1980, 1983; Anderson and May 1982c). The degree of coverage required for eradication (to reduce the effective reproductive rate, R, to less than unity in value) was discussed in the preceding chapter (see eqn (16.25)).

In practice, however, repeated mass treatment is expensive both with respect to drug purchase and the use of trained personnel. Furthermore, the goal of eradication appears difficult to achieve in the case of many helminths due to the ease with which travellers or immigrants can reintroduce infection into a control area (there is no naturally acquired or artificially induced protective immunity to reinfection) and the apparently low level of the breakpoint worm burden below which mating frequency is insufficient to maintain parasite transmission (see Fig. 16.4). This is especially true for the directly transmitted intestinal helminths (with comparatively short generation times and rapid times of return to equilibrium burdens), but less so for the indirectly transmitted schistosome flukes and filarial worms. There are exceptions in the case of intestinal nematodes, since in conjunction with greatly improved standards of hygiene, education, and sanitation induced by rapid economic growth, a nationwide programme for the control of *Ascaris* in Japan has produced a remarkable reduction in parasite abundance (Fig. 17.9). A similar programme

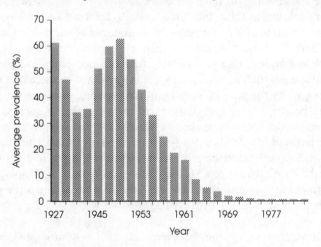

Fig. 17.9. Annual average prevalence of *Ascaris lumbricoides* infection in Japan from 1927 to 1982 (Yokogawa 1985).

in South Korea has also led to a dramatic impact on the prevalence of *Ascaris* infection in recent years (APCO 1980, 1983). In most developing countries, however, the resources are not available to mount such effective nation-wide programmes against intestinal nematode infection given other more urgent priorities in primary health care (e.g. mass vaccination against killing childhood viral and bacterial infections).

The availability of new and effective drugs for the treatment of schistosome and filarial infection (e.g. Praziquantal and Ivermectin) may mean that effective control can be achieved in endemic areas in the future by relatively infrequent mass treatment, given the longer generation times of these parasites and their slower rates of return to pre-control levels following a simple intervention. In all these cases, however, simple theory can help to gauge how frequently mass chemotherapy should be applied to suppress average worm loads to low levels when compared with pre-control burdens.

For the non-age-structured model (see eqn (16.21)) the rate of change in the overall mean worm burden with time under the impact of repeated or continuously applied mass chemotherapy which imposes an extra per capita parasite mortality c (see eqn (16.21)) is given by

$$\mathrm{d}M/\mathrm{d}t = M(\mu + \mu_1)[\phi R_0(1 + M(1 - z)/k)^{-(k+1)} - 1 - c/(\mu + \mu_1)]. \quad (17.5)$$

It is assumed here that density dependence acts solely on parasite fecundity and that the parasites are distributed in a negative binomial pattern. Numerical solutions of eqn (17.5) for varying values of c (and hence different rates of proportional coverage of the population—see eqn (16.27)) illustrate how the degree of suppression of worm abundance at levels above the critical unstable breakpoint depends on the magnitude of the basic reproductive rate, R_0 (see Fig. 17.10); the mating probability, ϕ, is as given earlier, with schistosomes assumed monogamous and intestinal nematodes assumed polygamous. In broad terms, permanently to suppress the abundance of short-lived species such as *Ascaris* and *Trichuris* in areas of endemic infection, mass treatment should be repeated at frequent intervals of the order of once every 2–3 months. For longer-lived species such as hookworm, the interval can be increased to perhaps yearly intervals. In the case of very long-lived species, effective suppression is predicted to be attained by fairly infrequent mass treatments such as every 2–3 years. These predictions are in broad agreement with observed trends. For example, a particularly detailed study of the impact of mass chemotherapy on the intensity of *Ascaris* infection repeated at various intervals in different villages (2, 4, 6, and 12 months) is reported by Seo *et al.* (1980). As displayed in Fig. 17.11, treatment at 2-month intervals was necessary to suppress the prevalence of infection in these South Korean villages to very low levels (i.e. 10 per cent or less).

Conclusions concerning the frequency of treatment are unaltered by an examination of the properties of the fully age-structured model (see eqn (16.44)). Provided the force of infection is independent of age, mass treatment must be

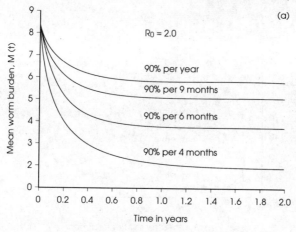

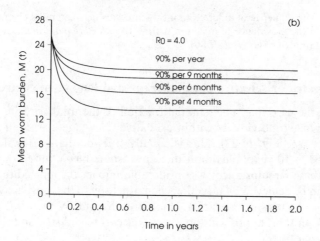

Fig. 17.10. Degree of suppression in the mean worm burden, $M(t)$, induced by various programmes of chemotherapy (mass treatment applied independently of worm load) as predicted by the numerical evaluation of eqn (17.5). The magnitude of the parameter c was set to mirror four levels of treatment; 90 per cent of the community per year, per 9 months, per 6 months, and per 4 months. Drug efficiency was set at 95 per cent and $R_0 = 2.0$ (graph (a)) and 4.0 (graph (b)). Other parameter values: $k = 0.1$, $\mu + \mu_1 = 11 \text{ yr}^{-1}$, $z = 0.99$. The mating function ϕ was chosen to represent a polygamous species distributed in a negative binomial manner in the host population.

applied uniformly across age classes at intervals related to the transmission potential of the parasite, R_0, its life expectancy, and its potential to return rapidly to the pre-control state following a single intervention (Fig. 17.12). All these properties are related; high transmission potential is linked with short life expectancy and rapid return times, and vice versa.

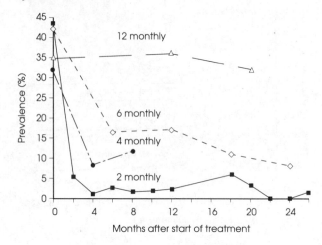

Fig. 17.11. The influence of different monthly intervals between mass chemotherapeutic treatment on the prevalence of infection with *Ascaris lumbricoides* in study populations in Korea (data from Seo *et al.* 1980).

17.4 Targeted or selective chemotherapy and long-term control

It is often the case that a substantial fraction of the total parasite population is harboured by individuals within a relatively few age classes of the human community (see Fig. 15.22). This is equally true for the intestinal nematodes (usually the 5–10 years olds) and the schistosome flukes (often the 5–15 year olds). In these circumstances a considerable impact on morbidity and transmission can be achieved by targeting chemotherapy to the most heavily infected age groups. As mentioned earlier, there are often many practical advantages associated with this approach, such as easy access to children on their assembly at schools, etc.

The age-structured model, eqn (16.44), can be adopted to describe this approach to control by assuming that contact with infective stages is age dependent (to reflect the unequal distribution of worm loads among age classes) and by adding an extra mortality term, $c(a)M(a, t)$, to the right-hand side of eqn (16.44). Here the drug-induced mortality rate, $c(a)$, is formulated as a function of age. For targeting the 5–10 year olds, we would assume that $c(a) = 0$ for $a < 5$ years and $a > 10$ years and $c(a) \neq 0$ for 5 years $< a < 10$ years. An example, generated by the numerical solution of eqn (16.44) (with the refinements outlined above), is presented in Fig. 17.13. The parameter values were chosen to correspond to the epidemiology of *Ascaris*, and as can be seen from the three-dimensional plot of changes in the mean worm burden across age classes and through time, the targeted approach (all 0–10-year-olds treated) is not necessarily effective in reducing transmission throughout the community as a whole. The value of this approach is very dependent on the age distribution of

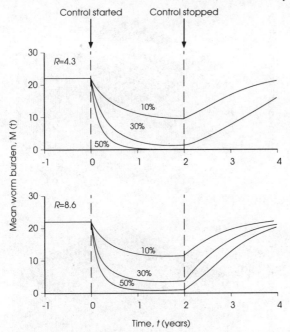

Fig. 17.12. The impact of the cessation of community-based chemotherapy on the rate at which average worm burdens return to pre-control levels, M^*. Two examples are presented, based on the numerical solution of the age-structured model defined by eqn (16.44) with the inclusion of an extra mortality term, c, to mimic the impact of drug treatment. Numerical solutions of changes through time mimic the dynamics of *Ascaris* transmission and show different levels of treatment in the community (10, 30, or 50 per cent per month). Control operates for 2 years, after which it ceases. The magnitude of the basic reproductive rate R_0 was set at 4.3 in graph (a) and at 8.6 in graph (b). Other parameter values: $k = 0.57$, $z = 0.96$, $\mu = 1 \, \text{yr}^{-1}$, $h = 0.9$.

worm loads prior to control. It is clearly beneficial if the age–intensity of infection profile is highly convex in form (see Fig. 15.20) but less so, with respect to the reduction of transmission, if this is not the case. However, even if convexity is not marked, targeting can still be of great value in the reduction of morbidity. Helminth infections are usually (except in the case of filarial worms) more a cause of morbidity in children than in adults. This is especially true in areas where malnutrition is prevalent, since it appears that under these circumstances heavy helminth burdens can seriously affect child growth and development (Crompton *et al.* 1989; Bundy and Golden 1987; Bundy 1988*b*; Nesheim 1989).

An alternative approach to age-group targeting is that of selectivity based on the intensity of infection within individuals. This approach rests on the observation that the majority of parasites are harboured by a relatively small fraction of people in areas of endemic helminth infection. Selectively treating

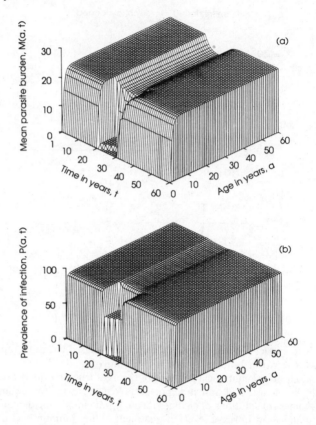

Fig. 17.13. Similar to Fig. 17.6, but with chemotherapy applied randomly only within the 0–10-year-old age classes. Parameter values as defined in the legend to Fig. 17.6 (from Anderson and May 1985*b*).

the 'wormy fraction' of a population has in principle great advantages with respect to the reduction of morbidity and transmission. Unfortunately, however, the deterministic models discussed in Chapter 16 are inappropriate for examining dynamic changes in parasite abundance under the impact of selective treatment. So far our models have been based on the assumption that the probability distribution of worm burdens per person is fixed in form (i.e. negative binomial) such that the degree of parasite aggregation is constant and independent of the mean worm burden. Repeated selective treatment of some proportion of the most heavily infected individuals clearly acts to alter the form of this distribution. Specifically, it will reduce the degree of parasite aggregation within the community (i.e. reduce the variance in worm load per person). Under these circumstances it is necessary to work with stochastic models which mimic changes in the full probability distribution of parasite numbers per person under the impact of different chemotherapy programmes. It is easy to formulate such models (see Bartlett (1960b) for examples in the field of population ecology), but the inclusion of simple non-linearities (such as density-dependent parasite fecundity) makes analytical investigation of their properties difficult, if not impossible, at present.

One way around this problem is to employ Monte Carlo simulation techniques (see Tocher 1963; Pielou 1969; Anderson and Gordon 1982) where chance variation in the timing and sequence of population events (i.e. infection, birth, or death in both host and parasite communities) is determined by the generation of pseudo-random numbers according to a set of assumptions that define the average rate at which each different event occurs. One advantage of this approach is that with the aid of modern digital computers, all events affecting each individual person in a large population (or within his or her parasite population) can be simulated, such that records can be generated of dynamic changes in the distribution of worm numbers per person. Some recent studies have employed this technique to investigate the impact of selective chemotherapy on helminth parasite abundance and distribution (Anderson and May 1985; Dietz and Renner 1985; Medley and Anderson 1991).

In one such study, the mathematical framework employed was essentially a stochastic version of the age-structured deterministic model defined by eqn (16.49) (see Anderson and Medley (1985) and Medley and Anderson (1991) for the detailed structure of the model). The principal assumptions made were as follows:

1. Contact with infection was assumed to depend on host age, such that the average rate rose to a maximum value in the 15–20-year-olds and declined thereafter.

2. Acquired immunity was assumed not to affect parasite establishment, survival, and fecundity. Convex changes in average worm load with age were generated solely by age-related changes in exposure to infection.

3. The demography of the human community was designed to mirror that of a typical developing country with a positive net growth rate and high mortality in the early years of life (i.e. up to 10 years of age). Mortality was assumed to be independent of parasite burden.

4. Parasite population regulation was assumed to act solely via density-dependent parasite fecundity (as defined in eqn (16.14)).

5. Heterogeneity (= aggregation) in parasite burdens per person within any given age class of the community was generated by two distinct mechanisms, namely, *predisposition* or *environmental heterogeneity*. Predisposition implies that each individual's susceptibility/exposure rate to infection was determined at birth, where its value is distributed as a gamma function (see eqn (16.64)) within each age group. The mean of the gamma function was weighted

differently among age classes to reflect age-related changes in contact with infective stages (rising to a maximum in the 15–20-year-olds—see (1) above). Differing susceptibilities can be envisaged as arising from genetically based variability in host immunocompetence, from variability in behavioural factors associated with the risk of exposure to infection, from heterogeneity in factors within the environment in which an individual lives that are relevant to transmission, or from any combination of these processes. Environmental heterogeneity was taken to imply that the rate of encounter with infective stages occurs at random (where the mean of the encounter rate varies between age classes but is constant within a class). On each encounter, however, it was assumed that the number of infective stages that established within a person followed a negative binomial distribution with clumping parameter k. This assumption was made to reflect spatial and temporal clumping of infective stages within the habitat of the community.

Simulation experiments based on this model shed light on two problems. First, how important is the mechanism generating heterogeneity in parasite numbers per host to the predicted impact of a selective chemotherapy programme. Second, what are the relative merits of selective treatment based on the identification of the heavily infected people at the start of the programme and the repeated treatment of the same people (labelled programme A) versus the input of selective treatment based on the repeated identification of the wormy people at each round of drug administration (labelled programme B). For the purpose of illustration we examine model predictions (based on the mean result from ten separate Monte Carlo runs, each seeded with a different sequence of pseudo-random numbers), with parameter values based on the epidemiology of *Ascaris* infection.

With respect to the first problem, Fig. 17.14 records changes in the overall mean worm burden and prevalence (over all age classes), over a period of 23 years for the treatment programme A (wormy people identified once and treatment continually focused on the same individuals). Control was initiated in year 9 and continued for 3 years, with treatment administered at 6-month intervals (a total of six rounds of selective treatment). After year 12 no further treatment was administered. The two projections denote predicted changes under the assumptions of heterogeneity generated by predisposition (labelled S) and environmental heterogeneity (labelled E). Selectivity was based on one round of identification of the 15 per cent most heavily infected individuals. Note that control programme A is predicted to have the greatest impact under the assumption that heterogeneity is generated by predisposition. This is to be expected on intuitive grounds. However, more importantly, once control ceases the rate of return of the overall mean to the pre-control level is predicted to be more rapid under the assumption of predisposition. This is a consequence of the fact that those predisposed to heavy infection more rapidly acquire parasites than the remaining individuals in the population, and thereby induce

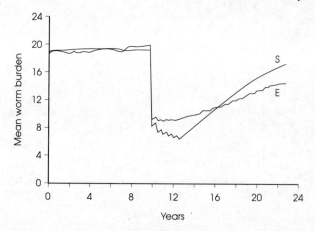

Fig. 17.14. Changes in the overall mean worm burden (over all age classes), over a period of 23 years, for treatment programme A (wormy people identified once and treatment continually focused on the same individuals) as predicted by the Monte Carlo simulation model outlined in the main text (see Anderson and Medley 1985). After year 12 no further treatment was administered. The two projections denote predicted changes under the assumptions of heterogeneity generated by predisposition (labelled S) and environmental heterogeneity (labelled E). Selectivity was based on one round of identifications of the 15 per cent most heavily infected individuals.

a quicker rise in the overall mean than is the case if parasite aggregation is determined solely by environmental heterogeneity (Anderson and Medley 1985).

A further set of results are recorded in Fig. 17.15 for a set of simulation experiments (ten runs per experiment) based on control programme B (the repeated identification of the 15 per cent most heavily infected individuals at each of the six rounds of selective treatment). The conditions of the experiment were otherwise identical to those described for Fig. 17.14. By comparison of Figs. 17.15 and 17.14 it can be seen that under both assumptions concerning the generative mechanism of heterogeneity, repeated identification of the wormy individuals leads to more effective suppression in the overall mean worm burden. The rate of return to the pre-control mean worm burden under programme B is again more rapid on the cessation of control under the assumption of predisposition. This point is more clearly illustrated in Fig. 17.16 which records the age profile of mean worm burdens under programme B for the predisposition assumption (17.16(a)) and the environmental heterogeneity assumption (17.16(b)) at three points in time during the course of the simulations. The profiles are shown for week 520 (prior to the start of control), at week 728 (at the end of the 3 years of selective treatment) and at week 1196 (after 10.5 years of reinfection following the cessation of control). Note the rapidity with which the parasite population recovers if heterogeneity is created by the predisposition assumptions. One final simulation concerned changes in

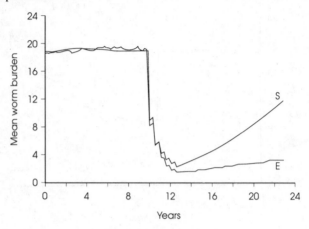

Fig. 17.15. Simulation experiments (ten runs per experiment) based on control programme B (the repeated identifications of the 15 per cent most heavily infected individuals at each of six rounds of selective treatment). The conditions of the experiment are otherwise identical to those described for Fig. 17.14.

the degree of parasite aggregation within the total community during the course of selective treatment. Variance-to-mean ratios of worm burdens per person for each of ten replicate simulation runs are recorded in Fig. 17.17, for mass treatment under the two different assumptions concerning the generation of parasite aggregation. Note that the degree of parasite contagion is only markedly reduced by mass treatment provided heterogeneity is generated by predisposition. This prediction could in principle be tested in communities in which mass treatment is applied, in order to improve current understanding of the factors that create parasite aggregation.

Many experiments are possible with this type of stochastic simulation model, and much remains to be done in this area. The central message to emerge, however, is that the generative mechanism of parasite aggregation can have an important influence on temporal changes in parasite abundance following perturbation induced by control measures. Their precise influence will depend on the type of chemotherapy programme, although such factors are likely to be of greatest significance if treatment is applied selectively. As discussed in Chapter 15, field data indicate that individuals heavily infected with helminth parasites are predisposed to this state by as yet undetermined factors. In these circumstances simulation studies suggest that the rate of return of parasite abundance to pre-control levels will be more rapid than would be the case if aggregation were largely determined by environmental factors.

More broadly, in ending this chapter on dynamics and macroparasite control, we return to the general insights produced by mathematical studies of parasite transmission. Our current understanding of macroparasite population biology seems sufficient to provide *qualitative* guidelines for the design of control based

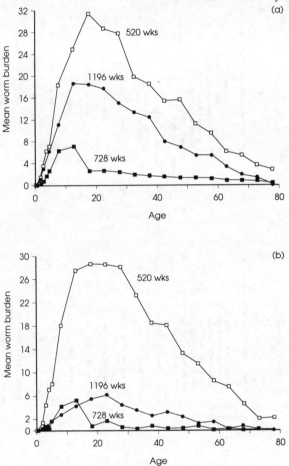

Fig. 17.16. The age profile of mean worm burden, under programme B for (a) the predisposition assumption and (b) the environmental assumption, at three points in time during the course of the simulations. The profiles are shown for week 520 (prior to the start of control), at week 728 (at the end of 3 years of selective treatment), and at week 1196 (after 10.5 years of reinfection following the cessation of control).

on chemotherapy programmes. There are some important gaps in our knowledge, such as an understanding of the factors that induce predisposition to heavy infection and the relevance (if any) of acquired immunity to helminth invasion (this topic will be examined in more detail in Chapter 18), but these are not of central importance. Since treatment confers no lasting protection to reinfection, and since eradication appears impractical unless intensive and long-lasting programmes are monitored on a national scale, the central issues in morbidity and transmission control are whom to treat, how many to treat, and how frequently should they be treated? The answers to these questions depend, to

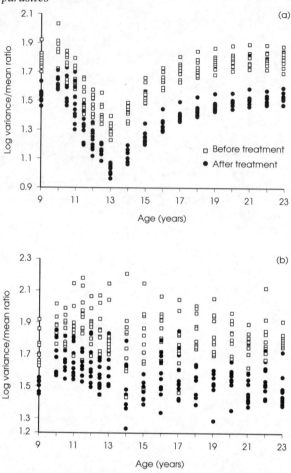

Fig. 17.17. Changes in the degree of parasite aggregation within the total community during the course of mass treatment. Variance to mean ratio of worm burdens per person, for each of 10 replicate simulation runs, are recorded under the two different assumptions concerning the generation of parasite aggregation (S = predisposition (graph (a)), E = environmental heterogeneity (graph (b))).

a large extent, on the intrinsic transmission potential of a particular helminth species. If the control of morbidity is the primary aim, selective or age-group targeted treatment should suffice; the latter is probably a more practically feasible approach. The interval between rounds of treatment should be short (3–4 months) for short-lived helminth species (i.e. *Ascaris* and *Trichuris*) in areas where the average intensity of infection increased rapidly with age before control. Greater intervals will suffice for long-lived species where intensity rises more slowly with age. For transmission control, mass treatment is clearly most beneficial, although age-group targeting is effective if changes in intensity with age are highly convex in form (such that the majority of parasites are harboured within a limited range of age groups). The choice of an interval between mass treatments is again governed by the force of transmission (i.e. the rapidity with which average intensity of infection increases with age prior to control).

The effective application of these principles, however, will depend on the availability of resources for community-based chemotherapy programmes. In terms of measurable morbidity and the risk of mortality, childhood viral and bacterial infections, such as measles and pertussis, clearly demand a high priority in health care programmes. It must be remembered, however, that helminth infections are persistent in character, such that a newborn child in an endemic area may expect to harbour helminth parasites for the majority of its life. The toll exacted by the lifelong presence of parasites is difficult to quantify at present, but commonsense argues that it must be of significance to overall community health, particularly in areas where malnutrition is prevalent.

18

Acquired immunity

18.1 Introduction

In this and the following four chapters, we turn to a series of biological complications that can have important influences on the transmission dynamics and population regulation of macroparasites. The first is that of acquired immunity. As mentioned in Chapter 15, this topic is one of much current debate. Unlike many microparasitic organisms, helminths do not induce sterile immunity to reinfection following primary exposure. Acquired host responses, however, can act to reduce rates of parasite establishment, fecundity, and survival as demonstrated by a large body of experimental work based on laboratory rodent–helminth systems (see Mitchell 1979; Dean 1983, Wakelin 1984). Current controversy centres on whether or not such laboratory work, being primarily based on rodent models, is of any relevance to what happens in human infections (see Warren 1973; Anderson and May 1985d). Convex patterns of change in the average intensity of infection with human age in areas of endemic helminth infection may be due to the build-up of acquired immunity in the older age groups or alternatively it may simply be a consequence of age-related changes in exposure to infection, or a combination of both processes (Figs. 15.20, 15.21). Following chemotherapeutic treatment rates of reinfection are often rapid, particularly in the case of directly transmitted nematodes such as *Ascaris* and *Trichuris*, even in the older age groups (Fig. 15.24). This argues against an important role for acquired immunity. Conversely, however, reinfection rates tend to be lower in the older as opposed to the younger age groups. But here again this may be due to acquired immunity or to age-related contact with infective stages.

We believe that acquired immunity does play an important role in human communities although it is probable that the observed convexity in age–intensity profiles arises via the concomitant action of immunological and ecological processes. The significance of immunity is probably related to the form of the parasite's life cycle. It is likely to be of greatest significance to those helminths that inhabit the circulatory systems of the human host at some stage in their life cycles (i.e. the schistosomes, filarial worms, and larval *Ascaris*) or feed on blood or the epithelial lining of the intestinal tract (i.e. hookworms and *Trichuris*).

Current evidence from laboratory host–macroparasite systems suggests that the severity of acquired responses (in their action to reduce parasite survival, establishment, or fecundity) is related in some manner to the host's accumulated experience of infection. In other words the constraints on survival, fecundity, and establishment are not simply related to current parasite load (which would give simple density dependence) but depend on the summed past experience of either exposure and/or worm load. The fact that a current response depends on past experience implies the existence of immunological memory. How perfect this is (i.e. whether all past experiences of infection are 'memorized' or only those that were experienced relatively recently) will vary according to the species of parasite and host. Humans appear, in general, to possess long-lasting memory of simple antigens (such as those expressed by many viral microparasites) but relatively short immunological memory (i.e. not lifelong) of more antigenically complex parasitic organisms such as helminths (Wakelin 1984; Roitt 1988). Any formal description of the dynamics of helminth transmission under the impact of acquired immunity must therefore encompass dependencies of parasite survival, establishment, and fecundity on past experience of infection plus the notion of immunological memory.

18.2 Models for immune suppression of parasite establishment

Recent research has begun to address the problem of formulating models. We base our analyses on this work (Anderson and May 1985*d*; Anderson 1985, 1986; Berding *et al.* 1986). We begin by assuming that acquired immunity acting to reduce the rate of parasitic establishment within the human host at time t, $\Lambda(t, M)$, is linearly related to the accumulated past experience of adult worms, $s(t, a)$ where

$$s(t, a) = \int_0^a M(a', t) \, \mathrm{d}a'. \tag{18.1}$$

Here $M(a, t)$ denotes the mean worm burden of hosts of age a at time t and $s(t, a)$ denotes the sum of all past worm loads experienced by hosts of age a at time t. For simplicity we initially assume that the relationship between Λ and s is of the form

$$\Lambda(t, a) = \Lambda_0(t)\left(1 - \varepsilon \int_0^a M(t, a') \exp[-\sigma(a - a')] \, \mathrm{d}a'\right). \tag{18.2}$$

Here Λ_0 denotes the pristine rate of infection at time t in the absence of past experience of infection, ε is a constant denoting the severity of the acquired immunological response, and the term $\exp[-\sigma(a - a')]$ describes immunological memory. Here memory is assumed to have an average duration of $1/\sigma$ time units ($\sigma = 0$ for lifelong immunity; $\sigma \to \infty$ for no acquired immunity).

Dynamic changes in $M(a, t)$ with respect to time and host age can be examined within the age-structured macroparasite model defined in Chapter 16 by replacing the $\Lambda(a)$ in eqn (16.44) by the $\Lambda(t, a)$ defined by eqn ((18.2) above. This gives

$$\partial M(t, a)/\partial t + \partial M(t, a)/\partial a = \Lambda(t, a) - \mu_1 M(t, a). \tag{18.3}$$

If we assume that, apart from the action of acquired immunity on parasite establishment, no other density-dependent constraints affect parasite population growth within a host, then the Λ_0 of eqn (18.2) is

$$\Lambda_0(t) = \left(R_0\mu_1 \int_0^\infty \ell(a)M(a, t)\, \mathrm{d}a\right)\left(\int_0^\infty \ell(a)\, \mathrm{d}a\right)^{-1}, \qquad (18.4)$$

where $\ell(a)$ is the probability that a person survives to age a and L is human life expectancy ($L = \int_0^\infty \ell(a)\, \mathrm{d}a$).

At equilibrium ($\partial M(a, t)/\partial t = 0$), the age distribution of mean worm loads, $M^*(a)$, is defined by

$$\mathrm{d}M^*(a)/\mathrm{d}a = \Lambda_0^*\left(1 - \varepsilon \int_0^a M^*(a')\exp[-\sigma(a - a')]\, \mathrm{d}a'\right) - \mu_1 M^*(a), \quad (18.5)$$

where

$$\Lambda_0^* = R_0\mu_1 \bar{M}^*. \qquad (18.6)$$

Here $\bar{M}^*$ is the equilibrium mean worm burden in the total population

$$\bar{M}^* = \left(\int_0^\infty \ell(a)M^*(a)\, \mathrm{d}a\right)\left(\int_0^\infty \ell(a)\, \mathrm{d}a\right)^{-1} \qquad (18.7)$$

For $(\mu_1 - \sigma)^2 > 4\varepsilon\Lambda_0^*$, the solution of eqn (18.5) is

$$M^*(a) = C + \frac{\Lambda_0^*}{\lambda}\left[\left(\frac{p_1 + \sigma}{p_1}\right)\exp(p_1 a) - \left(\frac{p_2 + \sigma}{p_2}\right)\exp(p_2 a)\right], \quad (18.8)$$

where $\lambda = [(\mu_1 - \sigma)^2 - 4\varepsilon\Lambda_0^*]^{1/2}$, $p_1 = -(\mu_1 + \sigma - \lambda)/2$, $p_2 = -(\mu_1 + \sigma + \lambda)/2$ and $C = \Lambda_0^*\sigma/(\sigma\mu_1 + \varepsilon\Lambda_0^*)$. Alternatively, when $(\mu_1 - \sigma)^2 < 4\varepsilon\Lambda_0^*$,

$$M^*(a) = C + \exp[-(\mu_1 + \sigma)a/2]$$

$$\times \left\{\frac{2\Lambda_0^*}{\theta}\left[1 - \frac{C(\mu_1 + \sigma)}{2\Lambda_0^*}\right]\sin\left(\frac{a\theta}{2}\right) - C\cos\left(\frac{a\theta}{2}\right)\right\}, \quad (18.9)$$

where $\theta = [4\varepsilon\Lambda_0^* - (\mu_1 - \sigma)^2]^{1/2}$ and C is as defined for eqn (18.8). The overall equilibrium worm burden $\bar{M}^*$ can be obtained from eqns (18.8) and (18.9) where, under the assumption of Type II human survivorship (death rate $\hat{\mu}$ constant and independent of age),

$$\bar{M}^* = \frac{\Lambda_0^*(\hat{\mu} + \sigma)}{[(\hat{\mu} + \mu_1)(\hat{\mu} + \sigma) + \varepsilon\Lambda_0^*]}. \qquad (18.10)$$

Thus with eqn (18.6) we obtain an expression for the pristine rate of infection at equilibrium, Λ_0^*, where

$$\Lambda_0^* = [(\sigma + \hat{\mu})/\varepsilon][R_0\mu_1 - (\hat{\mu} + \mu_1)]. \qquad (18.11)$$

Since parasite life expectancy $(1/\mu_1)$ is much less than human life expectancy $(1/\bar{\mu})$, eqn (18.11) reduces to

$$\Lambda_0^* \simeq \mu_1(\sigma + \bar{\mu})(R_0 - 1)/\varepsilon. \tag{18.12}$$

The solution defined by eqns (18.8), (18.9), and (18.12) enables us to explore the equilibrium profile of changes in mean worm load with age under various assumptions concerning the severity and longevity of acquired immunity. Before doing so, however, it is important to note that the assumption of a linear relation between the rate of establishment and the accumulated past experience of adult worms is rather crude. If ε is large in relation to Λ_0 this assumption could result in negative establishment rates! In biological terms this can be interpreted as very strong immunity which acts both to decrease parasite establishment and increase mortality. In practice, however, it seems likely that the value of ε will be very small such that this situation is unlikely to arise.

The model can mimic a wide range of patterns of change in worm load with age, including: monotonic increase in $M^*(a)$ to a stable plateau; $M^*(a)$ peaking within childhood, teenage, or early adult age groups, and then declining; and damped oscillations in intensity with age (Fig. 18.1). For a fixed severity of the acquired response, ε, the intensity profile tends to be convex if immunological memory is long, and/or transmission is intense (i.e. R_0 large), and/or worm life expectancy is long ($1/\mu_1$ large). The age at which a maximum average worm load is attained depends primarily on the life expectancy of the worm $1/\mu_1$, and the severity of acquired immunity, ε.

The damped oscillations in worm burdens that can be produced under appropriate circumstances derive from essentially the same mechanisms that can produce oscillations in the incidence of microparasitic infections, such as measles, within populations (see Chapter 6).

Although crude parameter estimates are available for R_0 and μ_1 (see Tables 16.2 and 16.3), virtually nothing is known about the possible values of ε and σ for the major helminth infections of humans. However, one qualitative prediction of the model, namely, that the convexity of an age–intensity profile for a given species should be related to the net intensity of transmission within a community is, in principle, testable against field observations. A series of average intensity versus age profiles for two different parasites, hookworm and *Schistosoma mansoni*, are displayed in Fig. 18.2. There appears to be a positive association between the form of transmission (as measured by rapidity with which intensity rises in the child age classes) and the degree of convexity in these examples. This observation provides some support for the notion that acquired immunity is of relevance to the transmission dynamics of human helminths (Anderson and May 1985d; Anderson 1986, 1987). Further tests of model predictions come from laboratory experiments with rodent–helminth systems where the hosts are continually exposed to repeated infection (termed trickle infections; see Crombie and Anderson (1985) and Slater and Keymer (1986)). This approach is examined in Chapter 21.

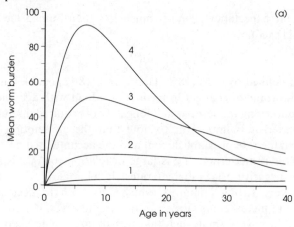

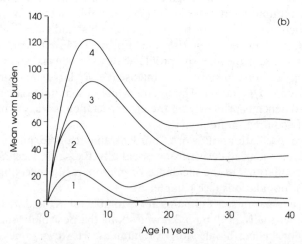

Fig. 18.1. Predicted changes in the average intensity of infection with age under varying assumptions concerning the severity and duration of acquired resistance to infection. (a) Predictions generated by eqn (18.8) with parameter values $\mu_1 = 0.33$ yr^{-1}, $\sigma = 0.001$ yr^{-1}, $\varepsilon = 0.005$, $\Lambda_0 = 6.6$ yr^{-1}, $1/\mu_2 = 50$ years. Four different simulations are recorded for varying values of R_0: in (4) $R_0 = 4$, in (3) $R_0 = 2.5$, in (2) $R_0 = 1.5$, and in (1) $R_0 = 1.1$. (b) Predictions generated by eqn (18.9) with parameter value $\mu_1 = 0.2$ yr^{-1}. Parameter values for trajectories (1) to (4) are: (1), $\sigma = 0.05$ yr^{-1}, $\varepsilon = 0.009$, $R_0 = 7.5$, $\Lambda_0 = 9.95$ yr^{-1}; (2), $\sigma = 0.1$ yr^{-1}, $\varepsilon = 0.004$, $R_0 = 6.0$, $\Lambda_0 = 30.0$ yr^{-1}; (3), $\sigma = 0.05$ yr^{-1}, $\varepsilon = 0.001$, $R_0 = 3.15$, $\Lambda_0 = 30.1$ yr^{-1}; (4), $\sigma = 0.09$ yr^{-1}, $\varepsilon = 0.001$, $R_0 = 3.0$, $\Lambda_0 = 44.0$ yr^{-1}.

How dependent are the patterns predicted by eqn (18.5) on the assumption concerning the mode of action of acquired immunity? This question can be examined either by changing the assumption of a linear dependency of the force of infection on past experience, by considering models in which acquired immunity acts on worm mortality as opposed to establishment, or by assuming

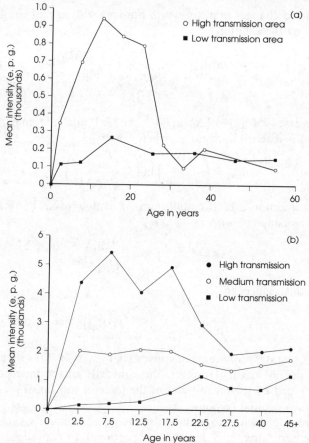

Fig. 18.2. Observed patterns of age-related change in the average intensity of infection (horizontal cross-sectional profiles). (a) Schistosome infection in areas of high and low transmission intensity. Intensity measured by eggs per gram of faeces (Kato technique). Source references provided in Anderson and May (1985*d*). (b) Hookworm infection in communities with high, medium, and low intensities of transmission. The indirect measure of hookworm burden (intensity) is mean eggs per gram of faeces. Source references provided in Anderson (1986). Note how in both (a) and (b) the intensity profiles become more convex in areas of high transmission intensity.

that immunity is related to past exposure as opposed to past adult worm loads. For example, we could assume that $\Lambda(t, a)$ decays linearly as the accumulated sum of past exposure to infection rises, such that

$$\Lambda(t, a) = \Lambda_0(t) \left(1 - \Delta \int_0^a \Lambda_0(t) \exp[-\sigma(a - a')] \, \mathrm{d}a' \right), \tag{18.13}$$

where Δ defines the severity of the acquired response.

The predicted changes in mean worm burdens with age, at equilibrium, are now defined by the solution

$$M^*(a) = \frac{\Lambda_0^*}{\mu_1}\left[[1 - \exp(-\mu_1 a)]\left(1 + \frac{\Delta\Lambda_0^*}{\mu_1 - \sigma}\right) - \frac{\Delta\Lambda_0^*\mu_1}{\sigma(\mu_1 - \sigma)}[1 - \exp(-\sigma a)]\right].$$

(18.14)

As age increases $M^*(a) \rightarrow [\Lambda_0^*/\mu_1][1 - \Delta\Lambda_0^*/\sigma]$ and the maximum mean parasite load is reached at age $a_{\max}$, where

$$a_{\max} = \left(\frac{1}{\mu_1 - \sigma}\right)\ln\left(1 - \frac{\mu_1 - \sigma}{\Delta\Lambda_0^*}\right).$$

(18.15)

The pristine infection rate at equilibrium Λ_0^* is now given by (for a Type II human survivorship curve)

$$\Lambda_0^* = \frac{\hat{\mu} + \sigma}{\Delta}\left(1 - \frac{\hat{\mu} + \mu_1}{R_0\mu_1}\right).$$

(18.16)

For $\mu_1 \gg \hat{\mu}$ this reduces to

$$\Lambda_0^* = \left(\frac{\hat{\mu} + \sigma}{\Delta}\right)[1 - (1/R_0)].$$

(18.17)

This model generates monotonic or convex changes in $M^*(a)$ with age; damped oscillations do not occur. However, the convexity of the intensity profile is again determined by the magnitudes of the force of transmission, R_0, and the severity of the acquired response, Δ.

A different approach is to assume that acquired immunity acts to increase adult worm mortality in a manner proportional to the accumulated past experience of adult parasites. In these circumstances the equilibrium age distribution of worm loads can be described by the following equation

$$dM^*(a)/da = \Lambda_0^* - \left(\mu_1\int_0^a \exp[-\sigma(a - a')]M^*(a')\,da'\right)M^*(a).$$

(18.18)

Numerical studies of this equation reveal that monotonic or convex patterns of change in average worm load with age occur for a wide range of parameter values (see Fig. 18.3).

More complex assumptions concerning the precise dependence of immunity on past experience of infection can of course be included in such models. An example is given by Berding *et al.* (1986) in a study of acquired immunity in mice to repeated exposure to an intestinal nematode, *Nematospiroides dubius*. For this experimental system, immunity appears to act to decrease adult worm survival in a manner non-linearly dependent on past exposure to infection by larval stages of the parasite. These authors argued that the function was S-shaped in form, such that the severity of the response had a threshold, being

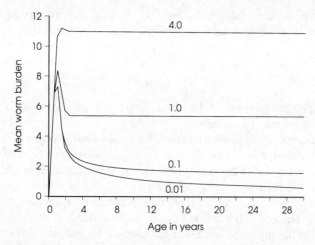

Fig. 18.3. Numerical evaluations of eqn (18.18) in which past experience of infection is assumed to increase the death rate of the parasite, in a manner related to the accumulated past experience of infection. Parameter values $\Lambda_0 = 12.0 \text{ yr}^{-1}$, $\mu_1 = 1.0 \text{ yr}^{-1}$ with the value of σ varied from 4.0, 1.0, 0.1 to 0.01 (all yr^{-1}).

absent for low levels of past exposure and rising rapidly to a maximum severity for high levels of past experience. The comparison of their model prediction with experimental data is briefly commented upon in Chapter 21.

The general conclusions to emerge from these approaches to describing acquired immunity to macroparasites is that convexity in change of mean worm burden with age can be generated by a wide variety of assumptions concerning the mode of action of the acquired response. Empirical evidence for which one of these assumptions is relevant to a particular parasitic infection of humans is not available at present. However, observations which show an association between the degree of convexity and transmission intensity (Fig. 18.1) suggest that they are of importance within human communities. The partial herd immunity created by such mechanisms can act as a very effective regulatory constraint on parasite population growth within the host community, even in the absence of other mechanisms such as density-dependent fecundity.

18.3 Acquired immunity and control

Under the belief that acquired responses to helminth infection are of epidemiological significance, we now briefly turn to the question of control by either mass chemotherapy or vaccination. In the case of mass chemotherapy, eradication requires the reduction of the effective reproductive rate, R, to less than unity. For example, in the case of the models in which acquired responses were assumed to decrease establishment in direct proportion to past worm loads (eqn (18.5)), chemotherapy will act to increase the adult worm mortality rate, say from μ_1 to $\bar{\mu}_1$. The relationship between $\bar{\mu}_1$ and the proportion of people treated per unit of time, g, and drug efficacy, h, is as defined by eqn (16.27) (where $\bar{\mu}_1$ replaces c). To reduce the effective reproductive rate below unity we simply require (given $\hat{\mu} \ll \mu_1$)

$$\bar{\mu}_1 = \mu_1 R_0. \tag{18.19}$$

Eradication is clearly more difficult to achieve if the parasite has a high transmission efficiency (R_0 large).

If chemotherapy is applied at a rate less than that required for parasite eradication, control may act perversely to increase average worm loads in the older age classes above the levels pertaining prior to treatment. This phenomenon is directly analogous to that described for the impact of mass vaccination on the age distribution of viral and bacterial infections (see Chapter 4). For helminths, the change in the shape of the profile under low to moderate levels of mass chemotherapy arises as a consequence of the induction of lower levels of acquired immunity in the older age classes due to a reduced intensity of transmission (i.e. less past experience of infection). Reduced immunity implies higher worm loads. This issue is illustrated graphically in Fig. 18.4 by a series

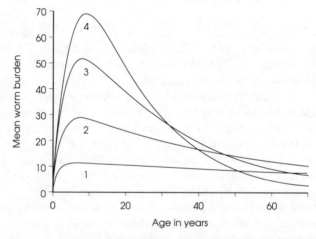

Fig. 18.4. Impact of chemotherapy on the intensity of infection in different age classes. The numerical simulations represent a homogeneous population (with respect to immunological responsiveness and exposure to infection) in which drug treatment is applied randomly (independent of parasite load) and repeatedly. The four curves denote the equilibrium age–intensity profile for the precontrol situation (curve 4) and three levels of drug application which increases the overall death rate of the parasite within the population from $\mu = 0.25$ (curve 4) to $\mu = 0.33$ (curve 3), $\mu = 0.5$ (curve 2) and $\mu = 0.75$ (curve 1) (all yr^{-1}). Other parameter values, $1/\mu_2 = 70$ years, $\varepsilon = 0.005$, $\sigma = 0.001$, $R_0 = 1.44$ (when $\mu = 0.75$), $R_0 = 2.15$ (when $\mu = 0.5$), $R_0 = 3.19$ (when $\mu = 0.33$), and $R_0 = 4.16$ (when $\mu = 0.25$). Note that at high levels of drug treatment (μ large) the intensity of infection in the older classes can exceed that prevailing in the pre-control curve.

of numerical examples based on changing the value of the death rate parameter in eqn (18.5). Note that for the higher levels of drug treatment (high values of $\bar{\mu}_1$) the average worm load at equilibrium in the older age classes (after many decades of mass treatment) rises above the level pertaining prior to control ($\bar{\mu}_1 = 0$). The overall mean, $\bar{M}^*$, is of course reduced by treatment. In practice this problem is unlikely to be of great significance to the control of morbidity induced by intestinal helminth infection since symptoms of disease are more common in young children as opposed to adults. However, it is as well to be aware of this possibility when designing or monitoring repeated mass treatment programmes in situations where infection normally induces a degree of acquired immunity in adults.

With respect to vaccination, theoretical analysis is very speculative at present since vaccines are unavailable for protection against infection by macroparasites. However, it is not unreasonable to assume that the first generation of products will only provide partial protection to reinfection (by reducing, but not preventing, parasite establishment or survival). We examine the potential impact of such vaccines by the use of the model defined in eqn (18.5), in which acquired immunity acts on parasite establishment in a manner linearly dependent on past worm burdens.

Suppose the vaccine consists of a quantity of parasite antigens (either genetically engineered or manufactured from live or killed parasites), which when injected act to reduce parasite establishment in a manner directly analogous to the action of past experience of adult worms in the unvaccinated individual. We define the immunogeneity of the vaccine as V, with units of single worm antigen equivalents. At equilibrium in a vaccinated community the rate of change in worm load with age, $M^*(a)$, can be defined as

$$dM^*(a)/da = \Lambda_0^* \left(1 - \varepsilon \int_0^a \exp[-\sigma(a - a')](M^*(a') + V(a')) \, da' \right) - \mu_1 M^*(a).$$

(18.20)

Assumed here is that the efficacy of the vaccine, ε, and the length of immunological memory it induces, $1/\sigma$, is identical to that created by an equivalent antigenic load acquired by natural infection. The term $V(a)$ is defined as a function of age to denote changes in the rate of vaccination with host age. We could also consider vaccination within discrete age classes (denoted by a_i) such that

$$\int_0^a V(a') \exp[-\sigma(a - a')] \, da' \rightarrow \sum_{i=1}^n V_i \exp[-\sigma(a_n - a_i)].$$ (18.21)

Here V_i denotes the age specific vaccination rate for individuals in age class i. Under these circumstances, the pristine rate of infection at equilibrium, Λ_0^*, is given (for Type II survival) by

$$\Lambda_0^* = \frac{(\hat{\mu} + \sigma)}{\varepsilon} \left[R_0 \mu_1 \left(1 - \frac{\varepsilon \hat{\mu}}{(\hat{\mu} + \sigma)} \sum_i V_i \exp(-\hat{\mu} a_i) \right) - (\mu_1 + \hat{\mu}) \right].$$ (18.22)

The effective reproductive rate will fall below unity, and eradication will be achieved, once the expression within the square brackets in eqn (18.22) becomes negative (corresponding to a negative infection rate). Consider two examples. Suppose vaccination is only given to individuals in their first year of life, at a rate V_1. Then for $\hat{\mu} \ll \mu_1$, we require

$$\varepsilon V_1 > \left(\frac{\hat{\mu} + \sigma}{\hat{\mu}}\right)[1 - (1/R_0)]. \qquad (18.23)$$

Alternatively, if vaccination takes place at random (independent of age) at a rate r, where the average time between inoculations is $1/r$, then

$$\varepsilon V r > (\hat{\mu} + \sigma)[1 - (1/R_0)]. \qquad (18.24)$$

Note the similarity of both expressions (18.23) and (18.24) to those derived for microparasites (Chapter 5). In the case of microparasites, vaccines were assumed to create lifelong protection and to generate sterile immunity, while for macroparasites the vaccine is assumed only partially to protect against parasite establishment and any protection achieved has a defined lifespan (of order $1/\sigma$). For microparasities the eradication criterion only involves R_0 and the proportion to be vaccinated p, while for macroparasites it involves the rate of vaccination, r, the strength, V, and the efficacy, ε, of the vaccine along with R_0 (eqn (18.24)).

When the properties of a potential macroparasite vaccine are known (Johnson et al. 1989), these types of models should help to define how best to create herd immunity within the community as a whole. To minimize the proportion to be vaccinated, or the rate of vaccination (for a given value of R_0), it is clearly desirable to maximize both the immunogeneity of the vaccine (the strength V and efficacy ε) and the duration of protection created ($1/\sigma$).

19

Heterogeneity within the human community

The importance of heterogeneity within the host community, with respect to the way in which individual people either are exposed to infection or respond to parasite invasion, has been alluded to in the three previous chapters. The overt manifestation of its relevance is aggregation in the frequency distribution of parasite numbers per person (see Fig. 15.17 and Table 15.5). We have already seen how a clumped distribution enhances the net impact of density-dependent constraints on parasite population growth, influences the likelihood that female worms find mates within hosts, affects the design of control programmes based on chemotherapeutic treatment to reduce morbidity and transmission, and determines the observed relationship between the two main epidemiological statistics, prevalence and average intensity of infection.

In this chapter we examine, in somewhat more detail, how heterogeneity affects the way in which we interpret observed epidemiological patterns. A hint of how variability in exposure to infection can be incorporated in model structure was given in Chapter 16. We now consider a more general approach to this problem.

19.1 Host heterogeneity and parasite clumping

To start, consider the simple immigration–death model of adult parasite recruitment and loss in an individual host, described by eqn (16.1). Suppose the human community (of constant size N) is divided into a series of groups (numbering s) such that the number in group i is N_i and the fraction in group i is f_i ($f_i = N_i/N$). Further assume that the immigration and death rates of the parasite are constant within a group but vary between groups, where Λ_i and μ_i define the rates for group i.

The rate of change in the worm burden in each individual in group i, $P_i(t)$, with respect to time is

$$dP_i(t)/dt = \Lambda_i - \mu_i P_i(t). \tag{19.1}$$

The equivalent stochastic model of this immigration–death process predicts that the probability distribution of parasite numbers per person at any time t is Poisson (=random) in form with equal mean and variance ($E\{P_i(t)\} = V\{P_i(t)\} = M_i(t)$), where

$$M_i(t) = [\Lambda_i/\mu_i][1 - \exp(-\mu_i t)]. \tag{19.2}$$

The probability distribution of parasite numbers within the total host community is formed from the mixture of a series of Poisson variates each with a different mean (eqn (19.2)). The probability generating function (p.g.f.) $\pi(i, z, t)$, for the distribution of parasites per person in group i at time t is simply

$$\pi(i, z, t) = \exp[M_i(t)(z - 1)]. \tag{19.3}$$

The p.g.f. for the total community, $H(z, t)$ is therefore

$$H(z, t) = \sum_{i=1}^{s} f_i \pi(i, z, t). \tag{19.4}$$

To take a simple case, if we let $s = 2$ where $N_1/N = f$ and $N_2/N = 1 - f$ then the mean and variance of the Poisson mixture distribution, $E\{P(t)\}$ and $V\{P(t)\}$ respectively, are

$$E\{P(t)\} = M_1(t)f + M_2(t)(1 - f), \tag{19.5}$$

$$V\{P(t)\} = E\{P(t)\} + f(1 - f)(M_1(t) - M_2(t))^2. \tag{19.6}$$

The variance to mean ratio, V/E, is therefore

$$V/E = 1 + \frac{f(1 - f)(M_1(t) - M_2(t))^2}{f M_1(t) + (1 - f)M_2(t)}. \tag{19.7}$$

The value exceeds unity and hence the parasites are aggregated or clumped within the total host community. This very simple example demonstrates that heterogeneity in exposure/establishment (Λ_i) and/or in adult parasite mortality (μ_i) within the host, can induce aggregated distributions of worm numbers per person. Such heterogeneity may be induced by environmental, behavioural, immunological, or genetic factors, or some combination of them.

Within an age-structured host community the simple immigration–death model of parasite abundance defined by eqn (19.1) can be adapted to mirror the equilibrium age distribution of worm loads by simply replacing the time variable t by the age variable a. This adaptation allows us to ask how the degree of parasite aggregation changes with age in a community with stable endemic infection.

First suppose that the death rate μ is constant and independent of host-group membership (i.e. heterogeneity is simply generated by variation in Λ_i among groups). In this case the degree of parasite aggregation, as measured by the variance to mean ratio, or the negative binomial clumping parameter k (where $k = VP(a)/(VP(a) - EP(a))$), remains *constant* and independent of age. Alternatively, if we hold Λ constant among groups and only allow μ to vary then the degree of parasite aggregation increases with age (k decreases with age). In general if both Λ and μ vary among groups then at $a \to 0$ (in the very young age classes)

$$k \to (E\{\Lambda\})^2/[E\{\Lambda^2\} - (E\{\Lambda\})^2], \tag{19.8}$$

while at $a \to \infty$ (the very old age classes),

$$k \to (E\{\Lambda/\mu\})^2/[E\{(\Lambda/\mu)^2\} - (E\{\Lambda/\mu\})^2]. \tag{19.9}$$

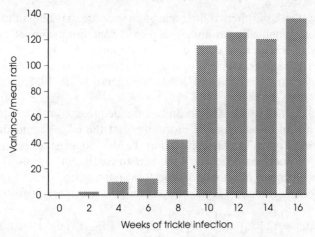

Fig. 19.1. The dynamics of *Nematospiroides dubius* in adult male MF1 mice subject to a trickle infection of 52 ± 3 larvae every 2 weeks. The graph records the change through time in the variance to mean ratio of worms per mouse (from Keymer 1985).

A rather nice illustration of the way in which aggregation changes with host age is provided by a series of experiments described by Keymer (1985) in which groups of mice were subjected to constant weekly rates of infection by the gut nematode *Nematospiroides dubius* over long periods of time. During the course of the 'trickle' exposure to infection, it was observed that the degree of parasite aggregation (measured by the variance-to-mean ratio) within samples of mice dissected at various intervals past the start of exposure to infection was increasing as the mice aged and the duration of exposure increased (Fig. 19.1). Subsequently, it was discovered that the outbred mice used in the experiment consisted, broadly speaking, of two genetic types: 'high responders' in which parasite life expectancy was short and 'low responders' in which the parasite survived well. The genetically based heterogeneity in the host's ability to influence parasite survival induced the observed changes in parasite aggregation, as predicted by our simple immigration–death model.

19.2 Acquired immunity and parasite distribution

We can easily extend these simple models of heterogeneous host exposure to infection and parasite survival, to discuss more complex situations that arise when acquired immunity plays a role in the regulation of parasite abundance. An important reason for doing so is the growing body of experimental evidence that points to the importance of the host's genetic background (sometimes mediated by nutritional status) as a determinant of the ability of mammalian species to mount effective immunological responses to macroparasitic invasion (see Wakelin 1978, 1986). Much of this work is based on rodent–helminth laboratory systems, but there is little reason to suppose that human populations will be any less genetically variable with respect to immunocompetence. Indeed a large body of research, in connection with human microparasitic infections, suggests that genetic factors are of major significance as determinants of the course of infection (Lindenmann 1964; Weatherall *et al.* 1988; Wakelin and Blackwell 1988).

The model defined by eqn (18.5) can be extended to encompass heterogeneity in exposure to infection, parasite mortality, and the efficacy and duration of acquired immunity. Such variability may be due to genetic, environmental, behavioural, or nutritional factors. If the human community consists of *s* groups when group *i* forms a fraction f_i of the total population, then at equilibrium the mean worm burden in people of age *a* in group *i*, $M_i(a)$, is given by

$$\mathrm{d}M_i^*(a)/\mathrm{d}a = \Lambda_{0i}^* \left(1 - \varepsilon_i \int_0^a M_i^*(a') \exp[-\sigma_i(a - a')]\, \mathrm{d}a' \right) - \mu_{1i} M_i^*(a).$$

(19.10)

It is assumed that acquired immunity acts to decrease parasite establishment in a manner directly proportional to the accumulated past experience of infection and that the exposure to infection, Λ_{0i}^*, the severity of the acquired response, ε_i, the duration of immunological memory, σ_i, and parasite mortality, μ_i, differ among groups of hosts. The exposure rate Λ_{0i}^* is obviously a function of the mean worm burden, $\bar{M}^*$, within all groups and age classes.

In a similar manner to that described in Chapter 18 (see eqns (18.6) and (18.10)) it is possible to derive an expression for $\bar{M}^*$ (and hence any one Λ_{0i}^*) in terms of the relevant basic reproductive rates within each group of the host population (the R_{0i}s) and the other population parameters incorporated in eqn (19.10). For example if we assume that parasite fecundity and the rate of contact with infective stages is constant and independent of group membership then

$$\Lambda_{0i}^* = R_{0i} \mu_{1i} \sum_{j=1}^s \frac{f_j \Lambda_{0j}^* (\sigma_j + \hat{\mu})}{(\hat{\mu} + \mu_{1j})(\hat{\mu} + \sigma_j) + \varepsilon_j \Lambda_{0j}^*}.$$

(19.11)

It is here assumed that human survivorship is Type II and that the rate of mortality μ is the same within all groups. Equation (19.11) can be expressed in terms of the overall mean $\bar{M}^*$ where

$$1 = \sum_{j=1}^s \frac{f_j R_{0j} (\hat{\mu} + \sigma_j)}{\hat{\mu} + \sigma_j + \varepsilon_j R_{0j} \bar{M}^*}.$$

(19.12)

19.3 Heterogeneity and control

With respect to control by vaccination (along the lines outlined in Chapter 18; see eqns (18.21), (18.23), (18.24)) or chemotherapy (which acts to increase the μ_is), eradication requires that the rates of infection, Λ_{0i}^*, all tend to zero simultaneously. This condition is reminiscent of that discussed in Chapter 10 on the control of microparasitic infections by vaccination in heterogeneous populations (caused by spatial, genetic, or other factors); see eqns (10.28)–(10.30).

In order to gain a more detailed understanding of how heterogeneity can influence either observed patterns of change in mean worm burden with age or the design of control programmes, we turn to a few simple numerical examples. Specifically, we consider two groups of people ($s = 2$) who are respectively 'wormy' ($i = 1$) and 'non-wormy' ($i = 2$), as a consequence of differences in the respective population parameters that control the magnitudes of the mean worm burdens. 'Worminess' or 'non-worminess' may be due to a variety of factors, such as genetic background or behaviour. However, there is no need to specify the precise cause in our deterministic models in order to gain a broad understanding of the consequences of heterogeneity. In line with observation (see Chapter 15), the wormy and non-wormy groups are predisposed to their respective states since the model assumes that group membership does not change as people age.

Numerical studies reveal that even a two-group model ($s = 2$) is able to generate a bewilderingly large array of different patterns of change in the overall mean $\bar{M}^*(a)$ with age. A few examples are recorded in Fig. 19.2 for various combinations of parameter values. Observation suggests that the wormy fraction of a population is usually of the order of 10–20 per cent of the total community (i.e. the percentage that harbours 70–80 per cent of the total worm population) (see Fig. 15.17). Our model suggests that the pattern of changes in $M_1^*(a)$ in this group can mask within the overall mean $\bar{M}^*(a)$ the build-up of strong acquired immunity (i.e. $M_2^*(a) \to 0$ as a becomes large) in the non-wormy majority of the population. Such patterns may induce complex changes in the degree of parasite aggregation as individuals age (Table 15.6). Depending on the values of the parameters, and the relative dominance of 'wormy' or 'non-wormy' people in the population, the tendency may be either for k (the negative binomial parameter) to increase or decrease with age. Observed patterns, which admittedly form a limited data base at present, suggest that k typically rises slightly in the older age groups (i.e. aggregation decreases) (Anderson 1980). Such patterns can arise if the dominant proportion of the population have low worm burdens, given that a degree of acquired immunity is built up in the older individuals who are predisposed to the 'wormy' state (Fig. 19.3).

With respect to control, these models provide some general insights into two particular issues. The first concerns selective chemotherapy aimed at the wormy fraction of the population. The model can be employed to assess just how beneficial this approach is, relative to mass treatment. A numerical example is presented in Fig. 19.4 in which the proportional reduction in the overall mean worm burden $\bar{M}^*$ (over both groups and all age classes) relative to its pre-control value is displayed as a function of the additional adult parasite death

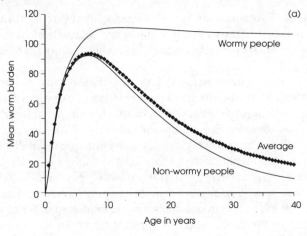

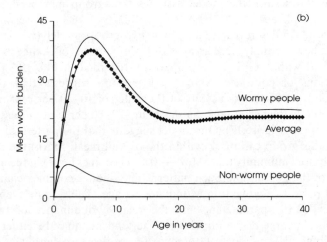

Fig. 19.2. Numerical studies of a two-group model ($s = 2$, see text) that record changes with age in the overall mean worm burden, $M^*(a)$, the mean burden in the wormy segment of the population, $M_1^*(a)$, and the mean burden in the non-wormy segment, $M_2^*(a)$. In graphs (a) and (b) the symbolled line denotes the overall mean, while the top line is the mean in the wormy segment and the bottom line is the mean in the non-wormy segment. (a) This example mirrors a population in which the wormy people constitute 10 per cent of the population ($f_1 = 0.1$) and are characterized by a short immunological memory ($\sigma_1 > \sigma_2$). Parameter values: $\mu_{12} = \mu_{11} = 0.33$, $\sigma_1 = 0.1$, $\sigma_2 = 0.00001$, $\varepsilon_1 = 0.001$, $\varepsilon_2 = 0.0005$, $\mu_{21} = \mu_{22} = 0.02$, $R_{01} = 1.1$, $R_{02} = 4.0$ (all yr^{-1}). (b) This example is similar to (a) but the dominant proportion of the population ($f_1 = 0.9$) are poor immunological responders to infection with a low rate of acquisition of immunity ($\varepsilon_1 = 0.003$) when compared with the small fraction ($f_2 = 0.1$) of good responders ($\varepsilon_2 = 0.02$). Parameter values: $\mu_{11} = 0.25$, $\mu_{12} = 1.0$, $\sigma_1 = \sigma_2 = 0.1$, $\mu_{21} = \mu_{22} = 0.02$, $R_{01} = R_{02} = 2.7$ (from Anderson and May 1985*d*).

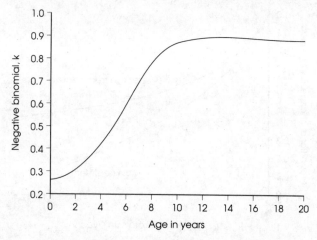

Fig. 19.3. Predicted changes with age in the negative binomial parameter k for the two-group model. Model parameters: $\mu_{11} = \mu_{12} = 1.0$, $\sigma_1 = \sigma_2 = 0.1$, $\varepsilon_1 = \varepsilon_2 = 0.01$, $\mu_{21} = \mu_{22} = 0.02$, $R_{01} = 1.1$, $R_{02} = 3.0$, $f_2 = 0.1$ (yr^{-1}). The differences in R_{0i} reflect differing rates of exposure to infection, perhaps induced by behavioural differences between the two groups of individuals. The smaller group ($f_2 = 0.1$) have a high rate of exposure to infection.

rate imposed by community drug treatment. The two curves in the graph shown in Fig. 19.4 show the proportional change for a selective programme aimed at the wormy 10 per cent of the community ($f_1 = 0.1$), and the change for a mass programme where individuals are treated at random irrespective of their group membership. Note that for an additional death rate of 0.3 per yr^{-1} (on μ_{11} in the case of selective treatment and on μ_{11} and μ_{12} in the case of mass application) selectively treating 10 per cent of the population gives a roughly 50 per cent reduction in mean worm load while treating the entire community only increases this by an additional 30 per cent. Selectivity is clearly very beneficial with respect to the trade-off between drug treatments administered and the degree of reduction in parasite population size. It is also advantageous if immunocompetence plays a role in determining parasite aggregation; the lightly infected, and hence immunocompetent, individuals may naturally acquire resistance via the maintenance of transmission in the untreated segment of the population. The second issue concerns vaccination in situations where 'worminess' arises due to lack of immunocompetence (if and when vaccines become available). Immunocompetence, perhaps genetically or nutritionally based, is measured within the model by two parameters: ε_i, which represents the severity of the acquired response; and σ_i, which measures the duration of 'immunological' memory of past exposure to infection. If the vaccine induces protection in a manner directly proportional to the protection acquired via natural exposure to live parasite antigens, then the chances of converting 'wormy' people to

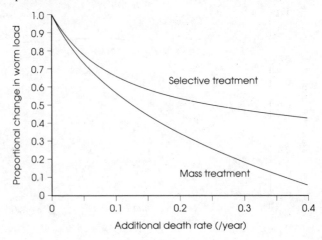

Fig. 19.4. Impact of chemotherapy on the intensity of infection. Proportional change at equilibrium (over that pertaining prior to control) in the overall population worm load, M (over all classes and all types of individual), in a population subject to varying degrees of treatment either targeted at a 'wormy fraction' (selective) or applied randomly to all the population (mass). In the selective programme the fraction of wormy people ($f_1 = 0.1$) were treated and the non-wormy fraction ($f_2 = 0.9$) were untreated. Parameter values $\mu_{21} = \mu_{22} = 0.0143$, $\varepsilon_1 = 0.00001$, $\varepsilon_2 = 0.0075$, $\sigma_1 = \sigma_2 = 0.1$, $\mu_{11} = 0.2$, $\mu_{12} = 0.6$ (all yr^{-1}), $R_{01} = 4.67$, $R_{02} = 1.63$. Horizontal axis denotes the extra death rate (above the pre-control value of μ_{11} and μ_{12}) resulting from chemotherapy. The top curve denotes the result of targeting in which only the wormy fraction are treated, and the bottom curve is for mass treatment (after Anderson and May 1985*d*).

non-wormy individuals by immunization are poor. Thus predisposition to heavy infection arising from heterogeneity in host immunocompetence, although beneficial to the operation of selective chemotherapy programmes, may present serious problems for the community-wide control of parasite transmission and morbidity by mass vaccination. A vaccine must be able to convert low responders (i.e. wormy people) into high responders (i.e. non-wormy people) if effective herd immunity is to be created. These comments are of course speculative at present, until more is understood both about the causes of predisposition to heavy infection and the properties of a potential helminth vaccine.

The central conclusion to emerge from this brief and perhaps rather superficial look at models that incorporate heterogeneity in exposure/suscep-tibility/responsiveness to macroparasite invasion concerns the design of future epidemiological studies in the field. The demonstration of predisposition (see Table 15.7), along with the predicted importance of heterogeneity in immuno-competence to resist helminth invasion, argue that much more attention should be directed towards longitudinal studies of parasite acquisition and loss in individual patients. In the vast majority of past field research, results are presented by reference to changes in average worm loads (or the average intensity of infection), either longitudinally or horizontally across age classes. Rarely is any reference made to the variance around the mean. Theory suggests that the means may mask interesting changes with age or time in worm loads within individual patients. Such changes could, in principle, help us to understand the factors which generate predisposition, and the role played by immunocompetence and acquired immunity. There are, of course, many statistical problems in interpreting the data connected with the study of trends in individuals as opposed to samples of people. However, at the very least, future work should focus more on attempts to record the variance as well as the average in stratified samples. A major priority should be the careful monitoring of nutritional state and parasite-specific antibody plus cellular responses, before drug treatment and during a period of reinfection, in patients who are predisposed to heavy and to light infection. Such work is under way for the schistosome parasites (Wilkins *et al.* 1984*a, b*; Butterworth *et al.* 1984, 1985; Bensted-Smith *et al.* 1989), but similar research is urgently required for the intestinal and filarial nematodes.

In summary, we stress the somewhat paradoxical point, that epidemiological research on macroparasitic infection must in the future turn to the study of trends in *individuals* as well as those within *populations*. It is likely that many important patterns at the community level derive ultimately from differences among individuals.

20

Indirectly transmitted helminths

The mathematical framework developed in Chapters 16 and 17 is of relevance to the study of directly and indirectly transmitted species of macroparasites. Although attention was focused on the directly transmitted helminths, the models can be adapted to take account of the biological details of transmission via more complex life cycles by appropriate parameter definitions of the basic reproductive rate, R_0. As discussed in Chapter 16, most intermediate hosts of indirectly transmitted macroparasites have very short life spans relative to that of the sexually mature parasite. Therefore it is usually sensible to consider the transmission dynamics of the parasite in human communities by collapsing (i.e. setting their time derivatives equal to zero) the equations which mirror changes in the abundances of free-living infective stages, or infected intermediate hosts, into a single equation for the mean parasite burden per person (Anderson and May 1982c).

For several reasons, we devote this chapter to describing models for the study of the transmission of two important indirectly transmitted infections, namely the schistosome flukes and the filarial nematodes. Their inclusion is in part due to a fascination with the complexity of their life cycles, which has resulted in much research on the biology of infection in human and snail populations, in part due to their historical significance in the development and use of mathematical models in the field of parasitology and tropical medicine, and in part for completeness.

20.1 Schistosomiasis

The human schistosomes or blood flukes are digenetic nematodes with indirect life cycles involving a molluscan intermediate host. Three major species infect humans: *Schistosoma mansoni*, *S. haematobium*, and *S. japonicum*. All three have similar life cycles that involve an alternation of generations, with the sexual generation of adult worms in people and an asexual stage in the molluscan host (various aquatic or amphibious species depending on the species of fluke and the geographical location). A very short-lived free-swimming stage, the miracidium, hatches from the egg that passes out of the human host via the faeces (*S. mansoni* and *S. japonicum*) or the urine (*S. haematobium*). The miracidium penetrates the snail host and develops into a first- and then a second-stage sporocyst. The latter gives rise, via asexual reproduction, to numerous cercariae which leave the snail to become free-swimming in the aquatic habitat. This stage is also very short-lived and is responsible for location and penetration of the human host. Their usual manner of entry is via direct

Table 20.1 Life expectancies of the hosts and various developmental states in the life cycle of *Schistosoma mansoni*

Host and parasite life cycle stage	Life expectancy
Human	40–60 years
Adult parasite in human	3–5 years
Biomphalaria glabrata (infected snail)	3–6 weeks
Cercarial stage	8–20 hours
Miracidial stage	4–16 hours

penetration of the skin, after which they are known as schistosomula. These juvenile worms migrate within the human host and develop into sexually mature adults in the blood system. A summary of the approximate time periods spent in each of these developmental states is shown in Table 20.1 (see also the diagrammatic flow chart shown in Fig. 15.2).

Mathematical models that describe parasite transmission from humans to snail and snail to humans have been described in numerous publications. The main papers are those of Hairston (1962, 1965a), Macdonald (1965), Nasell and Hirsch (1972a, b), Lewis (1975a, b), Nasell (1976a, b, 1977), May (1977a), Barbour (1978), Goddard (1978), Bradley and May (1978), Anderson and Crombie (1984), and Anderson and May (1979a, 1982c, 1985b, d).

We summarize the main themes of this research by reference to a general deterministic model whose structure, broadly speaking, underpins most of the published work. The flow chart shown in Fig. 15.2 gives the general structure of the model. We denote the mean number of worms per human host, the number of miracidia, the numbers of susceptible, infected but latent, shedding, and recovered snails, and the number of cercariae, respectively, by the following time-dependent (but host-age independent) variables: $M(t)$, $L_1(t)$, $X(t)$, $Z(t)$, $Y(t)$, $W(t)$, and $L_2(t)$. We assume that the human and snail populations are constant in size (N_1 and N_2 respectively) and let $x(t)$, $z(t)$, $y(t)$, and $w(t)$ denote the proportions of snails in the susceptible, latent, shedding, and recovered classes. Some authors assume that the host populations (human, snail, or both) are subject to immigration and mortality (see Nasell 1976a; Lewis 1975b), but such refinements make little difference to the dynamics of parasite transmission. Note that in the definition of variables we have adopted a mixed prevalence–density framework. We need to do this because the parasite can multiply asexually within the snail host. It is not possible (or sensible) to count parasite numbers per snail. Prevalence scores give a sufficiently accurate assessment of the potential parasite transmission within the molluscan population, because the output of cercariae by an infected snail appears to be independent of the number of miracidia that successfully penetrated it (see Jordan and Webbe 1982; Chu *et al.* 1966b).

20.1.1 *The snail population*

Models of change in the prevalence of infection with snail age (=size) have been used extensively to help interpret observed patterns in the field and in laboratory experimentation (see Sturrock and Webbe 1971; Cohen 1973b; Sturrock *et al.* 1975; May 1977a; Barbour 1978; Anderson and May 1979a; Anderson *et al.* 1982; Anderson and Crombie 1984, 1985; Crombie and Anderson 1985). We start by considering these so-called 'catalytic models', a title which derives from their development by Muench (1959) as an adaptation of equations employed to describe chemical reactions. Then we move on to examine transmission between snails and people.

Consider a cohort of newly born snails, numbering $N_2(0)$ at age $a = 0$, all of which are uninfected. The members of this cohort will progress through a sequence of categories at rates dependent on the force of infection, λ, the duration of snail latency, τ (period from infection to start of cercarial shedding), and the rate of loss of infection, γ. These categories are, as defined earlier, uninfected snails, infected snails not releasing cercariae, shedding snails, and recovered snails, denoted respectively as $X(a)$, $Z(a)$, $Y(a)$, and $W(a)$ at age (=time) a. We assume for now that λ is constant and independent of time or snail age (i.e. the adult worm population is at a stable equilibrium M^* such that the rate of input of eggs into the aquatic habitat is constant). A summary of the notation employed in the models described in this section is presented in Table 20.2. At equilibrium, changes in $X(a)$, $Z(a)$, $Y(a)$, and $W(a)$ with respect to snail age may be mirrored by four coupled first-order differential equations:

$$dX/da = (\lambda + \mu_3)X, \tag{20.1}$$

$$dZ/da = \lambda X - \mu_3 Z - \lambda X(a - \tau) \exp(-\mu_3\tau)\theta(t - \tau), \tag{20.2}$$

$$dY/da = \lambda X(a - \tau) \exp(-\mu_3\tau)\theta(t - \tau) - \mu_4 Y - \gamma Y, \tag{20.3}$$

$$dW/da = \gamma Y - \mu_3 W. \tag{20.4}$$

Here $\theta(u)$ is a step function such that $\theta(u) = 1$ if $u > 0$ and $\theta(u) = 0$ if $u < 0$. The variables X, Z, W, and Y have the initial values $X(0) = N_2$, $Z(0) = W(0) = Y(0) = 0$.

The solutions of eqns (20.1)–(20.4) can be easily derived where

$$X(a) = N_2 \exp[-(\lambda + \mu_3)a], \tag{20.5}$$

$$Z(a < \tau) = N_2 \exp(-\mu_3 a)[1 - \exp(-\lambda a)], \tag{20.6}$$

$$Z(a > \tau) = N_2 \exp[-(\lambda + \mu_3)a][\exp(\lambda\tau) - 1], \tag{20.7}$$

$$Y(a < \tau) = 0, \tag{20.8}$$

$$Y(a > \tau) = N_2(\lambda/\alpha) \exp[\lambda\tau - (\lambda + \mu_3)a]\{\exp[\alpha(a - \tau)] - 1\}, \tag{20.9}$$

$$W(a < \tau) = 0, \tag{20.10}$$

$$W(a > \tau) = N(\gamma\lambda/\alpha) \exp(-\mu_3 a)(\{\exp[s(a - \tau)] - 1\}/s$$
$$- \{1 - \exp[-\lambda(a - \tau)]\}/\lambda). \tag{20.11}$$

Table 20.2 Notation employed in the models of the transmission dynamics of schistosome species

Population variables	Definition
N_2	Total density of snails
X	Density of susceptible and uninfected snails
Z	Density of infected snails not yet shedding cercariae ($=$ latent)
Y	Density of infected and shedding snails
W	Density of snails that have recovered from infection
y	Prevalence of shedding snails
$\hat{y}$	Prevalence of infected snails
N_1	Total density of humans
M	Mean worm burden in human host
L_1	Density of miracidia
L_2	Density of cercariae
Snail	
μ_3	Per capita death rate of susceptible and latently infected snails
μ_4	Per capita death rate of shedding snails
γ	Per capital rate of recovery from infection
τ	Average latent period (infected but not shedding)
λ	Per capita force or rate of infection
Human	
μ_1	Per capita death rate of mature worms
β_1	Per capita rate at which cercariae establish within the human host
λ_1	Per capita fecundity of mature female worms
β_2	Per capita rate at which miracidia establish within the snail host
μ_2	Per capita death rate of miracidia
μ_5	Per capita death rate of cercariae
λ_2	Per capita rate of production of cercariae (per shedding snail)
ϕ	Probability that a female worm is mated
k	Negative binomial aggregation parameter

Here $\alpha = \lambda + \mu_3 - \mu_4 - \gamma$ and $s = \mu_3 - \mu_4 - \gamma$. The predicted changes in X, Y, Z, and W as the cohort of snails age is illustrated in Fig. 20.1 for a particular set of parameter values.

At age a, the prevalence of infection, $y(a)$, defined as the proportion of that age class releasing cercariae, is given by

$$y(a) = Y(a)/(X(a) + Y(a) + Z(a) + W(a)). \qquad (20.12)$$

In some instances, however, the proportion of infected snails within an age or size class is estimated by examining squashed snails for the presence of larval parasites. In these circumstances, the prevalence of infected snails $\hat{y}(a)$ is

$$\hat{y}(a) = (Y(a) + Z(a))/(X(a) + Y(a) + Z(a) + W(a)). \qquad (20.13)$$

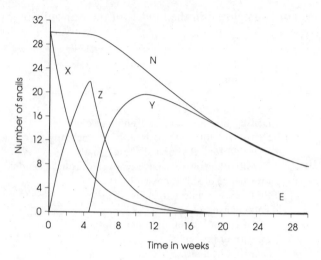

Fig. 20.1. Changes through time in the total numbers of snails alive (N), the number of uninfected snails (X), the number of latently infected snails (Z), the number of infected and shedding snails (Y), and the number of snails recovered from infection (W), as predicted by eqns (20.5)–(20.11). Parameter values: $N_2(0) = 30$, $\mu_3 = 0.00285$, $\mu_4 = 0.062$, $\lambda = 0.308$, $\gamma = 0.0$ (yr^{-1}), and $\tau = 4.5$ weeks (after Anderson and May 1979a).

Prevalence data based on cercarial release assessments underestimate the proportion of infected snails (latent plus shedding hosts) by a factor d where

$$d = 1 + [\exp(\mu_3\tau) - 1](\mu_4/\mu_3). \tag{20.14}$$

With respect to transmission to humans, however, it is the parameter $\hat{y}(a)$ that is of importance.

The predictions of the simple model described above have been compared with laboratory experiments in which cohorts of snails were exposed to a constant force of infection (a fixed number of miracidia introduced into the experimental areas per unit of time) over long periods of time (e.g. 40 weeks or more) (Anderson and Crombie 1984). These experiments were also designed to test the assumption that the magnitude of the force of infection λ is directly proportional to the rate of input of miracidia into the habitat of the snail population (as assumed in all published models; see Anderson (1978a), May (1977a), and Macdonald (1965)). Encouragingly, the relationship between λ and miracidial input was shown to be approximately linear (Fig. 20.2). Furthermore, observed age-dependent changes in the prevalence of infection were well mirrored by the model's predictions (Fig. 20.3).

The agreement between the model and the observations worsened, however, when more complex experimental designs were employed (Anderson and Crombie 1984, 1985). Specifically, when snail populations were allowed to vary in size and age structure via the input of new cohorts of young hosts and natural

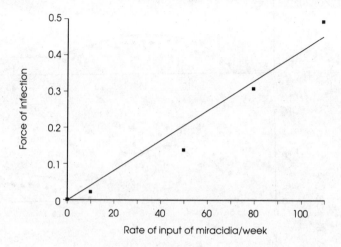

Fig. 20.2. Relationship between the per capita force of infection, λ, and the rate of input of miracidia (per week) into an experimental tank containing a population of the snail host, *Biomphalaria glabrata*, of defined size and age structure (Anderson and Crombie 1984). The full line is the best-fit linear model for the observed data, constrained to pass through the origin.

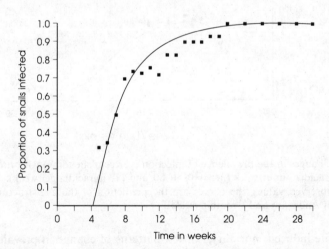

Fig. 20.3. Changes in the prevalence of infection, ($y(a)$, percentage of snails shedding cercariae) with time (= age) in a snail population exposed to infection by the miracidia of *Schistosoma mansoni*. The squares are observed values (see Anderson and Crombie 1984). The full curve represents the prediction of eqn (20.12). Parameter values: $\lambda = 0.308$ week^{-1}, $\mu_3 = 0.00285$ week^{-1}, $\mu_4 = 0.062$ week^{-1}, $\tau = 4.5$ weeks, $\gamma = 0$.

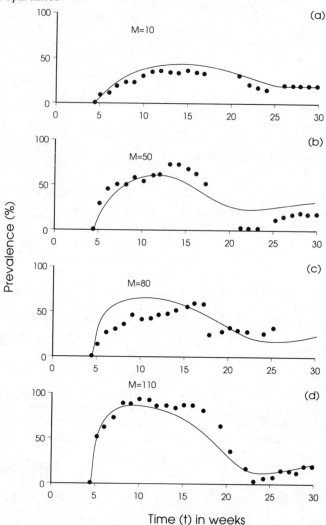

Fig. 20.4. Changes in the prevalence of infection (per cent shedding) with time for four levels of miracidial input/week (M = 10, 50, 80, and 110 miracidia per week). The points represent observed values; the curves are the prediction of the age-structured model described in Anderson and Crombie (1984).

and parasite-induced mortality, convex patterns of change in prevalence with age were recorded (Fig. 20.4). In our simple model convex relationships between prevalence and age arise only if the snails are able to recover from infection ($\gamma \neq 0$) (Fig. 20.5). Recovery was not observed in the experimental studies of Anderson and Crombie (1984) although other workers have reported this phenomenon within some strains of *Biomphalaria glabrata* after long intervals

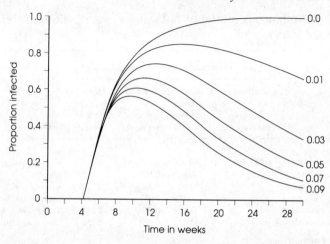

Fig. 20.5. The influence of different rates of snail recovery from infection (the magnitude of the parameter γ in eqns (20.3) and (20.4)) on the proportion of snails infected (of a cohort) from time of exposure to infection. The values of γ range from 0.0 to 0.09 week^{-1}. Other parameter values as defined in the legend of Fig. 20.3.

of infection (Teesdale 1962; Sturrock *et al.* 1975; Minchella and Loverde 1983). The relevance of snail recovery to transmission in field situations is very limited, however, given the short life expectancy of the intermediate host in most natural habitats (Table 20.3).

Other experimental studies have shown that convex age–prevalence curves can arise if the force of infection, λ, depends on snail age and size (Anderson *et al.* 1982; Anderson and Crombie 1984) (Fig. 20.6). These experiments also showed that the death rate of shedding snails, μ_4, depends on the length of time during which individual snails shed cercariae (Fig. 20.7). A more accurate description of the dynamics of snail infection by schistosome parasites is therefore attained by the use of age-structured models that incorporate these refinements and allow for the recruitment of uninfected snails to the population. For example, if we exclude the class of recovered snails, W, define $X(a, t)$ and $Z(a, t)$ as the numbers of susceptible and infected but latent snails of age a at time t, and denote $Y(a, t, s)$ as the number of shedding snails of age a at time t who have been shedding cercariae for s time units, then

$$\partial X(a, t)/\partial a + \partial X(a, t)/\partial t = -(\lambda(a) + \mu_3)X(a, t), \tag{20.15}$$

$\partial Z(a, t)/\partial a + \partial Z(a, t)/\partial t$

$$= \lambda(a)X(a, t) - \mu_3 Z(a, t) - \lambda(a)X(a, t - \tau)\theta(t - \tau)\exp(-\mu_3\tau), \tag{20.16}$$

$$\partial Y(a, t, s)/\partial a + \partial Y(a, t, s)/\partial t + \partial Y(a, t, s)/\partial s = -\mu_4(s)Y(a, t, s). \tag{20.17}$$

Here $\lambda(a)$ denotes the age-dependent force of infection (see Fig. 20.6) and $\mu_4(s)$ denotes the death rate of shedding snails as a function of the duration of

Table 20.3 Instantaneous mortality rates and expected life spans of infected and uninfected snails

Parasite and snail species	Uninfected snails		Infected snails		Reference
	Death rate, μ_3 (per snail per week)	Mean expected life span (weeks)	Death rate, μ_4 (per snail per week)	Mean expected life span (weeks)	
Schistosoma mansoni					
Biomphalaria glabrata	0.017–0.015	60–68	0.180	5.6	Barbosa (1962)
Biomphalaria glabrata	0.007	140.8	0.109	9.2	Pan (1965)
Biomphalaria glabrata	0.274	3.644	0.361	2.770	Sturrock (1973)
Biomphalaria glabrata	0.152	6.579	0.607	1.647	Sturrock and Webbe (1971)
Biomphalaria sudanica	0.252	3.968	0.448	2.232	Webbe (1962a,b)
Biomphalaria alexandria	0.301	3.222	0.392	2.551	Dazo et al. (1966)
Schistosoma haematobium					
Bulinus nasutus productus	0.175	5.714	0.294	3.401	Webbe (1962a,b)
Bulinus nasutus productus	0.276	3.623			Dazo et al. (1966)
Bulinus nasutus productus	0.178	5.600			Sturrock and Webbe (1971)
Bulinus truncatus	0.129	7.777			Barlow and Muench (1951)
Bulinus truncatus	0.029	35.000	0.087	11.471	Chu et al. (1966a)
Bulinus truncatus	0.280	3.570	0.385	2.600	Hairston (1965a)
Schistosoma japonicum					
Oncomelania quadrasi	0.064	15.618			Pesigan et al. (1958)
Oncomelania quadrasi	0.027	37.380	0.089	11.180	Pesigan et al. (1958)
Oncomelania quadrasi	0.094	10.582	0.161	6.211	Hairston (1965a)

shedding s (see Fig. 20.7). The initial and boundary conditions of eqns (20.15)–(20.17) depend on the demography of the snail population and the initial age structure. The patterns predicted by this more complex model show good agreement with the observed trends recorded in laboratory populations of snails constantly exposed to miracidial infection (Anderson and Crombie 1984, 1985) (Fig. 20.4). These experimental studies also show that under conditions of high exposure to infection, schistosome parasites can severely depress snail abundance below the level that would be attained in the absence of infection (Fig. 20.8). Field studies of schistosome infection in snail populations reveal a number of interesting points. First, observed patterns of change in prevalence with snail age (size) vary greatly depending on the species of snail and parasite, the intensity of transmission, and geographical locality (Fig. 20.9). Prevalence may rise monotonically to attain a stable plateau, or it may fail to attain a plateau or exhibit a decline in the older age classes. Where convexity is observed, the model outlined above suggests that this will be due to age dependency in the rate of acquisition of infection and shedding-snail mortality. The second point concerns the overall prevalence of infection (across age classes). As shown in Table 20.4, for the three major species of schistosomes, observed prevalences are characteristically low in endemic areas. Where large

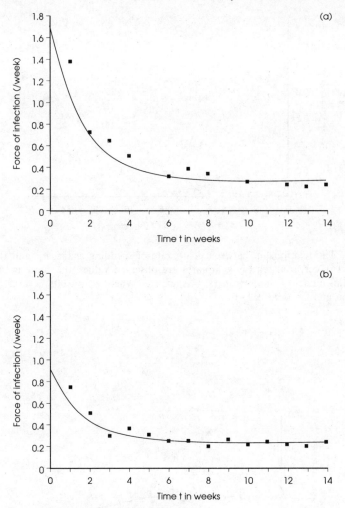

Fig. 20.6. The dependence of the force of infection, λ, on snail age ($=$size) for two levels of miracidial input. Squares are observed values and the curves are the best-fit model of the form $\lambda(a) = a + b \exp(ct)$ where a, b, and c are constants and t denotes age in weeks. (a) Miracidial input of 110 week^{-1}, $a = 0.29$, $b = 1.43$, $c = -0.63$. (b) Miracidial input of 80 week^{-1}, $a = 0.24$, $b = 0.69$, $c = -0.66$ (Anderson and Crombie 1984).

samples of snails have been examined the average prevalence of infection throughout a year, or over a large sampling area, tend to lie in the range 1–10 per cent, irrespective of the species of snail or schistosome, or of the geographical location (Anderson and May 1979*a*).

An understanding of the factors that influence this overall prevalence can be gained via simple prevalence models outlined in this section. For example, if

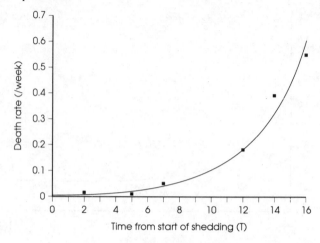

Fig. 20.7. The relationship between death rate of shedding snails, μ_4, and the period from start of cercarial release, s. Squares are observed values; the curve is the best-fit exponential model of the form $\mu_4(s) = \lambda_4 \exp(\gamma s)$, where $\lambda_4 = 0.005$, $\gamma = 0.3$ ($r = 0.98$) (Anderson and Crombie 1984).

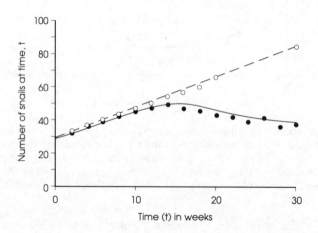

Fig. 20.8. Changes in snail abundance with time. Open circles, uninfected populations in control experiment with no exposure to infection. Full circles, infected population, in experiment where snail population was exposed to 80 miracidia per week. The curves are the predictions of the age-structured model as described in Anderson and Crombie (1984).

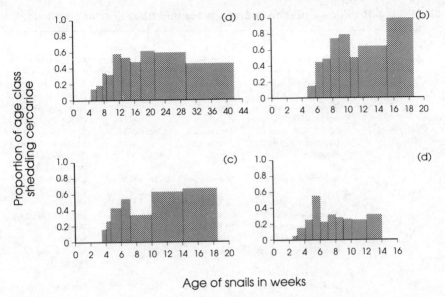

Age of snails in weeks

Fig. 20.9. Examples of observed age–prevalence data for *Schistosoma mansoni* in *Biomphalaria glabrata* (sampled in St Lucia). (a) Data from Sturrock and Webbe (1971). (b) Data from Sturrock (1973). (c) Data from Sturrock and Webbe (1971). (d) Data from Sturrock (1973).

we exclude the class of recovered snails, W, and ignore the complications introduced by age dependency in the rates of exposure to infection and shedding-snail mortality then eqns (20.5)–(20.11) provide an estimate of the overall equilibrium prevalence $\bar{y}^*$, where

$$\bar{y}^* = \bar{Y}^*/(\bar{Y}^* + \bar{X}^* + \bar{Z}^*). \tag{20.18}$$

Here the $\bar{Y}^*$, $\bar{X}^*$, and $\bar{Z}^*$ denote the integrals of $Y(a)$, $X(a)$, and $Z(a)$ over all age classes (e.g. $\bar{Y}^* = \int_0^\infty Y(a)\,\mathrm{d}a$). Provided the force of transmission is not very small eqn (20.18) reduces to the simpler expression

$$\bar{y}^* \simeq f/[f + (1 - f)(\mu_4/\mu_3)], \tag{20.19}$$

where $f = \exp(-\mu_3\tau)$. In the limit where the latent period τ tends to zero, $\bar{y}^*$ tends to unity, corresponding to essentially all snails releasing cercariae. If the death rates of susceptible, μ_3, latent, μ_3, and shedding, μ_4, snails are equal then eqn (20.19) reduces to $\bar{y}^* = f$. This has exactly the form $\exp(-\mu\tau)$ or p^τ as Macdonald (1965) showed when he took explicit account of the latent period that elapses between a mosquito becoming infected and its becoming infectious (see Chapter 14).

Empirical estimates of the parameters μ_3 (death rate of susceptible and latent snails), μ_4 (death rate of shedding snails), and τ (the latent or pre-patent period)

Table 20.4 Prevalence of schistosome species infections in snail populations

Schistosome species	Snail species	Location	Sample	Prevalence (per cent)	Reference
Schistosoma mansoni	*Biomphalaria glabrata*	N.E. Brazil		11.1	Barbosa and Oliver (1958)
	Biomphalaria glabrata	Puerto Rico		1–10	Harry and Aldrich (1958)
	Biomphalaria glabrata	Venezuela		5–10	Scott (1942)
	Biomphalaria glabrata	Puerto Rico		5–25	Ritchie *et al.* (1962)
	Biomphalaria glabrata	Brazil	1000	50–70	Pellegrino and de Maria (1966)
	Biomphalaria glabrata	St Lucia	10 736	1.09	Christie and Upatham (1977)
	Biomphalaria glabrata	St Lucia	14 526	1.1–1.5	Jordan (1977)
	Biomphalaria glabrata	St Lucia	47 526	1.4	Sturrock (1973)
	Biomphalaria glabrata	St Lucia		5.8–17.8	Wright (1973)
	Biomphalaria glabrata	Guadeloupe	2474	0.6	Wright (1973)
	Biomphalaria pfeifferi	Tanzania	889	27	Sturrock and Webbe (1971)
	Biomphalaria pfeifferi	Liberia		0.8–44	Wright (1973)
	Biomphalaria pfeifferi	Sierra Leone	1751	7.7	Gordan *et al.* (1934)
	Planorbis globosus	Sierra Leone	711	10.1	Gordan *et al.* (1934)
	Biomphalaria sudanica tangangensis	E. Africa	31 813	2.2	Webbe (1962*a*)
Schistosoma haematobium	*Bulinus nasutus productus*	Tanzania	273	57	Sturrock and Webbe (1971)
	Bulinus nasutus productus	Tanzania	17 293	3.1	Webbe (1962*b*)
	Planorbis globosus	Kenya	32	3.1	Teesdale (1962)
	Planorbis globosus	Sierra Leone		11	Gordan *et al.* (1934)
	Paludomus obesa	India		2.6	Kuntz (1955)
	Planorbis africanus	Kenya	70	7.1	Teesdale (1962)
	Bulinus jousseaumei	The Gambia	990	3.9	Smithers (1956)
	Bulinus quienei	The Gambia	132	1.5	Smithers (1956)
	Bulinus quienei	Senegal		2–8	Gretillat (1961)
	Bulinus truncatus	Chad		0.4	Wright (1973)
Schistosoma japonicum	*Oncomelania quadrasi*	Philippines	1011	0.9–17.4	McMullen (1947)
	Oncomelania quadrasi	Philippines		10.0–13.8	Bauman *et al.* (1948)
	Oncomelania quadrasi	Philippines	83 059	4.7	Pesigan *et al.* (1958)
	Oncomelania quadrasi	Japan	56 123	1.5	McMullen *et al.* (1951)
	Oncomelania quadrasi	Japan	200	1.5	Wright *et al.* (1947)
	Oncomelania quadrasi	Japan		0.3	Sugiura (1933)
	Oncomelania formosana	Taiwan		1.3	Hsu *et al.* (1955)

are presented in Tables 20.3 and 20.5. For example, *S. mansoni* has a pre-patent period, τ, of approximately 5 weeks at 25 °C and, in St Lucia, Sturrock and Webbe (1971) estimated the mortality rates μ_3 and μ_4 to be roughly 0.15 and 0.61 per snail per week, respectively. Putting these parameter values into eqn (20.19) yields the prediction that the equilibrium percentage of snails shedding cercariae will be around 18 per cent. This is slightly higher than the observations (Table 20.3 and Fig. 20.9). A lower prediction would result if age dependency

Table 20.5 Latent period from point of infection of snail to release of cercariae

Schistosome species	Snail species	Temperature (°C)	Latent period (days)	Reference
Schistosoma mansoni	*Biomphalaria glabrata*	21–24	42	Pan *et al.* (1965)
	Biomphalaria glabrata	23–25	30–37	Stirewalt (1954)
	Biomphalaria glabrata	26–28	22–23	Stirewalt (1954)
	Biomphalaria glabrata	31–33	18	Stirewalt (1954)
	Biomphalaria glabrata	23–24	31–38	Evans and Stirewalt (1951)
	Biomphalaria glabrata	25–28	25–45	Standen (1949)
	Biomphalaria glabrata	28–30	28–35	Schreiber and Schubert (1949)
	Biomphalaria glabrata	18	55	Sturrock and Webbe (1971)
	Biomphalaria glabrata	32	17	Sturrock and Webbe (1971)
	Biomphalaria glabrata	22–28	21–35	Sturrock and Sturrock (1970)
	Biomphalaria pfeifferi	21	42–43	Schiff *et al.* (1975)
	Biomphalaria pfeifferi	20	35	Gordan *et al.* (1934)
	Biomphalaria pfeifferi	26–28	21–28	Gordan *et al.* (1934)
	Biomphalaria pfeifferi	32–33	15–20	Gordan *et al.* (1934)
	Biomphalaria pfeifferi	16–23	40	Fain (1953)
	Biomphalaria pfeifferi	32–33	13–15	Fain (1953)
	Biomphalaria pfeifferi	30	18	Sturrock and Webbe (1971)
	Planorbis boissyi	25–28	45	Standen (1949)
Schistosoma haematobium	*Bulinus globosus*	18–20	119	Schiff *et al.* (1975)
	Bulinus globosus	22–23	43	Schiff *et al.* (1975)
	Bulinus globosus	28	26–27	Schiff *et al.* (1975)
	Bulinus globosus	21	70	Gordan *et al.* (1934)
	Bulinus globosus	26–28	35–42	Gordan *et al.* (1934)
	Bulinus globosus	32–33	25	Gordan *et al.* (1934)
	Bulinus nasutus productus	20–30	56–72	Sturrock (1967)
	Bulinus truncatus	22–24	40–46	Chu *et al.* (1966b)
Schistosoma japonicum	*Oncomelania hupensis*	24–26	56	Vogel (1948)
	Oncomelania hupensis	26–28	39–52	Vogel (1948)
	Oncomelania quadrasi	20–32	53–70	Pesigan *et al.* (1958)

in the rates of acquisition of infection and shedding-snail mortality were taken into account. The tendency for prediction to be slightly higher than observation could also be accounted for by the tendency of field studies to underestimate (rather than overestimate) snail mortality in natural habitats; this is a direct result of the failure to take fully into account poor survival by juvenile snails. As illustrated in Fig. 20.10, eqn (20.19) predicts very low equilibrium prevalences when μ_4 and μ_3 are high, or when τ is long. The important point revealed by the simple model, eqn (20.19), is that the standing prevalence of infectious (i.e. shedding) intermediate hosts will be low, irrespective of the intensity of transmission, if there is a long latent period of infection (long relative to snail life expectancy), and if the parasite has a significant impact on host survival (see Tables 20.3 and 20.5).

20.1.2 *The human community*
Our model for the mean worm burden per person, $M(t)$, is developed along lines similar to those set out in Chapter 16. If we ignore age structure and

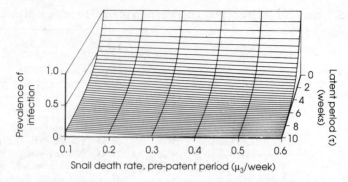

Fig. 20.10. The relationship between the prevalence of snail infection at equilibrium, and the parameters τ (pre-patent period of infection) and μ_3 (the death rate of uninfected and infected snails not releasing cercariae) predicted by eqn (20.19).

acquired immunity or other forms of density-dependent regulation of population growth within the human host, then the simplest equation to describe changes in $M(t)$ with respect to time is

$$dM/dt = \beta_1 L_2 - \mu_1 M. \qquad (20.20)$$

Here L_2 denotes the density of cercariae, β_1 defines the per capita rate at which infective stages establish within the adult worm population, and $1/\mu_1$ is the life expectancy of the mature worm; the term $\beta_1 L_2$ is then the per capita force of infection for the human host.

20.1.3 *Transmission from human to snail and snail to human*

A system of differential equations can be formulated to describe transmission between the two host populations. The simplest model (with the notation defined earlier (see Table 20.2) is of the form:

$$dM/dt = \beta_1 L_2 - \mu_1 M, \qquad (20.21)$$

$$dL_1/dt = \tfrac{1}{2}\lambda_1 M N_1 \phi - \mu_2 L_1 - \beta_2 N_2 L_1, \qquad (20.22)$$

$$dX/dt = \mu_3(X + Z) + \mu_4 Y - \beta_2 X L_1 - \mu_3 X, \qquad (20.23)$$

$$dZ/dt = \beta_2 L_1 X - \mu_3 Z - \beta_2 L_1(t - \tau)X(t - \tau)\exp(-\mu_3\tau)\theta(t - \tau), \quad (20.24)$$

$$dY/dt = \beta_2 L_1(t - \tau)X(t - \tau)\exp(-\mu_3\tau)\theta(t - \tau) - \mu_4 Y, \qquad (20.25)$$

$$dL_2/dt = \lambda_2 Y - \mu_5 L_2 - \beta_1 N_1 L_2, \qquad (20.26)$$

where $N_2 = X + Y + Z$ and θ is as defined for eqns (20.1)–(20.4). It is here assumed that the total human and total snail populations are of constant sizes, denoted by N_1 and N_2, respectively. In eqns (20.23)–(20.25), for example, the birth term in the equation for susceptible snails ($\mu_3(X + Z) + \mu_4 Y$) exactly balances the net death rate of the total population of snails. Human mortality is not represented in eqn (20.21).

The function ϕ represents the mating probability as discussed in Chapter 16 (see Table 16.1). For schistosome species, which are dioecious and probably monogamous, the appropriate function for a population in which the parasites follow a negative binomial distribution is (see May 1977a)

$$\phi(M, k) = 1 - \frac{1 - \alpha}{2\pi} \int_0^{2\pi} \frac{(1 - \cos \theta)\, d\theta}{(1 + \alpha \cos \theta)^{1+k}}, \tag{20.27}$$

where $\alpha = M/(k + M)$. Here the two parameters of the negative binomial are the mean worm burden M and the clumping parameter k. Note that for k small (as it usually is), $\phi \to 1$ for moderate to high values of M (see Fig. 16.2).

This rather messy set of equations can be reduced to a single equation for the mean worm burden $M(t)$, by methods similar to those described in Chapter 17 for the models of directly transmitted nematode infections. Relative to the life expectancy of the adult worm (see Table 20.1) the time-scales of the equations for L_1, X, Z, Y, and L_2 are all fast. Setting $dL_1/dt = dX/dt = dZ/dt = dY/dt = dL_2/dt = 0$, we get

$$Y^* = \frac{\beta_2 L_1^* f N_2}{\mu_4 + \beta_2 L_1^* [f + (1 - f)(\mu_4/\mu_3)]}, \tag{20.28}$$

where $f = \exp(-\mu_3\tau)$.

Since f is usually small, given that the life expectancy of the snail, $1/\mu_3$, is of similar magnitude (or a little bit greater) than the latent period τ, then eqn (20.28) simplifies to

$$Y^* = \beta_2 L_1^* f N_2/(1 + \beta_2 L_1^*/\mu_3)\mu_4. \tag{20.29}$$

The equilibrium densities of miracidia, L_1^*, and cercariae, L_2^*, are

$$L_1^* = \tfrac{1}{2}\lambda_1 M N_1 \phi/(\beta_2 N_2 + \mu_2), \tag{20.30}$$

and

$$L_2^* = \lambda_2 Y^*/(\beta_1 N_1 + \mu_5). \tag{20.31}$$

The equation for the mean worm burden, $M(t)$, is therefore

$$dM/dt = \mu_1 M\left(\frac{\tfrac{1}{2}T_1 T_2 \phi}{\tfrac{1}{2}T_2 \phi M + 1} - 1\right). \tag{20.32}$$

The factor $\tfrac{1}{2}$ arises from the assumed 1:1 sex ratio of male to female parasites. Here the parameters T_1 and T_2 characterize transmission from snail to human and human to snail respectively (in the terminology of Macdonald (1965)), where

$$T_1 = \beta_1 \lambda_2 N_2/[\mu_1(\beta_1 N_1 + \mu_5)] \tag{20.33}$$

and

$$T_2 = f\beta_2 \lambda_1 N_1/[\mu_4(\beta_2 N_2 + \mu_2)]. \tag{20.34}$$

Here λ_2 is the rate of cercarial shedding per infected snail, $\beta_1/(\beta_1 N_1 + \mu_5)$ is the probability for a cercaria to infect a given human (μ_5 is the cercarial death rate), μ_1 is the death rate of mature worms, and N_2 is the snail density. Similarly, λ_1 is the rate of egg laying per mated female, N_1 is human density, $\beta_2/(\beta_2 N_2 + \mu_2)$ is the probability for an egg to produce a miracidium which infects a susceptible snail, f is the proportion of latent snails that survive to release cercariae, and μ_4 is the death rate of shedding snails.

The basic reproductive rate R_0 of the schistosome parasite is therefore given by

$$R_0 = \tfrac{1}{2} T_1 T_2 \phi. \tag{20.35}$$

Equations (20.33), (20.34), and (20.35) clearly illustrate how the numerous population parameters involved in the two-host life cycle act concomitantly to determine reproductive or transmission success.

An analytical solution of eqn (20.32) for arbitrary ϕ is not feasible, given the complexity of the mating function (see eqn (20.27)). The qualitative dynamical properties can, however, be explored by phase plane analysis. For $\phi \simeq 1$, the model has two solutions: the trivial case $M^* = 0$ and a state of endemic infection where

$$M^* = (\tfrac{1}{2} T_1 T_2 \phi - 1)/(\tfrac{1}{2} T_2 \phi). \tag{20.36}$$

For this state to be positive, R_0 must exceed unity ($R_0 = 1$ defines the transmission threshold).

For $\phi \neq 1$, the analysis follows lines identical to those outlined for the directly transmitted helminth model (Chapter 16). When $R_0 > 1$ the system has two stable states $M^* = 0$ and M^* as defined by eqn (20.36). These states are separated by an unstable equilibrium point, M_μ^* (the breakpoint). As discussed earlier for the intestinal nematodes, the numerical value of the unstable state approaches zero worms per host as the degree of parasite aggregation increases. In the limit, when all the worms are harboured by one host, all others being uninfected, the unstable state M_μ^* disappears (Fig. 20.11). In practice schistosomes appear to be highly clumped within human communities, hence the breakpoint concept is again of limited significance to the design of control policies. Macdonald (1965), in an early study of the transmission dynamics of schistosome parasites, falsely assumed that the worms were randomly distributed. This led him to the incorrect conclusion that the unstable breakpoint lay some way from the stable state of zero worms per person.

A further conclusion drawn by Macdonald concerned the relative merits of altering the values of the transmission parameters T_1 and T_2 in attempting to reduce the net force of transmission below the threshold $R_0 = 1$ by control measures. He concluded that the threshold condition is more sensitive to changes in T_1 (snails to humans) than to changes in T_2 (humans to snails). This led him to conclude that 'safe water supplies are more important than latrines'. As discussed more fully elsewhere (May 1977a), Macdonald's conclusion tends

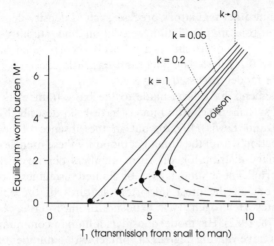

Fig. 20.11. The influence of worm aggregation on the value of the breakpoint worm burden, M_B. The equilibrium worm loads, M^*, are shown as a function of the transmission coefficient T_1 (snail to man), for T_2 (man to snail) fixed at a value of unity (May 1977a). The full curve to the far right is for a Poisson distribution of worms ($k \rightarrow \infty$). The broken line denotes the breakpoint and the solid curves the states of stable endemic infection (M^*). To the left of the Poisson line are curves for various degrees of parasite aggregation as measured inversely by the value of the negative binomial parameter k. Note that as aggregation increases ($k \rightarrow 0$) the breakpoint phenomenon becomes less conspicuous, finally disappearing in the limit $k \rightarrow 0$ (essentially all worms harboured in one individual).

to be true if T_1 is small; in this event the probability for a given host to harbour both a male and a female worm, and thus to be able to continue the cycle, is proportional to T_1^2, and thence R_0 varies roughly as $T_1^2 T_2$. But if T_1 is relatively large, as it is in most places where the infection is endemic, hosts possessing a worm of one sex tend to harbour one of the other sex (since the parasites are highly aggregated within human communities), and R_0 varies simply as $T_1 T_2$. In this circumstance, changes in T_1 are equally effective as changes in T_2 in reducing overall transmission success. In short, although Macdonald's conclusions were valid for the limited range of parameters he chose to explore in his numerical studies, they are not representative.

In the simple schistosome model outlined above, regulation of parasite abundance is achieved not via density-dependent constraints on adult worm establishment, fecundity, or survival (as in the models for intestinal helminths) but via constraints on cercarial production by infected snails. Implicit in the model defined by eqns (20.21)–(20.26) is the assumption that cercarial production by infected snails is independent of the number of miracidia that have penetrated the host. As noted earlier, empirical evidence is in agreement with this assumption (Jordan and Webbe 1982; Chu *et al.* 1966b). However, it appears likely that other regulatory process, such as density-dependent fecund-ity, also play a role in population regulation and stability (Medley and Anderson 1985). Such constraints can be easily incorporated in the structure of eqns (20.21)–(20.26), but their inclusion has little effect on the qualitative properties of the model discussed above.

Various refinements have been made to the basic framework of the model detailed in this system. Stochastic models have been described by Nasell and Hirsch (1972a) and Lewis (1975a), but in the absence of heterogeneity in exposure to infection within the human community these models simply predict that the stationary distribution of worm numbers per host will be Poisson (random) in form. These models are of limited usefulness, because worm aggregation is one of the most important features of the epidemiology of helminth parasites. Heterogeneity in exposure to infection has been examined by Barbour (1978, 1982). His model considers a human community subdivided into groups that have varying degrees of contact with a number of water bodies of differing transmission potentials. The conclusions to emerge from this study are similar to those outlined (Chapter 12) for microparasite transmission within human communities that are distributed in a spatially heterogeneous manner. In such cases, heterogeneity adds to the stability of the parasite population in response to perturbation (a further confirmation of the general ecological principle that heterogeneity is stabilizing). Control (with respect to the reduction in parasite abundance) is best achieved by treating the more heavily infected water bodies, or groups of people, more intensely than the lightly infected areas, or groups.

The topic of acquired immunity to infection has received little attention to date; the models of Barbour (1978) and Cohen (1977) make the unrealistic assumptions that sterile immunity follows recovery from infection. The most detailed discussion of this issue is that of Anderson and May (1985d), which considers the framework discussed earlier (see Chapter 18) in which parasite establishment decreases as an individual's accumulated past experience of infection rises. This type of assumption is more in accord with the current understanding of immunity to helminth infection. Furthermore, the models that incorporate this assumption are able to generate convex relationships between parasite burden and host age, where the degree of convexity is dependent on the intensity of transmission (as observed in endemic areas) (Fig. 18.2). However, the role of acquired immunity in the transmission dynamics of schistosomes remains controversial, and future refinements in model structure will depend on an improved biological understanding of this issue (Warren, 1973, 1984; Anderson and May 1985d).

20.1.4 *Prediction versus observation*

What can we say about the lessons to be learned from mathematical studies of the transmission of schistosome parasites, with respect both to the interpretation of observed trends and to the design of control programmes? In the context of parasite transmission within snail populations, the prevalence framework models provide predictions in reasonable agreement with the patterns recorded in the field and in the laboratory. Theory suggests that the low prevalences of cercarial-shedding snails observed in endemic areas are caused by the high death rates of infected snails, and the long latency period (relative to snail life expectancy) during which snails are infected but not yet releasing infective stages. More complex models, and experimental evidence, reveal that convex changes in prevalence within snails arise as a consequence of age-related changes in snail susceptibility to infection and the death rate of shedding hosts. For this segment of the parasite's life cycle there exists a nice balance between model structure, biological detail, and the availability of parameter estimates plus quantitative records of epidemiological patterns in the natural habitat.

This degree of harmony is not mirrored for the segment of the cycle involving transmission within the human community. The model detailed in eqn (20.32) is crude and offers only a few qualitative insights of practical value to epidemiologists. These may be summarized as follows:

1. Parasite aggregation has important dynamical effects, acting to enhance mating success and to lower the unstable breakpoint to close to zero worms per person.

2. The parasite's intrinsic reproductive potential is determined by a large number of population parameters that interact, in a manner defined by the parameter structure of the basic reproductive rate, R_0, to determine transmission success via the complete life cycle.

3. The parasite population is regulated by one or more density-dependent mechanisms (probably including fecundity and cercarial production by multiply infected snails) such that it is very stable to perturbations induced by control or other interventions.

4. The rate of return to the stable state of endemic infection, M^*, following perturbation will be related to the expected life span of the adult parasite, $1/\mu_1$ (for schistosomes the 'return time' will be longer than that for intestinal nematodes due to differences in life expectancies (see Table 15.2)).

The shortcomings of the model concern its lack of applicability in the interpretation of observed age-related changes in prevalence and average intensity of infection. For schistosome species such age-related patterns tend to be much more convex in form than for any of the other major helminth infections in man (Fig. 20.12). As in the case of intestinal helminths, convexity may be due to age-related changes in contact with infection and/or the build-up of acquired immunity in the older age classes. The relative significances of both factors remain unclear at present although data are available for the schistosome infection to confirm that contact with infected water bodies (termed 'water contact') is closely correlated with human age, in areas of endemic infection.

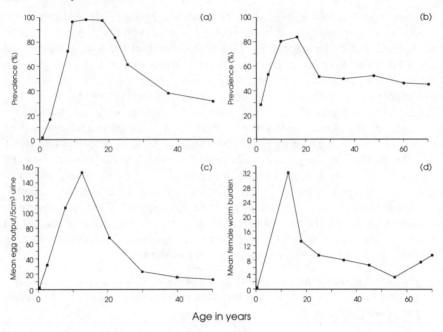

Fig. 20.12. Age–prevalence and age–intensity curves for schistosome infections. (a) *S. japonicum*, Philippines (Palo, coastal region) (Pesigan *et al.* 1958). (b) *S. haematobium*, Tanzania (Bradley and McCullough 1973). (c) *S. haematobium*, Ghana (Scott *et al.* 1982). (d) *S. mansoni*, Brazil (Cheever *et al.* 1977).

Some examples are recorded in Fig. 20.13 from which it can be seen that maximum water contact usually occurs in the child and teenage segments of the community (there are exceptions in areas where water contact is related to adult work practices) (Warren 1981). Recorded patterns of change in average intensity with age are often well mirrored by the associated patterns of change in water contact (Dalton 1976; Dalton and Poole 1978; Jordan *et al.* 1980; Jordan and Webbe 1982).

Evidence for the significance of acquired immunity as a determinant of infection intensity is much weaker at present. Analyses of a wide range of age–average intensity profiles show a positive association between the degree of convexity in the profile and the net intensity of transmission in the community (Crombie 1985; Anderson and May 1985*d*) (Fig. 20.14). This correlation is to be expected if acquired immunity plays a role (Fig. 18.2). Care must be exercised in interpretation, however, since it could also be caused by egg-induced pathology (independent of immunity to resist infection). Intensity of infection is measured by egg output, but egg output could decline independently of worm load in older patients, as a consequence of the pathology associated with long periods of egg production (Jordan and Webbe 1982).

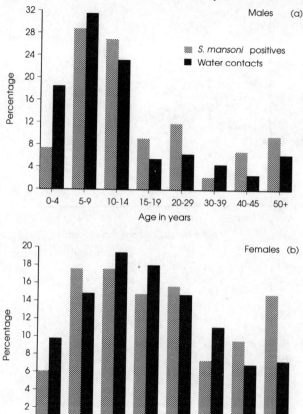

Fig. 20.13. Correlation between observed water contact and infection with *Schistosoma mansoni* in each age group and sex in a population in St Lucia. The number of *S. mansoni* positives and water contact in an age group are recorded as a percentage of the total number of *S. mansoni* positives and water contacts across all age classes (Jordan *et al.* 1980).

Recent studies of patterns of reinfection in individual patients following drug treatment are beginning to provide clues to the role of immunity (Wilkins *et al.* 1984*a*, *b*; Butterworth *et al.* 1984, 1985; Sturrock *et al.* 1987; Bensted-Smith *et al.* 1986). Work in Kenya, for example, suggests that heavily infected children appear to develop some immunity to reinfection by *S. mansoni*; the degree of protection seems to be related to the duration of past exposure to infection (Butterworth *et al.* 1984). Further studies in the same area have provided evidence for predisposition to heavy (or light) infection, but the strength of the statistical evidence is greatest in younger as opposed to older age groups

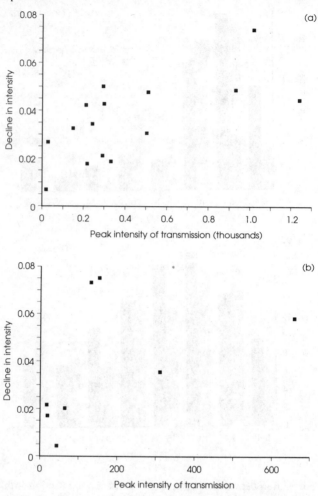

Fig. 20.14. The relationship between the rate of decline with age in intensity of infection post peak intensity, and the peak intensity reached in all age groups of the community. (a) *S. mansoni*. Spearman's rank correlation coefficient: 0.66 (significant at the 5 per cent level). (b) *S. haematobium*. Spearman's rank correlation = 0.64 (significant at the 5 per cent level) (see Anderson 1987).

(Bensted-Smith *et al.* 1989). This can be interpreted as suggesting that acquired immunity is important. Predisposition is associated with measures of water contact but a large proportion of the variance in intensity of infection between patients of a given age is not accounted for by behavioural scores.

The picture clearly remains confused at present. We need more evidence from carefully designed field studies to guide us in refining the structure of the model. The question of how best to control infection within a community, employing

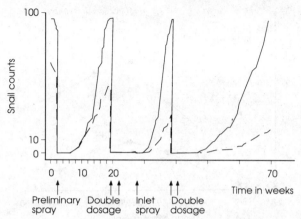

Fig. 20.15. Weekly snail counts in a small body of impounded water, Tengeru Dam, Tanzania, following treatment with high doses of N-tritylmorph: full curve, *Biomphalaria pfeifferi*; broken curve, *Lymnaea ratalensis* (Fenwick and Lidgate 1970).

the currently available methods (i.e. chemotherapy, the reduction of snail densities, and the provision of safe water supplies and sewage disposal facilities), is to a large extent independent of the resolution of the issue of acquired immunity. Current understanding of the ecology and population dynamics of the parasite provides important information for the design of effective control programmes. The short life expectancy of the snail host and its very high reproductive potential (relative to that of the human host) suggest that lasting suppression of snail abundance will require repeated and intensive use of molluscicides. Experience supports this conclusion (Fig. 20.15). Snail populations are often able to recover to their pre-control levels within 6 months or less from the time of intensive molluscicide application. Given the expected (3–5 years) or maximum (10–20 years) life spans of the adult worm (see Hairston 1965*a*, *b*; Warren *et al.* 1974; Wilkins and Scott 1978; Goddard and Jordan 1980), intermediate host abundance must be suppressed to very low levels over very long intervals of time (a decade or more) to have a major impact on parasite transmission within human communities. This point is well illustrated by research on the island of St Lucia involving the repeated application of molluscicides (Jordan 1977). Four years of intensive effort had relatively little impact on the overall prevalence of infection in both high- and low-transmission areas of the island (Fig. 20.16).

The distribution of worm burdens within human communities provides important clues as to how best to employ chemotherapeutic agents. First, even within an age class, the parasites are highly aggregated. Second, the very convex pattern of change in average intensity with age reveals that aggregation is also marked between age classes. Targeted chemotherapy aimed at the children and young teenagers would therefore seem to be a practical option, both for the

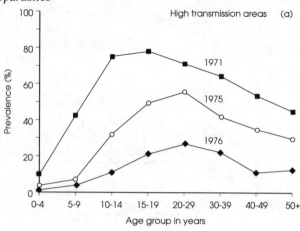

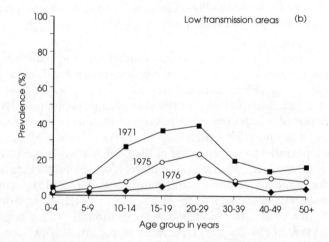

Fig. 20.16. Prevalence of *Schistosoma mansoni* infection in Cul-de-Sac Valley, St Lucia, 1971 and 1975 (before and four years after mollusciciding) and in 1976, one year after chemotherapy (Jordan 1977).

suppression of transmission and the control of morbidity (Warren and Mahmoud 1976, 1980; Mahmoud and Warren 1980). A recent study in the Machakos District, Kenya, of the control of *S. mansoni* by chemotherapy administered selectively to those individuals with $\geqslant 400$ eggs per gram of faeces produced encouraging results (Fig. 20.17). The heavily infected individuals were dominantly within the child and teenage segments of the population and hence a cruder targeted approach (simply based on membership in an age class, as opposed to egg-output class) would also have been highly effective. The theoretical prediction that rates of reinfection following treatment should be lower for schistosomes than for intestinal nematodes seems to hold in practice

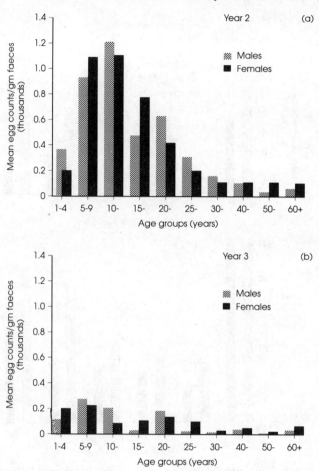

Fig. 20.17. Age versus intensity of infection (mean egg count per gram of faeces) with *Schistosoma mansoni* in low Nduu, Machakos District, Kenya prior to treatment (year 2) and one year after treatment (year 3) of 122 of 380 individuals with egg counts >400 eggs per gram of faeces (Mahmoud and Warren 1980).

(Fig. 20.18). This observation argues that targeted or mass treatment need only be applied at relatively infrequent intervals (2–3 years) in order to permanently suppress morbidity and transmission to low levels.

To conclude this section on schistosomiasis, we wish to emphasize the importance to control at a community level of an understanding of the population dynamics of the schistosome parasites. Mathematical models are obviously very crude at present but via their use as caricatures of parasite transmission, in conjunction with the careful interpretation of observed patterns of parasite distribution and abundance, it is possible to make testable predictions of population behaviour in response to different forms of intervention.

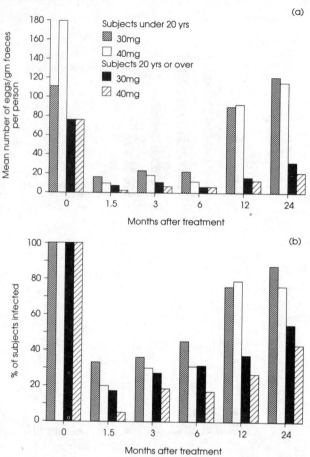

Fig. 20.18. Reinfection with *Schistosome mansoni* in Bulamata, Burundi, following treatment with different regimens of praziquantal showing: (a) the increase in prevalence of infection, and (b) the increase in mean egg load per person (uninfected and infected) (Gryseels and Nkulikyinka 1989).

20.2 Filariasis

The filarial nematodes have, until recently, attracted less attraction from epidemiologists and biomathematicians than the schistosome flukes and intestinal nematodes. This is in part owing to the difficulty of obtaining quantitative scores of worm burdens within individual patients. Indirect scores can be obtained by examining body tissues or fluids and recording the densities of larval nematodes (microfilaria). This procedure involves taking skin snips, in the case of *Onchocerca volvulus*, or blood samples, for *Wuchereria bancrofti*. To further complicate matters, the densities of microfilariae in the peripheral blood systems of patients can fluctuate in a regular daily cycle as in periodic bancroftian filariasis. Thus, the time at which samples are collected can bias the indirect assessment of worm load (Hawking 1967).

The filarial nematodes are tissue-dwelling parasites and are responsible for two of the most important helminth diseases of man. Bancroftian filariasis ('elephantiasis') causes much morbidity in large areas of Africa, Asia, the Pacific, the West Indies, and South America, while *Onchocerca volvulus* is responsible for 'river blindness' (Muller 1975). Both nematode species are transmitted indirectly by the bites of blood-sucking arthropods (various species of mosquito in the case of *W. bancrofti*, and flies of the genus *Simulium* (blackflies) in the case of *O. volvulus*). The adult worms in humans are dioecious and females give birth to early first-stage larvae, known as microfilariae, that are found in the blood or the skin. On ingestion by a suitable insect vector the larvae undergo development to an infective stage (the third-stage larvae). The principal populations and rate parameters involved in the life cycle of *O. volvulus* are depicted in Fig. 15.3.

Few attempts have been made to construct mathematical models of the transmission of filarial parasites. Past work includes an elegant study by Hairston and Jackowski (1968) in which the authors attempted to construct detailed life tables for *W. bancrofti* in order to estimate the basic reproductive rate of the parasite in defined communities. More recently, Dietz (1980, 1982a) has published a more formal account of the dynamics of *O. volvulus* transmission.

20.2.1 *An age-structured model*

We base this section on an adaptation of the mathematical framework developed by Dietz (1982a). Emphasis is placed on the relationship of the model's structure to our earlier models of the transmission of intestinal nematodes and schistosome flukes. We consider two epidemiological variables, namely $M(a, t)$, the mean worm burden per person, and $L(a, t)$, the mean number of infective larvae per arthropod vector. Both quantities are expressed as functions of host age a, and time t. These variables are of direct epidemiological significance since they are the measures most commonly recorded in surveys (adult worm burden is measured indirectly by microfilariae counts while infective larvae are counted by dissecting). Note that in contrast to the schistosome model, we here employ a density framework for describing parasite abundance in both host species.

A pair of coupled non-linear partial differential equations, for change in $M(a, t)$ and $L(a, t)$ with respect to age and time, can be formulated as follows (the dependencies of L and M on a and t are dropped for notational convenience):

$$\partial M/\partial t + \partial M/\partial a = T_1 \bar{L}(f_1(T_1, \bar{L})) - \mu_1 M(g_1(M)). \tag{20.37}$$

$$\partial L/\partial t + \partial L/\partial a = T_2 \bar{M}(f_2(T_2, \bar{M})) - \mu_2 L(g_2(L)). \tag{20.38}$$

The variables $\bar{M}$ and $\bar{L}$ represent average values of the parasite densities over all age classes weighted by the proportional representation of each class in the total population. For example, if the human and vector populations are of constant size (N_1 and N_2 respectively) with stable age distributions where survival in both is Type II (with constant per capita mortality rates $\hat{\mu}_1$ and $\hat{\mu}_2$ for humans and vectors respectively), then the weighted average values $\bar{M}(t)$ and $\bar{L}(t)$ are

$$\bar{M}(t) = \hat{\mu}_1 \int_0^\infty M(a, t) \exp(-\hat{\mu}_1 a) \, da, \tag{20.39}$$

$$\bar{L}(t) = \hat{\mu}_2 \int_0^\infty L(a, t) \exp(-\hat{\mu}_2 a) \, da. \tag{20.40}$$

The parameters T_1 and T_2 denote the rates of transmission from vector to human and human to vector respectively. Their definition follows lines similar to those described in the previous section for the schistosome transmission model (see eqn (20.32)). The term T_1 is a function of various parameters,

$$T_1 = (N_2/N_1)\bar{\beta}pd_1. \tag{20.41}$$

Here N_1 is human density, N_2 is vector density, $\bar{\beta}$ is the number of blood meals taken per vector per unit of time, p is the proportion of blood meals taken from humans (certain vectors of filarial parasites feed on a variety of different mammalian species), and d_1 is the proportion of the mean load of infective larvae in the vector that establish within the human host and develop to sexual maturity (defined per vector bite on the human host). The parameter T_2 is defined as

$$T_2 = \tfrac{1}{2}\phi\bar{\beta}p\lambda d_2. \tag{20.42}$$

Here ϕ is the mating probability (a function of the mean worm burden per person and the degree of parasite aggregation), $\bar{\beta}$ and p are as defined for T_1, λ is the per capita fecundity of the mature female worm, and d_2 is the probability that an inflective larva is ingested by the vector per bite and survives to attain infectivity in the arthropod host. The parameters μ_1 and μ_2 denote the death rates of mature worms and infective larvae, respectively, in the absence of density-dependent constraints.

The functions f_1 and f_2 denote density-dependent constraints on the input of infective larvae into the human host and vector, respectively. Similarly, the functions g_1 and g_2 denote density-dependent constraints on adult worm and infective larval survival, respectively.

An expression for the basic reproductive rate, R_0, may be obtained from the equilibrium equations ($\partial M/\partial t = 0$) of the model defined by eqns (20.37) and (20.38):

$$R_0 = T_1 T_2/[(\mu_1 + \hat{\mu}_1)(\mu_2 + \hat{\mu}_2)]. \tag{20.43}$$

Note that a term N_2/N_1 (see eqn (20.41)) is embodied in the above expression for R_0, denoting the ratio of vectors to humans. This is to be compared with the product N_1N_2 that arose in the expression for R_0 derived from the schistosome model (see eqns (20.33), (20.34), and (20.35)). The difference is a consequence of the differing modes of transmission: one by a biting vector (the filarial worms), the other by free-living infective stages (the schistosome flukes). As discussed in Chapter 14 in the context of malaria, for infections borne by biting arthropods, the intermediate host tends to make a fixed number of bites per unit time, independent of the number of human hosts available to feed on. Net transmission therefore depends on the ratio of vectors to humans (see May and Anderson 1979). This assumption is somewhat crude if the biting vector takes its fixed number of blood meals from several different mammalian species (as appears to be the case for vectors of certain filarial species). In this case the proportion taken from humans may be proportional to human density N_1. Then R_0 is again proportional to N_1N_2, rather than to the ratio N_2/N_1. Which is the better of these two assumptions will depend on the particular epidemiology of a given nematode species in a defined geographical location. In the absence of any detailed information for a particular case we work with the assumption that R_0 is proportional to the ratio N_2/N_1.

The dynamical properties of the partial differential equation model (eqns (20.37) and (20.38)) will depend to a large extent on the density-dependent functions f_1, f_2, g_1, and g_2. Empirical data on the forms of these functions are unavailable, so there is little point in studying the model's properties in detail. But in the hope that such data may soon appear, we pursue a few special cases.

On the assumption that density-dependent constraints do not affect infective larval survival and uptake (i.e. the production of microfilariae in the human host) by the vector (i.e. $f_2 = 1$, $g_2 = 1$) eqn (20.38) simplifies to

$$\partial L/\partial t + \partial L/\partial a = \Lambda_2 - \mu_2 L, \tag{20.44}$$

where $\Lambda_2 = T_2\bar{M}$. At equilibrium ($\partial L/\partial t = 0$), the weighted mean number of infective larvae over all age classes (i.e. the overall population mean), $\bar{L}^*$, is simply

$$\bar{L}^* = T_2\bar{M}^*/(\mu_2 + \hat{\mu}_2). \tag{20.45}$$

Note that T_2 is a function of the mating probability ϕ, which is itself a function of $\bar{M}^*$ (see eqn (20.42)). If we assume that filarial worms are polygamous and distributed (sexes together) in a negative binomial pattern with clumping parameter k (independent of host age), then

$$\phi(\bar{M}^*, k) = 1 - (1 + \bar{M}^*/2k)^{-(k+1)} \tag{20.46}$$

(see May (1977b) and Table 16.1.

In this simple case the relationship between $\bar{L}^*$ and $\bar{M}^*$ is predicted to be essentially linear for all but very small values of $\bar{M}^*$ (Fig. 20.19). A limited number of data are available to test this prediction. One example is for *O. volvulus* infections in humans and *Simulium* in a sequence of villages in West Africa (Dietz 1982a) (Fig. 20.20). The evidence for a linear association is

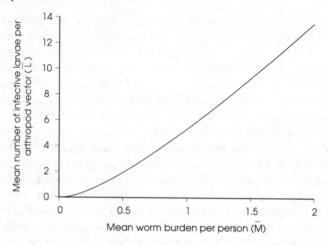

Fig. 20.19. The relationship between mean worm burden per person and the number of infective larvae per arthropod vector, as predicted by eqns (20.45) and (20.46).

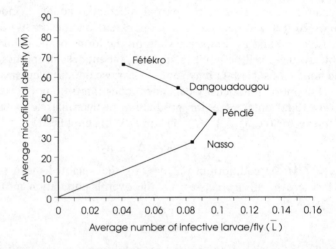

Fig. 20.20. The observed relationship between the average microfilarial density, $\bar{M}$, and the average number of infective larvae/fly, $\bar{L}$, based on four villages in the area of the Onchocerciasis Control Programme. The hypothetical line joining the points goes through the point $(\bar{M}, \bar{L}) = (0, 0)$ since this corresponds to a trivial equilibrium (Dietz 1982a).

somewhat inconclusive since the data hint at the presence of an asymptote in $\bar{M}^*$ as $\bar{L}^*$ increases.

An alternative approach is to consider what happens if the rate of vector mortality depends on parasite burden. Several experimental studies provide support for this suggestion (Rosen 1955; Christensen 1978). A study by Rosen (1955), which is discussed by Hairston and Jachowski (1968), provides

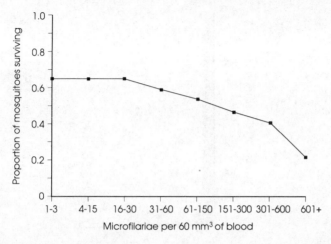

Fig. 20.21. Influence of microfilarial density (*Wuchereria bancrofti*) in the peripheral blood of the host upon which a vector feeds on the proportion of mosquitoes (*Aedes polynesiensis*) surviving to development of third-stage larvae (Hairston and Jachowski 1968).

particularly detailed information on the relationship between the survival of the mosquito *Aedes polynesiensis* and the burden of larval *Wuchereria bancrofti*. Information is also provided on the density of microfilariae in the blood of the patients used to infect the vectors within the experimental study. As illustrated in Fig. 20.21, vector survival declines as parasite burden following a blood meal rises. Even if we make the simplest assumption that the death rate of an infected vector is directly proportional to parasite burden, the net rate of loss of parasites in the equations for $L(a, t)$ (eqn (20.38)) will still depend on the distribution of parasite numbers per arthropod (Anderson and May 1978). Field data suggest that larval filarial worms are typically very highly aggregated within arthropod populations (Fig. 20.22) (see Cheke *et al.* 1982). The negative binomial distribution with a very small value of k is again a useful empirical model. Putting these two assumptions together (i.e. linear dependence of mortality on parasite burden and a negative binomial distribution) the loss term in eqn (20.38) is given by (see Anderson and May 1978)

$$\mu_2 L(g_2(L)) = \mu_2 L[c_1 + c_2(1 + 1/k)L], \tag{20.47}$$

where c_1 and c_2 are constants and k is the negative binomial dispersion parameter. In the derivation of eqn (20.47) it is assumed that vector density remains constant (i.e. its abundance is determined by factors other than the parasite) and that parasite-induced host mortality does not alter the form of the parasite's distribution (i.e. k independent of L).

Given eqn (20.47), it is again possible to derive an expression, at equilibrium,

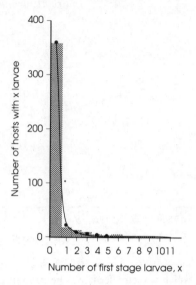

Fig. 20.22. Frequency distribution of the number of first-stage larvae of *Onchocerca* spp. per fly vector (*Simulium damnosum*) (data from Cheke *et al.* 1982). The histogram bars are observed values and the full curve denotes the best-fit negative binomial model. Parameter values: $k = 0.073$, mean $= 0.29$.

for the relationship between $\bar{L}^*$ and $\bar{M}^*$ (given that $f_2 = 1$):

$$\bar{L}^* = T_2 \bar{M}^* \hat{\mu}_2 \int_0^\infty \exp(-\hat{\mu}_2 a) h(a) \, da, \tag{20.48}$$

where

$$h(a) = (1 - e^{-\alpha a})/(A_1 + A_2 e^{-\alpha a}). \tag{20.49}$$

Here $\alpha = [(\mu_2 c_1)^2 + 4\mu_1 c_2(1 + 1/k)T_2\bar{M}^*]^{1/2}$, $A_1 = \frac{1}{2}(\alpha + \mu_2 c_1)$ and $A_2 = \frac{1}{2}(\alpha - \mu_2 c_1)$. The relationship between $\bar{L}^*$ and $\bar{M}^*$ is convex if $\bar{L}^* \to 0$ as $\bar{M}^* \to \infty$.

To produce the sort of pattern portrayed in Fig. 20.20, it is necessary to place a density-dependent constraint on the population growth of adult worms in the human host. For example, if the human death rate is proportional to parasite burden, as we assumed in eqn (20.47) and as is reasonable for *O. volvulus*, which is a cause of blindness in adults and concomitant mortality (Prost and Prescott 1984), then by replacing L by M in eqn (20.47) and $\bar{L}^*$ by $\bar{M}^*$ in eqn (20.48), via eqn (20.37) with $f_1 = 1$, we can arrive at a mimic of the relationship observed for *O. volvulus* (Fig. 20.20).

These rather abstract manipulations of the density-dependent functions defined in eqns (20.37) and (20.38) support the view that regulatory constraints on adult worm abundance are likely to be of greater significance to parasite flow via the entire life cycle than those acting on infective larvae in the vector

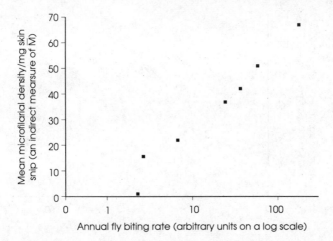

Fig. 20.23. The relationship between the mean density of *Onchocerca volvulus* micro-filariae per milligram skin snip (an indirect measure of $\bar{M}$) and the annual fly biting rate (Dietz 1982*a*).

population, given the observation that $\bar{M}^*$ tends to a maximum value for intermediate or high values of $\bar{L}^*$. In the absence of additional data, we are unable to pursue this issue further.

The data shown in Fig. 20.20, concerning the relationship between $\bar{M}^*$ and $\bar{L}^*$, were collected by the Onchocerciasis Control Project (OCP) in the Volta River Basin which was initiated by the World Health Organization in 1974 (see WHO 1985). This project also focused on entomological studies which enabled estimates to be made of the relationship between a measure of the net biting rate of the insect vector, estimated from observations of fly attacks on volunteer human baits, and the mean infective filarial density in the human populations (Fig. 20.23). This measure of biting activity is roughly proportional to the term $\bar{\beta}N_2/N_1$ in eqn (20.41) of the model. If the annual biting rate drops below a certain level, the basic reproductive rate of the parasite will fall below the transmission threshold $R_0 = 1$ (see eqns (20.41) and (20.43)). Evidence for a transmission threshold is clearly revealed in the data collected on $\bar{M}^*$ and the annual biting rate in the OCP project (Fig. 20.23). Dietz (1982*a*) used this observation to estimate the basic reproductive rate of *O. volvulus* in different villages in the Volta River Basin. He based these estimates on the assumptions that adult worms have a life expectancy of roughly 8 years (see Roberts *et al.* 1967) and that the *Simulium* vector has a life expectancy of a few weeks (Dalmat and Gibson 1952). Dietz's estimates are summarized in Table 20.1, as are other epidemiological records from the OCP project in the Volta River Basin area. The estimates vary greatly between villages, as do age-related changes in the average intensity of infection in the human communities (measured indirectly by microfilarial skin snip counts) (Fig. 20.24). The observed convexity in the

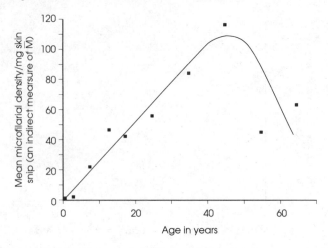

Fig. 20.24. The relationship between the mean density of *Onchocerca volvulus* micro-filariae per milligram skin snip (an indirect measure of $\overline{M}$) and human age in years (Dietz 1982*a*).

relationship between intensity of infection and age may be due to a variety of factors. Age-related changes in contact with the vector, along with differences in survival between lightly and heavily infected people, are thought to be the main processes at work (Dietz 1982*a*).

20.2.2 *Epidemiological patterns and control*

Epidemiological studies of age-related patterns of infection with filarial worms reveal a number of interesting points. First, the prevalence and intensity of infection typically rise much more slowly with age in endemic areas than do the same statistics for intestinal nematode and schistosome infections (Fig. 20.25). This is largely owing to the long life expectancies of the filarial species compared with the other major helminths (see Table 15.2). This implies longer generation times and lower reproductive potential (per unit time). Note, for example, that R_0 is defined per generation of the parasite such that a value of, say, 5, for both *Ascaris* and *Onchocerca* in a given community (with respective life expectancies of 1 and 8 years) implies very different rates of parasite transmission for the two species (as measured by the rapidity with which intensity rises with host age). It should also be noted, however, that the available data on worm life expectancies are very limited for the filarial species. Hairston and Jachowski (1968), in a study of *Wuchereria bancrofti* in Samoa, obtain estimates of mature worm life expectancy of between 2.5 and 3 years, and they estimate the latent period in humans at roughly 14 months. For *Onchocerca volvulus*, estimates range between 8 and 11 years for mature worm life expectancy and between 12 and 18 months for the latent period (Chartres 1955; Roberts *et al.* 1967; Duke 1970; Muller 1975).

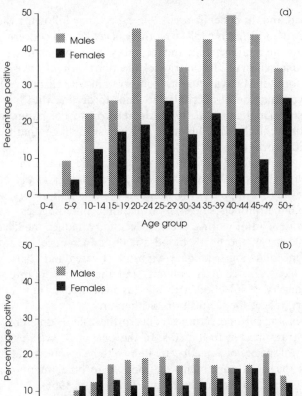

Fig. 20.25. Age and sex distribution of the microfilarial rate (prevalence) of (a) *Wuchereria bancrofti* in Anami, Japan (Sasa *et al.* 1970) and (b) *Onchocerca volvulus* in Ethiopia (Oomen 1969).

Another pattern concerns the maximum prevalence of infection attained in any age class within endemic areas. For filarial species, the upper asymptote rarely approaches 100 per cent (Fig. 20.25). This may be due to very high degrees of parasite aggregation, or more likely, to a combination of moderate reproductive potential combined with the early death of heavily infected people when compared with lightly infected people.

Many uncertainties still remain concerning the life cycles of filarial worms. We have already mentioned the role of density-dependent constraints on population growth. These certainly act on vector survival which is inversely related to worm load, and for *O. volvulus* also on human survival. The occurrence of blindness as a result of *Onchocerca* infection is related to parasite load and, in endemic areas, life expectancy following the loss of sight is short (Prost and Prescott 1984). Nothing is yet known concerning constraints on adult parasite establishment and fecundity. An experimental study involving the repeated infection of cats (a 'trickle' infection) with infective larvae of *Brugia pahangi* (a form of Malayan filariasis observed in wild carnivores) suggests that the rate of production of microfilariae tends to decline with increases in adult worm density (Denham *et al.* 1972). In relation to the patterns observed for other helminth infections of humans, it would seem likely that worm fecundity declines with worm density.

With respect to acquired immunity, the chronic nature of filarial infection implies either that protective responses are absent or weak, or that worms somehow evade or suppress the immune system. Laboratory studies with a variety of animal models suggest that acquired immunity can act to increase the death rate of adult worms, decrease fecundity, reduce the life expectancy of the microfilariae in the host's blood stream, and reduce the rate of parasite establishment following secondary exposure (Evered and Clark 1987). Similar effects are likely to occur in humans, and the convex nature of changes in average intensity of infection with age (as measured by microfilarial counts) may, in part, reflect the acquisition of immunity.

Further biological uncertainties concern the role of different vector species in parasite transmission to humans. In the case of *O. volvulus*, for example, a wide variety of species of *Simulium* are known to be involved, but the frequencies with which they feed on humans as opposed to other mammalian species in endemic areas are unknown at present (Duke *et al.* 1966).

Given these uncertainties, mathematical models of filarial infection remain in their infancy. Certain qualitative conclusions do emerge, however, from the simple formulation discussed at the beginning of this section. Most importantly, theory shows how important it is to gather quantitative data on the relationship between mean infective larval burdens in the vector and mean microfilarial counts in humans, and on the relationship between the vector biting rates, and mean intensity of infection in the human community (see Figs. 20.20 and 20.23). Such information can help to identify the most important density-dependent constraints on parasite population growth. It can also help to reveal the level to which vector density must be reduced if transmission is to be interrupted (Fig. 20.23).

All the vectors of filarial parasites have short life expectancies relative to those of the adult parasites in humans (Table 20.2). Thus, vector density would have to be depressed below the critical level for the maintenance of transmission ($R_0 = 1$) for very long periods of time to have a substantial impact on worm loads within the human community. A simple numerical example serves to illustrate this point. Consider an area in which onchocerciasis is endemic and where vector control by the widespread application of larvicides in aquatic habitats has interrupted transmission. Suppose that prior to control the mean worm burden was 40 parasites per person, distributed as a negative binomial

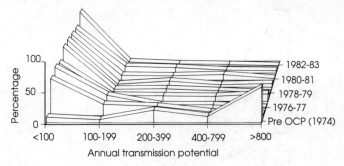

Fig. 20.26. Percentage of catching points for each category of annual transmission potential (the estimated total number of infective larvae indistinguishable from *Onchocerca volvulus*, that would be received by a subject stationed at a capture point over a 1-year period) in the initial programme area, before the start of the Onchocerciasis Control Programme (OCP) and in subsequent years (WHO 1985).

with clumping parameter $k = 0.2$ (a value appropriate for many helminth species, see Table 15.5). Given that *O. volvulus* has a life expectancy of roughly 10 years, then after 8 years of perfect vector control (i.e. no new infections), the mean worm load will have decayed from 40 to 18 worms per person (assuming a constant death rate μ_1 of $1/10 \text{ yr}^{-1}$) and the prevalence will have fallen from 65 to 59 per cent (assuming that k remains constant). This example is not just of academic interest since it mirrors the situation that has arisen under the WHO Onchocerciasis Control Project (OCP) in the Volta River Basin of West Africa. Intensive and repeated application of larvicides over an 8-year period (1975–83) interrupted transmission within many regions in the control project area (Fig. 20.26). Over this period the mean intensity of infection (as measured by microfilarial counts) showed a consistent but slow decline (Fig. 20.27). Prevalence decayed much more slowly than intensity, as would be expected given an aggregated distribution of parasite numbers within the human population. Although the achievements of the OCP have been impressive with respect to the reduction of morbidity from infection, it remains true that long-term suppression of parasite abundance will require continual and intensive vector control. If this ceased for any reason, or if insecticide resistance became prevalent within the vector population, the remaining adult parasites in the human community would be able to bring about the slow return of mean worm loads to their pre-control levels.

The rate of return of parasite abundance following a cessation in control will depend on a variety of factors. The reproductive potential of the vector species is of obvious significance and is greater for the mosquito vectors of *Wuchereria* than it is for the longer lived *Simulium* vectors of *Onchocerca*. In addition, *Onchocerca* has a longer life expectancy in humans than does *Wuchereria*. Both factors together suggest that *O. volvulus* would recover more slowly than would *W. bancrofti*.

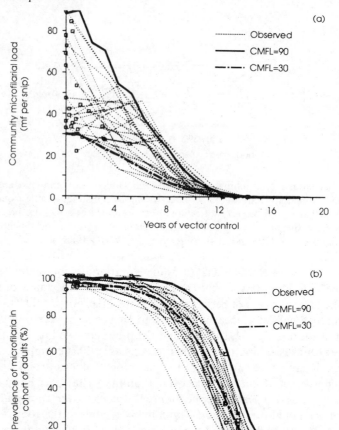

Fig. 20.27. Observed trends in (a) intensity and (b) prevalence of *Onchocerca volvulus* infection during the control period of the Onchocerciasis Control Project in villages where the community microfilarial level (CMFL) was greater than 30 microfilaria per skin snip, prior to the instigation of control. The heavier curves are the predicted trends for starting values of CMFL of 30 and 90 under the impact of control (see Remme 1989). Note the sigmoid decay in prevalence and exponential decay in parasite mean intensity.

The OCP was based on the reduction of vector density, because in the early 1970s there were no chemotherapeutic agents suitable for treating infection in humans. Today a number of promising drugs are undergoing trials and community-based chemotherapy programmes should soon be feasible (the drug Ivermectin looks particularly promising but new compounds are also being tested). Community-based programmes should have a substantial impact owing to the long life expectancy of the worm in untreated individuals and the predicted slow rate of recovery of the parasite population following perturbation. The factors determining the frequency and intensity of drug treatment required within a community to interrupt transmission are identical to those outlined earlier for intestinal nematode and schistosome infections (see Chapter 17).

21

Experimental epidemiology

21.1 Introduction

We have seen in the previous three chapters that much uncertainty surrounds the epidemiological interpretations of changes in average worm loads with respect to human age. The importance of acquired immunity, or other density-dependent constraints on parasite establishment, survival, or fecundity, in shaping observed patterns is not at all clear at present. To a very large extent this gap in our knowledge arises from the simple fact that, for obvious ethical reasons, it is rarely possible to obtain quantitative measures of the population processes influencing the abundance of an endoparasite within a human patient. Rapid advances in research on human immune responses to infectious agents raised the hope in the 1970s that new techniques would facilitate quantitative measurement of parasite abundance and effective immunity within human communities. In the case of macroparasites this hope has not as yet been realized, although recent advances in immunology and molecular biology may yet provide the epidemiologist with the practical tools required for the rapid quantification of parasite abundance and distribution under field conditions.

Current ignorance of the factors that control helminth abundance in individual patients can to some extent be offset by recourse to experimental studies that employ rodent host–helminth parasite models. There are of course many problems inherent in drawing conclusions about human infections on the basis of laboratory work with rodents. However, provided these limitations are kept in mind, the precision of laboratory experiments can provide valuable clues to the link between process and pattern. This is especially true in the interpretation of dynamic changes in parasite abundance both within individuals and populations of hosts. For example, it is possible within the laboratory to expose groups of hosts of known age, sex, nutritional status, and genetic background to repeated infection, over long periods of time, under defined and controlled conditions. Such experiments, often referred to as 'trickle' exposure studies, are thought more closely to mimic human exposure to helminth infection in endemic areas than the primary and challenge experiments which are a feature of much immunological research in parasitology (Anderson and Crombie 1984, 1985; Sturrock et al. 1984; Wakelin 1984; Crombie and Anderson 1985). In the latter type of study, experimental designs are geared to eliciting a measurable immunological response and usually involve a primary infection and subsequent challenge (often entailing exposure of a host to large numbers of infective stages); resistance is recorded as the percentage reduction in parasite establishment, survival, or fecundity in challenged hosts when compared with that in naive hosts (primary infection). Little research has focused on the dynamic nature of helminth establishment and mortality, and their presumed dependence on the rate of current and past experience to infection, in hosts repeatedly exposed to low levels of infection (as human populations are thought to be exposed in areas of endemic infection).

In this chapter we examine some recent research on the repeated exposure of rodent hosts to helminth infection, with the dual aims of sharpening current debate on the factors responsible for age-related changes in helminth abundance within human communities and testing model predictions concerning the regulatory impact of acquired immunity. We refer to work on two particular laboratory models, namely the human blood fluke *Schistosoma mansoni* and a directly transmitted intestinal nematode, *Heligmosomoides polygyrus*. Both parasites can establish within and develop to sexual maturity in the laboratory mouse.

21.2 Schistosomes and mice

Before turning to the patterns generated by repeated exposure to infection, it is helpful to examine what happens in a primary infection. Observed trends in parasite establishment, survival, and mortality depend on a variety of host characteristics such as age, sex, nutritional status, and genetic background (Dean 1983). Within inbred mice (having uniform genetic make-up) of known age and sex, maintained on a defined diet, parasite establishment (defined as the attainment of sexual maturity) is directly proportional to the density of infective stages to which the mice are exposed (Fig. 21.1). Sexual maturity of the parasite is attained within 4–6 weeks from entry into the host. For a variety of mouse strains, approximately 40–50 per cent of the density of cercariae to which the host is exposed attain maturity. Within inbred strains the distribution of worm numbers per mouse in a sample where each mouse is exposed to the same number of cercariae tends to be Poisson in form. In outbred strains the distribution may be slightly aggregated in pattern. Under conditions of exposure to infected water bodies in the field, the distribution of parasites in samples of mice may be highly aggregated, having the form shown in Fig. 21.2. Following maturation, parasite survival is approximately Type II in form (i.e. a constant per capita death rate) where life expectancy is of the order of 20–30 weeks (to some extent dependent on mouse strain; see Fig. 21.3). Parasite survival may be density dependent at high levels of infection owing to parasite-induced mouse mortality (see Fig. 21.4). At moderate to low levels of infection (5–30 parasites per mouse) the rates of mortality of many strains of mice differ little from those pertaining in uninfected animals. Egg production by mature female worms is age dependent and attains a peak roughly 10–16 weeks after maturation (Fig. 21.5).

Under conditions of constant and repeated exposure to infection, where rates of parasite establishment, maturation, and survival remain unchanged, average

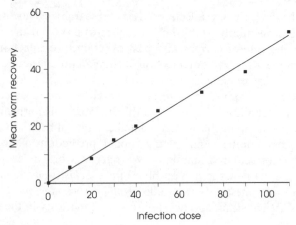

Fig. 21.1. Recovery of *S. mansoni* 6 weeks post-infection from naive mice exposed to a single infection of varying intensity (10–100 cercariae). The squares record observed mean burdens (per 10 mice) and the solid line records the best-fit linear model with slope $b = 0.4711$ ($r^2 = 0.99$) (from Crombie and Anderson 1985).

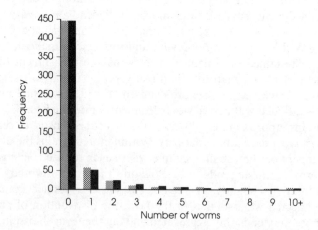

Fig. 21.2. Frequency distribution of numbers of mice harbouring different numbers of *S. mansoni* resulting from the exposure of the mice to water contact in eight field sites on St Lucia (from Sturrock 1973). The graph records the observed distribution (stippled bars) and the best-fit negative binomial model (mean = 0.614, $k = 0.152$) (solid bars).

parasite burdens per host will rise monotonically as the duration of exposure increases (i.e. with mouse age) to a stable equilibrium ($M^* = \Lambda/\mu_1$ where Λ is the rate of infection and $1/\mu_1$ is worm life expectancy), in the manner discussed at the beginning of Chapter 17 (a simple immigration–death process).

A series of experiments described by Crombie and Anderson (1985) were designed to test how such age-related (equivalent to duration of exposure)

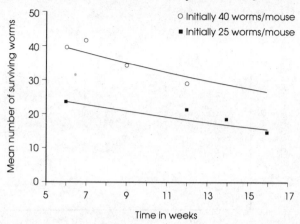

Fig. 21.3. Survival of adult *S. mansoni* in CBA/Ca mice over a 10-week period post worm maturation. Two examples are shown where initial adult worm densities at week 6 of infection (average time to maturation) were 40 and 25 parasites per mouse. Symbols denote observed means (per mouse for a sample size of 10) and the lines denote the fit of an exponential decay survival model with constant death rate $\mu = 0.045$ per week (from Crombie and Anderson 1985).

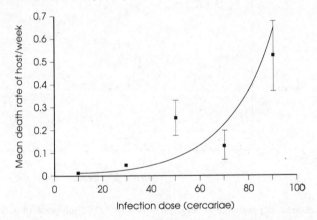

Fig. 21.4. Estimated mean death rate (per week) of mice (with 95 per cent confidence limits) infected with varying doses of the cercariae of *S. mansoni*. The curve denotes the best-fit model of the form $y = a \exp(bx)$ (y = death rate, x = infection dose) where $a = 0.00523$ and $b = 0.05387$ (from Crombie 1985). As recorded in Fig. 21.1 parasite density per host is directly proportional to the infective dose to which the mice are exposed.

trends in worm burden changed under different levels of exposure to infection. Four groups of 10 mice were exposed to 10, 30, 100, and 300 cercariae per group per week. Worms were recovered at intervals after infection by perfusion of the hepatic portal system and general dissection of the host. The results of

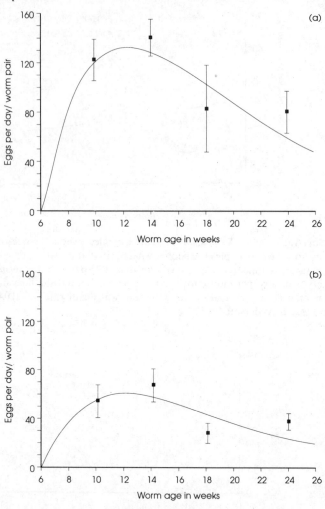

Fig. 21.5. Age dependence in egg production by *S. mamsoni* in CBA/Ca mice. Egg production is recorded as eggs per day per worm pair. The squares record mean values (per 10 mice) with 95 per cent confidence limits. In (a) mice were exposed to 10 cercariae/mouse and in (b) mice were exposed to 40 cercariae/mouse (from Sithithaworn 1986). The curves denote the best-fit model of the form $y(x) = ax \exp(-bx)$, where y = egg production and x = worm age.

those experiments are presented in Fig. 21.6. The severity of the initial rise in mean worm burden with age of the host, and the maximum worm burden attained, are dependent on the density of cercariae to which the host is exposed. At the lowest infection dose, mice survived well and the experiment ran for 50 weeks with worm burdens attaining a stable plateau of about 4–6 parasites per

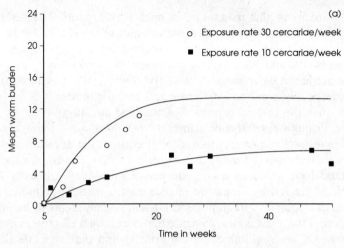

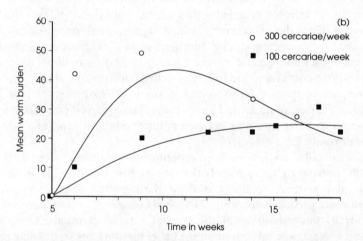

Fig. 21.6. The recorded mean burdens of *S. mansoni* in mice exposed to 10 and 30 cercariae per group of 10 mice per week (a) and 100 and 300 cercariae per group of 10 mice per week (b). Groups of 10 mice were exposed to infection at weekly intervals by paddling for 30 minutes in tanks containing a suspension of cercariae (of age < 2.5 hours) in 200 ml dechlorinated tap water at 25 °C (from Crombie and Anderson 1985). Note that the abscissae start at 5 weeks because of the maturation delay (of 5 weeks) of *S. mansoni* in laboratory mice. The curves denote predicted worm recoveries calculated from an immigration–death model, described in Anderson and May (1985*b*), where parasite establishment decays in direct proportion as the summed past experience of infection rises (see Crombie and Anderson 1985).

mouse. Burdens of this magnitude in mice may produce diseases that most closely resemble human hepatosphenic schistosomiasis (Dean 1983). At higher exposure levels some host mortality occurred. In the two highest exposure experiments (100 and 300 cercariae per mouse per week) there was a decline in parasite burden in older mice, the severity of which was not accounted for by a dependence between host death rate and parasite burden.

Given that the rate of exposure of the host to infective stages was kept constant through time (hence constant with host age), these observations suggest that hosts acquire resistance to infection as the duration and intensity of exposure increases (Crombie and Anderson 1985). The convex pattern (Fig. 21.6) could have arisen as a consequence of time-delayed density-dependent mechanisms created by limitation of resources or pathology induced by past infection, as opposed to immunological defences. This seems to be unlikely for two reasons. First, there is clear evidence that mice mount effective immunological responses to *S. mansoni* infection from primary and challenge infection experiments (Dean 1983). Second, the experiments generated comparatively low burdens of mature and juvenile worms when compared with the much higher worm loads that can be harboured in the mesenteric veins (Dean 1983).

Perfusion of infected mice led to the recovery of juvenile worms throughout the course of all the experiments, which suggests that parasites can become established in hosts despite long durations of past experience of infection and the presence of mature adult worms. This observation is in direct contradiction of past dogma concerning the role of so-called concomitant immunity, in which the presence of mature schistosomes is supposed to prevent larval parasite establishment (see Smithers and Terry 1969). The observed patterns of infection represent a dynamic interplay between parasite establishment (at a rate $\bar{\Lambda}$) and worm mortality (at a rate μ_1).

A more detailed analysis of these experimental results and some unpublished work (Sithithaworn 1986) reveals that the numbers of juvenile worms within the population tends to decay both as the duration of past exposure, and exposure intensity, increase (Fig. 21.7). This observation is in agreement with our current understanding of the mechanisms of immunity to *S. mansoni* infection in mice, which is based on the belief that host resistance acts primarily to restrict parasite establishment (as opposed to increased adult worm mortality or decreased fecundity) (Dean 1983).

The assumptions of the model of acquired immunity to helminth infection described in Chapter 18 (by eqn (18.5)) therefore seem to be an appropriate description of the main biological processes acting within these trickle infection experiments. The model contains four adjustable parameters: $\bar{\Lambda}$, the rate of parasite establishment in the absence of host resistance; μ_1, the death rate of adult parasites; ε, the severity of acquired responses that limit parasite establishment; and $1/\sigma$, the duration of immunological memory (see Chapter 18). Estimates are available for $\bar{\Lambda}$ and μ_1 (see Figs. 21.1 and 21.3) on the basis of the experimental design and information from primary infections in mice,

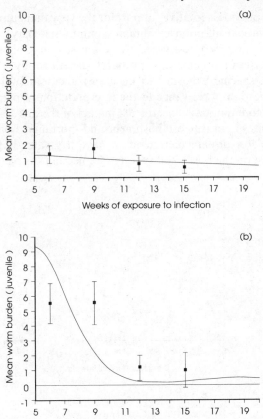

Fig. 21.7. The change in the mean number of juvenile *S. mansoni* with time of exposure to repeated infection in mice (sample size of 20 mice per mean) exposed to 1.4 cercariae per week (a) and 9.4 cercariae per week (b). The vertical bars denote 95 per cent confidence limits. The lines denote the predictions of a simple model based on parasite recruitment and maturation (see Sithithaworn 1986).

and a crude estimate of ε can be obtained via the observations on the rate of decline in juvenile worm establishment as a function of past worm loads. However, the experimental results provide no information on the duration of immunological memory (the parameter σ). A fit of the model to the experimental results, with no adjustable parameters other than $\bar{\Lambda}$, which is set by the experimental design (the density of cercariae to which the mice are exposed times the proportion that establish in primary infections), and σ, was obtained via a non-linear least squares technique (see Crombie and Anderson 1985; Crombie 1985). Model predictions and observed patterns are compared in Fig. 21.6. The model is able to reflect monotonic growth to a stable parasite burden for low rates of exposure to infection and convex curves for high rates of exposure. This provides tentative support for the view that convex age–intensity curves of *S. mansoni* infection in human communities may in part arise as a consequence of acquired resistance. As discussed in Chapter 20, however, observed patterns in humans are probably generated by a combination of ecological (age-specific exposure to infection) and immunological processes.

A further question of relevance to the interpretation of patterns of infection within human communities concerns the impact of the host's nutritional status on the dynamics of parasite establishment and mortality. For the *S. mansoni*–mouse system, low-protein diets tend to have a greater impact on parasite abundance than on the host's ability to resist infection. As recorded in Fig.21.8,

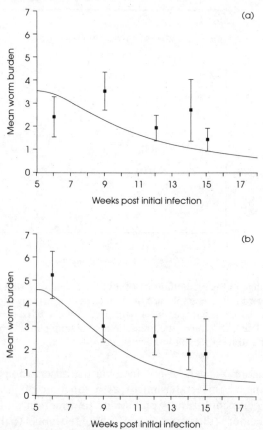

Fig. 21.8. Changes in burdens of juvenile *S. mansoni* in mice fed on diets containing varying levels of dietary protein. The mice were exposed to 3.6 cerceriae per week in (a) and fed on a diet with 4 per cent protein. In (b) the mice were exposed to 4.7 cercariae per week and fed on a 12 per cent protein diet (from Sithithaworn 1986). The curves denote the predictions of a model in which parasite establishment decays in proportion to the summed past experience of infection. The vertical bars denote 95 per cent confidence limits.

trickle experiments involving two batches of mice, one maintained on a high-protein diet and one on a low-protein diet, revealed that poor host nutritional status (as revealed by host growth during the course of the experiment) acts to depress the abundance of the parasite (Sithithaworn 1986). The parasite's niche in the blood system of the host probably has a direct bearing on this observation.

Further experiments have been performed to explore the significance of immunological memory using curative chemotherapy after a period of repeated exposure to infection and monitoring what happens when exposure is resumed at various intervals after treatment (Sithithaworn 1986; Crombie and Anderson 1985). Some results from these experiments are displayed in Fig. 21.9. They reveal that at low rates of exposure to infection memory is non-existent, such that following treatment mice acquire parasites at similar rates to those observed at the beginning of the period of trickle infection. At higher rates of exposure, however, a degree of resistance is retained (as measured by the reduction in parasite establishment) for some weeks (about 6 weeks) after treatment. Resistance is not dependent on the presence of adult worms within the mice.

The relationship between the results of these experimental studies of *S. mansoni* in mice and infection in human communities is of course uncertain. However, they do suggest that the degree of acquired resistance in mammalian hosts may be dependent on both the duration and intensity of past exposure to infection. In addition they provide quantitative evidence that 'immunological memory' of past experience is dependent on the intensity of past exposure and is of relatively short duration in relation to adult worm and host life expectancy. It is not implausible that such processes are of direct relevance in the transmission dynamics of schistosomes within human communities.

21.3 Intestinal nematodes and mice

Gastrointestinal nematodes invoke a complex immunological response from their mammalian hosts. Antibody and cell mediated events are involved, although present understanding of their respective roles is incomplete (Wakelin 1984). A variety of laboratory models involving mice and nematodes have been used to explore immunity to intestinal helminths. One system of particular convenience (because the parasite is easily cultured) is *Heligmosomoides polygyrus* (formerly called *Nematospiroides dubius*). Infective nematode larvae exsheath after penetration of the mouse host, developing into tissue-dwelling larvae which moult into the adult worms found within the lumen of the alimentary canal. Each stage is characterized by specific surface and secretory antigens (Phillip *et al.* 1980; Pritchard *et al.* 1984) and in turn can invoke a distinct immunological response from the host. Typically, the tissue-dwelling larvae are the most immunogenic stage in the parasite life cycle. This is thought to reflect the increased exposure of tissue-dwelling larvae, as compared with adult worms in

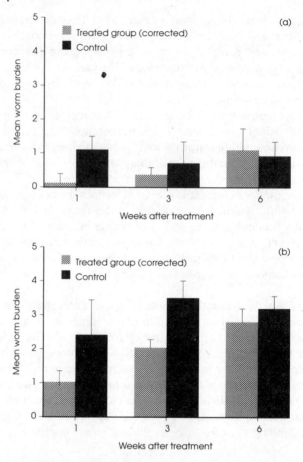

Fig. 21.9. Persistence of residual resistance (acquired immunity) to *S. mansoni* infection in mice given curative chemotherapy. The histogram bars represent the mean parasite burden (square root transformation) and 95 per cent confidence limits of the treated (=infected) group and a 'naive' control group (age matched) determined at varying time intervals (weeks) post curative chemotherapy. Two levels of infection were employed; (a) 30 cercariae/10 mice/week; and (b) 200 cercariae/10 mice/week (from Sithithaworn 1986).

the gut lumen, to the surveillence of the host's immune system, coupled with the immunosuppressive and evasive actions of the adult worms (Behnke 1987).

Effective immunity appears to depend on the degree to which the host is exposed to infective larvae (Wakelin 1984). For example, in the case of the nematode *Nippostrongylus brasiliensis*, laboratory rats rapidly expel a single large infection (> 1000 infective larvae), but repeated low-level infections (five larvae per day) fail to elicit immunologically mediated worm expulsion (Jenkins and Phillipson 1971) (Fig. 21.10). Rats given five larvae per day for 12 weeks

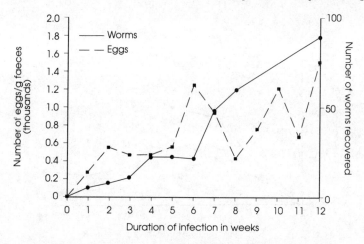

Fig. 21.10. Egg counts (eggs per gram of faeces) and worm burdens from rats that had been infected with five larvae of *Nippostrongylus brasiliensis* per rat per day over a 12-week period (from Jenkins and Phillipson 1971).

accumulated approximately 30 per cent of the total number of larvae that were administered. When rats were infected with 50 larvae per day a smaller total proportion established but worms were able to survive in the partially immune hosts (Jenkins and Phillipson 1971).

More detailed work on the dynamics of nematode establishment and survival has been described by two research groups. This work involves studies of trickle infections, employing the *H. polygyrus*–mouse model (Keymer 1985; Maema 1986; Berding *et al.* 1986; Keymer and Hiorns 1985; Slater and Keymer 1986). One particular set of experiments by Slater and Keymer (1986) involved groups of 30 outbred CD1 mice which were repeatedly infected with 5, 10, 20, or 40 infective larvae of *H. polygyrus* every 2 weeks. Experiments were performed with mice fed on purified, artificial diets containing either 2 per cent ('low protein') or 8 per cent ('high protein') weight for weight protein. As protein deprivation is known to impair the function of the mammalian immune system (Chandra and Newberne 1977; Keusch *et al.* 1983), this design allows a comparison to be made of parasite establishment and survival in the presence or absence of an effective acquired immune response.

Acquired immunity to *H. polygyrus* is primarily triggered by exposure to larval antigens (Jacobsen *et al.* 1982). In genetically resistant inbred strains of mice (termed 'high responders'), this immune response induces a high mortality rate among the tissue-dwelling larvae of *H. polygyrus*. However, in susceptible inbred and outbred strains of mice ('low responders') the immune response is less capable of preventing larval development (Behnke and Robinson 1985). Two trickle infection experiments described by Maema (1986) well illustrate the different patterns of parasite population growth in high-responder

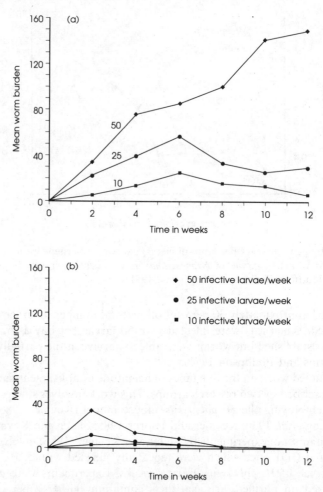

Fig. 21.11. Changes in the mean burdens of *Heligmosomoides polygyrus* in mice repeatedly exposed to varying doses of infective larvae per week. In (a), mice (10 per group) were exposed to 10, 25, and 50 L3 larvae per week. The mouse host was the 'low responder' CBA/Ca strain. In (b), mice were exposed to 10 (squares), 25 (circles) amd 50 (diamonds) L3 larvae per week. The mouse host was the 'high responder' NIH strain (from Maema 1986).

('non-wormy') and low-responder ('wormy') mouse strains (Fg. 21.11). In the low responders, mean parasite burdens rise monotonically to a stable plateau at which the net mortality rate exactly balances the net input rate of parasites (the immigration–death model described at the beginning of Chapter 17). Convex changes in worm burdens with mouse age (equivalent to duration of exposure) arise in the high responders, since parasite establishment and survival declines in the older hosts that have built up a degree of immunity to infection.

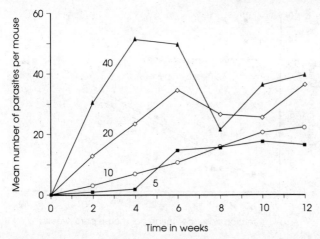

Fig. 21.12. Mean burdens of *Heligmosomoides polygyrus* in mice repeatedly infected with 5, 10, 20, and 40 larvae per 2-week period, and fed on an 8 per cent (by weight) protein diet (from Slater and Keymer 1986).

The severity of the acquired response is related to the degree to which the mice are exposed to infection (the magnitude of the input term).

Returning to the experiments of Slater and Keymer (1986), the mice employed were of the high-responder strain. On high-protein diets the patterns of change in mean worm burden with age varied from monotonic growth at low rates of exposure to convex patterns at high exposure rates (Fig. 21.12). In the malnourished mice on low-protein diets, however, worm burdens increased approximately linearly as the duration of exposure increased, with slope proportional to the rate of exposure to infection (Fig. 21.13). The appropriate

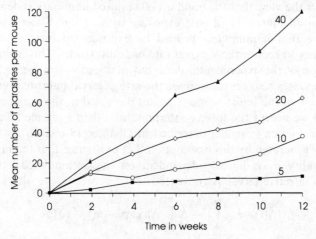

Fig. 21.13. Identical to Fig. 21.12 but with mice fed on a 20 per cent (by weight) protein diet (from Slater and Keymer 1986).

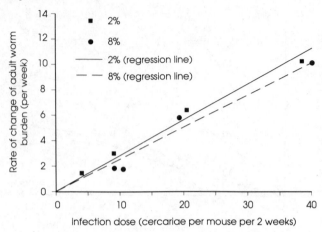

Fig. 21.14. The observed rate of change of adult worm burden in naive mice exposed to varying doses of infective larvae of *H. polygyrus*. Adult parasite worm establishment is proportional to infection dose (from Slater and Keymer 1986).

model consistent with this latter pattern is that adult parasite establishment is proportional to infection dose as recorded in primary infection studies (Fig. 21.14), and that adult parasite mortality is essentially zero. These assumptions lead to the prediction that the mean worm burden $M(t)$ will rise linearly as time t increases (i.e. $M(t) = \Lambda p t$ where $\Lambda =$ biweekly dose of infective larvae and p is proportional establishment, measured by the slope of the graph in Fig. 21.14).

The patterns generated by repeated exposure in the mice fed on high-protein diets support the view that the build up of acquired immunity is dependent on the duration and intensity of past exposure to infection. Slater and Keymer (1986) argue that immunity is primed by exposure to infective larvae but effectively acts to reduce the survival rate of adult worms. This is one possible interpretation of the experimental data, but in addition it appears likely that immune responses also act to decrease the rate of larval parasite establishment (as in the case of the schistosome parasites discussed in the previous section). However, if we accept the former interpretation, then a simple adaptation of the acquired immunity model described in Chapter 18 enables us to explore the patterns generated by this assumption. Let us assume that the rate of adult worm mortality μ_1 is linearly dependent on the accumulated sum of past exposure to infective larvae $\bar{\Lambda}(t)$, where

$$\mu_1(\bar{\Lambda}(t)) = \mu_1\left(1 + \Delta \int_0^t \Lambda p \exp[-\sigma(t - t')]\mathrm{d}t'\right). \qquad (21.1)$$

Here μ_1 denotes the rate of adult worm mortality in naive mice, $1/\sigma$ is the duration of immunological memory of past exposure, Λ is the dose of infective larvae (held constant in time within the experimental design), p is the proportional establishment (the slope of the graph in Fig. 21.14), Δ denotes the severity of the acquired response, and $\bar{\Lambda}(t) = \int_0^t \Lambda p \, dt'$. The rate of change in the mean burden of parasites is then given by

$$dM/dt = \Lambda p - \mu_1 \left(1 + \Delta \int_0^t \Lambda p \exp[-\sigma(t - t')] \, dt' \right) M. \qquad (21.2)$$

The solution of this equation is

$$M(t) = \Lambda p \int_0^t \exp(H(t, t')) \, dt' \qquad (21.3)$$

where

$$H(t, t') = -(t - t')\mu_1 \left[1 + \frac{\Delta p \Lambda}{\sigma} \left(1 - \frac{\exp(-\sigma t') - \exp(-\sigma t)}{\sigma(t - t')} \right) \right].$$

For plausible parameter values ($\sigma = 0$ over the duration of the experiments, $\mu_1 = 0.0056$ day^{-1} and Λp set by the experimental design; see Berding *et al.* (1986)), the model generates patterns in broad agreement with those observed. A rather more complex model is proposed by Berding *et al.* (1986) to describe these experimental results, involving an equation to describe the dynamics of the larval parasites and a threshold effect in the immune response. Both models, however, provide reasonable descriptions of the observed trends and, at present, the data do not allow a finer analysis of the respective assumptions of the two models.

These trickle infection studies of recruitment and mortality in intestinal nematode infections of mammals reveal a number of points relevant to the interpretation of observed patterns in human communities. First, and most importantly, acquired resistance can generate convex changes in average intensity with host age where the degree of convexity is dependent on the duration and intensity of past exposure. As noted in the chapters on intestinal infections in humans (Chapters 17 and 18), the convexity of observed changes in human communities appears to depend on the intensity of transmission in a given habitat (the magnitude of R_0) (see Fig. 18.2). Second, the degree of acquired resistance to infection is very dependent on both the genetic background of the host and its nutritional status. With respect to genetic background, it appears likely that the observed aggregation of parasite numbers per person in human communities will, in part, be determined by differing levels of immuno-competence to resist helminth invasion mediated by the genetic background of the host. Interestingly, protein malnourishment in mice has a very different effect on the population abundance of intestinal nematodes compared with that recorded for schistosome parasites in the preceding section. The trickle experiments suggest that protein deficiency is beneficial to the intestinal nematodes but detrimental to the schistosome flukes (see Figs. 21.8 and 21.12).

More research is needed in the area of experimental epidemiology since, as we have seen in this chapter, experiments that are based on the repeated exposure of hosts to low levels of helminth infection produce patterns of persistence of the parasite population. In the more classical immunoparasitological experiments, involving a primary infection and challenge with large numbers of infective stages, parasite persistence is not the usual outcome in immunocompetent host strains. Helminth infections are clearly persistent within human communities in endemic areas, and hence we feel that much can be learned about the processes controlling parasite abundance within individual hosts from experimental studies that attempt to mimic long-term exposure to infection as experienced by people in endemic regions.

22

Parasites, genetic variability, and drug resistance

22.1 Introduction

Much of conventional theory and practice in epidemiological and ecological research is based on the premise that an understanding of observed patterns and processes can be achieved by reference to the average phenotypic characteristics of a group or sample of individuals and to some measure of variance. This approach is widely adopted despite the certain knowledge that populations of organisms are genetically heterogeneous. It is clearly an 'economy of thought' which often works well in practice when the genetical structure of the population under study is relatively stable and not subject to strong directional selection. In other instances the failure to recognize the variable genetical constitution of a population can lead to erroneous conclusions concerning the factors responsible for observed trends. This is particularly true when strong selective pressures are applied by intensive efforts to control parasite or vector abundance. The evolution of genetic resistance to insecticides induced by attempts to control malaria and onchocerciasis via the suppression of mosquito or black fly abundance are poignant examples of the problems that can arise (Molineaux and Gramiccia 1980; Kurtak 1986). Similarly, the recent and rapid spread of drug-resistant strains of *Neisseria gonorrhoeae* (gonorrhoea) and *Plasmodium falciparium* (falciparium malaria) throughout large areas of the world emphasize the potential of parasite populations for rapid genetic change (Martin *et al.* 1970; Peters 1985) (Fig. 22.1).

The experimental scientist studying the relationship between infectious disease agents and hosts is very familiar with the need to employ inbred strains of laboratory hosts and standard cultures of parasites in order to minimize the variation within an experimental design. Implicit in this practice is the recognition that the genetic background of the host and disease agent is of central importance to the outcome of the interaction between the two species. All too often, however, such laboratory practice is not translated into the procedures employed in the interpretation of events in field situations. In part, this is a consequence of the many practical problems inherent in the study of genetic variability of host and parasite within natural habitats. As we have seen in earlier chapters, the simple measurement of temporal and spatial changes in parasite abundance, without reference to genetic structure, presents many problems in the case of human hosts and endoparasitic organisms. However, in addition to practical issues, there is often a failure to recognize the importance of mechanisms of population genetics in maintaining or disrupting the stability of host–parasite interactions. In past research on infectious diseases, for

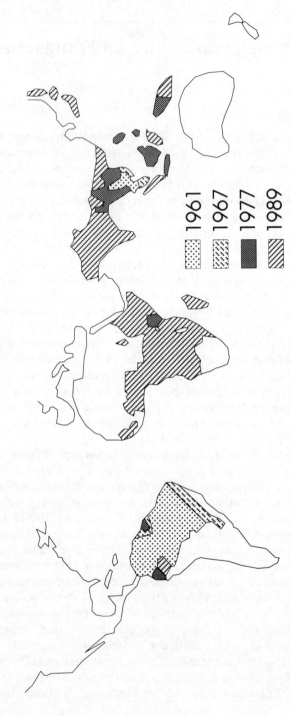

Fig. 22.1. The current world-wide distribution of reports of confirmed resistance of *Plasmodium falciparum* to the drug chloroquine (C. Facer, personal communication).

example, geneticists have usually considered changes in gene frequency without reference to changes in parasite or host abundance, population ecologists and epidemiologists have tended to study changes in abundance without reference to changes in genetic structure, and immunologists have focused on the mechanisms of resistance to infection without reference to population or genetic change. Encouragingly, recent advances in molecular biology and biochemistry offer a powerful range of new techniques (e.g. DNA probes) with which to address questions concerning genetic variation of host and parasite. Their application in epidemiological surveys has already revealed, for example, that populations of *Plasmodium falciparium* within human communities are highly genetically heterogeneous with respect to antigenic characteristics (Forsyth *et al.* 1988). This therefore holds much promise, although the interpretation of what such variability implies for the interaction between host and parasite populations raises a different set of problems.

This chapter stems from our belief that no book on the epidemiology and transmission dynamics of infectious disease agents could be regarded as comprehensive without some reference to population genetics. We have already alluded to the influence of heterogeneity (perhaps genetically based within host populations) on the generation of aggregated distributions of parasite numbers per host (Chapters 16 and 17), on the interpretation of age-related changes in average intensity of infection or the proportion seropositive (Chapters 10 and 17), and on transmission dynamics among groups of differing immunocompetence (Chapters 10, 18, and 19). We now consider a rather miscellaneous selection of topics which relate to the consequences of genetic variability within parasite populations.

22.2 The evolution of resistance

The discussion in this section applies equally to the evolution of drug resistance within parasite populations and the evolution of pesticide resistance in populations of insects or molluscan intermediate hosts. For clarity we restrict our attention to situations where the genetics of resistance involves only one locus with two alleles, in a diploid parasite or insect (and is therefore not directly applicable to certain microparasites such as viruses). This is a very simple assumption but it does appear to be realistic for many recorded instances where a detailed understanding of the mechanisms of resistance is available. We initially consider a closed population in which the selective effects of the drug or pesticide act homogeneously in space.

Following customary usage (see Crow and Kimura 1970), we denote the original susceptible allele by S, and the resistant allele by R. In generation t, the gene frequencies of R and S are p_t and q_t, respectively, with $p + q = 1$. The genotype RR is taken to be resistant, SS to be susceptible and the heterozygotes RS in general to be of intermediate fitness (i.e. resistance partially dominant). In the presence of the application of a drug at a specified (and constant) intensity, the fitnesses of the three genotypes are denoted by w_{RR}, w_{RS}, and w_{SS}. We assume that $w_{RR} > w_{RS} > w_{SS}$.

The equation relating the gene frequencies of R in successive generations of the parasite (or intermediate host) is then the standard expression (see Crow and Kimura 1970)

$$p_{t+1} = \frac{w_{RR}\,p_t^2 + w_{RS}\,p_t q_t}{w_{RR}\,p_t^2 + 2w_{RS}\,p_t q_t + w_{SS}\,q_t^2}. \tag{22.1}$$

In the early stages of drug application, the resistant allele will invariably be very rare (it usually confers a selective disadvantage in the absence of the selective pressure exerted by control measures), so that $p_t \ll 1$ and $q_t \simeq 1$. A numerical example of the change in p_t through time predicted by eqn (22.1), for specified fitness functions, is displayed in Fig. 22.2. Note that the curve is S-shaped (with $p_t \to 1$ as $t \to \infty$ in the absence of heterozygous advantage, i.e. $w_{RR} > w_{RS} > w_{SS}$), such that the appearance of significant (or observable) levels of resistance depends on the period of time over which control measures have been applied to the population. The practical implication of this prediction is that resistance problems may emerge suddenly after many years of control during which the resistant genotype was rare.

The initial ratio p_t/q_t will, as mentioned earlier, be very small (resistant gene very rare) such that in most situations its value will be significantly less than the ratios w_{RS}/w_{RR}, or w_{SS}/w_{RS}. In these circumstances, to a good approximation (see May and Dobson 1986), eqn (22.1) reduces to

$$p_{t+1}/p_t \simeq w_{RS}/w_{SS}. \tag{22.2}$$

Suppose the allele R is present in the pristine population at frequency p_0.

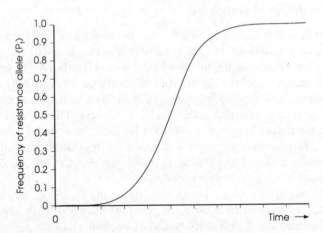

Fig. 22.2. A numerical example of the change in the gene frequency of a resistance gene, R, as defined by eqn (22.1), following selection by drug application ($w_{RR} = 1$, $w_{RS} = 0.5$, $w_{SS} = 0.25$).

Further assume that the recognition of a significant and observable degree of resistance in the parasite population occurs at the frequency p_f (for example say $p_f \sim \frac{1}{2}$). By compounding eqn (22.2) we see that the number of generations of the parasite, n, that must elapse before an observable degree of resistance appears is given roughly by

$$p_f/p_0 = (w_{RS}/w_{SS})^n. \tag{22.3}$$

If T_R is the absolute time taken for a significant degree of resistance to appear, and T_g is the cohort generation time (the average time from birth to reproductive maturity; see, for example, Krebs (1978)) of the parasite or vector in question, then $n = T_R/T_g$. Thus the approximate relation of eqn (22.3) may be rewritten as

$$T_R \simeq T_g \frac{\ln(p_f/p_0)}{\ln(w_{RS}/w_{SS})}. \tag{22.4}$$

It is to be remembered that eqn (22.4) is only an approximation, since if R is recessive such that $w_{RS} = w_{SS}$ then eqn (22.2) is clearly an inadequate description of the details in eqn (22.1). However, even the crude approximation represented by eqn (22.4) is useful in providing a qualitative understanding of what is happening, namely th at T_R is very long when R is recessive (taken literally, eqn (22.4) gives $T_R \to \infty$).

Equation (22.4) demonstrates that the absolute time taken for an observable (or significant) degree of resistance to occur, T_R, depends directly on the parasite's generation time, T_g, but only logarithmically on other factors. Specifically, T_R depends only logarithmically on: the initial frequency of the resistant allele, p_0, prior to control; the choice of the threshold at which resistance is recognized, p_f; and the selection strength, w_{RR}/w_{SS}, which in turn is determined by the intensity of drug or pesticide application and by the degrees of dominance of the resistance allele R. Research on the development of resistance by insects to insecticides suggests that p_0 values may range from 10^{-2} to 10^{-13} (the frequency of the resistance allele prior to widespread insecticide application) (Rousch and Croft 1986). This enormous range, however, collapses to a mere factor of six separating highest from lowest, when logarithms are taken. Likewise, fitness ratios of w_{SS}/w_{RS} ranging from 10^{-1} to 10^{-4} or less all make similar contributions to the denominator in eqn (22.4), which involves only the logarithm of this ratio. These observations simply emphasize the point that parasite or vector generation time is the central factor in determining the rate of appearance of observable levels of resistance.

Table 22.1 sets out values of T_R for a variety of parasites of vertebrates and vectors of infectious diseases, under the selective forces exerted by various chemotherapeutic agents or insecticides. We see that for the great variety of organisms embraced by Table 22.1, T_R lies in the surprisingly narrow range of around 5–100 generations. It is suggested by May and Dobson (1986) that such relative constancy of T_R, despite enormous variablity in p_0 and w_{RS}/w_{SS}, is because T_R depends on all these factors, except T_g, only logarithmically.

Table 22.1 Characteristic times for the appearance of resistance, T_R, in some specific systems

Species	Control agent	Generations[a]	Years	Reference
Avian coccidia				
Eimeria tenella	Buquinolate	6 (<6)	1	Chapman (1984)
	Glycarbylamide	11 (9)	<1	
	Nitrofurazone	12 (5)	7	
	Clopidol	20 (9)	6	
	Robenicline	22 (16)	10	
	Amprolium	65 (20)	14	
	Zoalene	11 (7)	22	
	Nicarbazin	35 (17)	27	
Gut nematodes in sheep				
Haemonchus contortus	Thiabendazole	3	<1	LeJambre *et al.* (1979)
	Cambendazole	(4)	<1	Kages *et al.* (1973)
Ticks on sheep				
Boophilus microplus	DDT	32	4	Stone (1972), Tahori (1978)
	HCH-dieldrin	2	<1	
	sodium arsenite		40	
Black flies (Japan)				
Simulium aokii	DDT + Lindane		6	Brown and Pal (1971)
Simulium damnosum	DDT		5	
Anopheline mosquitoes (different localities)				
Anopheles sacharovi	DDT		4–6	Brown and Pal (1971)
	Dieldrin		8	
An. maculipennis	DDT		5	
An. stephansi	DDT		7	
	Dieldrin		5	
An. culicifacies	DDT		8–12	
An. annuaris	DDT		3–4	
An. sundaicus	DDT		3	
	Dieldrin		1–3	
An. quadrimaculatus	DDT		2–7	
	Dieldrin		2–7	
An. pseudopunctipennis	DDT		>20	
	Dieldrin		18 weeks	

[a] The figures give the number of generations before a majority (>50 per cent) of the individuals in the population are resistant to the control agent. In brackets are the number of generations before resistance is first observed (usually >5 per cent of individuals resistant).

The above discussion assumed pesticides or chemotherapeutic agents to be applied uniformly to a closed population of vectors or parasites. In natural habitats, the next generation of vectors or parasites will usually include some immigrants from untreated or more lightly treated regions, particularly in the case of mobile insect vectors such as mosquitoes. This flow of susceptible genes will work against the spread of resistance. This observation relates to one of the more interesting questions of evolutionary biology: under what circumstances will gene flow (via migration) wash out the selective forces that are tending to adapt an organism to a particular local environment? It was originally held that very small amounts of gene flow would be sufficient to prevent local differentiation, so that geographical isolation was usually necessary before local adaptation could lead to new strains, races, or species (Mayr 1963). More recently, population geneticists have shown that the occurrence of local differenti- ation (or 'clines' in gene frequency) depends on the balance between the strength and the steepness of the spatial gradient of selection versus the amount and spatial scale of migration (Slatkin 1973; May *et al.* 1975; Endler 1977).

Migration is of direct relevance to the rate of evolution of drug and pesticide resistance and it is important to understand the essential mechanisms involved. Suppose that there is an infinite reservoir of untreated parasites or vectors in which the gene frequency of the resistant allele R is constant at the pristine value which we denote by $\bar{p}_R$. In the control area, the next generation of vectors or parasites will come partly from the previous generation that have survived drug or insecticide application, and partly from those among the previous generation in the untreated area that have migrated into the control zone. As shown in detail by Comins (1977b), and as discussed by May and Dobson (1986), the rate of evolution of resistance in the control area will, under the above circumstances, depend on: the gene frequency of the resistant allele, R, in the untreated reservoir, $\bar{p}_R$; the degree of dominance of R, as measured, say, by a parameter d; and the magnitude of migration in relation to selection, as measured by a parameter m. We may define the migration/selection parameter m to be (see Comins 1977b),

$$m = v/[(1 - v)(1 - w)]. \qquad (22.5)$$

Here v is the migration rate (i.e. the fraction of parasites or vectors in a given area that migrate rather than 'staying at home'), and w measures the strength of selection ($w = w_{SS}/w_{RR}$).

Comins (1977b), in an important paper, shows that if d is low enough (resistance sufficiently recessive), then gene frequencies in the control area will settle to a stable equilibrium in which the frequency of the resistant allele, R, remains low provided migration is high (m large). Conversely, for low rates of migration (m small), selection overcomes gene flow and the system settles to an equilibrium at which the frequency of the resistant allele, p_R, is close to unity.

More generally, the untreated region will of course be finite such that a more symmetrical situation will arise. To begin with, preponderately resistant (R) genes will migrate out of the control area into the untreated zone, while at the same time preponderately susceptible (S) genes will flow from the untreated to the control area. For any specific value of the migration parameter m (see eqn (22.5)), the gene frequency of the resistant allele will increase in the untreated zone.

22.3 Implications for parasite and vector control

The conceptual issues discussed above have a series of practical implications for the design of control policies. We begin by considering a situation in which gene flow between control and non-treated areas is absent (i.e. a closed population). The expression defined in eqn (22.4) for the time taken for the evolution of a significant (or observable) level of resistance mixes factors that are under the direct control of the public health manager (such as dosage levels), with factors that are intrinsic to the genetic system underlying the resistance phenomenon (such as T_g, p_0, and the degree of dominance of the resistance allele, R). Comins (1977a) suggests a useful partitioning of these two kinds of factors. First, let the relative fitnesses of the genotypes RR, RS, and SS, be $1:w^{1-d}:w$. Here w is the fitness of the susceptible homozygote relative to the resistant homozygote ($w = w_{SS}/w_{RR}$); intensive chemotherapy or pesticide application imply low w values. The parameter d measures the degree of dominance of the resistance allele R: if R is perfectly dominant, $d = 1$; if R is completely recessive $d = 0$; and in general d will take some numerical value intermediate between 0 and 1.

Equation (22.4) can now be written

$$T_R = T_0/\ln(1/w). \tag{22.6}$$

This separates the parameter w, which measures the selection pressure as determined by the intensity of the control effort, from the parameter T_0, which conflates intrinsic genetic factors. The quantity T_0 is defined as

$$T_0 = T_g \ln(p_f/p_0)/d. \tag{22.7}$$

We can see from eqns (22.6) and (22.7) that the rate of evolution of a significant level of resistance, T_R, depends logarithmically on the intensity of the control effort (the magnitude of w).

The ideas discussed above also apply to 'back-selection' or the decay in resistance following cessation in control. It is possible that a drug or pesticide may have cycles of useful life (Comins 1984). The frequency of the gene R first increases under the selection pressure exerted by the control programme until it reaches a level where resistance becomes a problem such that the use of the drug or pesticide is discontinued. In the absence of pesticide application, it will usually be that the fitness of the homozygote susceptible genotype is greater than that of the resistant genotype ($w_{SS} > w_{RR}$). Applying eqn (22.4) to this 'back-selection' process, we note that the time elapsed before the population is again effectively susceptible to the drug or pesticide will depend on: the fitness ratios $w_{RR}:w_{RS}:w_{SS}$, which measure the strength of back-selection or regression to susceptibility in the absence of control; the frequency of the resistance allele R when control ceases; and how low a frequency of R is required before re-use of the drug or pesticide becomes practically sensible. In the area of pesticide resistance, several authors have shown that back-selection does indeed occur (Ferrari and Georghiou 1981; Roush 1985). However, the rate of back-selection or regression is typically weaker than the corresponding rate of evolution of resistance. This is presumably due to the fact that the difference in the fitnesses of the resistant and susceptible genotypes is greater when control is operating than when it is absent.

With respect to the practical question of when to stop the use of a particular drug or pesticide, clearly regression will be faster if control ceases before the frequency of the resistance allele R gets too high. In other words, once resistance becomes an observable problem alternative forms of control should immediately be sought.

At what frequency of the resistant allele is it safe to reapply the drug or pesticide after a period of regression? In pristine populations before control, the frequency of R may typically be around 10^{-6} to 10^{-8} (Rousch and Croft 1986). After drug or pesticide use is stopped, resistance will be unobservable and effectively unmeasurable long before it attains levels as low as those pristine ones. A frequency of R of around 10^{-2}, for example, could easily be consistent with the population being regarded as having regressed to effective susceptibility. Taking the above numbers as illustrative, we see that resistance to the recycled drug or pesticide is likely to appear significantly more quickly than it did in the first instance (T_R depends on $\ln(1/p_0)$, giving a factor of three for the difference between $p_0 = 10^{-6}$ to 10^{-8} versus 10^{-2}).

All three factors outlined above suggest that the time interval before a parasite or vector population recovers susceptibility, so that a drug or pesticide may be reintroduced, is likely to be significantly longer than the initial time to acquire resistance, and also that resistance is likely to re-emerge significantly faster following such reintroduction. With respect to gene flow (migration), simple population genetic models suggest that management or control strategies can delay the appearance of significant levels of resistance by keeping the magnitude of the migration parameter m in eqn (22.5) as high as possible. Such strategies include maximizing the area of untreated regions (or refugia) as much as possible, as well as keeping the intensity of the selective pressure exerted by control as low as is practically possible.

These latter two points are of direct relevance to the design of community-based chemotherapy programmes for the control of macroparasitic infections (particularly helminths). One way in which to maximize the 'untreated areas' is of course to apply chemotherapy selectively to those individuals who harbour high worm loads. The majority of the population who harbour low parasite burdens remain untreated and thus their parasite populations continue to dilute the total parasite gene pool with genes for drug susceptibility. How much this approach will slow the evolution of resistance, compared with mass chemo-therapy, depends essentially on two factors. First, and most obvious, a reasonable fraction of the total parasite population must be harboured by the untreated segment of the human community such that the 'migration rate' of susceptibility genes is maintained at a reasonable level. Second, and perhaps less immediately obvious, is the role of density-dependent constraints on parasite fecundity. If such constraints are severe, then even if a relatively small fraction of the total parasite population is harboured by the untreated ('non-wormy') individuals, this fraction may make a disproportionate contribution to the total production of transmission stages. If this is the case (as seems to be true for the major helminth infections of man) then the small population of parasites in the large group of untreated people will produce a good supply of offspring with susceptibility genes, to dilute the total gene pool. A precise assessment of the relative advantages of selective versus mass chemotherapy in the slowing of the rate of evolution of drug resistance will depend on the quantitative details of the distribution of parasite numbers per host both within the total community and within those to be treated, and upon the severity of density-dependent constraints on worm fecundity. Aside from helminths, these general arguments also apply to certain microparasitic infections such as malaria. The rate of evolution of drug resistance by *Plasmodium falciparium*, for example, could be retarded by selectively treating those with high parasitaemias.

More broadly, resistance to antibiotics and antihelminthics poses growing problems in the control of infectious disease among human and other animals. Resistance is always likely to appear in the long run, given that the selective pressures imposed by control are sufficiently intense relative to other selection factors. Rational management, given this observation, therefore involves the avoidance of too much reliance on a single .method of control involving one drug or one pesticide. Integrated approaches, involving a combination of methods or drugs, have many advantages in this context. In the case of malaria, for example, Peters (1985) concludes that in order to retard the evolution of resistance a mixture of drugs should be used, combined with high dosage rates in those most susceptible to disease. These lessons have rarely been applied in practice, either in drug or in pesticide usage. As a result, the prospects for malaria control are bleak at present (unless a vaccine is developed in the not-too-distant future), owing to widespread drug resistance in parasite populations and insecticide resistance in vector populations.

The foregoing discussion has dealt exclusively with biological aspects of the evolution of drug or pesticide resistance. Such a discussion, however, only makes sense if embedded in a larger economic context. The costs associated with infectious diseases are broadly of three kinds: the cost of disease to the individual and to the community (loss of working days and the cost of health care); the cost of drug and/or pesticide application (for vector-transmitted diseases); and the more subtle costs arising from the need to develop new drugs or new pesticides as the appearance of resistance retires old ones. Common sense and formal theory (see Comins 1979) both say that, as the intensity of control effort increases, the cost associated with disease to the individual and the community decreases, but the cost of application increases, as does the cost associated with developing new drugs or pesticides (because this task becomes more frequent). In weighing up these relative costs, different groups of individuals may come to different decisions. For example, a pharmaceutical company or the political party in power (and responsible for the health care of the population) may favour short-term benefits versus gain from effective long-term control. An international agency such as the World Health Organization, however, may favour long-term gains as opposed to short-term benefits. Thus even with good biological understanding of the factors that control the rate of evolution of resistance, it can be that different sectors have different aims in the design of control policy. Scientific study can clarify these tensions but it cannot resolve them.

22.4 The maintenance of genetic variability

The study of the degree of genetic variability within populations, and how it is shaped by selective pressures in the course of evolution, is the subject matter of the field of population genetics. Host–parasite interactions present a fascinating example of how ecological interaction between species may act to maintain genetic diversity. In this section we consider some topics that have relevance to an understanding of observed epidemiological patterns.

The maintenance of polymorphisms and genetic variability within populations has been the focus of much attention in the genetical literature. Genetic polymorphism is here defined as the occurrence, in the same locality, of two or more strains of a species in such proportions that the rarest of them cannot be maintained merely by recurrent mutation. Mutation rates are difficult to measure in practice but convention holds that it is reasonable to assume that a gene is polymorphic when it is found in at least 1 per cent of the population. The major histocompatibility complex of genetic loci in humans (MHC), for example, which codes for cell surface molecules that seem to be a vital element of the immune system, is characterized by a high degree of both polymorphism and heterozygosity (Bodmer 1980). The MHC is involved in most reactions of immune recognition. It is pertinent at this point to speculate on the enormous amount of variation observed in the HLA region (the histocompatibility locus antigens, the MHC of humans, occupies about 1/3000th of the total genome). Although the reason is not known, it has been suggested that by carrying a large number of different MHC molecules there is less likelihood that a parasite could evade the body's immune system by imitating one of the self-recognition molecules of the system. Moreover, when viewed at the population level, the self–non-self recognition systems of individuals are all different, though working on the same principles. The 'perfect pathogen' which mimics particular host antigens cannot, therefore, evolve to spread through a host population, because patterns of immune recognition differ among different hosts. This is all very well in principle, but it is known that the possession of particular MHC antigens

Table 22.2 Infections in which HLA-linkage of susceptibility in response to infection or pathology has been demonstrated (from Wakelin and Blackwell 1988)

Infectious agent	Infection
Bacteria	Tuberculosis
	Leprosy
Protozoa	Giardiasis
	Malaria
Helminths	Schistosomiasis
	Filariasis
Anthropod	Scabies

renders people more (or less) susceptible to particular infectious diseases. Some examples are listed in Table 22.2.

Polymorphism ensures that in an outbred population of hosts every individual's immune system is different (by varying degrees dependent on the genetic relatedness of individuals). We might expect that such variability within the host population creates strong selective pressures for the maintenance of genetic variability within the parasite population. How does this influence the interaction between host and parasite populations? Might we expect genetic variability within both populations to attain some stable interactive state? Or, conversely, is the system constantly evolving under mutations in a very dynamic but unstable manner? Both situations probably arise, but empirical evidence on concomitant dynamic changes in genetic diversity within human and parasite populations is rarely available.

One example that has the appearance of instability is that of the interaction between the influenza virus and man. As a consequence of genetic 'shift' and 'drift', new antigenic types of the virus are constantly evolving so that epidemics occur in communities that have built up substantial herd immunity to earlier variants of the parasite (Stuart-Harris 1982). Viral strains are classified on the basis of very labile surface haemagglutinin (H) and neuraminidase (N) antigens which undergo major 'shifts' (e.g. from H_1 to H_2 to H_3, and from N_1 to N_2; infection by one strain confers little immunity to infection by another strain) and more frequent minor 'drifts' (identified by minor differences in serological tests) (Pereira 1979). Major 'shifts' in the antigenic character of the virus facilitate persistence in a population with a high degree of herd immunity to earlier antigenic variants (Nakajima *et al.* 1978). Such instability is difficult to describe in neat mathematical terms due to the unpredictable nature of the 'birth' of a major new antigenic variant. However, a qualitative understanding of the major factors invoked in promoting genetic change can be aimed at by

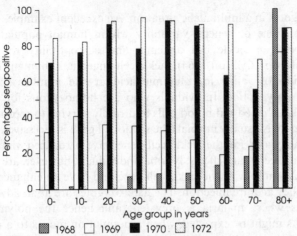

Fig. 22.3. Age-stratified serological profiles (haemagglutination test) for the percentage of sera collected from individuals in the city of Sheffield, with antibody to A/Hong Kong/68 influenza virus. Four profiles are displayed, for samples collected in 1968, 1969, 1970, and 1972, to show the creation of herd immunity to the viral strain during three successive epidemics (1968–9, 1969–70, 1971–2). The virus disappeared in 1972, and was replaced by the A/Eng/72 influenza virus strain (from Stuart-Harris 1982).

heuristic arguments. The influenza virus is highly transmissible within high-density human communities and it has a very short generation time (incubation and infectious periods are in general of a few day's duration). In a susceptible population (having no experience of the new variant) the virus spreads rapidly and a high level of herd immunity is built up across all age classes within a few years (Fig. 22.3). The effective reproductive rate of the virus may therefore fall below unity after the first major epidemic, thus creating strong selective pressures for genetic change of the virus within the largely immune host community. Inherent ability for genetic change (i.e. high mutation rates during replication within a host cell or during sexual or asexual reproduction) can therefore be of great selective value to a parasite that induces a strong and effective immunological response from the host. This principle applies to parasite population growth both within an individual (e.g. the expression of variable antigenic types (VATs) by the trypanosone protozoan parasites (Vickerman 1978; Cross 1979) and within a population of hosts (e.g. the influenza virus).

The mechanisms that promote stable polymorphisms within host and/or parasite populations are somewhat more amenable to theoretical study. They can be categorized under two general headings.

22.4.1 *Frequency- and density-independent processes*
The best known mechanism of this type is heterozygous advantage (or overdominance). This arises when heterozygotes enjoy a selective advantage

over homozygotes in a multiallelic situation. An excellent example, with respect to the maintenance of genetic variablity within human populations, is the interaction between sickle cell anaemia and susceptibility to *Plasmodium falciparium* infection (Allison 1964). Sickle cell anaemia in humans is caused by the substitution of valine for glutamic acid at site number six of the β-haemoglobin polypeptide. Individuals who are homozygous for this altered gene have sickle-shaped red blood cells and rarely survive to reproductive age. The heterozygote is usually normal (the sickle cell gene is recessive). Individuals who are homozygous for the sickle cell gene have a reduced viability due to anaemia and its secondary effects. Normal individuals, however, are more prone to malaria than those with the sickle cell gene and have an enhanced mortality as a result if they acquire infection. The heterozygotes are at an advantage over both in areas where malaria is prevalent and hence the polymorphism is maintained. As might be expected, when a population moves to a malaria-free area, or when the incidence of malaria declines due to control measures or climatic change, there is a decrease in the frequency of the sickle cell genes in ensuing generations. The situation is now one of directional selection against the sickle cell gene homozygote (Allison 1964).

The frequency of a particular gene at a polymorphic equilibrium, created by heterozygous advantage, may be calculated via the standard expression (for a single locus with two alleles in a diploid host) defined in eqn (22.1). For heterozygous advantage $w_{RR} < w_{RS} > w_{SS}$, where S denotes the susceptibility gene and R the gene that confers resistance to infection (in the sickle cell example R is the sickling gene). For algebraic convenience we define the relative fitnesses of the different genotypes as $w_{RR} = 1 - s$, $w_{RS} = 1$ and $w_{SS} = 1 - t$, where s and t lie between zero and unity. Then a non-trivial (i.e. $0 < q^* < 1$) stable equilibrium exists for the frequency of the sickle cell gene, q^*, at

$$q^* = s/(s + t). \qquad (22.8)$$

In regions where malaria has been endemic for some time the frequency of the sickling gene is in the region of 5–20 per cent, depending on the intensity of disease transmission (i.e. the relative selection advantage enjoyed by the heterozygote) (Mears and Lachman 1981).

Resistance to infection among populations of the mosquito vectors (*Aedes aegypti*) of certain filarial parasites (e.g. *Brugia malayi*) appears to provide a further example of polymorphism maintained by heterozygous advantage (Macdonald 1976). Innate resistance in mosquitoes to larval nematode infection is a dominant character controlled by a single gene or a small group of genes. In resistant homozygotes, reproductive performance (as measured within laboratory experiments) is poor by comparison with uninfected susceptible homozygotes. Under the pressure of infection, the heterozygote appears to enjoy a fitness advantage (Macdonald 1976).

Within invertebrate and vertebrate host populations the genetic trait of resistance (whether innate or immunologically based) often appears to be a dominant character. The reason why host populations do not rapidly evolve to become completely resistant under selection from infection is in part due to the fact that the trait of resistance often carries some fitness cost with respect to the survival and reproduction of the host in the absence of the parasite. One of the most detailed studies of this phenomenon is that of Minchella and Loverde (1983) who demonstrated that strains of the molluscan host *Biomphalaria glabrata*, susceptible to infection by *Schistosoma mansoni*, had, in the absence in infection, a higher intrinsic reproductive potential than resistant strains of the host. The difference in the net reproductive rate was approximately twofold. In such circumstances, the heterozygote may often enjoy a fitness advantage over both homozygotes in the presence of parasitic infection.

Other mechanisms that can maintain stable polymorphisms include migration (i.e. the gene flow example discussed in the section on drug and pesticide resistance), sex linkage, and unequal selection on the different sexes of an organism (see Crow and Kimura 1970). However, the relevance of these mechanisms to the maintenance of genetic variability within populations of humans and infectious disease agents is poorly understood at present.

22.4.2 *Frequency- and density-dependent processes*

Theory tells us that stable polymorphic equilibria can arise if the fitnesses of the different genotypes within a population depend on their relative or absolute abundances. This point is easily established from eqn (22.1) if we represent the fitnesses of the different genotypes as functions of their respective densities or relative abundances (henceforth referred to as their 'frequencies'). With appropriate choices of these functions, it is possible to generate a single stable polymorphic equilibrium ($0 < p^* < 1$ and $0 < q^* < 1$), multiple stable equilibria, or even cyclic and chaotic trajectories in changes of frequency from generation to generation. For example, a study by May and Anderson (1983a) of models of host–parasite interactions that incorporates both genetic and ecological factors reveals that chaotic changes in gene frequencies can arise when the fitness functions of the different host and parasite genotypes are not chosen arbitrarily (as has been usually the case in past theoretical work in population genetics), but are derived from the epidemiological principles that govern the population interaction. In particular, the simple equations in Chapter 3 which describe changes in the densities of susceptible, infected, and immune hosts (the prevalence framework of the microparasite models) can generate highly non-linear frequency- and density-dependent fitness functions for the different genotypes of both host and parasite (Gillespie 1975; May and Anderson 1983a). In these circumstances the interaction between host and parasite populations can lead to very complex patterns of change in gene frequencies.

We believe that frequency- and density-dependent selection is of great importance in the maintenance of genetic diversity within populations of human infectious disease agents. This observation is especially relevant for microparasitic organisms that induce mortality or lasting immunity to infection in those individuals that recover (see Haldane 1949; Clarke 1975; May and Anderson 1983*a,b*). The example of the influenza virus has been discussed earlier in the context of unstable or unpredictable changes in genetic type. The pressure for antigenic change is undoubtedly dependent on the frequency and density of the viral strain. When a particular strain is abundant, the virus will create a high degree of herd immunity in the human community and, as such, will lower its own reproductive fitness. Conversely when a strain is rare within a population that has no past experience of infection by that particular antigenic variant, reproductive fitness is high.

Among certain groups of viruses such as the coxsackie viruses, the adenoviruses and the echoviruses, many antigenically different strains persist within a single host community (Fig. 22.4). Little is understood at present concerning the antigenic cross-reactivities between different strains of a given virus. For example, infection by one variant may create a degree of immunity against infection by antigenically similar variants. Thus the reproductive potential of one strain may depend on the abundance of a closely related strain via the action of heterologous herd immunity.

Simple population models can help to further our understanding of the persistence of many viral strains within the same human community. Consider two strains of the same virus within a host population of constant size N. We denote the densities of susceptible, infected, and immune individuals by the variables X, Y_i and Z_i where the subscript i adopts the values of 1 and 2 to represent the two different strains. Following the notation and model framework laid out in Chapter 2 for compartmental models of the dynamics of microparasites we can formulate a system of differential equations for X, Y_i, and Z_i as follows:

$$\mathrm{d}X/\mathrm{d}t = \mu N - X(\beta_{11}Y_1 + \beta_{22}Y_2 + \mu), \tag{22.9}$$

$$\mathrm{d}Y_1/\mathrm{d}t = Y_1(\beta_{11}X + \beta_{12}Z_2) - (\gamma_1 + \mu)Y_1, \tag{22.10}$$

$$\mathrm{d}Y_2/\mathrm{d}t = Y_2(\beta_{22}X + \beta_{21}Z_1) - (\gamma_2 + \mu)Y_2, \tag{22.11}$$

$$\mathrm{d}Z_1/\mathrm{d}t = \gamma_1 Y_1 - Z_1(\mu + \beta_{21}Y_2), \tag{22.12}$$

$$\mathrm{d}Z_2/\mathrm{d}t = \gamma_2 Y_2 - Z_2(\mu + \beta_{12}Y_1). \tag{22.13}$$

It is here assumed that immunity arising from recovery from infection by one strain is fully protective against future reinfection by that strain but not against infection by the other antigenic types of the virus. The degree of cross-reactive immunity is determined by the magnitudes of the transmission parameters β_{ij} (the coefficients of transmission of strain i to susceptibles and immunes of strain j, resulting from contact with infectives of strain i). The rates of recovery from infection from strain 1 and 2 are denoted by γ_1 and γ_2, respectively. The total population size N is assumed to be constant ($N = X + Y_1 + Y_2 + Z_1 + Z_2$), with net mortality, μN, being exactly balanced by the net rate of input of new susceptibles. It is assumed for simplicity that a person cannot be infected with two strains concurrently. The model can of course be easily extended to encompass n different strains of the virus.

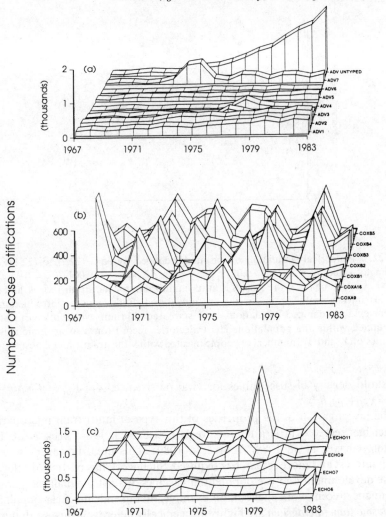

Fig. 22.4. Temporal changes in the number of cases of infection with different antigenic strains of (a) adenovirus; (b) coxsackie virus and (c) echovirus, based on reports to the Public Health Laboratory Service, Communicable Disease Surveillance Centre in England and Wales between 1967 and 1983.

Analytical and numerical studies reveal that the stable coexistence of both viral strains (in this simple 'two-species' model) depends critically on the degree of cross-transmission from infecteds of type i to immunes of type j (Fig. 22.5). In the simplest case, where cross-transmission does not occur ($\beta_{12} = \beta_{21} = 0$), the two strains are unable to coexist. The strain that wins is the one with the greatest basic reproductive rate, R_{0i} (that is, the one with the lowest

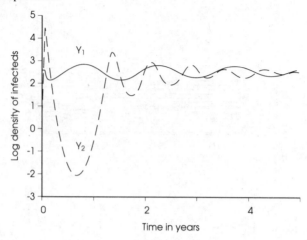

Fig. 22.5. Numerical simulation of the model defined by eqns (22.9) to (22.13), with parameter values $N = 10^6$, $\mu = 0.02$, $\gamma_1 = \gamma_2 = 52$, $\beta_{11} = \beta_{12} = 0.001$, $\beta_{22} = 0.05$, $\beta_{21} = 0.0$ (yr^{-1}). At time $t = 0$ the system is at its equilibrium for the strain 1 virus, and a few persons infected with strain 2 virus are introduced. Following the introduction, the system exhibits damped oscillations to a stable equilibrium, with both virus strains maintained within the population. The trajectories record (on a logarithmic axis) the densities of Y_1 and Y_2 (numbers of people infected with viral strain 1 and 2, respectively).

threshold density of susceptibles for viral persistence, X_{Ti}; $R_{0i} = \beta_i N/(\gamma_i + \mu)$, $X_{Ti} = (\gamma_i + \mu)/\beta_i$.

The investigation of the properties of this type of multistrain microparasite model has received little attention to date (see Beck 1984; Beck *et al.* 1984; Castillo-Chavez *et al.* 1988; Andreasen 1989). This area, however, is one of much interest and more research is required. Such work has particular relevance to the development and use of potential vaccines against the malarial parasites of humans. Recent work suggests, for example, that in endemic areas populations of *Plasmodium falciparium* are highly antigenically heterogeneous, so that many different strains of the parasite are present at any one time (Forsyth *et al.* 1988). This may present great problems in the development of an effective vaccine since it will probably be necessary to formulate a 'cocktail' which incorporates antigens from the different development stages of the parasite (i.e. merozoite, sporozoite, and gametocyte) and from the dominant strains of the parasite in the locality in which immunization is to take place. Strain composition, however, may well vary from one geographical locality to another. Moreover, the community-wide use of a vaccine could apply a frequency-dependent selection pressure in favour of those strains that were initially rare before immunization, and consequently were not incorporated in the vaccine cocktail. In future epidemiological research on malaria, it would therefore appear sensible to acquire detailed and quantitative information about strain variability within different locations and about how such genetic heterogeneity changes through time. Furthermore, as noted in Chapter 14 in the discussion on malaria, age-related changes in the prevalence of infection within endemic regions may well, in part, reflect repeated exposure to different antigenic variants of the malarial parasite that possess different transmission potentials.

In summary, this section has simply hinted at a range of interesting problems at the interface between the fields of epidemiology and population genetics about which we understand little at present. It offers a fascinating and important area for future research.

23

The ecology and genetics of host–parasite associations

Our interest in the work described in this book originally grew out of our attempts to understand the extent to which parasites—broadly defined to include viral, bacterial, protozoan, and fungal pathogens along with the more conventionally defined helminth parasites—regulate the numerical abundance or geographical distribution of non-human animal populations. This is an area that ecologists have tended to neglect. A growing number of field, laboratory, and theoretical studies have focused on the possibility that predators may influence animal numbers or affect the geographical distribution of species, but only very recently have the 'predatory' effects of parasites begun to receive similar attention. Although all ecology texts have at least one chapter on prey–predator interactions, the first ecology text to give significant attention to the population biology of host–parasite interactions was published in 1986 (Begon *et al.* 1986). We suspect that part of the explanation is that ecologists prefer to study four- or six-legged creatures that are visible to the naked eye (and that preferably have engaging behaviour and live in romantic places). Conversely, the growing body of research on the transmission and maintenance of infectious diseases understandably tends to focus on individual hosts, these being the units of concern for medical or veterinary practitioners.

In this concluding chapter, therefore, we lift our sights and aim at a more general discussion of the ecology and population genetics of host–parasite interactions. We begin with a broad outline of the conditions under which parasites—defined broadly, as above—may provide density-dependent regulation of their host populations, and of the dynamical character of the regulated state (stable points, stable cycles, chaos). Next, we combine epidemiology with population genetics, to discuss gene-for-gene associations between hosts and parasites; the main conclusions are that such interactions tend to generate and to maintain polymorphisms (again either stably, or cyclically, or even chaotically), and that whether or not parasites evolve toward 'harmlessness' depends on the relationship among parasite virulence and transmissibility and the cost of host resistance. Having reviewed these issues in general terms, with examples drawn from the world of non-human animals, we then turn briefly to sketch some examples of the impact of diseases upon human demography. We conclude with a messianic plea for more deliberate attention to population-level aspects of infections of humans: we need both more measurements of the epidemiological and demographic parameters that characterize interactions between infectious agents and their host populations, and a better understanding of the complex, and often counter-intuitive, effects that may be produced by the non-linearities that are inherent in such interactions.

23.1 Dynamics of host–parasite associations

The following abbreviated summary of work on the dynamical behaviour of particular kinds of host–parasite systems provides some striking examples of central themes in present day ecology, including chaos and the stabilizing effects that patchiness and aggregation can have. Although we focus mainly on general principles, there is some discussion of specific associations between hosts and parasites in the field and laboratory.

23.1.1 *Microparasites: host population with discrete generations*

Many populations, such as univoltine insects in temperate regions, have discrete generations that do not overlap. For such populations, the census data may be taken to be the number of adults emerging in each generation t, N_t. Suppose such a population is regulated by a lethal pathogen that spreads in epidemic fashion throughout each generation before reproductive maturity is attained; the survivors then go on to reproduce, each producing on average λ offspring that survive to emerge as adults at the start of the next generation. The numbers of adults in successive generations are then related by a first-order non-linear difference equation,

$$N_{t+1} = \lambda N_t(1 - I(N_t)).$$ \hfill (23.1)

Here $I(N_t)$ represents the fraction of the population infected by the epidemic in generation t: $1 - I$ is thus the fraction surviving to reproduce. This fraction I is given by a simple extension of the Kermack–McKendrick (1927) equation that was discussed in Chapter 6:

$$1 - I = \exp(-IN_t/N_T).$$ \hfill (23.2)

Here N_T is a threshold density, as discussed in Chapter 6. In this particular instance, N_T is determined by the transmissibility, β, and the virulence, α, of the pathogen ($N_T = \alpha/\beta$). It is often convenient to express eqns (23.1) and (23.2) in dimensionless form by defining the variable X_t to be the ratio of N_t to N_T, $X_t = N_t/N_T$. If N_t is below threshold magnitude ($N_t < N_T$; $X_t < 1$), the pathogen cannot spread, and essentially nobody is infected: $I = 0$. If, on the other hand, N_t is above threshold ($N_t > N_T$; $X_t > 1$), the pathogen does spread, infecting a larger and larger fraction as N_t increases: eqn (23.2) has a non-trivial solution $I \neq 0$.

The 'map' relating the host population densities in successive generations is shown in Fig. 23.1, for the representative value $\lambda = 2$. The essential features of this figure hold for all values of λ: for N_t below threshold ($X_t < 1$) there is density-independent growth at the rate λ; for N_t above threshold ($X_t > 1$) the

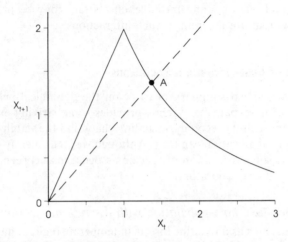

Fig. 23.1. The full line depicts the functional relationship or map determining the (dimensionless) population density in generation $t + 1$, X_{t+1}, in terms of that in generation t, X_t, for a population regulated by a pathogen: specifically, the map is for eqn (23.1) with $\lambda = 2$. The spikey hump in the map derives from the discontinuous nature of the threshold phenomenon, whereby a deterministic epidemic spreads if and only if the host population exceeds a critical value. The broken line corresponds to an unchanging population, $X_{t+1} = X_t$, so that the point A represents a possible equilibrium point (after May 1985).

pathogen inflicts pre-reproductive mortality that increases in severity as host density increases.

Clearly this lethal pathogen provides density-dependent regulation of its host population, and it appears possible from Fig.23.1 that the population may be regulated around the point $N_{t+1} = N_t = N^*$ which is labelled A in Fig. 23.1. The dynamics of this simple and natural model for a population regulated by disease are, however, astonishing. The system has no stable point nor any stable cycles for any value of $\lambda > 1$ (and for $\lambda < 1$ the population of course declines to extinction). Instead, the purely deterministic relation described by eqns (23.1) and (23.2), or equivalently by Fig. 23.1, leads always to the 'deterministic randomness' that has come to be called 'chaos'. That is, the dynamical behaviour of the host population is always like the sample function of some random process.

Figures 23.2 and 23.3 illustrate this chaotic dynamical behaviour. Figure 23.2 was obtained by plotting long runs of iterations of eqn (23.1) for specific values of λ. It gives some idea of the probability distributions for host densities thus obtained. For relatively small values of λ, the host population alternates between a band of relatively high values and a band of relatively low values; these bands are narrow for λ close to unity (and indeed there are four bands, which correspond to trajectories looking rather like a four-point cycle, for λ less than about 1.68). For $\lambda > 2.91$ the two bands coalesce, and the population

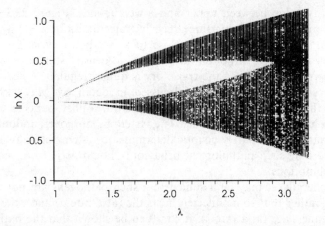

Fig. 23.2. This figure is constructed by plotting the population values (on a logarithmic scale, ln X) generated by iterating the difference equation (23.1) many times, for each of a sequence of λ values. The diagram gives an impression of the probability distribution of population values generated by this purely deterministic difference equation; for a fuller discussion see May (1985).

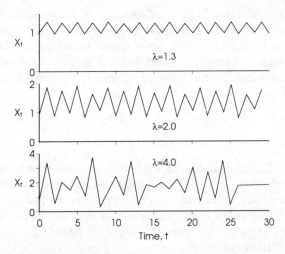

Fig. 23.3. This figure shows the variation in the population, X, with time, t, as described by eqn (23.1) for three particular values of λ. These three population trajectories further illustrate the character of the chaotic dynamical behaviour noted in Fig. 23.2 and discussed more generally in the text: (top) for $\lambda = 1.3$, the trajectory—although strictly aperiodic—is close to a two-point cycle; (middle) for $\lambda = 2$, the trajectory is obviously aperiodic, but still alternates up and down in successive generations; (bottom) for $\lambda = 4$, the trajectory is quite ragged.

can take any value between upper and lower bounds. Figure 23.3 illustrates these properties by displaying three specific trajectories: for $\lambda = 1.3$ the trajectory—although in fact chaotic—is close to a two-point cycle; for $\lambda = 2$ the aperiodicity is marked, although the population density still clearly alternates up and down; and for $\lambda = 4$ the trajectory is quite irregular.

These results are derived and discussed in detail by May (1985). It is surprising that this simple and sensible model for a host–parasite interaction should not have been studied earlier. The system is, moreover, undoubtedly the simplest example of a purely chaotic deterministic system yet known, and it is remarkable that such pathological behaviour should arise from natural biological assumptions.

More generally, it may be assumed that such pathogens are not invariably lethal, but rather that some infected hosts die (at a rate α) and others recover to an immune state (at a rate v). It can then be shown that the pathogen can regulate its host population if, and only if, it is sufficiently virulent

$$\alpha > v(\lambda - 1). \tag{23.3}$$

This equation represents the commonsense requirement that the pathogen be able to inflict sufficient mortality to overcome the host population's propensity to growth (for $\lambda > 1$). The regulated state may be a stable point, or a stable cycle if v is sufficiently large in relation to α (while still obeying eqn (23.3); May (1985)).

At the opposite extreme from the above case of an epidemic infection is an endemic infection, in which all infected hosts simply recover to the susceptible state. This could be relevant to some insect populations, where acquired immunity is rare. Suppose all infected hosts recover ($\alpha = 0$), but do not reproduce while infected. The analogue of eqns (23.1) and (23.2) can then be seen simply to be

$$X_{t+1} = \lambda X_t \qquad \text{if } X_t < 1, \tag{23.4a}$$

$$X_{t+1} = \lambda \qquad \text{if } X_t > 1. \tag{23.4b}$$

This relation is illustrated in Fig. 23.4, where it is seen that an endemic infection of this kind will always regulate the host population to a stable equilibrium value. More generally, we can assume that some infected hosts die, while others recover to their susceptible state. The results are relations intermediate between Figs. 23.1 and 23.4, with dynamics ranging from stable equilibrium points to apparently chaotic trajectories.

23.1.2 *Microparasites: host population with continuously overlapping generations*

At the opposite extreme from populations with discrete, non-overlapping generations, are those where generations overlap completely so that population growth is a continuous process. The basic model for the interaction between

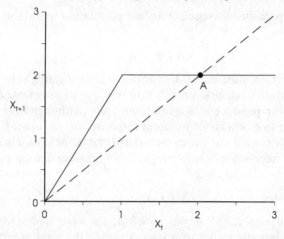

Fig. 23.4. This map differs from that of Fig. 23.1 in that it shows the relation between X_{t+1} and X_t for a host population regulated by an endemic infection: infected hosts recover directly back into the susceptible class; infected hosts are not killed by the infection, but they do not reproduce while infected. As in Fig. 23.1, the broken line corresponds to an unchanging population, $X_{t+1} = X_t$. Here the equilibrium point A is globally stable.

such a host population and a microparasitic infection takes the familiar form of differential equations describing the rate of change of the numbers of susceptible, infected and infectious, and recovered and immune hosts, $X(t)$, $Y(t)$, $Z(t)$, respectively:

$$dX/dt = a(X + Y + Z) - \mu X - \beta X Y + \gamma Z, \qquad (23.5)$$

$$dY/dt = \beta X Y - (\mu + v + \alpha)Y, \qquad (23.6)$$

$$dZ/dt = vY - (\mu + \gamma)Z. \qquad (23.7)$$

This is the basic model of Chapter 4, but with explicit recognition given to the effects of disease-induced mortality (at a rate α) and to the possible loss of immunity (at a rate γ: $\gamma = 0$ if immunity is lifelong). The other features are as discussed earlier on several occasions: the host population is assumed to be homogeneously mixed, with new infections appearing at a rate proportional both to the number of susceptibles and the number of infecteds, $\beta X Y$; β is the transmission parameter; a represents the per capita birth rate; μ is the per capita death rate from causes other than the disease in question; and v is the recovery rate. Unlike the situations considered throughout this book (except in Chapter 13), the total host population, $N = X + Y + Z$, is not taken to be constant, but rather increases exponentially at the rate $r = a - \mu$ in the absence of this infection.

Such a microparasite will regulate its host population to a stable equilibrium value provided

$$\alpha > r[1 + v/(\mu + \gamma)]. \qquad (23.8)$$

That is, the infection must be virulent enough (α large enough) to prevail over the host population's intrinsic growth rate ($r = a - \mu$) augmented by a factor that allows for the presence of acquired immunity. Although invertebrates are capable of mounting cellular or humoral responses to microparasitic infection, they rarely if ever manifest acquired immunity (that is, for invertebrates $\gamma \to \infty$); in this case, the infection will stably regulate its host population provided only that

$$\alpha > r. \qquad (23.9)$$

Conversely, if eqn (23.8) is not satisfied, the system described by eqns (23.5)–(23.7) eventually settles to a state in which the total population grows exponentially at a rate ρ given by

$$\rho = [B^2 - (\mu + \gamma)(\alpha - r) + rv]^{1/2} - B, \qquad (23.10)$$

with $B \equiv \frac{1}{2}(\alpha + \mu + v + \gamma - r)$. This population growth rate is necessarily less than the disease-free one, $\rho < r$.

In either event, the infection is unable to establish itself so long as the host population, $N(t)$, lies below the threshold value, $N_T = (\alpha + \mu + v)/\beta$. Under the disease-free conditions, however, the population will grow exponentially at the rate r, and must eventually exceed the threshold density. The infection can then establish itself within the population, and the system either converges—steadily or with damped oscillations—to a stable equilibrium level (if eqn (23.8) is satisfied), or else continues to grow exponentially at the diminished rate ρ of eqn (23.10) (if eqn (23.8) is not satisfied).

Although the nature of immunological responses by individual hosts to specific pathogens has received much attention in recent years, comparatively little thought has been given to the population consequences of acquired immunity (sometimes called 'herd immunity'). The general insights just culled from eqns (23.5)–(23.10) can be illuminated by a numerical example. Figure 23.5 shows the growth of a fictitious human population (from an initial size of 50 000) that is subject to a virus disease, under various assumptions about the duration of immunity. The vital rates and transmission parameter values are as detailed in the figure caption. In more homely terms, they represent a growth rate of the disease-free population of around 3 per cent per annum, a case mortality of about 30 per cent (similar to measles in malnourished human populations with no previous exposure), duration of the infection around 4 weeks, and a transmission coefficient β that implies a threshold population density of $N_T \simeq 400\,000$ people.

In all cases in Fig. 23.5, the disease is not maintained and the population grows at its intrinsic 3 per cent rate if it is below the threshold value N_T. Above

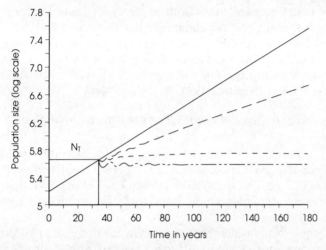

Fig. 23.5. Illustrating the effects of disease-induced mortality on the dynamics of host population growth $N(t)$. The figure is for a hypothetical disease in a hypothetical population, with the various demographic and epidemiological parameters (as defined in the text) being $r = 0.03$, $\mu = 0.015$, $v = 13.0$, $\alpha = 6.0$, $\beta = 5 \times 10^{-5}$ (all yr^{-1}), and $N(0) = 50\,000$. The full line depicts the population growth in the absence of the infection. The three broken lines depict the effects of immunity of varying duration, namely (from top to bottom): lifelong immunity, $\gamma = 0$ (long dashes); immunity of average duration 5 yr, $\gamma = 0.2$ (short dashes); and no immunity, $\gamma = \infty$ (dot-dot-dash). Notice that the effects of the disease do not become manifest until the population exceeds a threshold size; for further discussion see the text.

this point, the population's fate depends on the nature of the immune response. If the duration of the immunity to reinfection, $1/\gamma$, is of short to medium length (less than about 20 years), the disease is able to regulate the host population to a stable level. If the disease induces hardly any immunity (γ large), this equilibrium level will be close to the threshold N_{T} for maintenance of the disease. Conversely, if the duration of immunity is above 20 years, the population continues to grow exponentially at some rate lower than 3 per cent; lifelong immunity ($\gamma = 0$, as for measles) results asymptotically in 1.6 per cent per annum growth. This example makes plain the important part immunity plays in determining the population consequences of a disease.

The above results have been derived, and a variety of possible refinements and applications discussed, by Anderson and May (1979*b*, 1981). Among the possible complications which may be included are: a latent, infected but not yet infectious, class (which makes regulation of the host population more difficult); vertical transmission, whereby some offspring of infected hosts are born infected (making regulation easier); diminished reproduction or even castration of infected hosts (again making regulation easier); and various complexities associated with indirect transmission via intermediate hosts (which can lead to sustained oscillations both in the incidence of infection and even in the magnitude of the host population). In particular, many viral or protozoan infections of forest insects have free-living transmission stages with long life spans, which can produce marked cyclic oscillations in the abundance of the host, with periods ranging from a few years to a few decades (Anderson and May 1981; Getz and Pickering 1983; Regniere 1984).

23.1.3 *An example: regulation of laboratory mice populations by pathogens*

Laboratory studies have shown that microparasitic infections are indeed able to regulate populations of bacteria (Levin and Lenski 1983), beetles (Park 1948), coelenterates (Stiven 1962), and mice (Greenwood *et al.* 1936; Fenner 1948). The simple ideas presented above can, moreover, be used to analyse these laboratory experiments.

As an example, we consider the studies of Greenwood *et al.* (1936) and Fenner (1948) on populations of laboratory mice infected with the bacterial 'mouse plague', *Pasteurella muris*, or with a pox-virus, ectromelia. In these experiments, the cage space available to the mice was adjusted to keep the population density constant as absolute levels changed, thus avoiding complications arising from density-dependent effects having nothing to do with disease transmission.

The mathematical model defined by eqns (23.5)–(23.7) can be used to analyse these host–parasite systems, with one important modification. In the experiments, adult mice were introduced by the hand of the experimenter, at a constant rate of A adult mice per day, rather than by natural birth processes (at some constant per capita rate); the result is that the term $a(X + Y + Z)$ on the right-hand side of eqn (23.5) should be replaced by the experimentally determined constant A.

In the absence of infection, A mice are added each day and μN are lost by natural deaths. The system therefore will settle to an equilibrium population density, N^*, at which births balance deaths: $N^* = A/\mu$. When the *P. muris* or ectromelia infection is introduced, it will spread among the mice if its basic reproductive rate (which from eqn (23.6) is $R_0 = \beta N/(\alpha + \mu + v)$) exceeds unity. That is, the infection will establish itself once the mouse population exceeds a threshold value, $N_T = (\alpha + \mu + v)/\beta$. It follows that, if the introduction rate A is low enough to keep the disease-free equilibrium population, $N^* = A/\mu$, below N_T, then the infection will not establish itself. But once the introduction rate A does exceed this critical level, $A > \mu N_T$, the disease will spread and will eventually control the mouse population to densities below that which would pertain in the absence of infection:

$$N^* = (A + \hat{\alpha} N_T)/(\mu + \hat{\alpha}). \tag{23.11}$$

Here $\hat{\alpha}$ has been defined, for notational convenience, as $\hat{\alpha} = \alpha/[1 + v/(\mu + \gamma)]$. Notice that this disease-regulated population density, N^*, increases linearly with increasing rates of introduction of new mice, A.

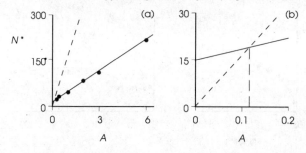

Fig. 23.6. (a) The equilibrium population in a colony of laboratory mice, N^*, is shown as a function of the daily rate of input of susceptible mice, A. The full circles represent the observed equilibrium populations infected with *P. muris*; the full line is the best linear fit, obtained using the theoretical relation (23.11); and the broken line shows the expected relation between N^* and A in the absence of infection (the slope is $1/\mu$, where $\mu = 0.006 \text{ yr}^{-1}$). (b) The intersection between the full line and broken line—the disease-regulated and disease-free dependence of N^* on A, respectively—gives the critical rate of introduction, μN_{T}, below which *P. muris* cannot be maintained. This enlargement of the lower left-hand corner of (a) suggests that the critical rate is 0.11 mice per day, corresponding roughly to an equilibrium population of 19 mice (after Anderson and May 1979*b*).

In their experiments with *P. muris*, Greenwood and his co-workers introduced new mice at rates ranging from 0.33 (one mouse every 3 days) to six mice per day. As can be seen in Fig. 23.6(a), the ensuing equilibrium populations of mice indeed depended linearly on A, as suggested by the simple model. In fitting the theoretical line to the observed data points, the transmission parameter β has been treated as an adjustable parameter. Figure 23.6(b) is an enlargement of the lower left corner of Fig. 23.6(a), showing the region where disease-free population levels, $N^* = A/\mu$, and disease-regulated ones, eqn (23.11), cross. The critical rate of introduction, $A = \mu N_{\text{T}}$, below which *P. muris* cannot be maintained, appears to be 0.11 mice per day, corresponding roughly to an equilibrium population of 19 mice. Unfortunately, the experiments were never conducted at so low a rate, so this conclusion remains untested.

Greenwood *et al.* (1936) also investigated the dynamical behaviour of the infected mouse populations, $N(t)$, as a function of time, t, for two particular introduction rates, six and 0.33 mice per day (Fig. 23.7). The theoretical curves here contain no adjustable parameters: the rates α, μ, v, and γ are estimated from independent studies of individual mice, while β (although it concatenates many biological and epidemiological factors in a way which defies direct estimation) is determined from Fig. 23.6 as explained above. The agreement between the data and the theoretical curves, thus constructed, is encouraging.

Similar analyses can be made of experiments on ectromelia infections of mice, and of the other laboratory studies referred to at the beginning of this subsection. We have given this one example in some detail because it adds specificity to the otherwise abstract analysis, and because it shows that simple

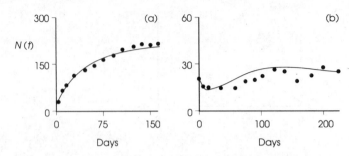

Fig. 23.7. (a) Changes in the number of mice in an experimental colony which was infected with *P. muris* are shown as a function of time, for an introduction rate of six mice per day. The full circles represent experimental observations, and the full curve is the result of the simple theoretical model outlined in the text (in which all the parameters are estimated from other kinds of data). (b) As for (a), except here the introduction rate is 0.33 mice per day. The agreement between theory and experiment suggests that the simple model does indeed capture the essentials of such a host parasite association (after Anderson and May 1979*b*).

mathematical models can give a satisfactory account of observed facts, at least in the laboratory.

23.1.4 *Macroparasites: host population with discrete generations*

Crofton (1971*a*,*b*) was the first to analyse models for hosts with discrete generations, whose densities are regulated by macroparasites. The basic model parallels that for microparasites. In each generation, host individuals acquire a burden of parasites as they advance to reproductive maturity. Hosts which are relatively heavily infected die, and their parasites—whose generation time is synchronized with that of the hosts—die with them. Hosts which are relatively lightly infected reproduce, to give on average λ offspring in the next generation, and their parasites also reproduce, each to give on average Λ free-living transmission stages that will infect the next generation of hosts. Specifically, Crofton assumed hosts with fewer than a lethal level of L parasites would survive to reproduce, while those with more than L parasites would die. Guided by observed patterns of parasite distribution within host populations, Crofton (1971*a*) did not assume that parasites are acquired independently randomly by host individuals, but rather assumed the parasite distribution to be a negative binomial. That is, the parasite distribution was taken to be clumped, with most hosts having relatively light burdens and a few having relatively heavy burdens; the degree of clumping is characterized by the familiar parameter k of the negative binomial, as discussed extensively earlier. Table 23.1 summarizes the degree of such clumping seen in a variety of associations between macroparasites and non-human hosts.

Crofton's numerical simulations (1971*b*) suggest that macroparasites can regulate their host populations in a steady way, provided parasite-induced

Table 23.1 Values of the negative binomial clumping parameter, k, observed for distributions of macroparasites in natural populations of non-human animal hosts (excerpted from Anderson and May 1978, 1982c)

Taxonomic group	Parasite	Host	Range of k values
Platyhelminthes	*Diclidophora denticulata*	*Gadus virens*	0.7
	Diplostomum gasterostei	*Gasterosteus aculeatus*	0.1–0.7
	Caryophyllaeus laticeps	*Abramis brama*	0.1–0.5
	Schistocephalus solidus	*Gasterosteus aculeatus*	0.7–2.4
Nematoda	*Chandlerella quiscoli*	*Culicoides crepuscularis*	0.5
	Toxocara canis	*Vulpes vulpes*	0.5
	Ascaridia galli	*Gallus gallus*	0.7
Acanthocephala	*Polymorphus minutus*	*Gammarus pulex*	0.6–3.1
	Echinorhynchus clavla	*Gasterosteus aculeatus*	0.07–0.5
Arthropoda	*Lepeophtheirus pectoralis*	*Pleuronectes platessa*	0.3–10.0
	Chondracanthopsis nodosus	*Sebastes marinus*	0.6
	Chondracanthopsis nodosus	*Sebastes mentella*	0.2
	Ixodes trianguliceps	*Apodemus sylvaticus*	0.04–0.4
	Liponysue bacoti	*Rattus rattus*	0.2

mortality is severe enough and k small enough. For k too large (parasite distribution insufficiently clumped), Crofton found diverging oscillations of a kind familiar in many models of interactions between hymenopteran or dipteran 'parasitoids' and their insect hosts (Hassell 1978). May (1977b) subsequently refined Crofton's model, replacing Crofton's step-function host survival (with its lethal level of L parasites) by a more continuously varying survival function (with the lethal level still roughly characterized by L parasites). May also made more realistic assumptions about the rate at which parasites are acquired by hosts. It can then be shown that, provided the critical worm burden L is significantly in excess of unity, the host population is regulated by the parasitic infection if, and only if (May 1977b),

$$\lambda < \Lambda^{k/(1+k)}. \tag{23.12}$$

That is, the basic reproductive rate of the parasite (discounted to a degree that depends on the amount of parasite clumping, k) must exceed that of the host for regulation to be possible. As found by Crofton, this equilibrium is a stable point provided that k is small enough in relation to λ, and is always a stable point if $k < 1$. In some situations, the equilibrium may be such that the system recovers from small disturbances, but is unstable (undergoing diverging oscillations) to large perturbations (May 1979).

Notice that clumping or overdispersion of parasites among host individuals is important for the persistence of these systems. This re-echoes a major theme of much recent theoretical and empirical research on prey–predator systems in general. If the system is homogeneous (that is, if predators or parasites attack independently at random) it cannot persist, undergoing wild oscillations. But if there is sufficient heterogeneity (patchiness and differential aggregation, as in the Crofton model), there can be global persistence, produced by local differences. For a review of work relating to this theme see Hassell and May (1984).

23.1.5 *Macroparasites: host population with continuously overlapping generations*

The corresponding differential equations modelling the interaction between a macroparasitic infection and a host population with continuously overlapping generations were first constructed and studied by Anderson and May (1978).

A crucial aspect of such host–macroparasite systems, for which good data are available, is again the clumped or aggregated way in which the parasites are distributed among hosts (Table 23.1). As has been the case in other contexts, these observed distributions are usually described well by a negative binomial, with the parameter k characterizing the degree of aggregation.

In constructing these host–macroparasite models, it is assumed that sufficiently high parasite burdens do indeed contribute to host deaths, with the mortality rate increasing either linearly or exponentially with increasing parasite numbers within a host. Such macroparasites are then capable of regulating their host population, provided

$$\Lambda - (\mu' + \mu + \alpha) > (a - \mu)(k + 1)/k. \qquad (23.13)$$

Here, Λ is the rate of production of transmission stages (eggs, spores, or cysts) per parasite; μ' is the per capita parasite death rate; α is the proportionality constant such that αi is the parasite-induced mortality rate in a host harbouring i parasites; a and μ, as before, are the birth and disease-free death rates per host; and k is the clumping parameter in the negative binomial parasite distribution. The criterion (23.13) for hosts with continuously overlapping generations is broadly comparable to eqn (23.12) for hosts with discrete generations: the left-hand side represents the parasite population growth rate (births, Λ, minus deaths from all causes—parasite death, natural host death, parasite-induced host death—$(\mu' + \mu + \alpha)$), which must be able to outrun the host population growth rate, $a - \mu$, corrected for parasite clumping. If eqn (23.13) is satisfied, the parasite will always be capable of regulating its host population. On the other hand, if parasite-induced mortality effects are not substantial (α insufficiently large), this parasite-regulated host population level is likely to be so high that other density-dependent regulatory effects intervene before it is reached. In short, regulation of a host population by macroparasites in general requires both that eqn (23.13) be obeyed, and that α be large enough.

Macroparasites may regulate their host population to a stable equilibrium value, or in stably sustained cycles (Anderson and May 1978; May and Anderson 1978). Factors tending to produce a stable point are parasite aggregation (small k), parasite-induced host mortality that rises steeply with parasite load, and density-dependent constraints on parasite numbers per host or on egg output per parasite. Factors tending to produce cyclic oscillations in host and parasite abundance are parasite-induced reduction in host reproduction, direct reproduction of parasites within hosts, and time delays in parasite reproduction and transmission.

Notice that macroparasites may be the sole agents providing density-dependent regulation of the host population, even though very few hosts harbour a lethal load of parasites. It is a common misconception that the effects of a density-dependent regulatory agent must be apparent in most host individuals. This simply is not so.

23.1.6 *Regulation of natural populations by parasites*

Parallel to the laboratory studies of the regulatory effects of microparasites that were briefly reviewed above, there are an increasing number of laboratory studies which demonstrate that helminth parasites can regulate populations of invertebrate hosts (Keymer 1981; Anderson and Crombie 1984) and of lower vertebrates (Scott and Anderson 1984). Moving up to mammals, Scott (1988) has shown that the nematode parasite, *Heligmosomoides polygyrus*, has the potential to regulate a freely breeding population of outbred laboratory mice.

It is much more difficult to evaluate the effect of a microparasitic or macroparasitic infection upon its host population in a natural field setting, because such effects are always embedded in a web of other biological and environmental complications. It is, however, clear that parasites cause many deaths in natural populations of non-human animals.

Thus Delyamure's (1955) survey shows that helminths contribute significantly to the mortality rate in many populations of pinnipeds and cetaceans. One particularly careful study, for example, suggests that 11 to 14 per cent of deaths among spotted dolphins (*Stenella* spp.) are caused by nematode infections in the brain (Perrin and Powers 1980). Lanciani (1975) has demonstrated that an ectoparasitic mite influences the population dynamics of the aquatic insect *Hydrometra myrae*. Lloyd and Dybas (1966) have suggested that the ultimate determinant of the population densities of the spectacular 13- and 17-year periodical cicadas is a fungal infection, *Massospora cicadina*. Many studies have shown that infectious diseases are an important, and possibly the predominant, mortality factor in bird populations (Davis *et al.* 1971). Other examples are reviewed by Edwards and McDonnell (1982), Dobson and May (1986), and, with particular emphasis on implications for conservation, by Scott (1988).

Parasites can also affect the outcome of competition among species. This was shown in Park's (1948) classic laboratory experiments on competition between two species of flour beetles; when the sporozoan parasite *Adelina* was present it dramatically reduced the population density of *Tribolium casteneum*, and in some situations reversed the outcome of its competition with *T. confusum*. The simian malarial parasite, *Plasmodium knowlesi*, is highly pathogenic for the rhesus monkey, *Macaca mulatta*, but produces a chronic and much less lethal infection in *M. fascicularis*; *M. mulatta* is distributed widely throughout central, northern, and western India, where the malarial mosquito vector, *Anopheles leucosphyrus*, is absent, but is replaced by *M. fascicularis* in eastern India and parts of Bangladesh where *A. leucosphyrus* is present (Allison 1982). On a grand scale, it seems that the geographical distribution of most artiodactyl species in East Africa today is determined largely by a pandemic of rinderpest virus that occurred toward the end of the nineteenth century.

In many cases, different species of parasites combine to kill the host. Thus among bighorn sheep in North America the main cause of death is probably infection by the lungworms *Prostostronglylus stilesi* and *P. rushi*, which then predispose the hosts to pathogens causing pneumonia (Forrester 1971). More generally, it may be that the interplay between parasitic infections and the nutritional state of the host contributes importantly to the density-dependent regulation of natural populations.

Despite these illustrations of the devastating effects that diseases can have on natural populations, it is hard to assess the extent to which diseases are the primary regulators of such populations, as opposed to acting as occasional or incidental sources of mortality. For example, among certain species of wild fowl in North America some 80 to 90 per cent of the individuals not shot by hunters die of diseases each year, yet it remains arguable that the essential factor regulating population density is the availability of breeding sites (Holmes 1982) (for a thoughtful appraisal of these issues see Scott (1988)). In a study with implications for many insect populations, both temperate and tropical, Wolda and Foster (1978) have documented outbreaks of the larvae of a tropical moth, *Zunacetha annulata*, which cause severe defoliation and are ended by a fungal infection; the key determinants of the overall population dynamics of this moth, however, remain enigmatic. Delyamure (1955) sums it up in his lament that 'unfortunately, so far the influence of helminths on the population dynamics of pinnipeds and cetaceans has not been investigated at all, despite its likely importance'.

These uncertainties and complexities have, indeed, resulted in some wildlife biologists holding the extreme view that disease plays no regulatory role in natural host populations, or even that disease rarely occurs in wild animal populations. An intermediate position is articulated by Holmes (1982), who suggests that invertebrate populations and vertebrate populations in disturbed situations may more typically be regulated by parasitic infections than are natural populations of vertebrates.

As Scott (1988) has emphasized, part of the problem derives 'from the tremendous difficulties associated with observing the effects of infection and disease in wild animal populations. Animals that are born must die, but how many of these dead animals are ever seen?' Moreover, it is not as widely appreciated as it should be that a particular factor—a predator, a resource, a pathogen, etc.—may cause only a tiny fraction of all deaths, yet can be the factor ultimately responsible for regulating population levels if all other mortality factors are essentially density independent. This can be seen more precisely by asking what fraction of all host deaths must be attributable to a particular microparasite or macroparasite, if the parasite is truly the regulator? A simple yet general answer can be given, provided only that we assume the per capita birthrate, a, and the per capita death rate from all other causes, μ, are density-independent constants (which, of course, is not usually so):

$$\frac{\text{parasite-induced host deaths}}{\text{total host deaths}} = \frac{a - \mu}{a}. \tag{23.14}$$

The result holds for both microparasites and macroparasites, independent of the mode of transmission and the nature of immune processes. If a and μ are not too disparate, so that $(a - \mu)/a$ is small, the parasite can be responsible for regulating the host population, even though few deaths will be laid at its door; this situation may pertain to many vertebrate populations. Conversely, if $a \gg \mu$ (as is the case for many invertebrates), the infection needs to be responsible for most of the observed mortality before it can be a candidate for consideration as the regulatory agent.

In short, empirical evidence about the extent to which parasitic infections determine the numerical abundance or geographical distribution of wild populations remains equivocal. Experimental studies of the effects of viral, bacterial, protozoan, and helminth parasites on laboratory populations of hosts, however, demonstrate the regulatory potential of such parasites, and confirms the dynamical behaviour suggested by mathematical models. More generally, we emphasize that—in contrast with many other biological and environmental effects—the effects of mortality and morbidity associated with parasitic infection tend always to be strongly density dependent; infections spread better in dense populations. Such density-dependent effects are often compounded by the reduced nutritional state of hosts and increased stress associated with high-density situations.

23.2 Population genetics of host–parasite associations

With the exceptions of Chapters 10 and 18, this book has focused on the dynamics of infections within host populations that are genetically homogeneous. Yet there is abundant evidence, mainly coming from blood-group polymorphisms, that individual hosts differ in their response to many infections and that these differences have an explicit genetic basis. It would be surprising if this were not so. As Haldane (1949) pointed out, in a paper which seems to us to be more often cited than read, infectious diseases have surely been the most significant agents of natural selection acting on human populations since the dawn of the agricultural revolution, and possibly earlier. Such selective forces would be expected to interact with the genetic variability found in all natural populations to produce, over time, genetic differences among different sub-populations in response to local differences in patterns of disease (the sickling trait and G6PD in regions where anophelene mosquitoes transmit malaria being the canonical example).

Moreover, it is in the nature of host–parasite interactions that the selective forces they exert are frequency dependent. If different strains or genotypes of the parasite are present, and if different host genotypes respond differently to the various parasite genotypes, then in general the host genotype that is most abundant at any one time will be differentially exposed to the adverse effects of infection (remember, infection spreads more efficiently among larger host populations, other things being equal). As the abundance of the most common host genotype declines, the abundance of some other genotype will correspondingly increase, and this host genotype will in turn suffer increasing depredation from the pathogen strains that most afflict it. And so on. Haldane, indeed, presented a simple mathematical model for this process in his 1949 paper, using two strains of a host attacked by two strains of a parasitic wasp (and using the simple Nicholson–Bailey (1935) equation to model the system; unfortunately, the plethora of typographical errors in the mathematics in this paper make it very hard to comprehend).

Following the early work of Mode (1958), Day (1974), and Van der Plank (1975), there now exists a substantial literature on the population genetics of 'gene-for-gene' interactions between hosts and pathogens. In these studies, specific associations between individual genotypes of hosts and corresponding genotypes of pathogens are assumed. The work is primarily directed toward pathogens of plants, especially crop plants, where there are documented instances of such gene-for-gene associations (for a critical review of the biological facts see Barrett (1983, 1985)). Constant values are assigned to the fitnesses of each host genotype when attacked by a specific parasite genotype, and the ensuing net fitnesses of the various host genotypes are weighted sums over the appropriate fitnesses (weighted according to the relative abundances of the parasite genotypes). Similar calculations give the fitnesses of the various parasite genotypes. The outcome is a system in which the host fitnesses depend on the relative gene frequencies within the parasite population, and parasite fitnesses on host gene frequencies. The simplicity of these assumptions is, however, such that threshold and other important density-dependent effects associated with epidemiological processes are omitted.

These mathematical models for gene-for-gene associations between hosts and pathogens suggest that polymorphisms in the gene frequencies of both hosts and pathogens can easily be maintained. The polymorphisms may be stable, or cyclic, or even chaotic. In an exceptionally lucid review of these mathematical models, Levin (1983) emphasizes that many of the simpler models can be seen to be neutrally stable, although this fact is often obscured by round-off errors and the proliferation of parameters in numerical studies.

The essential mechanism responsible for maintaining polymorphism in these models, whatever the dynamical details, is the interplay between parasite virulence and the costs of host resistance.

23.2.1 *Genetics and epidemiology*

More recent studies take the earlier gene-for-gene framework, but now calculate the various fitness functions from epidemiological analyses that take account of the non-linear nature of transmission processes. The pioneering study here is by Gillespie (1975) who, however, only considered the statics and not the dynamics of his model. Studies of the full dynamics of such combined genetic and epidemiological models reveal interesting biological and mathematical features (Hamilton 1980; May and Anderson 1983*a*; Beck 1984).

These models are notable, *inter alia*, as the first examples to our knowledge where a population genetic analysis has employed fitness functions whose frequency and density dependences are derived from an explicit ecological model, rather than being constructed in an *ad hoc* way. The essential character of the models can be appreciated by considering a haploid host with discrete, non-overlapping generations. We focus on a single locus with two alleles, A and a: genotype A is susceptible to pathogen genotype 1 (but resistant to pathogen genotype 2), and conversely host genotype a is susceptible to pathogen 2 (and resistant to pathogen 1). In the usual way, the gene frequency of A in generation $t + 1$, p_{t+1}, is related to that to generation t, p_t, by

$$p_{t+1} = p_t w_1 / \bar{w}_t. \tag{23.15}$$

The fitnesses of host genotypes A and a are labelled w_1 *and* w_2, respectively, and $\bar{w}_t$ is the mean fitness in generation t:

$$\bar{w}_t = p_t w_1 + (1 - p_t) w_2. \tag{23.16}$$

In this simplest model, we assume that the pathogens spread epidemically through the populations of susceptible hosts, eventually infecting a fraction I_i of the hosts of genotype i ($i = 1, 2$); these infected hosts either die (at the disease-induced death rate α_i) or recover (at a rate v_i). The survivors then each produce on average λ_i offspring. It follows that the fitness of hosts of genotype i ($i = 1, 2$) is

$$w_i = \lambda_i (1 - s_i I_i). \tag{23.17}$$

Here, s_i is the fraction of those infected who die, $s_i = \alpha_i/(\alpha_i + v_i)$, and I_i is given by the usual extension of the Kermack–McKendrick result, eqn (23.2), for each genotype.

For an initial analysis, we can assume the pathogen serves only to determine the *relative* proportions of the various host genotypes, with some other ecological factor holding the total number of hosts to a constant density, K, in each generation. That is, the pathogen affects the gene frequencies in each generation, but not the total host numbers. In this case, the number of hosts

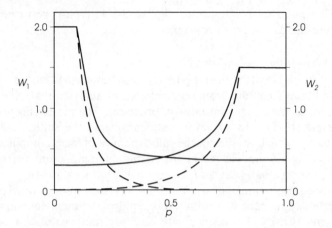

Fig. 23.8. For a haploid host, this figure shows the fitnesses w_1 and w_2 of the genotypes A and a, respectively, as functions of the gene frequency p. The fitnesses are given by eqns (23.17) and (23.18), with the parameter values $\lambda_1 = 2$, $\lambda_2 = 1.5$, $R_1 = 10$, $R_2 = 5$; the full curves are for $s_1 = s_2 = 0.8$, and the broken curves are for $s_1 = s_2 = 1$.

of genotype i, N_i, can be written $N_i = f_i K$ (with $f_1 = p$ and $f_2 = 1 - p$), and eqn (23.2) takes the form

$$1 - I_i = \exp(-I_i R_i f_i). \tag{23.18}$$

The reproductive rate R_i for pathogens of genotype i $(i = 1, 2)$ is given as $R_i = K/N_{T.i}$, where $N_{T.i}$ is the threshold density for host genotype i.

Figure 23.8 illustrates the kind of frequency dependence exhibited by the fitness function of eqns (23.17) and (23.18) for this haploid host. When p is small (frequency of the allele A small; genotype A or 1 relatively rare), the density of the host genotype A is below the threshold for maintaining the parasite $(R_1 p < 1)$, and $w_1 = \lambda_1$. Once p is sufficiently large $(R_1 p > 1)$, the epidemic can 'take off', and thereafter the fitness w_1 falls as p increases. For values of the parasite reproductive rate, R_1, significantly in excess of unity, the fitness w_1 will tend to saturate to $w_1 \to \lambda_1 (1 - s_1)$ unless s_1 is very close to unity; for an invariably lethal infection $(v_1 = 0, s_1 = 1)$, w_1 will not saturate, but will decline exponentially as p increases. The fitness of the other host genotype (labelled a or 2) exhibits similar behaviour as p decreases from 1 to 0. Obviously, the details depend on the relative magnitudes of the demographic and epidemiological parameters λ_i, s_i, and R_i, but with the rarer genotype enjoying an advantage there is the possibility of a polymorphic equilibrium at an internal point where $w_1 = w_2$.

By substituting the fitness functions of eqns (23.17) and (23.18) into eqns (23.15) and (23.16), we obtain non-linear 'maps' relating p_{t+1} to p_t:

$$p_{t+1} = F(p_t). \tag{23.19}$$

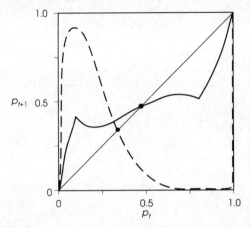

Fig. 23.9. The map relating p_{t+1} to p_t, as given by eqn (23.15), is shown for a haploid host with the fitness functions illustrated in Fig. 23.8: the full and broken curves correspond to the full and broken curves, respectively, in Fig. 23.8. The stability of the fixed points where the map $p_{t+1} = F(p_t)$ intersects the 45° line, $p_{t+1} = p_t$, are as discussed in the text (after May and Anderson 1983*a*).

These mapping functions $F(p)$ depend explicitly on genetic and epidemiological assumptions about the host–parasite association. Figure 23.9 displays a typical such map, corresponding to the fitness functions of Fig. 23.8.

As discussed in detail elsewhere (Levin *et al.* 1982; Levin and Lenski 1983; May and Anderson 1983*a*), the situation depicted in Fig. 23.9 is typical, in that there exists an 'interior fixed point' or polymorphism, $p_{t+1} = p_t \neq 0$ or 1. The dynamics of this system are, however, not trivial. If non-linearities are not too severe, the map shown in Fig. 23.9 can give a stable equilibrium or balanced polymorphism. But, with sufficient non-linearity, there can easily arise stable cycles in which host gene frequencies alternate high and low in successive generations, or there can even be chaotic fluctuations in gene frequency. This range of possibilities—stable point, cycles, or chaos—is illustrated in Fig. 23.10. The underlying mathematics is in some ways similar to, but in other ways more complicated than, that found in simple population models (May (1976): the familiar population models have 'maps with one hump'; the maps in Fig. 23.9 are messier in possessing 'two humps'). The details of this array of dynamic behaviour are presented elsewhere (May 1979; May and Anderson 1983*a*).

The above discussion dealt only with frequency-dependent selection, with the parasites affecting the relative proportions of the host genotypes but not the total number of hosts (which was taken to be constant, $N_t = K$). More generally, we may return to eqns (23.15)–(23.17), and let the parasites alone be responsible for regulating the density of the host population. In this case, the fitnesses w_i of eqn (23.17) will all depend—via the infected fraction I_i—both on the gene frequency, p_t, and on the total host density at the start of generation t, N_t.

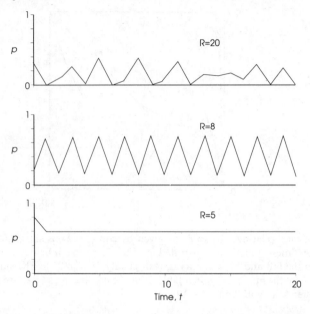

Fig. 23.10. The gene frequency, p, of the A allele in the host population can exhibit a range of dynamical behaviour, as illustrated here. As shown, increasing R values tend to take the system from a stable point, through stable cycles, to apparently chaotic dynamics. The example shown here is for a haploid host system whose fitnesses are given by eqns (23.17) and (23.18) with $R_1 = 5, 8, 20$ (as labelled), $R_2 = 0$ (so that host genotype a or 2 is resistant to infection, $I_2 = 0$), $s_1 = 1$, and $\lambda_2 = 0.95\lambda_1$. For a fuller discussion see May and Anderson (1983a).

For hosts of genotype i, I_i is given from eqn (23.2) by

$$1 - I_i = \exp(-I_i f_i N_t / N_{T.i}). \tag{23.20}$$

Here, as before, $f_1 = p_t$ and $f_2 = 1 - p_t$ for this haploid system. Equation (23.15) now gives, via eqns (23.17) and (23.20), an expression for p_{t+1} in terms of p_t and N_t. It remains to obtain a parallel relation for N_{t+1} in terms of p_t and N_t. Such a relation comes from the basic definition of the fitness functions, and is

$$N_{t+1} = \sum_i N_i w_i = N_t \bar{w}_t. \tag{23.21}$$

This frequency- and density-dependent system can now be studied, both analytically and numerically (May and Anderson 1983a). As in the purely frequency-dependent case, polymorphism usually exists unless resistance can arise with essentially no cost, or unless parasite virulence can become very low with no loss in transmissibility. Such polymorphisms are more likely to exhibit cyclic or chaotic oscillations than are the corresponding cases with no parasite-induced density dependence. Figure 23.11 illustrates a typical example,

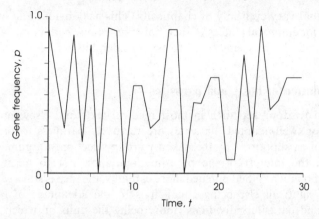

Fig. 23.11. This figure shows the highly chaotic dynamic behaviour in the gene frequency, p, that can arise once the selective forces exerted by the pathogen are both frequency and density dependent. The figure is for a haploid host, where the fitness functions are given by eqn (23.20) in conjunction with the density-dependent eqn (23.21): $\lambda_1 = \lambda_2 = e^2$; $s_1 = s_2 = 1$; and $N_{T.1} = N_{T,2} = 2$.

which in some ways is a direct extension (to a genetically polymorphic system) of the population interactions studied earlier in this chapter between a host with discrete generations and a microparasite.

Thus the phenomenon noted above, whereby gene-for-gene associations between hosts and parasites may promote the maintenance of genetic diversity (either stably, or cyclically, or with chaotic dynamics), is also manifested when the parasites are the regulators of host population density.

All the above studies are for single-locus systems. The work can be extended to two-locus systems that include the effects of recombination, which can be important in reshuffling both host and parasite gene pools each generation. The conclusions are broadly as we have just found, in that frequency- and density-dependent effects again lead to polymorphisms which can be stable, cyclic, or chaotic. In particular, Seger (1988) has used computer simulations to explore the coevolutionary properties of a model in which two loci in the host determine a strain-specific defence against parasites. Seger finds that intermediate rates of recombination tend to produce cyclically varying polymorphisms (while extreme recombination rates do not). Seger's model suggests that parasites can, in effect, act as a fluctuating environment which favours the evolution of intermediate rates of recombination in the host population.

In short, it has long been recognized that the frequency- and density-dependent selective effects exerted by viral, bacterial, protozoan, and helminth parasites on their host populations are likely to create and maintain genetic polymorphisms. But essentially all earlier work, both theoretical and empirical, has implicitly assumed that such polymorphisms will be at some steady level. It now seems likely that host–parasite interactions will often produce polymorphisms that vary cyclically or chaotically. This has obvious and important implications for empirical studies of such polymorphisms, both in the laboratory and in the field. There seems to us to be considerable need for such studies.

23.3 Coevolution of hosts and parasites

The received wisdom, set forth in most medical texts and elsewhere, is that 'successful' or 'well-adapted' parasites are relatively harmless to their hosts. The idea is often supported by the nakedly group-selectionist argument that it is clearly in the interest of the parasite population not to harm its host population too much. When pursued more carefully, the idea is still a reasonable one at first sight: all else being equal, it is to the advantage of both host individuals and parasite individuals (those being the units on which selection usually acts) to inflict little damage.

This view is, moreover, supported by a certain amount of anecdotal information. Thus in regions of Africa where trypanosomiasis is endemic, indigenous ruminants suffer mild infections with insignificant morbidity, while domestic ruminants that have been bred for a long time in the region suffer more severely, and recently imported exotic ruminants suffer virulent infections which are usually fatal if untreated (Allison 1982). The fact that parasitic infections appear to be more effective as regulatory agents among newly introduced species of plants and animals, or when the parasites are introduced into new regions, further supports this conventional view (Holmes 1982).

On theoretical grounds, it would indeed appear that parasites evolve to be avirulent, provided that the transmissibility and duration of infectiousness are entirely independent of virulence. This assumption, however, is not generally valid. The damage inflicted on their hosts by viral, bacterial, protozoan, and helminth parasites is often directly associated with the mechanism by which the organism produces its transmission stages. Once these complications are introduced into the theoretical models, it appears that many coevolutionary paths are possible, depending on the details of the interplay between the virulence and the transmissibility of the parasite (Anderson and May 1978, 1981, 1982e; Levin and Pimentel 1981; Levin et al. 1982).

One very simple way of making these complications explicit is to write down the simple formula for the basic reproductive rate of a microparasite that was obtained in Chapter 3:

$$R_0 = \frac{\beta(\alpha, N)N}{\alpha + \mu + v(\alpha)}.$$ (23.22)

Here, as discussed in Chapter 3, α is the disease-induced host mortality rate, μ is the per capita host mortality rate from all other causes, v is the recovery rate, β is the transmission coefficient, and N is the total population size. We have, however, written β as $\beta(\alpha, N)$ to give explicit recognition to the fact that overall transmission probability is generally dependent both on the virulence, α, and on population density, N (not necessarily linearly, as discussed in Chapter 13). Similarly, the recovery rate, $v(\alpha)$, will in general be related to the virulence, α.

If neither transmission, βN, nor recovery rate, v, depend on α, then clearly the parasite's basic reproductive rate, R_0, is maximized by having $\alpha \to 0$. That is, the evolutionary pressures on the parasite are toward avirulence. This is essentially the basis of the conventional argument that parasites will evolve to be harmless. But if $v(\alpha)$ and/or $\beta(\alpha)$ has some functional relation to α, the value of α which maximizes R_0 will depend on the details of this relationship. For instance, if β tends to increase faster than linearly with α (nastier strains being more-than-linearly more communicable), then R_0 would increase without bound as α increased, and—on the basis of this simple argument—the evolutionary pressures on the parasite would be to ever-increasing virulence!

Equation (23.22) makes it clear that the extent to which parasites will tend to evolve toward avirulence depends on the degree to which transmissibility and recovery rates are linked with harmful effects on host physiology or behaviour. Unfortunately, virtually no information is available about these kinds of linkages. Yet, without such information, studies of the evolution of virulence are doomed to sterile abstraction.

23.3.1 *An example: myxoma virus in Australian rabbits*

There is one example where enough data are available to attempt a crude assessment of the interrelationships in eqn (23.22), and thence to say something about the likely course of evolution of virulence. The people who studied myxoma virus in rabbit populations in Australia, after the introduction of the virus in 1950, adopted experimental protocols designed to maximize our understanding of the system (Fenner and Ratcliffe 1965; Fenner and Myers 1978; Fenner 1983). In particular, reference strains of the original rabbit population were kept, so that the virulence of newly appearing strains of the myxoma virus in the field could be monitored. Similarly, reference strains of the originally introduced virus were kept, for assaying the susceptibility of subsequent field populations of rabbits.

The data compiled by Fenner and co-workers suggest the functional relationship between recovery rate and virulence shown in Fig. 23.12 (here the points show the data for the six observed strains of myxoma virus, and the two curves represent functions fitted to these data, as discussed in more detail by Anderson and May (1982*e*). The relation between transmission, βN, and α is harder to determine for this system. On the one hand, there is evidence (Fenner and Ratcliffe 1965; Fenner 1983) that transmission is somewhat greater for rabbits infected with more virulent strains, mainly because there are a greater number of open lesions. On the other hand, mortality is greater and rabbit populations relatively smaller when the predominant strains of the virus are highly virulent; smaller N makes for lower βN. There are not sufficient data to estimate how these countervailing effects balance out in natural myxoma–rabbit associations,

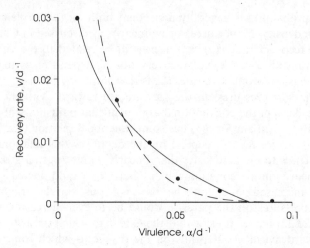

Fig. 23.12. This figure shows the empirical relationship between virulence, α, and recovery rate, v, for various strains of myxoma virus in wild populations of rabbits in Australia. The full circles are the observed values, and the two functional fits are as described in detail in Anderson and May (1982*e*).

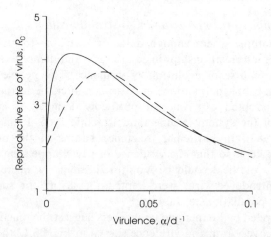

Fig. 23.13. The relationship between the basic reproductive rate, R_0, of eqn (23.22) and virulence, α, for the various grades of myxoma virus in wild populations of rabbits in Australia, for the two functional relations between v and α displayed in Fig. 23.12. The disease-free death rate is $\mu = 0.011$ day^{-1}, and βN is arbitrarily set constant at 0.2 day^{-1} (after Anderson and May 1982*e*).

and for a first estimate we arbitrarily take βN to be independent of α.

With $v(\alpha)$ depending on α as shown in Fig. 23.12, and βN taken to be constant, eqn (23.22) leads to the relation between R_0 and α that is shown in Fig. 23.13. Our rough analysis thus suggests that R_0 for the parasite is maximized by an *intermediate* grade of virulence (specifically, virulence grade IV): too big an α

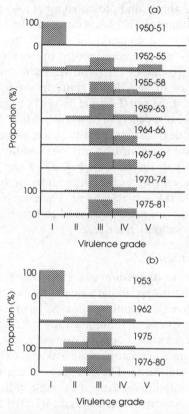

Fig. 23.14. (a) This figure shows the proportions in which the various grades of myxoma virus have been found in wild populations of rabbits in Australia, at different times from 1951 to 1981. The data are those compiled by Fenner (1983), and come from various sources. (b) The proportions of the various grades of myxoma virus recovered from wild populations of rabbits in Britain are shown, for different times from 1953 to 1980. The data again come from a variety of sources, as summarized by Fenner (1983).

kills off hosts too fast, leading to lower transmission of the infection; too small an α leads to hosts recovering too fast, again resulting in lower transmission efficiency.

Figure 23.14 shows what has actually happened in field populations of rabbits in Australia. Following the introduction of the virulence grade I of myxoma virus in 1950, successively less virulent strains rapidly appeared. The system appears, however, to have settled to a steady equilibrium, with the predominant strain of myxoma virus being the intermediate grades III–IV (although all grades are still found, with I, II, and V being relatively uncommon). As shown in Fig. 23.14, the history of the myxoma–rabbit association in Britain appears to be similar to that in Australia, even though the ecological details (such as the intermediate vector being fleas rather than mosquitoes) are different.

The analysis outlined above, and presented more fully in Anderson and May (1982*e*) and May and Anderson (1983*a*), is crude in many ways. The imprecision of the assumption that βN is constant has already been noted. Evolution of resistance by the rabbits has also been ignored in this study, which has centred on the basic reproductive rate of the parasite. There are some arguments for expecting such resistance to be a less significant aspect of the parasite–host evolution, at least in the short run (Levin *et al.* 1982). Fenner (1983) summarizes evidence for the existence of a degree of resistance in field populations of rabbits; this resistance varies in degree from place to place, accounting for shifts in the predominant grade of myxoma virus in any one location that may vary up to about half a grade (that is, the peak in Fig. 23.14 can vary by about half a grade, depending on the geographical locality under study). Clearly the analysis summarized in Fig. 23.13 is a very rough one. The example does, however, serve to show that parasites do not necessarily tend to become avirulent, and shows why this may be so in one particular case.

23.3.2 *Other complications*

In essentially all the above discussion, any given host individual was assumed to harbour at most one genotype of parasite at any one time. Bremermann and Pickering (1983) have given a preliminary discussion of the additional complications that arise when hosts can be simultaneously infected with several different strains or genotypes of parasite. Focusing on single hosts, these authors show that the most virulent strain of microparasite will tend to be favoured by natural selection within individual hosts. The essentials of the analysis can be made intuitively clear by considering an explicit example with two strains or clones of a parasite: the more virulent strain 1 kills an infected host after *m* days, and produces transmission stages at a constant rate, λ; the less virulent strain 2 kills hosts after $2m$ days, and produces transmission stages at a rate 0.6λ. The less virulent strain 2 has reproductive success 1.2 times that of the more virulent strain 1, provided we compare singly infected hosts. But in hosts infected with both strains, strain 1 kills the host before strain 2 can reap its longer term advantage, and the reproductive success of strain 2 is effectively only 0.6 that of strain 1. This particular complication is only one of several which further muddy the theoretical waters.

Looking to the empirical evidence, we can find many examples where transmissibility and damage to the host are so entwined that a parasite can find it hard, if not impossible, to evolve toward 'harmlessness'. Moore (1984), for example, has reviewed many instances where parasites with indirect life cycles modify the behaviour of their vertebrate or invertebrate host in such a way as to facilitate transmission to the next stage in the parasite's life cycle, even though this behaviour increases host mortality. Many invertebrate hosts have relatively short lives anyway, and such pressures toward avirulence as do exist are correspondingly weak; thus many baculoviruses kill their insect hosts and, by so doing, effectively turn them into masses of viral transmission stages.

Our central conclusion is that 'successful' parasites need not necessarily evolve to be harmless. Both theory and some empirical evidence indicate that the coevolution between parasites and hosts can follow many paths, depending on the relation between virulence and transmissibility of the parasite, and the cost to the host of evolving resistance.

23.4 Parasites and the population biology of humans

During most of the million or so years that humans have existed, their numbers have been low and relatively constant. The processes of fertility and mortality that kept this rough balance among hunter–gatherer populations are still far from understood.

Figure 23.15 shows a survival curve, deduced from skeletal evidence (Acsadi and Nemeskeri 1970), for a group of Mediterranean hunter–gatherers who lived about 15000 years ago. This curve is probably fairly typical for such pre-agricultural groups (Hassan 1981). There is little doubt that disease contributed to the mortality patterns exemplified by Fig. 23.15, but precise knowledge of the extent of the contribution is impossible. Although some parasitic infections leave traces on early human skeletons—usually the only remains available for examination—most, particularly those caused by viruses and bacteria, do not.

Certain conclusions may, however, be drawn from the ideas about threshold host densities that have been developed throughout this book. Bands of

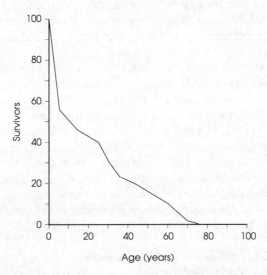

Fig. 23.15. This figure shows the survival curve for a group of hunter–gatherers who lived approximately 15000 years ago on the Mediterranean coast. The curve shows high child mortality, with only about 50 per cent of the population surviving past age 10 (after Acsadi and Nemeskeri 1970).

hunter–gatherers probably ranged in size from around 20 to at most 100 individuals (Hassan 1981), and these populations may have been sufficient to maintain many macroparasites as well as microparasites with long periods of infectiousness or (as is the case with hepatitis, herpes simplex, gonorrhoea, and other infections) with asymptomatic carriers (Cockburn 1971). Pathogenic organisms whose normal habitat is a host other than man or that are able to multiply and survive successfully in the soil and other inanimate environments (such as tetanus, gas gangrene, and other *Clostridiae*) could also have played a role among these sparse early populations. But the directly transmitted microparasites responsible for much mortality in historical times—smallpox, measles, cholera, and the like—have very high host threshold densities, and could not have been present in the pre-agricultural era.

Starting about 10 000 years ago in the Old World, nomadic cultivation began to give way to true agriculture, leading to denser and denser aggregations of people. Many macroparasites now undoubtedly began to attain infection levels that could produce morbidity and mortality. Zoonoses associated with domestic animals (such as tuberculosis) probably became significant. More important, population levels now became high enough for the virulent microparasitic infections to establish themselves. We notice, in passing, that the problem of 'where the AIDS virus came from' is not a new one; most of the microparasitic infections of childhood have appeared in human populations only in the last 10 000 years or so, which is a blink of an eye in evolutionary time.

Many authors have discussed the various consequences of these changing patterns in the relation between 'plagues and people' (Haldane 1949; Armelagos and McArdle 1975; McNeill 1976). A brief review of some of the epidemiological traumas of historical times, and of their social and political consequences, was given in Chapter 1.

One large pattern deserves more attention than it has received. According to Deevey's (1960) necessarily rough estimates, which are illustrated in Fig. 23.16, the first 5000 years after the beginning of the Agricultural Revolution saw human numbers increase about twentyfold, from about 5 million to about 100 million. A second, roughly equal period, from about 5000 years ago to around 300–400 years ago, saw only a fivefold increase, to approximately 500 million. One among several possible explanations is that human conglomerations gradually rose to levels capable of maintaining directly transmitted microparasitic diseases, whose effect was then to slow population growth. That is to say, the kind of demographic effects illustrated in the abstract in Fig. 23.15 may actually be manifest in the post-Agricultural Revolution phase of Fig. 23.16.

A more familiar application of these ideas about threshold population sizes lies in the history of the Western European conquest of the New World and Oceania, which was accomplished largely with biological weapons: smallpox, tuberculosis, measles, and others. It seems likely the people of the New World and Oceania had no similarly virulent microparasites of their own with which

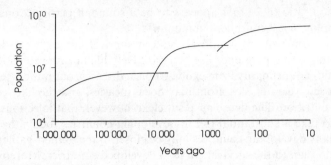

Fig. 23.16. A rough estimate of the total population of humans is shown on a doubly logarithmic plot, from around 1 million years ago to around 10 years ago. There are three broad phases of population growth: the pre-agricultural or hunter–gatherer phase, when total human numbers increased slowly for something like 1 million years; the Agricultural Revolution, beginning around 10 000 years ago, which led initially to a rapid rise in numbers that later slowed somewhat; and the Scientific–Industrial Revolution, beginning around 300–400 years ago, which has led to ever-increasing rates of population growth. This figure is based on the necessarily approximate estimates given by Deevey (1960).

to counter because they were, or until recently had been, at densities too low to maintain such infections. A notable exception that may have been exported to the Old World (although even this is debatable) is syphilis, which is well adapted to persist at low host densities. The dramatic magnitude of the mortality caused among indigenous New World peoples by first contact with European diseases is still emerging from revisionist analysis of the fragmentary evidence (Dobyns 1966; Myers 1974, 1981; May 1984). For Central Mexico, Dobyns estimates a population reduction by a factor in excess of 20 over the 130 years following the Spanish Conquest. For the Coastal Mexicans, he gives a depopulation ratio of about 10:1 in less than 60 years. For the Incan Empire in the Andes, rough ratios are assessed at several sites: 16:1 for Rimac (the modern Lima) area, and 25:1 for Chincha in less than 50 years after conquest; 9:1 over 115 years in Andean highland mines; over 100:1 from very crude estimates made by the Marques de Varinas in 1695 around Lima. In California, Indian depopulation ratios are around 17:1 to 25:1 over the 140 year span from the first Spanish missions in the 1770s to the population nadir in 1910. In Tierra del Fuego, where the natives seem to be headed for biological extinction, the total Indian population had declined from around 7000–9000 in 1871 to around 200 in 1950; a single measles epidemic in 1884 played a key role in this 40:1 depopulation. Anecdotes about groups of Amazonian Indians first contacted in the 1920s give depopulation ratios ranging from around 20:1 to around 200:1 over periods of less than 50 years. Pooling these variegated New World data, Dobyns concludes that over the 100 years following first contact, 'the depopulation ratio of 20 to 1 appears to be a sound, if perhaps ·conservative, tool to employ as a hemispheric minimum'.

Figure 1.4 (on page 5) contrasts modern survival curves for a developed country and a developing one. The comparatively high death rate in the Third World comes not primarily from exotic tropical diseases, but rather—especially in the first few years of life—from diarrhoea, measles, and the like, combined with poor nutrition. The figure makes it clear, however, that infectious diseases continue to take a substantial toll in developing countries today; the survival curve in many developing countries may be closer to the hunter–gatherer curve of Fig. 23.15 than to the survival curve in developed countries. Moreover, both present day curves would tell a gloomier story if they were plotted for somewhat earlier times. The increases in life expectancy in the developed world over the past two centuries, and in the developing world since World War II, are due almost wholly to reduced mortality from infectious diseases (Hassell *et al.* 1982).

Although this broad conclusion is plain, the details are difficult to elucidate. In Western Europe, mortality from microparasitic infections fell throughout the late eighteenth and the nineteenth centuries, long before the advent of modern drugs or vaccines (excepting that for smallpox). There is an unresolved argument about the relative contributions made by better nutrition, improved hygiene due to innovations ranging from more use of soap to better sanitation, and other factors (McKeown 1976; Razzell 1974). Similarly complex is the debate about the contribution made to overall population growth in European countries from 1750 to 1850 by this decreased mortality, versus that made by increased fertility. Recent analyses suggest no single answer (Wrigley and Schofield 1981): in England, population grew mainly as a result of increased fertility, but with some help from declining mortality; in Sweden, population grew almost entirely as a result of decreased death rates, partly associated with smallpox vaccination; and in France, population remained roughly steady as mortality and fertility fell together.

In short, infectious diseases have been important sources of mortality throughout human history. In any epoch, however, their exact contributions to demographic trends are hard to pin down.

Appendix A

Static properties of models for host–microparasite interactions

This appendix presents results for the static properties of the model with classes of hosts who are protected by maternal antibodies, susceptible, latent, infectious, and immune ($I(a)$, $X(a)$, $H(a)$, $Y(a)$, $Z(a)$, respectively), as described by eqns (4.44)–(4.48). As throughout Chapters 4 and 5, the force of infection, λ, is taken to be an age-independent constant.

The terms involving the age-dependent death rate, $\mu(a)$, on the right-hand side in eqns (4.44)–(4.50) can be removed by writing the equations in terms of the proportions in the various classes, $x(a) = X(a)/N(a)$ and so on. The total number of hosts of age a is still given by eqns (4.7) and (4.8), which we repeat for convenience:

$$N(a) = N(0)\ell(a), \tag{A.1}$$

$$\ell(a) \equiv \exp\left(-\int_0^a \mu(s)\, ds\right). \tag{A.2}$$

The set of eqns (4.44)–(4.48) translate into an elementary set of linear, first-order differential equations with constant coefficients:

$$di/da = -di, \tag{A.3}$$

$$dx/da = di - \lambda x, \tag{A.4}$$

$$dh/da = \lambda x - \sigma h, \tag{A.5}$$

$$dy/da = \sigma h - vy, \tag{A.6}$$

$$dz/da = vy. \tag{A.7}$$

The boundary conditions are $i(0) = 1$, and $x(0) = h(0) = y(0) = z(0) = 0$. The solutions to these equations are trivial (though tedious for the later classes):

$$i(a) = e^{-da}, \tag{A.8}$$

$$x(a) = [d/(d-\lambda)][e^{-\lambda a} - e^{-da}], \tag{A.9}$$

$$h(a) = \left(\frac{\lambda d}{d-\lambda}\right)\left(\frac{e^{-\sigma a} - e^{-\lambda a}}{\lambda - \sigma} - \frac{e^{-\sigma a} - e^{-da}}{d - \sigma}\right), \tag{A.10}$$

$$y(a) = \sigma\lambda d\left(\frac{e^{-va} - e^{-\sigma a}}{(\lambda-\sigma)(d-\sigma)(\sigma-v)} + \frac{e^{-va} - e^{-\lambda a}}{(\lambda-d)(\lambda-\sigma)(\lambda-v)}\right.$$
$$\left. + \frac{e^{-va} - e^{-da}}{(d-\lambda)(d-\sigma)(d-v)}\right). \tag{A.11}$$

From this, $z(a)$ is given simply as $z = 1 - (i + x + h + y)$.

Relations among R_0, λ, A, β

Type II survival

By integrating $X(a) = x(a)N(a)$ over all ages, we get:

$$\bar{X} = dN(0)/[(\lambda + \mu)(d + \mu)]. \tag{A.12}$$

As those protected by maternal antibodies are never candidates for infection, the appropriate factor by which R_0 should be discounted to reduce the effective reproductive rate to unity at equilibrium is $x^* = \bar{X}/(\bar{N} - \bar{I})$. Here $\bar{N} = N(0)/\mu$ and $\bar{I} = N(0)/(\mu + d)$, whence

$$R_0 = (\lambda + \mu)/\mu. \tag{A.13}$$

This is eqn (4.25) for the basic SIR model.

Substituting from eqns (A.1) and (A.9) into eqn (4.27) for A leads, for Type II survival, to

$$A = \frac{d + \lambda}{(\lambda + \mu)(d + \mu)}. \tag{A.14}$$

Alternatively, if the average age at infection is calculated on the basis of proportions infected in each age class, $\hat{A}$ (rather than absolute numbers), eqn (4.31) leads to

$$\hat{A} = (d + \lambda)/d\lambda. \tag{A.15}$$

That is,

$$\hat{A} = M + (1/\lambda). \tag{A.16}$$

Inverting these expressions, we obtain

$$\lambda \simeq 1/(A - M). \tag{A.17}$$

This expression is approximate for A defined as above, and exact if 'A' is actually assessed as $\hat{A}$.

To relate R_0 to A, we eliminate λ between eqns (A.13) and (A.14). This gives

$$R_0 = \frac{d - \mu}{\mu[A(d + \mu) - 1]}. \tag{A.18}$$

This reduces approximately to

$$R_0 = (L - M)/(A - M), \tag{A.19}$$

if we replace the factor $A(1 + M/L)$ by A (which, since M/L is less than 1 per cent, is a correction beyond the practical accuracy of measurement of A). This eqn (A.19) is eqn (4.54) of the main text.

Finally, if we integrate over $Y(a)$, as given by eqns (A.1) and (A.11), we get

$$\bar{Y} = \frac{N(0)\lambda\sigma d}{(v + \mu)(d + \mu)(\sigma + \mu)(\lambda + \mu)}. \tag{A.20}$$

Writing $\lambda = \beta\bar{Y}$, and solving for λ, we arrive at

$$\lambda = \mu\left[\left(\frac{\beta\bar{N}}{v + \mu}\right)\left(\frac{d}{d + \mu}\right)\left(\frac{\sigma}{\sigma + \mu}\right) - 1\right]. \tag{A.21}$$

By the argument given earlier in Chapter 4, the first term inside the square brackets may be identified with R_0, to give the relation, eqn (4.55), between R_0 and β that is discussed in the main text.

Type I survival

The corresponding set of calculations with Type I survival are similarly straightforward, although the results are more untidy because of factors like $\exp(-\lambda L)$ draped over the landscape. Since $1/d$, $1/\sigma$, $1/v$ are at longest of the order of a few months, while L is 50 years or more, we consistently omit terms of relative order $\exp(-dL)$, $\exp(-\sigma L)$, and $\exp(-vL)$ in what follows. To this order of accuracy, integration of eqn (A.9) gives

$$\bar{X} = (N(0)/\lambda)[1 - d\,e^{-\lambda L}/(d - \lambda)]. \tag{A.22}$$

As noted above, the effective factor by which R_0 is to be discounted at equilibrium is $x^* = \bar{X}/(\bar{N} - \bar{I})$. Here $\bar{N} = LN(0)$ and $\bar{I} = N(0)/d$, so that

$$R_0 = \frac{\lambda L(1 - 1/dL)}{1 - [d/(d - \lambda)]\exp(-\lambda L)}. \tag{A.23}$$

The average age at infection A (or $\hat{A}$, which is identical with A for Type I survival) is given from eqns (4.27) and (A.9) as

$$A = \left[\left(\frac{d + \lambda}{d\lambda}\right)\left(1 - \frac{d^2(1 + \lambda L)\,e^{-\lambda L}}{(d^2 - \lambda^2)}\right)\right]\left(1 - \frac{d\,e^{-\lambda L}}{(d - \lambda)}\right)^{-1}. \tag{A.24}$$

As ever, terms of relative order $\exp(-dL)$ have been discarded. Eliminating λ betweens eqns (A.23) and (A.24), and ignoring terms of relative order $\exp(-\lambda L)$, we again get eqn (A.19), as discussed in the main text.

Integrating eqn (A.11) over all ages leads to the result

$$\bar{Y} = (N(0)/v)\left(1 - \frac{v\sigma d\,e^{-\lambda L}}{(v - \lambda)(\sigma - \lambda)(d - \lambda)}\right). \tag{A.25}$$

Writing $\lambda = \beta\bar{Y}$ in eqn (A.25) and comparing with eqn (A.23), we get

$$R_0 \simeq \beta\bar{N}/v. \tag{A.26}$$

Here the terms of relative magnitude $\exp(-\lambda L)$ have also been neglected, as discussed in the main text.

Appendix B

Static aspects of a programme of immunization according to a general age-dependent schedule

Consider an immunization programme described by some age-specific rate, $c(a)$, at which susceptibles are successfully immunized. At equilibrium, the numbers of susceptibles, infecteds, and immunes as functions of age will obey the equations

$$dX'/da = -(\lambda'(a) + c(a) + \mu(a))X'(a), \tag{B.1}$$

$$dY'/da = \lambda'X' - (v + \mu(a))Y'(a), \tag{B.2}$$

$$dZ'/da = vY' + c(a)X' - \mu(a)Z'(a). \tag{B.3}$$

Here immunization is taken to have the effect of transferring susceptibles directly into the immune class. As explained in the main text, we have also included (albeit in a crude way) the possibility that λ' is age dependent, with the relation

$$\lambda'(a) = \beta(a)\bar{Y}'. \tag{B.4}$$

The transmission parameter β is assumed to have some fixed age dependence.

As outlined in the main text, this set of four equations in the four unknowns $X'(a)$, $Y'(a)$, $Z'(a)$, and $\lambda'(a)$ may be solved—in general numerically—once $c(a)$ and $\mu(a)$ are specified; $\beta(a)$ is deduced from the pre-immunization data. As usual, the boundary conditions are $X'(0) = N(0)$ and $Y'(0) = Z'(0) = 0$.

Two comments may be made here. First, categories of hosts who are latent and/or who are protected by maternal antibodies can clearly be included in an extended version of the above calculations. Second, if a proportion *p of girls only* (or of boys only) is immunized, the results will be as if a proportion $p/2$ of both girls and boys were immunized under the same schedule (assuming a 1:1 sex ratio of girls to boys, which is an excellent approximation at early ages). This is an important point in connection, for example, with some vaccination schemes against rubella.

Equation (B.1) for $X'(a)$ can be integrated, to get

$$X'(a) = N(0)\ell(a) \exp\left(-\int_0^a [\lambda'(s) + c(s)]\, ds\right). \tag{B.5}$$

Here $\ell(a)$ is the usual age-specific survivorship function. We now indicate some explicit applications of this formalism.

Proportion p immunized at age b

Here the immunization rate, $c(a)$, is a discontinuous function (being zero everywhere except at age b, where it is infinite), which can be treated by standard techniques using Dirac delta-functions. Alternatively, we can observe that at age b a fraction of the susceptibles are transferred directly to the immune class, so that

$$X'(a) = N(0)\ell(a) \exp(-\lambda'a), \qquad a \leqslant b, \tag{B.6a}$$

$$X'(a) = (1 - p)N(0)\ell(a) \exp(-\lambda'a), \qquad a > b. \tag{B.6b}$$

For any specified mortality curve, $\mu(a)$, we can now calculate $R_0 = \bar{N}/\bar{X}$, as a function of λ', p, and b.

For Type I survival, we have

$$\bar{X} = N(0)[1 - p \exp(-\lambda'b) - (1 - p) \exp(-\lambda'L)]/\lambda'. \tag{B.7}$$

With $\bar{N} = N(0)L$, this gives eqn (5.8) of the main text. This in turn leads to the eradication criterion (5.12).

For Type II survival, we have

$$\bar{X} = N(0)\{1 - p \exp[-(\lambda' + \mu)b]\}/(\lambda' + \mu). \tag{B.8}$$

This gives eqn (5.9) for R_0, and thence eqn (5.14) for p_c.

Notice that we have taken λ' to be independent of age in these calculations.

Proportion p immunized at a constant rate c

In this case, a fraction $1 - p$ of the population are never immunized, while the remaining fraction p undergo immunization at the constant per capita rate c. The average age at immunization, for that fraction who indeed experience it, is $V = 1/c$. Here eqn (B.1) gives, for constant λ',

$$X(a) = N(0)\ell(a)\{(1 - p) \exp(-\lambda'a) + p \exp[-(\lambda' + c)a]\}. \tag{B.9}$$

We now take the short-cut of relating λ' to R_0, as used throughout Chapter 5 (rather than the equivalent procedure of expressing λ' in terms of β, and thence in terms of R_0).

For Type II survival, we get

$$\bar{X} = N(0)\left(\frac{p}{\lambda' + c + \mu} + \frac{1 - p}{\lambda' + \mu}\right). \tag{B.10}$$

As ever, $\bar{N} = N(0)/\mu$. It follows that

$$R_0 = \frac{(\lambda' + \mu)(\lambda' + \mu + c)}{\mu[\lambda' + \mu + c(1 - p)]}. \tag{B.11}$$

The actual proportion, p, to be immunized at the rate c in order to eradicate the infection is found by taking the limit $\lambda' \to 0$ in eqn (B.11):

$$p_c = [1 - (1/R_0)](1 + \mu/c). \tag{B.12}$$

Using the previously obtained result $R_0 = L/A$, and writing $\mu = 1/L$ and

$c = 1/V$, we have

$$p_c = (1 - A/L)(1 + V/L). \tag{B.13}$$

The corresponding result for Type I survival can be seen to be

$$p_c = \frac{1 - (1/R_0)}{1 - (V/L)[1 - \exp(-L/V)]}. \tag{B.14}$$

Equation (B.12) or (B.14) can be compared with eqn (5.14) or (5.12), respectively. As noted in the main text, the results are essentially identical with those for immunization at exactly age b (so long as b/L and V/L are small, as they usually will be). Eradication is only possible for $A > V$, and it becomes difficult (p_c approaches unity) for V close to A.

Appendix C

Dynamic properties of models for host–microparasite interactions

In this appendix, we discuss a miscellany of mathematical technicalities, all having to do with the dynamical behaviour of our basic model for microparasitic infections (as developed in Chapters 6 and 7). We first deal with the derivation of dynamical equations for total numbers of susceptibles, infectives, etc. from equations for the age- and time-dependent variables $X(a, t)$, $Y(a, t)$, etc. Next, the analytic results presented in Chapter 6 (Fig. 6.1 and surrounding discussion) for the dynamics of epidemic and endemic oscillations are established. The dynamic consequences of immunization programmes are then discussed, and we outline the derivation of various results that are quoted in Chapter 7. The appendix ends with the stability analysis of the 'pedagogic preliminary' model defined by eqns (6.22) and (6.23).

Integrating over age to obtain equations for total numbers

As defined in the text, $X(a, t)$, $H(a, t)$, $Y(a, t)$, and $Z(a, t)$ are the number (or density) of susceptible, latent, infectious, and recovered-and-immune individuals, respectively, of age a at time t. We include the latent class because it is present in many of the numerical computations shown in Chapters 6 and 7. A class of individuals protected by maternal antibodies could similarly be included, but in the computations these effects are usually handled by simply assuming that susceptibles appear at age M (typically around 6 months); that is, one boundary condition is $X(M, t) = N(M, t)$. The set of partial differential equations describing this system is (as described in Chapter 3):

$$\partial X(a, t)/\partial t + \partial X(a, t)/\partial a = -(\lambda(t) + \mu(a))X, \qquad (C.1)$$

$$\partial H(a, t)/\partial t + \partial H(a, t)/\partial a = \lambda X - (\sigma + \mu(a))H, \qquad (C.2)$$

$$\partial Y(a, t)/\partial t + \partial Y(a, t)/\partial a = \sigma H - (v + \mu(a))Y, \qquad (C.3)$$

$$\partial Z(a, t)/\partial t + \partial Z(a, t)/\partial a = vY - \mu(a)Z, \qquad (C.4)$$

$$\partial N(a, t)/\partial t + \partial N(a, t)/\partial a = -\mu(a)N. \qquad (C.5)$$

As usual, $N = X + H + Y + Z$; the parameters λ, $\mu(a)$, σ, v have the meanings defined in the main text; and the standard boundary/initial conditions apply. In particular, the latent class can be removed by assuming that the latent period is zero, whereupon $\sigma \to \infty$ (and $H \to 0$) and the right-hand side of eqn (C.3) for $Y(a, t)$ is the familiar $\lambda X - (\mu + v)Y$.

To collapse eqns (C.1)–(C.5) into a set of ordinary differential equations for the total numbers in the various epidemiological classes, we integrate over all ages, remembering the boundary condition $X(0, t) = N(0, t)$, $H(0, t) = Y(0, t) = Z(0, t) = 0$ (in the absence of maternal antibody protection):

$$d\bar{X}(t)/dt = N(0) - \lambda(t)\bar{X}(t) - \int_0^\infty \mu(a)X(a, t)\,da, \tag{C.6}$$

$$d\bar{H}(t)/dt = \lambda(t)\bar{X}(t) - \sigma\bar{H}(t) - \int_0^\infty \mu(a)H(a, t)\,da, \tag{C.7}$$

$$d\bar{Y}(t)/dt = \sigma\bar{H}(t) - v\bar{Y}(t) - \int_0^\infty \mu(a)Y(a, t)\,da. \tag{C.8}$$

Here $N(0)$ is the total number born into age class zero, per unit time, which is independent of time, t, because the total population is assumed to be unchanging (births balancing deaths according to constant fertility and mortality schedules); for a discussion that departs from this conventional but unrealistic assumption, see Chapter 13. Because $\bar{N}$ is constant, we do not need an equation for $\bar{Z}(t)$: $\bar{Z}(t) = \bar{N} - (\bar{X}(t) + \bar{H}(t) + \bar{Y}(t))$.

In eqns (C.6)–(C.8), we see that the messy terms involving $\mu(a)$ have prevented us from, in fact, obtaining equations for the total numbers in each category. Dealing with this problem requires specific assumptions about the dependence of $\mu(a)$ on a.

1. Type II survivorship: $\mu = $ constant. In this case, the integral on the right-hand side of eqn (C.6) gives simply $\mu\bar{X}$, and so on. The equations for total numbers then have the simple form given by eqns (6.1)–(6.3) where there is no latent class ($\sigma \to \infty$), with an obvious extension if $\bar{H}(t)$ *is* involved. These equations are essentially always used in discussions of epidemiological dynamics, usually with little emphasis on the mild swindle involved in assuming Type II survival (age-independent mortality rate) in developed countries.

2. Type I survivorship: $\mu = 0$ for $a < L$, $\mu = \infty$ for $a > L$ (that is, everyone lives L years). Equations (C.6)–(C.8) now take the form:

$$d\bar{X}(t)/dt = N(0) - \lambda(t)\bar{X}(t) - X(L, t), \tag{C.9}$$

$$d\bar{H}(t)/dt = \lambda(t)\bar{X}(t) - \sigma\bar{H}(t) - H(L, t), \tag{C.10}$$

$$d\bar{Y}(t)/dt = \sigma\bar{H}(t) - v\bar{Y}(t) - Y(L, t). \tag{C.11}$$

The quantities $X(L, t)$, $H(L, t)$, and $Y(L, t)$ represent the numbers of susceptibles, latents, and infectious in the age class L, at time t, respectively. The quantities could, of course, be calculated (along lines made explicit below) from the fully age-structured equations, but here we want equations that avoid age complications. We can, however, note that $H(L, t)$ will be of order $H(t)/L$, and this will be smaller than $\sigma H(t)$ by a factor of order $1/\sigma L$, which is the ratio between the duration of the latent period and the life expectancy; since $1/\sigma$ is of order days and L is of order decades, the term $H(L, t)$ may usually, to an excellent approximation, be neglected. Similarly, the ratio of $Y(L, t)$ to $vY(t)$ is of order $1/vL$, which likewise is usually negligibly small. The term $X(L, t)$ in eqn (C.9) is more problematic, in that its ratio to $\lambda X(t)$ is of order $1/\lambda L$, where $1/\lambda$ (the average age at infection) is not usually negligibly small compared with L ($1/\lambda$ is usually a few years, rather than the few days of $1/\sigma$ and $1/v$). But, as discussed more fully below (see also Anderson and May (1983*a*)), the $X(L, t)$ term in eqn (C.9) is less of a problem that the $H(L, t)$ and $Y(L, t)$ terms, because it can be expressed fairly directly in terms of $\lambda(t)$.

In most of what follows, and in most of the analytic (as opposed to numerical) results in Chapters 6 and 7, we avoid these problems by assuming Type II survivorship.

Dynamics following the first introduction of an infection

If we assume $\mu = $ constant, and neglect latency, we obtain a pair of differential equations for $\bar{X}(t)$ and $\bar{Y}(t)$, or, equivalently, for $x(t) = \bar{X}(t)/\bar{N}$ and $\lambda(t) = \beta \bar{Y}(t)$. These eqns (6.5) and (6.6) are repeated here for convenience:

$$dx/dt = \mu - (\mu + \lambda(t))x(t), \qquad (C.12)$$

$$d\lambda/dt = (v + \mu)\lambda(t)(R_0 x(t) - 1). \qquad (C.13)$$

Here R_0 is defined by eqn (6.8).

Since for most infections $v \gg \mu$, essentially all analyses of the dynamics of the epidemics that follow the initial introduction of an infection into a wholly susceptible population put $\mu = 0$ in eqns (C.12) and (C.13). This is sensible so long as discussion is restricted to the epidemic itself, but it fails to describe the next phase of slow recovery *en route* to the next epidemic wave, as shown in Fig. 6.1; this figure is not to be found in epidemiological texts, but we think it helps to illuminate the relation between epidemic and endemic phases of infections.

In the very earliest phase following the appearance of the infection, we have $x(t) \simeq 1$ (almost everyone is still susceptible), and thus

$$d\lambda/dt \simeq v(R_0 - 1)\lambda. \qquad (C.14a)$$

That is, λ grows at first exponentially,

$$\lambda(t) \simeq \lambda(0)\, e^{\Lambda t}, \qquad (C.14b)$$

where $\lambda(0)$ is the initial 'seed' value of the force of infection, and $\Lambda = v(R_0 - 1)$ as defined by eqn (6.9). As the epidemic grows, $x(t)$ falls significantly below unity, and the sequence of dynamical events summarized by eqns (6.16)–(6.21) unfolds, on the 'fast' time-scale $1/v$. This is all standard stuff (see, for example, Bailey (1975)), although we believe that the results in eqns (6.16)–(6.21) are expressed in a somewhat unfamiliar, yet simple, form. A full description of this first phase can be obtained by writing $x(t) = \exp(-\phi(t))$, where $\phi(t) = \int_0^t \lambda(s)\,ds$, and then using eqns (6.19) and (6.4) to arrive at

$$\int_0^\phi \frac{d\phi'}{R_0[1 - \exp(-\phi')] - \phi' + (\varepsilon/v)} = vt. \qquad (C.15)$$

Here ε is the initial value of λ, $\lambda(0) = \varepsilon$. Equation (C.15) is a much-discussed result, giving the details of this first phase, which clearly takes place on a time-scale $1/v$, or even $1/(R_0 v)$ (Bailey 1975).

This 'first wave' ends with the fraction susceptible given by eqn (6.21), which for R_0 significantly in excess of unity leads to $x \simeq \exp(-R_0)$. The force of infection, λ, is also small at this end of the first wave, and it continues to fall (because $R_0 x - 1$ is now negative, indeed close to -1). In the aftermath of the epidemic, we can no longer neglect μ in eqn (C.12): births will now be crucial in rebuilding the population of susceptibles. Thus in the 'second phase', shown by the roughly linear regrowth of susceptibility in Fig. 6.1, we may neglect λx in comparison with μ in eqn (C.12), to get

$$dx/dt \simeq \mu(1 - x). \qquad (C.16)$$

On this 'second phase' time-scale of $1/\mu$, we may regard the initial epidemic as taking place in effectively zero time ($v \gg \mu$), to write the initial condition for eqn (C.16) as $x(\text{'}0\text{'}) \simeq 0$. Integrating eqn (C.16) with this initial condition, we find susceptibility growing throughout the 'second phase' approximately as

$$x(t) \simeq 1 - e^{-\mu t}. \qquad (C.17)$$

So long as μt, and thence $x(t)$, are significantly less than unity, this gives

$$x(t) \simeq \mu t - (\mu t)^2/2 + \cdots. \qquad (C.18)$$

This roughly linear growth in $x(t)$ with time, following the 'first wave' epidemic, is seen clearly in Fig. 6.1 (where the first indications of saturation, described by the more accurate eqn (C.17), can also be seen).

This 'second phase' of rebuilding susceptibility lasts so long as $\lambda(t)x(t)$ remains significantly less than μ. Eventually, however, $x(t)$ increases to the point where $R_0 x > 1$ (as shown below, this happens approximately at time $t \simeq 1/\mu R_0$), whereupon $\lambda(t)$ stops decreasing and begins to increase (cf. eqn (C.13)). The 'second phase' ends, and a second epidemic is triggered (again on the fast time-scale $1/v$), once the value of $\lambda(t)x(t)$ significantly exceeds μ.

To get a rough estimate of when this happens, we substitute the 'second phase' approximation (C.17) or (C.18) for $x(t)$ into eqn (C.13) for $\lambda(t)$:

$$d\lambda/dt \simeq v[R_0(1 - e^{-\mu t}) - 1]\lambda. \qquad (C.19)$$

Integrating, we get

$$\ln(\lambda(t)/\lambda(\text{'}0\text{'})) \simeq v[(R_0 - 1)t - (R_0/\mu)(1 - e^{-\mu t})]. \qquad (C.20)$$

Here $\lambda(\text{`0'})$ is the value of λ at the end of the 'first wave' epidemic, when $x(t)$ has attained its minimum value (as seen in Fig. 6.1). Recognizing that $\mu t < 1$ throughout this 'second phase', we rewrite eqn (C.20) as

$$\ln(\lambda(t)/\lambda(\text{`0'})) \simeq -vt[(1 - (1/2)R_0\mu t + (1/6)R_0\mu^2 t^2 - \cdots]. \quad (C.21)$$

As long as the quantity inside the square brackets on the right-hand side of eqn (C.21) is positive, $\lambda(t) < \lambda(\text{`0'})$. But once the quantity inside the square brackets becomes negative, $\lambda(t)$ exceeds $\lambda(\text{`0'})$. Indeed, given that $v \gg R_0\mu$, once the right-hand side of eqn (C.21) is positive, $\lambda(t)x(t)$ will increase on the time-scale $1/v$, to become significantly greater than μ, triggering the 'second wave' epidemic. In short, the duration of the 'second phase' of regrowth in susceptibility is essentially determined by the time it takes before the right-hand side of eqn (C.21) becomes positive, which is to say $t \simeq 2/\mu R_0$. This is just what is seen in Fig. 6.1: after a time $t \simeq 1/\mu R_0$ we have $x > 1/R_0$ (i.e. susceptibility in excess of the endemic equilibrium fraction); but it takes a second period of roughly the same duration before λ has built up to the point where λx can launch the next epidemic.

Noting that the average age at infection in the endemic situation is approximately $A = 1/\mu R_0$, we see that the duration of the slow 'second' phase is roughly $t \simeq 2A$.

Inter-epidemic oscillations in the endemic state

As explained in Chapter 6, each successive epidemic wave is less severe than its predecessor, until the distinction between the fast, epidemic, $1/v$ time-scale and the slow, re-growth, $1/\mu R_0$ time-scale blurs, giving way to damped oscillations with a period roughly equal to the geometric mean of fast and slow scales. We now derive this result (which is standard) for eqns (6.5) and (6.6), or equivalently (C.12) and (C.13), and then discuss some extensions (which represent new results).

Equations (C.12) and (C.13) have the much-discussed equilibrium solutions $x^* = 1/R_0$ and $\lambda^* = \mu(R_0 - 1)$, corresponding to endemic levels of infection. Small perturbations about this equilibrium may be described by writing $x(t) = x^* + \zeta(t)$ and $\lambda(t) = \lambda^* + \xi(t)$, where ζ and ξ are assumed small. In the standard way, we can now substitute these expressions in eqns (C.12) and (C.13), expand in Taylor series keeping only terms linear in ζ or ξ, and factor out the time dependence in the ensuing linear differential equations as $\exp \Lambda t$. The dynamics are now characterized by the eigenvalues Λ, which are found from the pair of equations

$$\Lambda\zeta = -\mu R_0\zeta - (1/R_0)\xi, \quad (C.22)$$

$$\Lambda\xi = v\mu R_0(R_0 - 1)\zeta. \quad (C.23)$$

These two equations are consistent if Λ obeys the quadratic

$$\Lambda^2 + \mu R_0 \Lambda + v\mu(R_0 - 1) = 0. \tag{C.24}$$

Recalling that the average age at infection in the endemic state (for Type II survivorship) is $A = 1/[\mu(R_0 - 1)]$, and that $A \gg D = 1/v$, we have

$$\Lambda \simeq -(1/2A) \pm i/(AD)^{1/2}. \tag{C.25}$$

That is, any disturbance to the endemic equilibrium will damp back, with decaying oscillations. However, the oscillatory period, $T \simeq 2\pi(AD)^{1/2}$, will be significantly shorter than the characteristic damping time, $T_D \simeq 2A$, if $A \gg D$ (as usually is the case). We now indicate several extensions of this familiar analysis.

For one thing, suppose a latent class is also included, as described by eqns (C.6)–(C.8) with $\mu = $ constant and with $\lambda = \beta \bar{Y}$. Equations (6.5) and (6.6) are then replaced by the set of three differential equations

$$dx/dt = \mu - (\mu + \lambda)x, \tag{C.26}$$

$$dh/dt = \lambda x - (\sigma + \mu)h, \tag{C.27}$$

$$d\lambda/dt = (v + \mu)[R_0(\sigma + \mu)h - \lambda]. \tag{C.28}$$

Here $h \equiv \bar{H}/\bar{N}$ and R_0 is appropriately redefined as

$$R_0 = \frac{\beta \bar{N}}{v + \mu}\left(\frac{\sigma}{\sigma + \mu}\right). \tag{C.29}$$

The equilibrium state is now $x^* = 1/R_0$, $h^* = [\mu/(\sigma + \mu)][1 - (1/R_0)]$ and $\lambda^* = \mu(R_0 - 1)$. The linearized stability analysis proceeds exactly as before, except that now Λ can be seen to be given by the roots of the cubic equation

$$\Lambda^3 + (v + \sigma + \mu R_0 + 2\mu)\Lambda^2 + \mu R_0(v + \sigma + 2\mu)\Lambda$$
$$+ \mu(R_0 - 1)(v + \mu)(\sigma + \mu) = 0. \tag{C.30}$$

If, as usually is the case, both σ and $v \gg \mu$ and μR_0, this cubic equation has one fast-decaying root, $\Lambda \simeq -(v + \sigma)$, and two other roots given approximately by the quadratic

$$\Lambda^2 + \mu R_0\Lambda + \mu(R_0 - 1)[v\sigma/(v + \sigma)] \simeq 0. \tag{C.31}$$

This is identical with eqn (C.24), except that in the final term of eqn (C.24) we have $v \to v\sigma/(v + \sigma)$. That is, we again have the damped oscillations of eqn (C.25), except that $D = 1/v$ has to be replaced by $D + D' = (1/v) + (1/\sigma)$. This establishes the result for the oscillatory period that was quoted in Chapter 6, as eqn (6.14) or eqn (6.15).

Notice that the oscillations are weakly damped (T_D significantly longer than T; $T_D/T \sim (A/D)^{1/2}$) essentially because the coefficient of Λ in the quadratic eqn (C.24) or (C.31) does not contain v. There are, however, various kinds of modifications to the basic model that result in the fast time-scale (i.e. the fast rate, v) appearing in the coefficient of Λ, with the consequence that perturbations are swiftly and smoothly damped. Three such modifications will now be briefly sketched.

First, suppose that infectious individuals, instead of recovering into an immune class, Z, move into an uninfectious state from which they episodically move briefly back into the infectious state. Such a situation is described by the equations

$$d\bar{X}/dt = \mu\bar{N} - (\mu + \lambda)\bar{X}, \tag{C.32}$$

$$d\bar{Y}/dt = \lambda\bar{X} - (v + \mu)\bar{Y} + w\bar{Z}, \tag{C.33}$$

$$d\bar{Z}/dt = v\bar{Y} - (w + \mu)\bar{Z}. \tag{C.34}$$

Here, everything is as before (with $\lambda = \beta\bar{Y}$) except that w measures the rate at which uninfectious individuals move back into the infectious class (out of which they continue to move at the rate v). Genital herpes is one example of an infection which appears to behave this way. Equations (C.32)–(C.34) are, of course, really only two equations, because $\bar{X} + \bar{Y} + \bar{Z} = \bar{N}$, which is constant. The result is that eqns (6.5) and (6.6), or (C.12) and (C.13), are replaced by

$$dx/dt = \mu - (\mu + \lambda)x, \tag{C.35}$$

$$d\lambda/dt = (v + w + \mu)[\mu R_0(\lambda x + w - wx)/(w + \mu) - \lambda]. \tag{C.36}$$

Here the definition of R_0 is $R_0 = \beta\bar{N}(w + \mu)/[\mu(v + w + \mu)]$. All this reduces back to eqns (C.12) and (C.13) if $w = 0$. The equilibrium solution is still $x^* = 1/R_0$, $\lambda^* = \mu(R_0 - 1)$, with the appropriate definition of R_0. The usual linearized stability analysis shows the eigenvalues, Λ, to be given by the quadratic equation

$$\Lambda^2 + [\mu R_0 + w + vw/(w + \mu)]\Lambda + \mu(R_0 - 1)(v + \mu + w) = 0. \tag{C.37}$$

The essential difference between eqn (C.37) and eqns (C.24) or (C.31) is that the fast rate, v, has appeared in the coefficient of Λ; unless w is so small that $wv/(w + \mu) \sim \mu R_0$ (which would mean that the characteristic time to return to the infectious state is significantly longer than the average life span), we would expect fast damping, and no oscillations, for such an infection with episodic return to infectiousness.

Second, suppose immunity is not life-long, but rather that recovered individuals lapse back into the susceptible state at a rate of γ. Gonorrhoea, or any other infection where individuals recover (after treatment or otherwise) directly back into the susceptible class, would be an extreme example (with $\gamma \to \infty$). Equation (C.13) or eqn (6.6) for λ remains unaltered, but eqn (C.12) or (6.5) for x can be seen now to read

$$dx/dt = \mu - (\mu + \lambda)x + \gamma\{1 - x - \lambda/[R_0(v + \mu)]\}. \tag{C.38}$$

Here R_0 is still as defined by eqn (6.8). The endemic equilibrium is $x^* = 1/R_0$ and $\lambda^* = (v + \mu)(R_0 - 1)(\gamma + \mu)/(\gamma + v + \mu)$; all this reduces back to the simpler, earlier results of eqns (C.12) and (C.13) *et seq.* if $\gamma = 0$. The usual stability analysis again boils down to a quadratic for Λ:

$$\Lambda^2 + (\gamma + \mu)[1 + (R_0 - 1)(v + \mu)/(\gamma + v + \mu)]\Lambda + (\gamma + \mu)(v + \mu)(R_0 - 1) = 0.$$

(C.39)

Again the fast time-scale, $1/v$, has been brought into the coefficient of Λ (unless γ is significantly smaller than μ!), and there are no longer weakly damped oscillations.

As shown in Chapter 9, the presence of 'carriers', which is to say long-lived infectiousness, also destroys the weakly damped oscillations.

All this accords with common sense. Episodic infectiousness, or reversion to the susceptible state following recovery, or long-lived infectiousness, all—in their different ways—add up to the steady input of fresh infectives. This undercuts the propensity to oscillate which occurs when each wave of infection depletes the pool of susceptibles, with a subsequent pattern of overshoot, overcompensation, and so on. It is pleasing to notice that the phenomenon of inter-epidemic periodicity is found among those infections where a brief period of infectiousness seems followed by lifelong immunity (measles, rubella, mumps, pertussis, smallpox), and is not found when there is recurring infectiousness (herpes, possibly chickenpox), or reversion to susceptibility (gonorrhoea), or where the infectious period is long, at least for some (HBV, typhoid, HIV).

A third circumstance which can preclude weakly damped oscillations arises when the force of infection does not depend linearly on the number of infections (Mollison, private communication). Suppose we have $\lambda = \beta \bar{Y}^v$, where v is some number close to unity. Then eqns (6.5) and (6.6), or (C.12) and (C.13) may, for the purposes of a stability analysis, be replaced by

$$d\bar{X}/dt = \mu\bar{N} - \beta \bar{Y}^v \bar{X},$$

(C.40)

$$d\bar{Y}/dt = \beta \bar{Y}^v \bar{X} - v\bar{Y}.$$

(C.41)

Here μ has been neglected in comparison with v or λ. We now write perturbations to the endemic equilibrium in the form $\bar{X}(t) = \bar{X}^* + \zeta(t)$ and $\bar{Y}(t) = \bar{Y}^* + \xi(t)$, linearize, and factor out the time dependence as $\exp \Lambda t$, to arrive at

$$\Lambda\zeta = -\lambda^*\zeta - (v\lambda^*\bar{X}^*/\bar{Y}^*)\zeta,$$

(C.42)

$$\Lambda\zeta + \Lambda\xi = -v\xi.$$

(C.43)

Recalling that $\lambda^* = 1/A$, and that $v = 1/D$, we arrive at a quadratic for Λ:

$$\Lambda^2 + \left(\frac{1}{A} + \frac{1 - v}{D}\right)\Lambda + \frac{1}{AD} = 0.$$

(C.44)

This differs from eqn (C.24) by virtue of the term $(1 - v)/D$ in the coefficient of Λ. But as $A \gg D$, this difference is crucial, and results in smooth and fast damping instead of weakly damped oscillations, unless v is so close to unity that $|1 - v| < D/A$. That is, the result whereby the damping time exceeds the oscillatory period by a factor of order $(A/D)^{1/2}$ depends sensitively on v being very close to unity; on the other hand, it does usually seem reasonable to assume that the force of infection will be linearly proportional to the fraction of the population who are infectious.

Perturbations induced by vaccination

This brief section outlines how the approximate eqns (7.4) and (7.5) are obtained from (7.1) and (7.2) by a linearized analysis.

We first write $x(t) = x(0) + \zeta(t)$ and $\lambda(t) = \lambda(0) + \xi(t)$, where $x(0) = 1/R_0$ and $\lambda(0) = \mu(R_0 - 1)$ are the initial, pre-immunization values. Terms of second or higher order in ζ and ξ are then discarded in a Taylor series expansion, to arrive at the pair of linear equations

$$d\zeta(t)/dt = -\mu p - \mu R_0 \zeta - \xi/R_0, \tag{C.45}$$

$$d\xi(t)/dt = \mu(v + \mu)R_0(R_0 - 1)\zeta. \tag{C.46}$$

This gives a standard second-order differential equation for $\zeta(t)$:

$$d^2\zeta/dt^2 + (\mu R_0)\, d\zeta/dt + \mu(v + \mu)(R_0 - 1)\zeta = 0. \tag{C.47}$$

The initial conditions are $\zeta(0) = 0$ and $d\zeta(0)/dt = -\mu p$. The solution of eqn (C.47) is routine, and is

$$\zeta(t) = -(\mu p/\omega)\, e^{-\alpha t} \sin \omega t. \tag{C.48}$$

Here the damping rate α, and the frequency ω, are as defined by eqn (C.25) and discussed in Chapter 6: $\alpha = 1/2A$ and $\omega = 2\pi/(AD)^{1/2}$, with A and D as defined above. Substituting eqn (C.48) into eqn (C.45), we find $\xi(t)$ to be

$$\xi(t) = -\mu R_0 p(1 - e^{-\alpha t} \cos \omega t). \tag{C.49}$$

These results now lead directly to eqns (7.4) and (7.5) in the main text; the features of these results are shown in Fig. 7.1 and the accompanying discussion.

The effects of age-dependent immunization

Here we summarize results that are presented more fully elsewhere (Anderson and May 1983a), and which are the basis for the numerical results presented in Chapter 7.

If the age-specific rate of immunization is $c(a)$, then the partial differential equation for $X(a, t)$ takes the form given by eqn (7.6), which differs from eqn (C.1) by the added term $-c(a)X(a, t)$. Equations (7.11) and (7.12) represent the solution to eqn (7.6), as can be verified by back-substitution (for those not versed in Green's functions).

In the often-met special case where a proportion p of each cohort are immunized at age b, eqns (7.11) and (7.12) take the following explicit form: for $a > t$, then if $t > a - b > 0$

$$X(a, t) = (1 - p)N(0)\ell(a) \exp\left(- \lambda_0(a - t) - \int_0^t \lambda(s) \, ds \right), \qquad \text{(C.50)}$$

but if $b > a$, or $a > t + b$,

$$X(a, t) = N(0)\ell(a) \exp\left(- \lambda_0(a - t) - \int_0^t \lambda(s) \, ds \right); \qquad \text{(C.51)}$$

for $t > a$, we have for $a > b$

$$X(a, t) = (1 - p)N(0)\ell(a) \exp\left(- \int_{t-a}^t \lambda(s) \, ds \right), \qquad \text{(C.52)}$$

and for $b > a$,

$$X(a, t) = N(0)\ell(a) \exp\left(- \int_{t-a}^t \lambda(s) \, ds \right). \qquad \text{(C.53)}$$

Here λ_0 is the value of λ before any immunization, and the mortality factor is contained in the quantity $\ell(a) \equiv \exp(-\int_0^a \mu(s) \, ds)$.

The above formulae give $X(a, t)$ in terms of known demographic and epidemiological parameters, along with the (unknown) time-dependent force of infection, $\lambda(t)$. As explained in the text of Chapter 7, if we assume $\lambda(t) = \beta \bar{Y}(t)$, the system of equations can be closed by integrating eqns (7.6)–(7.8) over all ages. The discussion in the first part of this appendix showed that two of the three ordinary differential equations (for $\bar{X}(t)$, $\bar{H}(t)$, and $\lambda(t) = \beta \bar{Y}(t)$) are:

$$d\bar{H}/dt = \lambda(t)\bar{X}(t) - \sigma\bar{H}(t), \qquad \text{(C.54)}$$

$$d\lambda/dt = \beta\sigma\bar{H}(t) - v\lambda(t). \qquad \text{(C.55)}$$

Here we have neglected terms of relative order $1/\sigma L$ and $1/vL$, as discussed earlier (for either Type I or Type II survivorship). The equation for $\bar{X}(t)$ must be treated with more respect, because $1/\lambda L$ is not necessarily negligible: for Type I survivorship we have

$$d\bar{X}/dt = - \lambda(t)\bar{X}(t) + N(0, t) - pX(b, t) - X(L, t); \qquad \text{(C.56)}$$

and for Type II survivorship we have

$$d\bar{X}/dt = -(\lambda(t) + \mu)\bar{X}(t) + N(0, t) - pX(b, t). \qquad \text{(C.57)}$$

In summary, the dynamical consequences of implementing a programme of immunizing a fraction p of each successive cohort at age b is determined by the triplet of ordinary differential equations (C.54)–(C.56) for Type I survivorship, or (C.54), (C.55), and (C.57) for Type II survivorship, with the awkward quantities $X(b, t)$ and $X(L, t)$ evaluated in terms of $\lambda(t)$ by using eqns (C.50)–(C.53).

A pedagogical example: neutral stability in a discrete-time model

We end this appendix by outlining the derivation of the stability properties of the discrete-time model defined by eqns (6.22) and (6.23). This model is of pedagogic use in illustrating, in a simple way, the propensity of host–pathogen systems to oscillate. As emphasized in the text, however, this dynamical behaviour is structurally unstable; we believe that biological insights need ultimately to be based always on structurally stable models (May 1974).

In eqns (6.22) and (6.23), the equilibrium numbers susceptible and infected are, respectively, $X^* = N/R_0$ and $Y^* = B = \mu DN$ (obtained by putting $X_{t+D} = X_t = X^*$ and similarly for Y). Writing $X_t = X^* + \zeta_t$ and $Y_t = Y^* + \xi_t$, and linearizing in the usual way, we obtain

$$\zeta_{t+D} = \zeta_t - \xi_{t+D},\tag{C.58}$$

$$\xi_{t+D} = \xi_t + (\mu R_0 D)\zeta_t.\tag{C.59}$$

The time-dependence in these linear equations can now be factored out as Λ^n, with $n = t/D$ being the number of steps from 0 to t. The eigenvalues Λ are consequently given by the quadratic equation

$$\Lambda^2 - 2(1 - \varepsilon)\Lambda + 1 = 0.\tag{C.60}$$

Here ε is defined as $\varepsilon = \tfrac{1}{2}\mu R_0 D = D/2A$; since the duration of infection, D, is typically a few days, while the average age at infection, A, is several years, we see that usually $\varepsilon \ll 1$.

The solution of eqn (C.60) is

$$\Lambda = (1 - \varepsilon) \pm i[1 - (1 - \varepsilon)^2]^{1/2}.\tag{C.61}$$

So long as $\varepsilon < 2$ (and we have just noted that usually $\varepsilon \ll 1$), Λ is a complex number, with modulus exactly unity. Indeed, we may rewrite eqn (C.61) as

$$\Lambda = \exp(i\omega D),\tag{C.62}$$

with ω defined as

$$\omega \equiv [\cos^{-1}(1 - \varepsilon)]/D.\tag{C.63}$$

That is to say the time dependence of the perturbations ζ_t and ξ_t is characterized by the behaviour of the function $\Lambda^{t/D} = \exp(i\omega t)$. The perturbations oscillate endlessly, showing no change in amplitude (corresponding to the eigenvalues lying exactly on the unit circle in the complex plane). The period of the oscillations is $T = 2\pi/\omega$; for $\varepsilon \ll 1$, eqn (C.63) gives $\omega \simeq (2\varepsilon)^{1/2}/D$, whence (given that $\varepsilon \equiv D/2A$) the oscillatory period is

$$T \simeq 2\pi(AD)^{1/2}. \tag{C.64}$$

This, of course, is the same result as was derived for the weakly damped oscillations in the continuous-time models.

Appendix D

Age-dependent transmission and WAIFW matrices

This appendix outlines the analysis underlying the results presented in Chapter 9. We begin by showing how the WAIFW matrix elements, β_{ij}, may be calculated from data about the age-specific force of infection, λ_i. We then show how to calculate the response of the system to a defined programme of immunization, and obtain a general expression for evaluating the critical coverage to achieve eradication of an infection which has age-specific transmission coefficients. The appendix ends by sketching the mathematical details of the new model, where transmission is concentrated within age cohorts, presented at the end of Chapter 9.

Throughout the appendix, much of the presentation is telegraphic, aimed at those who may be likely to retrace or extend our calculations.

Basic relationships, with age a continuous variable

Equation (9.5), which we repeat for ease of exposition, gives a relation between $\lambda(a, t)$ and $Y(a, t)$ once the age-specific transmission function $\beta(a, a')$ is specified

$$\lambda(a, t) = \int_0^\infty \beta(a, a') Y(a', t) \, da'. \tag{D.1}$$

As explained in the text, the set of partial differential equations (3.11)–(3.15) or (C.1)–(C.4) allows us to compute $Y(a, t)$ once $\lambda(a, t)$ is known; we can then use eqn (D.1) to compute the value of $\lambda(a, t)$ for the next time step, and thus compute the dynamical trajectories under any specified regime of changes (such as the introduction of an immunization programme). But, as emphasized in Chapter 9, the problem is that $\beta(a, a')$ is usually not known, and must be deduced from data about $\lambda(a)$ in the equilibrium state before any immunization.

The number of susceptible, latent, and infectious individuals of age a at this equilibrium ($X(a)$, $H(a)$, $Y(a)$, respectively) are found by dropping all time dependence in eqns (3.11)–(3.15) or (C.1)–(C.4), to get (see also eqns (4.3)–(4.5) or (4.44)–(4.48)):

$$dX/da = -(\lambda(a) + \mu(a))X(a), \tag{D.2}$$

$$dH/da = \lambda X - (\sigma + \mu(a))H(a), \tag{D.3}$$

$$dY/da = \sigma H - (v + \mu(a))Y(a). \tag{D.4}$$

These equations, which are linear if λ is treated as a parameter, can be integrated to get

$$X(a) = N(0)\ell(a) \exp(-\phi(a)), \tag{D.5}$$

$$H(a) = N(0)\ell(a) \int_0^a \lambda(a') \exp[-\sigma(a - a') - \phi(a')] \, da', \tag{D.6}$$

$$Y(a) = \sigma\ell(a) \int_0^a (H(a')/\ell(a')) \exp[-v(a - a')] \, da'. \tag{D.7}$$

Here, as always, $\ell(a) = \exp(-\int_0^a \mu(a') \, da')$, and $\phi(a)$ is defined as

$$\phi(a) = \int_0^a \lambda(a') \, da'. \tag{D.8}$$

We can now substitute eqn (D.7) for $Y(a)$ into eqn (D.1), to obtain an integral equation for $\lambda(a)$:

$$\lambda(a) = \sigma N(0) \int_0^\infty B(a, a') \lambda(a') \exp(-\phi(a')) \, da'. \tag{D.9}$$

Here $\phi(a)$ is given by eqn (D.8), and the kernel, $B(a, a')$, is defined as

$$B(a, a') = \int_t^\infty ds \int_{a'}^\infty dt \, \beta(a, s)\ell(s) \exp[-\sigma(t - a') - v(s - t)]. \tag{D.10}$$

Once the transmission function $\beta(a, a')$ and the parameters σ, v, $\mu(a)$, and $N(0)$ are specified, eqn (D.9) can be solved to find $\lambda(a)$, and thence the complete solution follows from eqns (D.5)–(D.7).

A useful approximation

The above programme of computation can often be simplified by noting that—for most childhood infections—the latent and infectious periods ($1/\sigma$ and $1/v$) are around a week or so, whereas the average age at infection ($A \simeq 1/\lambda$) is several years. If we use this biological fact to put $\sigma, v \gg \lambda$ in eqns (D.2)–(D.4), we obtain the approximate result given as eqn (9.8):

$$Y(a) \simeq \lambda(a)X(a)/v. \tag{D.11}$$

This result is obtained by evaluating the integrals in eqns (D.6) and (D.7) approximately, by noting that the functions $\ell(a')$ and $\phi(a')$ in general change more slowly than either $\sigma(a - a')$ or $v(a - a')$ in the exponents (provided $v, \sigma \gg \lambda$). For constant λ, in particular, it can be seen that the approximation of eqn (D.11) is correct up to terms of relative order λ/σ, λ/v, $\exp[-(\sigma - \lambda)a]$, and $\exp[-(v - \lambda)a]$; see May (1986).

With this approximation, the integral equation for $\lambda(a)$, eqn (D.9), takes the much simpler form

$$\lambda(a) = (N(0)/v) \int_0^\infty \beta(a, a')\lambda(a')\ell(a') \exp(-\phi(a')) \, \mathrm{d}a'. \tag{D.12}$$

Finite age classes: the β_{ij} matrix

In all practical applications, it makes sense to group individuals into some finite set of age classes, as discussed in Chapter 9. We define 'age class i' to include those individuals in the range of age from a_{i-1} to a_i: the force of infection is treated as a constant, λ_i, within an age class. We thus move from the above analysis of continuous functions to matrix algebra.

In what follows, we assume, for specificity, that survivorship is Type I: $\mu = 0$ for $a < L$, $\mu = \infty$ for $a > L$; $\ell(a) = 1$ for $a < L$, $\ell(a) = 0$ for $a > L$. This implies $N(0) = \bar{N}/L$, before any immunization. Extensions to any other functional form for $\mu(a)$ are straightforward, along the lines laid down below.

At equilibrium, eqn (D.5) now shows that the number of susceptibles of age a, in the age class i, is

$$X_i(a) = N(0) \exp[-\psi_{i-1} - \lambda_i(a - a_{i-1})]. \tag{D.13}$$

Here ψ_i is defined as the age-independent constant

$$\psi_i = \sum_{j=1}^{i} \lambda_j(a_j - a_{j-1}). \tag{D.14}$$

The index i runs over the n age classes, $i = 1, 2, \ldots, n$ (and $\psi_0 = 0$). The total number of susceptibles in the age class i, $\bar{X}_i$, is obtained directly by integrating eqn (D.13) to get

$$\bar{X}_i = N(0)[\exp(-\psi_{i-1}) - \exp(-\psi_i)]/\lambda_i. \tag{D.15}$$

The total number of infectives in the age class i is given by the approximate eqn (D.11) as

$$\bar{Y}_i \simeq \lambda_i \bar{X}_i/v. \tag{D.16}$$

Substituting eqns (D.15) and (D.16) into the basic eqn (D.1) for λ (now in matrix form), we arrive at an equation relating λ_i to the WAIFW matrix, β_{ij}, that is defined and discussed in Chapter 9:

$$\lambda_i = \sum_{j=1}^{n} \tilde{\beta}_{ij} \Psi_j. \tag{D.17}$$

Here we have, for notational convenience, defined Ψ_j as

$$\Psi_j \equiv \exp(-\psi_{j-1}) - \exp(-\psi_j), \tag{D.18}$$

and $\tilde{\beta}_{ij}$ is a constant multiple of β_{ij},

$$\tilde{\beta}_{ij} \equiv (\bar{N}/vL)\beta_{ij}. \tag{D.19}$$

If the elements of the WAIFW matrix, β_{ij}, were known, we could use eqn (D.17) to determine the λ_i, and all else would follow. As discussed more fully in Chapter 9, the more usual situation is that we know the set of n quantities λ_i before immunization (from serology or otherwise), and we seek to estimate β_{ij} from them. The special structures imposed on the WAIFW matrix in Chapter 9 are chosen so that β_{ij} has only n distinct elements, which can then indeed be estimated from the known, pre-immunization values of λ_i.

Specifically, once the n quantities λ_i have been found from data, we first calculate ψ_i from eqn (D.14), then calculate Ψ_j from eqn (D.18), and in this way compute the n distinct elements of β_{ij} from eqn (D.17).

Some other relevant quantities are computed as follows.

The total fraction of the population remaining susceptible, at equilibrium, is given by $x = \sum_i \bar{X}_i/\bar{N}$, which reduces to

$$x = \sum_{i=1}^{n} \Psi_i/\lambda_i L. \tag{D.20}$$

The average age at infection, A, is given by eqn (4.27). Substituting eqn (D.13) for $X_i(a)$ into this definition, and performing the integrals, we arrive at the result

$$A = \sum_{i=1}^{n} [(1 + \lambda_i a_{i-1}) \exp(-\psi_{i-1}) - (1 + \lambda_i a_i) \exp(-\psi_i)]/\{\lambda_i[1 - \exp(-\psi_n)]\}. \tag{D.21}$$

The age-specific value of the basic reproductive rate, $R_{0,i}$, for an infective in age class i, follows from the definition given by eqn (9.10), and is

$$R_{0,i} = \sum_{j=1}^{n} \tilde{\beta}_{ji}(a_j - a_{j-1}). \tag{D.22}$$

Equation (D.22) gives the explicit results in eqns (9.11) when there are only two age classes.

Criterion for eradication by immunization

Suppose a fraction p of each cohort is successfully immunized, essentially at birth. As discussed in Chapter 9, the new equilibrium (if it exists) under this programme can be evaluated along the above lines, with just two changes: the effective birth rate into the susceptible category is reduced from $N(0)$ to $N(0)(1 - p)$; and the force of infection has some new set of values, λ_i'.

The eradication criterion corresponds to the limit $\lambda_i' \to 0$ for all i. In this limit, the quantities Ψ_i of eqn (D.18) reduce to

$$\Psi_i \to \lambda_i'(a_i - a_{i-1}). \tag{D.23}$$

Thus, at the margin of eradication, eqn (D.17) for $\{\lambda_i'\}$ reduces to a set of n

simultaneous linear equations:

$$\lambda_i' = (1 - p) \sum_{j=1}^{n} \tilde{\beta}_{ij}(a_j - a_{j-1})\lambda_j'. \tag{D.24}$$

Here, $\tilde{\beta}_{ij}$ is a constant multiple of β_{ij}, as defined by eqn (D.19) (for Type I survivorship). These matrix elements will in general be evaluated from the pre-immunization forces of infection, λ_i, by the procedures just described. Equations (9.12) in Chapter 9 are a special case of eqn (D.24), when there are only two age classes.

The set of homogeneous eqns (D.24) will be satisfied if and only if

$$\det\|\tilde{\beta}_{ij}(a_j - a_{j-1})(1 - p) - \delta_{ij}\| = 0. \tag{D.25}$$

That is, the critical level of immunization, p_c, is given by

$$p_c = 1 - (1/\Lambda), \tag{D.26}$$

where Λ is the dominant eigenvalue of the matrix whose elements are $\tilde{\beta}_{ij}(a_j - a_{j-1})$.

Notice that essentially all the WAIFW matrices used in Chapter 9 are symmetric, $\beta_{ij} = \beta_{ji}$ ('WAIFW 3' is an exception). In this case, it can be seen from eqn (D.22) that if all $R_{0,i}$ are the same ($R_{0,i} = R_0 = $ constant), then $\Lambda = R_0$ and $p_c = 1 - (1/R_0)$; this is the familiar result for a homogeneously mixed population.

Notice also that, in the limit as $\lambda_i' \to 0$, the average age at infection, A, is given by the appropriate limiting form of eqn (D.21):

$$A = \left(\frac{1}{2} \sum_{i=1}^{n} (a_i^2 - a_{i-1}^2)\lambda_i'\right)\left(\sum_{i=1}^{n} (a_i - a_{i-1})\lambda_i'\right)^{-1}. \tag{D.27}$$

Here the λ_i' are computed from eqn (D.24); they are the eigenvectors of the matrix in eqn (D.25).

Suppose a fraction p are immunized not at birth, but at age b (where b lies in the age class k: $a_k > b > a_{k-1}$). The above analysis can be carried through, with appropriate modifications, to obtain the eradication criterion

$$\det\|\tilde{\beta}_{ij}\theta_j - \delta_{ij}\| = 0. \tag{D.28}$$

Here $\tilde{\beta}_{ij}$ is as defined by eqn (D.19), and the quantities θ_j are defined to be

$$\theta_j = a_j - a_{j-1} \qquad\qquad \text{if } j < k; \tag{D.29a}$$

$$\theta_j = (1 - p)(a_k - b) + (b - a_{k-1}) \qquad \text{if } j = k; \tag{D.29b}$$

$$\theta_j = (1 - p)(a_j - a_{j-1}) \qquad\qquad \text{if } j > k. \tag{D.29c}$$

Computation of the critical value of p is now straightforward. Other, more complex, age-dependent immunization schedules can clearly be evaluated by appropriate extensions of the above analysis.

The presence of maternal antibodies is one further complication that is relevant to detailed calculations. Such complications correspond to an additional age class, labelled '0', which cannot be infected and cannot transmit infection: $\beta(a, a') = 0$ if either a or $a' < D$, where maternal antibodies protect new-borns up to age D. These features can be included by defining the 'zeroth' age class, with $\beta_{0i} = \beta_{i0} = 0$, for all i. The calculations go forward as above, except now the entering age is D rather than zero; $a_0 = D$, and $\psi_1 = \lambda_1(a_1 - D)$ rather than $\psi_1 = \lambda_1 a_1$. Obviously the complications associated with maternal antibodies can be combined with immunization at age b (rather than zero). Some further discussion is in Anderson and May (1985a).

Analytic results for the simple model with transmission concentrated within cohorts

This section provides some mathematical details (including graphical solutions of eqns (9.29) and (9.32)) for the model in which the transmission coefficient, $\beta(a, a')$, is defined by eqn (9.14).

For the 'endemic equilibrium' situation, in the simple case when $g(a) = 1$, the fraction susceptible at age a, $x(a)$, is given by eqn (9.29), which we repeat here:

$$G(x) \equiv x \exp[R_a(1 - x)] = \exp(-\lambda_0 a). \qquad (D.30)$$

Here R_a is essentially the basic reproductive rate of the infection for within-cohort transmission; the 'endemic equilibrium' situation corresponds to $R_a < 1$. A pictorial way of understanding the solution of eqn (D.30), to get $x(a)$ as a smooth function of age a, is shown in Fig. D.1. This graphical analysis is straightforward, essentially because $R_a < 1$.

In contrast, for the 'mixed epidemic and endemic equilibrium' that arises when $R_a > 1$, the fraction susceptible at age a is given by eqn (9.32), which we also repeat here:

$$H(x) \equiv (R_a x) \exp(1 - R_a x) = \exp(-\lambda_0 a). \qquad (D.31)$$

Figure D.2 illustrates the solution of this equation; the picture is more complicated, essentially because $H(x)$ attains its maximum value for $x = 1/R_a < 1$. The result, as shown in Fig. D.2, is that x moves discontinuously (in fact, on the fast time-scale $1/v$) from its initial value $x(0) = 1$ to a 'post-mini-epidemic' value of $x(0+) = 1/R_a$. Thereafter the graphical solution is akin to that in Fig. D.1, and $x(a)$ decreases smoothly as age, a, increases (and $\exp(-\lambda_0 a)$ decreases).

As discussed in the text of Chapter 9, the above analysis is easily modified to take account of the more realistic circumstance where $g(a) = 1$ for $a_2 > a > a_1$, and $g(a) = 0$ otherwise (that is, the within-age-class component of transmission only operates within the age range a_1 to a_2).

The Epidemic Phase: To complete the analysis of the above system when $R_a > 1$, we return to eqn (9.21) to outline the dynamics of the epidemic in

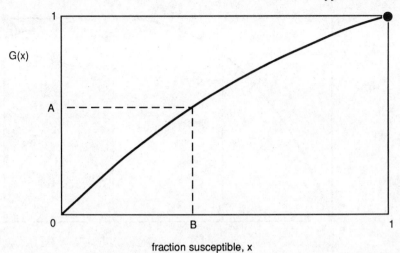

Fig. D.1. This figure illustrates the solution of eqn (D.30), for the case $R_a < 1$ (specifically, $R_a = 0.5$). The function $G(x) = x \exp[R_a(1 - x)]$ attains its maximum value for $x = 1/R_a > 1$, which is outside the meaningful range of x values. At age $a = 0$, we have $x = 1$ and $G(1) = 1$ as required by eqn (D.30). For finite a, $x(a)$ is given by the solution of $G(x) = \exp(-\lambda_0 a)$: if $\exp(-\lambda_0 a) = A$, then $x(a) = B$ can be found graphically as illustrated. Clearly $x(a)$ falls smoothly as age, a, increases (and $\exp(-\lambda_0 a)$ decreases).

age-class zero (and to justify the statement that these dynamics take place on the time-scale $1/v$).

As discussed in Chapter 9, the argument for discarding the left-hand side of eqn (9.21)—because $1/v$ is very small—breaks down if Ψ (as defined by eqn (9.19)) is changing very fast. Writing $d\Psi/da = \dot{\Psi}$, and using the identity $\ddot{\Psi} \equiv \dot{\Psi}(d\dot{\Psi}/d\Psi)$, we can rewrite eqn (9.21) as

$$(1/v)\dot{\Psi}(d\dot{\Psi}/d\Psi) = \dot{\Psi}(R_a e^{-\Psi} - 1) + \lambda_0. \tag{D.32}$$

If Ψ is changing so fast that terms of order $1/v$ cannot be neglected, then λ_0 can be disregarded, and eqn (D.32) reduces to

$$d\dot{\Psi} = v(R_a e^{-\Psi} - 1)\, d\Psi. \tag{D.33}$$

Performing the integration, with $\Psi(0) = 0$ and $\dot{\Psi}(0) = \lambda_0$, we arrive at

$$\dot{\Psi}(a) = \lambda_0 + v[R_a(1 - e^{-\Psi}) - \Psi]. \tag{D.34}$$

Recalling that $\Psi = -\ln x$ (from eqn (9.18), $x = e^{-\Psi}$), we can rewrite eqn (D.34) as

$$\int_{1/R_a}^{1} \frac{dx}{x[(\lambda_0/v) + R_a(1 - x) + \ln x]} = vT_f. \tag{D.35}$$

Here we have used the discussion in Chapter 9, or equivalently Fig. D.2, to

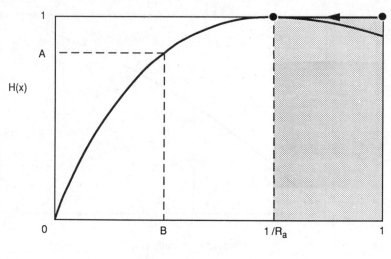

fraction susceptible, x

Fig. D.2. This figure illustrates the solution of eqn (D.31), for the case $R_a > 1$ (specifically, $R_a = 1.5$). The function $H(x) = R_a x \exp(1 - R_a x)$ attains its maximum value (which is $H(\max) = 1$) at $x = 1/R_a < 1$; in contrast with Fig. D.1, this x value is below the initial value of $x(0) = 1$. The solution of eqn (D.31) at age $a = 0$ is given by $H(x) = 1$. This solution is attained by x falling on the fast time-scale $(1/v)$ from $x = 1$ to $x = 1/R_a$. The nature of this 'singular perturbation' is discussed more fully in the text. After this initial discontinuity, the solution proceeds as in Fig. D.1, with $x(a)$ obtained from $H(x) = \exp(-\lambda_0 a)$: as in Fig. D.1, if $\exp(-\lambda_0 a) = A$ then $x(a) = B$ can be found graphically, as illustrated.

determine the value of x before $(x = 1)$ and after $(x = 1/R_a)$ the within-cohort epidemic. The duration of the epidemic is defined to be T_f. Equation (D.35) is related to standard results in the theory of epidemics (see Chapter 6 or Bailey (1975)): in general we have $\lambda_0/v \ll 1$, and thus $T_f \sim c/v$, where c is some constant of the order of $[\ln(v R_a/\lambda_0)]/R_a$.

Eradication Criterion. Finally, we evaluate the integral in eqn (9.40), to obtain the critical level of coverage, p_c, when $g(a) = 1$ for $a_2 > a > a_1$ and $g(a) = 0$ otherwise. That is, we generalize the result of eqn (9.41) to the case where within-cohort transmission is confined to the age range a_1 to a_2.

For this form of $g(a)$, the integral in eqn (9.40) has the value

$$L + (a_2 - a_1)R_a(1 - p_c)/[1 - R_a(1 - p_c)]. \qquad (D.36)$$

Substituting this expression into eqn (9.40) results in a quadratic equation for the quantity $1 - p_c$:

$$R_a R_b(1 - \varepsilon)(1 - p_c)^2 - (R_a + R_b)(1 - p_c) + 1 = 0. \qquad (D.37)$$

Here ε is defined as $\varepsilon = (a_2 - a_1)/L$. It follows that p_c is given by

$$p_c = 1 - \{(R_a + R_b) - [(R_a - R_b)^2 + 4\varepsilon R_a R_b]^{1/2}\}/[2R_a R_b(1 - \varepsilon)]. \quad \text{(D.38)}$$

This more general result reduces to eqn (9.41) in the limit $\varepsilon \to 1$ (which corresponds to $g(a) = 1$ for all a).

Appendix E

Aspects of heterogeneities in host–microparasite interactions

In this appendix, we derive various epidemiological results for populations that are genetically, culturally, behaviourally, geographically, or otherwise heterogeneous (in the specific sense that there are different categories of individuals, with β_{kl} representing the probability, per unit time, that an infective in class l will infect a susceptible in class k). We first derive expressions for the forces of infection, fraction susceptible, and other quantities, at equilibrium. Next, criteria for eradication of infection by immunization are obtained. Finally the dynamics of epidemics in such heterogeneous populations are explained. These analyses underpin results used in Chapters 9, 10, and 11.

Equilibrium results

Throughout this appendix, overbars are omitted, so that X_k and Y_k represent total numbers of susceptibles and infectives, respectively, in the kth class.

The equilibrium number of susceptibles in the kth class, X_k^*, is obtained from eqn (10.18) as

$$X_k^* = \mu N_k / (\mu + \lambda_k). \tag{E.1}$$

If we define f_k to be the fraction of the total population in the kth class, $f_k \equiv N_k/N$, we obtain eqn (10.21) for the overall fraction susceptible at equilibrium, simply by summing over all k in eqn (E.1). The corresponding equilibrium version of eqn (10.19) relates Y_k^* to X_k^*, which in combination with eqn (E.1) gives

$$Y_k^* = \mu N_k \lambda_k / [(\mu + v_k)(\mu + \lambda_k)]. \tag{E.2}$$

Substitution of eqn (E.2) into eqn (10.14) leads directly to eqn (10.22), which enables λ_k to be calculated once β_{kl} is specified.

The average age at infection, A, is given by the appropriate extension of the definition of eqn (4.27):

$$A = \left(\sum_k \int_0^\infty a \lambda_k X_k(a) \, \mathrm{d}a \right) \left(\sum_k \int_0^\infty \lambda_k X_k(a) \, \mathrm{d}a \right)^{-1}. \tag{E.3}$$

With the equilibrium solution for $X_k(a)$ given by eqn (10.15), and assuming Type II survivorship ($\mu = \text{constant}$), eqn (E.3) leads directly to eqn (10.23).

For infections such as gonorrhoea, where infectives recover directly back into the susceptible state, eqns (10.18) and (10.19) are replaced by (11.5) and (11.6), respectively. At equilibrium we now have

$$X_k^* = N_k(\mu + v_k)/(\mu + v_k + \lambda_k), \tag{E.4}$$

and

$$Y_k^* = \lambda_k N_k/(\mu + v_k + \lambda_k). \tag{E.5}$$

Substitution of eqn (E.5) into the basic eqn (10.14) that defines λ_k gives eqn (11.7).

Eradication criterion

If a fraction $p(k)$ of each cohort of new-borns in class k is immunized, the force of infection in the kth class will eventually settle to a new equilibrium value, λ_k', given by eqn (10.22) with N_k replaced by $N_k(1 - p(k))$:

$$\lambda_k' = \sum_{l=1}^{n} \left(\frac{\mu \beta_{kl} N_l(1 - p(l))}{\mu + v_l} \right) \left(\frac{\lambda_l'}{\mu + \lambda_l'} \right). \tag{E.6}$$

The eradication criterion is obtained as the limit when $\lambda_k' \to 0$ for all k. In this limit, eqn (E.6) reduces to

$$\sum_{l=1}^{n} [(1 - p_c(l)) \beta_{kl} N_l/(\mu + v_l) - \delta_{kl}] \lambda_l' = 0. \tag{E.7}$$

This set of n homogeneous, linear equations will have a consistent solution if, and only if, the determinant of the $n \times n$ matrix A_{kl} vanishes; A_{kl} is the matrix whose elements are given by the expression inside the square brackets in eqn (E.7). This establishes eqn (10.25) and (10.26) in the main text.

A useful result about a special class of matrices

The result $\det\|\mathbf{A}\| = 0$ can be put into a much simpler form whenever the coefficients of the transmission matrix can be factored, $\beta_{kl} = g_k h_l$. As discussed in Chapters 10, 11, and 12, there are many interesting situations where such factorization is biologically reasonable.

We begin by considering a case somewhat more general than the above A_{kl} with $\beta_{kl} = g_k h_l$, namely the matrix whose elements are

$$A_{kl} = a_k b_l - c_k \delta_{kl}. \tag{E.8}$$

That is, A_{kl} is obtained by multiplying a column vector $\{a_k\}$ by a row vector $\{b_l\}$, and then subtracting the diagonal matrix whose diagonal elements are $\{c_k\}$. In the equation $\det\|\mathbf{A}\| = 0$, we can now divide the kth row by a_k (for $k = 1$ to n) and the kth column by b_l (for $l = 1$ to n), to obtain the equivalent equation $\det\|\mathbf{B}\| = 0$; here the matrix $\mathbf{B}$ has elements

$$B_{kl} = 1 - \kappa_k \delta_{kl}, \tag{E.9}$$

with the definition $\kappa_k = c_k/a_k b_k$. This $n \times n$ determinant can now be expanded in powers of the κ terms. The product of all n diagonal κ terms gives $\prod_{k=1}^{n} (-\kappa_k)$. Omission of any one κ term gives n contributions of the form $[\prod_{k=1}^{n} (-\kappa_k)]/(-\kappa_1)]$. If two (or more) κ terms are omitted, we have 2×2 (or higher) minors where all elements are unity, giving zero. The result is that $\det\|\mathbf{A}\| = \det\|\mathbf{B}\| = 0$ leads to the relation

$$\left(\prod_{k=1}^{n} \kappa_k \right)\left(1 - \sum_{k=1}^{n} (1/\kappa_k) \right) = 0. \tag{E.10}$$

In the simple and general case when all $\kappa_k \equiv c_k/a_k b_k \neq 0$, eqn (E.10) gives

$$1 = \sum_{k=1}^{n} a_k b_k/c_k. \tag{E.11}$$

This result, eqn (E.11), has many useful applications, as we shall see throughout Chapters 9, 10, 11, and 12.

In particular, if $\beta_{kl} = g_k h_l$ in eqn (E.7), we have the situation of eqn (E.8) with $a_k = (1 - p_c(k))g_k N_k$, $b_l = h_l/(\mu + v_l)$, and $c_k = 1$. Substituting these expressions into eqn (E.11), we obtain eqn (10.30) for the eradication levels, $\{p_c(k)\}$. Equation (E.11) is employed in various contexts in Chapters 9–12, to simplify equations of the form $\det\|\mathbf{A}\| = 0$ when the matrix $\mathbf{A}$ obeys eqn (E.8).

Other applications of the formula (E.11) are found in Chapter 12, where it is used to derive both eqn (12.10) and eqn (12.19), as conditions for the vanishing of the determinants of two different matrices, both of which have the form given by eqn (E.8).

Epidemics in inhomogeneous populations: fraction ever infected

As discussed in Chapter 6, for infections where $v \gg \mu$ we may put $\mu \to 0$ in studying the dynamics of an epidemic. For an inhomogeneous population, the appropriate versions of eqns (10.18) and (10.19) are then

$$dX_k/dt = -\lambda_k X_k, \tag{E.12}$$

$$dY_k/dt = \lambda_k X_k - v_k Y_k. \tag{E.13}$$

As always, λ_k and Y_l are related by eqn (10.14), $\lambda_k = \sum_l \beta_{kl} Y_l$. We now generalize the Kermack–McKendrick (1927) results, to obtain an expression, eqns (10.31) and (10.32), for the fraction ever infected by such an epidemic in a closed population (that is, ignoring births and immigration).

First, we integrate eqn (E.12) (with the initial condition $X_k(0) = N_k$) to get

$$X_k(t) = N_k \exp(-\phi_k(t)). \tag{E.14}$$

Here ϕ_k is defined as

$$\phi_k(t) = \int_0^t \lambda_k(s)\, ds. \tag{E.15}$$

Second, we add eqns (E.12) and (E.13) and integrate, to get

$$X_k(t) + Y_k(t) = N_k - v_k \int_0^t Y_k(s)\, ds. \qquad (E.16)$$

In the limit $t \to \infty$ (the end of the epidemic), we have $Y_k \to 0$ and $X_k/N_k \to 1 - I_k$, where I_k is the overall fraction of the kth class to experience infection during the course of the epidemic. Thus, in this limit, eqn (E.16) gives

$$N_k I_k/v_k = \int_0^\infty Y_k(s)\, ds. \qquad (E.17)$$

Third, an integration over eqn (10.14) for λ_k gives the result

$$\phi_k(\infty) = \sum_{l=1}^n \beta_{kl} \int_0^\infty Y_l(s)\, ds. \qquad (E.18)$$

Combining eqns (E.17) and (E.18), we have

$$\phi_k(\infty) = \sum_{l=1}^n \beta_{kl} N_l I_l/v_l. \qquad (E.19)$$

Substituting from eqn (E.14), in the limit $t \to \infty$, for I_l, we arrive at

$$\phi_k(\infty) = \sum_{l=1}^n \beta_{kl}(N_l/v_l)[1 - \exp(-\phi_l(\infty))]. \qquad (E.20)$$

This represents a set of n non-linear equations for the n quantities $\phi_k(\infty)$. Once these quantities are found, the fractions ever infected in each class, I_k, and other epidemiologically interesting quantities are easily calculated.

In the commonly met case when $\beta_{kl} = g_k h_l$, eqn (E.20) takes a much simpler form. We see that the k dependence in $\phi_k(\infty)$ is contained solely in the factor g_k. We can therefore write

$$\phi_k(\infty) = g_k \alpha, \qquad (E.21)$$

and I_k obeys eqn (10.31), $I_k = 1 - \exp(-g_k \alpha)$. The constant α itself is found from the single eqn (10.32), which follows trivially from eqn (E.20) with eqn (E.21) for $\phi_k(\infty)$.

For the simple model for the transmission dynamics of HIV/AIDS in Chapter 11, eqns (11.31)–(11.36), we have in effect $\beta_{ij} = ij\beta/\sum_i iN_i$; see eqn (11.3). This transmission matrix has elements that factorize, and so the fraction in the ith class, I_i, is found by replacing g_i by $i\beta/\langle i \rangle N$ and h_j by j (and the constant α by $\alpha\langle i \rangle N/\beta$) in eqns (E.20) and (E.21) to get:

$$I_i = 1 - \exp(-i\alpha), \qquad (E.22)$$

with α determined by

$$\alpha = (\beta/v) \sum_i iN_i[1 - \exp(-i\alpha)] \Big/ \sum_i iN_i. \qquad (E.23)$$

Equation (E.22) is eqn (11.40), and eqn (E.23) leads directly to eqn (11.41) with R_0 defined by eqn (11.30).

More generally, we need to take account of deaths from AIDS, as such deaths deplete the pool of infectives and can have a pronounced effect on the probability that a given partner is infected ($\sum_i i Y_i / \sum_i i N_i$), particularly in the later stages of the epidemic. In Chapter 11, we have tended to move from analytic estimates to numerical computations once these, and other, complications are included. The above expressions for the fraction of the ith class ever to be infected, I_i, can, however, be further extended to the somewhat more realistic case where a fraction (possibly 100 per cent) of the infected individuals are removed by death. Specifically, suppose a fraction f of those infected die (at the rate v), while the remaining fraction, $1 - f$, move at the same rate into an uninfectious state; the number of individuals in the ith class then declines, $dN_i/dt = -fvY_i$. The asymptotic fraction to be infected in the ith class, I_i, again obeys eqn (10.40) or (E.22), but α is now given by the more general expression

$$\alpha = -(\beta/fv) \ln\left\{1 - f \sum_i iN_i[1 - \exp(-i\alpha)] \Big/ \sum_i iN_i\right\}. \tag{E.24}$$

This reduces to eqn (E.23), as it should, when $f \to 0$. This and other analytic results are derived and discussed in May and Anderson (1988).

Epidemics in inhomogeneous populations: early exponential growth rates

As explained in Chapters 6 and 11, in the early stages of the epidemic most individuals are still susceptible, and a linearized approximation is obtained by putting $X_k \simeq N_k$ in eqn (E.13). Factoring out the time dependence as $\exp \Lambda t$, in the usual way, we obtain from eqn (E.13) the relation

$$(\Lambda + v_k)Y_k \simeq \lambda_k N_k. \tag{E.25}$$

Substituting eqn (E.25) into the basic eqn (10.14) for λ_k, we obtain the set of n linear equations

$$\lambda_k = \sum_{l=1}^{n} \left(\frac{\beta_{kl} N_l}{\Lambda + v_l}\right)\lambda_l. \tag{E.26}$$

This is equivalent to eqn (10.33); the set of equations has a consistent solution if, and only if, the appropriate determinant vanishes:

$$\det\| \beta_{kl} N_l - (\Lambda + v_l)\delta_{kl}\| = 0. \tag{E.27}$$

This is eqn (10.34) of the main text.

If β_{kl} factorizes, $\beta_{kl} = g_k h_l$, then the matrix in eqn (E.27) is of the form defined in eqn (E.8), and the determinantal equation (E.27) reduces to the simpler form given by eqn (E.11)

$$\sum_{k=1}^{n} \frac{g_k h_k N_k}{\Lambda + v_k} = 1. \tag{E.28}$$

This is eqn (10.35), and—with appropriate definitions for $g_k h_k$ ($=\beta_{kk}$)—eqn (11.28).

Appendix F

Behavioural heterogeneity and the transmission dynamics of HIV/AIDS and other STDs

This appendix establishes a miscellany of analytic results, all pertaining to the dynamical behaviour of relatively realistic models for the transmission of HIV/AIDS, as discussed in Chapter 11.

Variability in levels of sexual activity characterized by a gamma distribution

Most of the numerical results presented in Chapter 11 were derived using a gamma distribution, eqn (11.42), to describe the variability in rates of acquiring new sexual partners, within the population being studied. As defined by eqns (11.42) and (11.43), this distribution is characterized by the mean rate of acquiring partners, $\langle i \rangle = m$, and by a parameter k that essentially measures the range of behaviour found in the population, $(CV)^2 = [\langle i^2 \rangle - \langle i \rangle^2]/\langle i \rangle^2 = 1/k$; also notice that the epidemiologically relevant rate of acquiring new partners, eqn (11.9) or (11.39), is $c = m(k + 1)/k$. Here the 'angular brackets' represent averages over the distribution: in general, $\langle F(i) \rangle \equiv \sum_i F(i)P(i)$ or $\int F(i)P(i)\,di$.

The overall fraction of the population to be infected during the course of the epidemic is now $I = \langle I_i \rangle$, where I_i is given by eqn (11.40) and the average is over the gamma distribution of eqn (11.42). We thus have

$$I = (k^k/m^k\Gamma(k)) \int_0^\infty i^{k-1} \exp(-ikm)[1 - \exp(-i\alpha)]\,di. \tag{F.1}$$

Here α is defined by eqn (11.41). Evaluating the integral in eqn (F.1) we have

$$I = 1 - \left(\frac{k/m}{\alpha + k/m}\right)^k. \tag{F.2}$$

Alternatively, we may define $\theta \equiv m\alpha/k$, to get eqn (11.44) for I. With θ, thus defined, replacing α in eqn (11.41) we have

$$\theta = (mR_0/k)\langle i[1 - \exp(-ik\theta/m)]\rangle/\langle i^2 \rangle. \tag{F.3}$$

Evaluating these averages over the above gamma distribution, we arrive at

$$\theta = [R_0/(1 + k)][1 - (1 + \theta)^{-k-1}]. \tag{F.4}$$

This is equivalent to eqn (11.45) for θ, as set out in Chapter 11.

We conclude this subsection by giving some analytic results for the dynamical behaviour of the model for HIV/AIDS transmission (in a behaviourally heterogeneous population) that is defined by eqns (11.31)–(11.36). We simplify somewhat by assuming $v_1 = v_2$, $\beta_1 = \beta_2$, and $\alpha \to \infty$. This corresponds to the assumption that all infected individuals are equally infectious, and that all move out of the infectious class at the same rate; a fraction f, however, then develop AIDS and are thereby assumed to be effectively removed from the population, while the remaining fraction, $1-f$, are assumed to continue being sexually active (asymptomatically infected and no longer infectious; an increasing amount of evidence suggests that, in fact, it may be that $f \simeq 1$). In these circumstances, eqns (11.31)–(11.36) take the somewhat simpler form

$$dX_i/dt = -i\lambda X_i, \tag{F.5}$$

$$dY_i/dt = i\lambda X_i - vY_i, \tag{F.6}$$

$$dN_i/dt = -fvY_i. \tag{F.7}$$

We have further assumed that deaths from causes other than AIDS can be neglected on the time-scales of interest for the epidemic ($\mu \to 0$), as can inputs of new susceptibles ($B_i \to 0$). The force of infection, per contact, is given by eqn (11.37), which reduces to

$$\lambda = \beta \sum_i iY_i \left(\sum_i iN_i \right)^{-1}. \tag{F.8}$$

As discussed more fully by May and Anderson (1988), studies of the dynamics of this set of equations are facilitated by defining the quantity $\phi(t)$:

$$\phi(t) = \int_0^t \lambda(s)\,ds. \tag{F.9}$$

Equation (F.5) can be integrated directly to get

$$X_i(t) = NP(i)\exp(-i\phi(t)). \tag{F.10}$$

Here $P(i)$ is the proportion of the population in the ith class of sexual activity. Substituting from eqn (F.7) for Y_i into the right-hand side of eqn (F.8), and integrating over time, we get the useful result

$$\sum_i iN_i(t) = \left(\sum_i iNP(i) \right) \exp(-fv\phi/\beta). \tag{F.11}$$

Now, we add eqns (F.5), (F.6), and $1/f$ times (F.7) to get

$$d(X_i + Y_i - N_i/f)dt = 0. \tag{F.12}$$

Integrating this to get an expression for $Y_i(t)$, and then multiplying by i and summing over all i, we arrive at the expression

$$\sum_i iY_i(t) = -N\langle i \rangle(1-f)/f + \sum_i iN_i(t)/f - \sum_i iX_i(t). \tag{F.13}$$

Finally, we can use eqn (F.10) for $X_i(t)$ and eqn (F.11) for $\sum_i iN_i(t)$, along with eqn (F.8) for $\lambda(t)$ and the definition (F.9)—which says $\lambda(t) = \mathrm{d}\phi/\mathrm{d}t$—to get a first-order differential equation for $\phi(t)$:

$$\mathrm{d}\phi/\mathrm{d}t = (\beta/f)[1 - \exp(fv\phi/\beta)] +$$
$$\beta \exp(fv\phi/\beta)\{\langle i[1 - \exp(-i\phi)]\rangle/\langle i\rangle\} + \lambda(0). \quad \text{(F.14)}$$

Here $\lambda(0)$ is the initial, 'seed' value of the force of infection.

Equation (F.14) can now be routinely integrated by numerical methods, once the distribution in degrees of sexual activity is specified, and the parameters β, f, and v defined. Once $\phi(t)$ is calculated, all other epidemiologically interesting quantities (such as the fraction remaining susceptible, incidence of HIV infection and of AIDS cases, and so on) can be easily found. Obviously the basic set of differential equations (F.5)–(F.8) can be integrated directly for any specified distribution $\{P(i)\}$, but this can be a very elaborate computation (because the distribution changes as those in the more sexually active classes are differentially removed, as indicated by eqn (F.11) above).

For the specific choice of a gamma distribution for $\{P(i)\}$, as discussed above, eqn (F.14) takes the explicit form

$$(\mathrm{d}\psi/\mathrm{d}t) \exp(-f\psi/R_0)$$
$$= vR_0\{1 - [1 + \psi/(1 + k)]^{-k-1} - [1 - \exp(-f\psi/R_0)]/f\} + c\lambda(0). \quad \text{(F.15)}$$

Here $\psi(t) = c\phi(t) = [m(k + 1)/k]\phi(t)$. The dynamics are now fully determined by the epidemiological parameters R_0, v, and f, along with the parameter k that characterizes the CV of the gamma distribution. Explicit expressions for the fraction infected with HIV by time t, the incidence of AIDS, the total number of cases of AIDS up to time t, and so on, are derived and discussed in more detail by May and Anderson (1988).

Early, exponential growth rate when infectiousness and incubation period depend on time since infection

This subsection derives the 'dispersion relation', eqn (11.57), for the exponential rate, Λ, at which the epidemic grows in its initial stages (i.e. under the linearized approximation $X_i \simeq N_i$), for the time-dependent infectiousness and incubation defined by eqns (11.49)–(11.51).

Equation (11.49) is linear in Y_i, so we may make a Laplace transform to

$$\tilde{Y}_i(p, \tau) \equiv \int_0^\infty Y_i(t, \tau)\, \mathrm{e}^{-pt}\, \mathrm{d}t. \quad \text{(F.16)}$$

This gives (with μ, as usual, neglected)

$$(p + v(\tau))\tilde{Y}_i + \mathrm{d}\tilde{Y}_i/\mathrm{d}\tau = Y_i(0, \tau). \quad \text{(F.17)}$$

Here $Y_i(0, \tau)$ is some specified distribution of infectiousness at time $t = 0$. Equation (F.17) can now be integrated over τ, to get

$$\tilde{Y}_i(p, t) \exp\left(p\tau + \int_0^\tau v(s) \, ds \right) - \tilde{Y}_i(p, 0)$$

$$= \int_0^\tau Y_i(0, \tau') \exp\left(p\tau' + \int_0^{\tau'} v(s) \, ds \right) d\tau'. \quad \text{(F.18)}$$

Here $\tilde{Y}_i(p, 0)$ is the Laplace transform of the initial condition, eqn (11.50), which in its linearized approximation is $\tilde{Y}_i(p, 0) = iN_i\tilde{\lambda}(p)$. The Laplace transform $\tilde{\lambda}$ can be obtained from the linearized version of eqn (11.51), and is

$$\tilde{\lambda}(p) = \sum_i i \int_0^\infty \beta(\tau) \tilde{Y}_i(p, \tau) \, d\tau / \langle i \rangle N. \quad \text{(F.19)}$$

Substituting from eqn (F.18) for $\tilde{Y}_i(p, \tau)$ into eqn (F.19) for $\tilde{\lambda}(p)$, we get

$$\tilde{\lambda}(p) = \sum_i i \int_0^\infty \beta(\tau) \, d\tau (iN_i\tilde{\lambda}(p) + \mathscr{F}_i(p, \tau)) \exp(-\Psi(p, \tau)) / \langle i \rangle N. \quad \text{(F.20)}$$

Here $\mathscr{F}_i(p, \tau)$ is the quantity on the right-hand side of eqn (F.18), which depends only on specific quantities (such as the initial values, $Y_i(0, \tau)$, and the distribution of incubation times, related to $v(\tau)$), and $\Psi(p, \tau)$ is defined as

$$\Psi(p, \tau) \equiv p\tau + \int_0^\tau v(s) \, ds. \quad \text{(F.21)}$$

Rearranging eqn (F.20), and recalling the definition $c \equiv \langle i^2 \rangle / \langle i \rangle$, we have

$$\tilde{\lambda}(p) = G(p)\left(1 - c \int_0^\infty \beta(\tau) \exp(-\Psi(p, \tau)) \, d\tau \right)^{-1}. \quad \text{(F.22)}$$

Here $G(p)$ is the term involving $\mathscr{F}$ on the right-hand side of eqn (F.20), which depends only on specific initial conditions.

Inverting the Laplace transform, we have

$$\lambda(t) = (1/2\pi i) \oint \tilde{\lambda}(p) \, e^{pt} \, dp. \quad \text{(F.23)}$$

The time dependence will thus (apart from early transients) be dominated by $e^{\Lambda t}$, where Λ is the pole in the denominator of eqn (F.22) with the largest real part; that is, Λ is the dominant root of

$$1 - c \int_0^\infty \beta(\tau) \exp(-\Psi(\Lambda, \tau)) \, d\tau = 0. \quad \text{(F.24)}$$

Recalling the definition of Ψ, eqn (F.21), we thus have eqn (11.57).

A more detailed and more realistic discussion, with the infectiousness at time τ since first infection, $\beta(\tau, T)$, being conditionally dependent on the incubation period, T, is given elsewhere (May and Anderson 1988).

Early, exponential growth rate for the model defined by eqns (11.60)–(11.64)

In this subsection, we derive the cubic eqn (11.66) for the early rate of growth, Λ, of HIV infection in a model where the time-dependent course of infectiousness for any one infected individual is described by the flow-among-compartments model of eqns (11.60)–(11.64).

In the early stages, we may, as always, put $X_i \simeq N_i$, and factor out the time-dependence in the ensuing, linear equations as $\exp \Lambda t$. The set of equations (11.60)–(11.62) then give

$$\Lambda Y_1 = \lambda N - v_0 Y_1, \tag{F.25}$$

$$\Lambda Y_2 = v_0 Y_1 - s Y_2, \tag{F.26}$$

$$\Lambda Y_3 = s Y_2 - v_1 Y_3. \tag{F.27}$$

Here, as defined in Chapter 11, Y_1, Y_2, and Y_3 represent the number of individuals in the first phase of infectiousness, the intervening 'silent phase', and the second, AIDS, phase of infectiousness, respectively. Equations (F.25)–(F.27) can be solved to express Y_1 and Y_3 in terms of λ:

$$Y_1 = \lambda N/(v_0 + \Lambda), \tag{F.28}$$

$$Y_3 = \lambda v_0 s N/[(v_0 + \Lambda)(s + \Lambda)(v_1 + \Lambda)]. \tag{F.29}$$

Substituting these expressions into eqn (11.64) for λ, we find the growth rate, Λ, in this linearized approximation obeys the cubic equation

$$(v_0 + \Lambda)(s + \Lambda)(v_1 + \Lambda) = c\beta_0(s + \Lambda)(v_1 + \Lambda) + c\beta_1 v_0 s. \tag{F.30}$$

Some trivial rearrangements bring this to the form (11.66).

Numerical solutions of eqns (F.30) or (11.66) are given in Fig. 11.25. Some analytic insight can be obtained by observing that, if v_0 and v_1 are significantly greater than s (infectious periods shorter than the typical 'silent' period, as they may well be; the numerical example uses $v_0 = v_1 = 1 \text{ yr}^{-1}$ and $s = 1/6 \text{ yr}^{-1}$), then

$$\Lambda \simeq (c\beta_0 - v_0)(1 + O(\Delta)). \tag{F.31}$$

Here the correction terms are of order $\Delta = (c\beta_1)sv_0/[(c\beta_0 - v_0)^2(c\beta_0 - v_0 + v_1)]$. In essentials, the initial growth rate will be determined mainly by the first episode of infectiousness, unless β_1/β_0 is sufficiently large to compensate for the relative smallness of s. The biological implications are discussed more fully in Chapter 11.

Appendix G

Optimal immunization programmes in heterogeneous populations

In this appendix, we outline the solution of the constrained optimization problem of Chapter 12, leading to eqn (12.20) for the optimum fraction remaining unimmunized in the ith group. A fuller discussion is given in May and Anderson (1984).

If we define $s_i \equiv q_i f_i$, then the problem is to maximize

$$Q \equiv \sum_i s_i, \tag{G.1}$$

subject to the constraint

$$1 - \sum_i \varepsilon \rho s_i / [1 - (1-\varepsilon)\rho s_i] = 0. \tag{G.2}$$

The problem itself, and the various symbols, are as defined in Chapter 12. There is an additional set of constraints, $f_i \geqslant s_i \geqslant 0$, which derive from the obvious requirement that $1 \geqslant q_i \geqslant 0$.

This problem can be solved by using Lagrange multipliers. For each i, we require

$$\partial Q/\partial s_i + \gamma \, \partial F/\partial s_i = 0. \tag{G.3}$$

Here γ is a Lagrange multiplier, and $F(s_1, s_2, \ldots, s_n)$ is the function defined by the left-hand-side of eqn (G.2). Using eqns (G.1) and (G.2) in eqn (G.3), we get

$$1 - \gamma \varepsilon \rho [1 - (1 - \varepsilon)\rho s_i]^{-2} = 0. \tag{G.4}$$

That is, choosing the positive square root so that eqn (G.2) may subsequently be satisfied, we get

$$s_i = [1 - (\gamma \varepsilon \rho)^{1/2}]/[1 - \varepsilon]. \tag{G.5}$$

Finally, the Lagrange multiplier, γ, may be determined by substituting the s_i values of eqn (G.5) into the constraining eqn (G.2), to get

$$(\gamma \varepsilon \rho)^{1/2} = n\varepsilon/(1 - \varepsilon + n\varepsilon). \tag{G.6}$$

We thus arrive at the result for the value of s_i ($\equiv q_i f_i$) that maximizes Q subject to the constraint of eqn (G.2):

$$s_i = 1/[\rho(1 - \varepsilon + n\varepsilon)]. \tag{G.7}$$

This is the result, eqn (12.20), that is discussed in the text. Problems that arise when the s_i of eqn (G.7) exceeds f_i are dealt with briefly in Chapter 12 (see Fig. 12.4), and more fully in May and Anderson (1984).

Appendix H

Mating probabilities and egg output for macroparasites

Here we indicate how to calculate the average egg output per female macroparasite, as discussed in Chapter 16, allowing both for density dependences in egg output and for mating effects.

Suppose $p(n)$ is the probability to find a total of n worms in a given host, and that $\Pi(j; n)$ is the probability to find j mated female worms given that n worms are present in total. May (1977a) has given expressions for $\Pi(j)$, under various assumptions about the worms' sexual habits (and allowing for male and female worms to be distributed jointly or separately). Suppose further that the egg output per mated female worm is $\lambda(n)$ when a total of n worms is present. The quantity λ could alternatively depend only on the number of females, or of mated females; the consequent calculations are variations on that below.

Under these assumptions, the average egg output from any one host is

$$\langle \text{egg output} \rangle = \sum_{n=o}^{\infty} \sum_{j=0}^{n} j\lambda(n)p(n)\Pi(j; n). \tag{H.1}$$

This is the probability to have n worms, $p(n)$, of which j are mated females, $\Pi(j; n)$—thus producing $j\lambda(n)$ eggs—summed over all n and j.

Now let us be more specific and assume $\lambda(n)$ to have the form of eqn (16.14). If the worms are promiscuous, we may further assume *all* females are mated so long as at least one male is present. But for a 1:1 sex ratio, the probability to have j female worms in a host with a total of n worms is $[n!/j!(n-j)!]2^{-n}$; this, then, is the expression for $\Pi(j; n)$ so long as $j < n$. For $j = n$, there can be no male worms, and so $\Pi(n; n) = 0$. Substituting all this into eqn (H.1), we get the specific expression

$$\langle \text{egg output} \rangle = \lambda_0 \sum_{n=0}^{\infty} 2^{-n}z^{n-1}p(n) \sum_{j=0}^{n-1} jn!/j!(n-j)!. \tag{H.2}$$

Here, as usual, $z \equiv \exp(-\gamma)$. When the summation over j is performed, this equation simplifies to

$$\langle \text{egg output} \rangle = \tfrac{1}{2}\lambda_0 \sum_{n=o}^{\infty} nz^{n-1}p(n)(1 - 2^{-n+1}). \tag{H.3}$$

Finally, we assume that male and female worms are distributed jointly in a negative binomial (with mean worm burden M and clumping parameter k), whereupon the summation in eqn (H.3) can be performed by differentiating the probability generating function:

$$\langle \text{egg output} \rangle =$$
$$\tfrac{1}{2}\lambda_0 M\{[1 + M(1-z)/k]^{-k-1} - [1 + M(1 - z/2)/k]^{-k-1}\}. \tag{H.4}$$

The average egg output per worm is thus $\frac{1}{2}\lambda_0$ times the factor in the curly brackets, which is the $\mathscr{F}(M)$ of eqns (16.21) and (16.22). The combination $\frac{1}{2}\lambda_0$ is absorbed in the definition of R_0 in eqn (16.19), with here $s = \frac{1}{2}$ (as usually will be the case). Obviously other formulae can be obtained along these lines, for other assumptions about how the worms are distributed, how they mate, and how egg output depends on density.

We conclude this appendix by indicating how eqn (H.4) may be used, in conjunction with the equilibrium relation $R_0\mathscr{F}(M^*) = 1$, to calculate the maximum value of the 'breakpoint' worm burden, $M_B(\max)$, that is illustrated in Fig. 16.4. From Fig. 16.3 and the accompanying discussion in Chapter 16, we see that the equilibrium relation $R_0\mathscr{F}(M^*) = 1$ will produce two solutions for M^* if R_0 is above the threshold value, and no solution if R_0 is below threshold. The maximum breakpoint density, $M_B(\max)$, therefore occurs at the point where $\mathscr{F}(M)$ is stationary:

$$\mathrm{d}\mathscr{F}/\mathrm{d}M = 0 \qquad \text{for } M = M_B(\max). \tag{H.5}$$

If $\mathscr{F}(M)$ is given by the factor in curly brackets in eqn (H.4), then eqn (H.5) leads to the result

$$M_B(\max) = \frac{k}{1-z}\left\{\left(\frac{z}{2-z}\right)\left[1 - \left(\frac{1-z}{1-z/2}\right)^{(k+1)/(k+2)}\right]^{-1} - 1\right\}. \tag{H.6}$$

This is the relation between $M_B(\max)$ and k that is illustrated in Fig. 16.4.

References

References with more than six authors are listed according to the names of the first three authors *et al.*

Aaby, P., Bukh, J., Lisse, I. M., and Smits, A. J. (1981). Measles vaccination and child mortality. *The Lancet*, **ii**, 93–4.

Aaby, P., Bukh, J., Lisse, I. M., and Smits, A. J. (1983). Measles mortality, state of nutrition and family structure: A community study from Guinea-Bissau. *J. Infect. Dis.*, **147**, 693–701.

Abbey, H. (1952). An examination of the Reed–Frost theory of epidemics. *Hum. Biol.*, **24**, 201–33.

Abdel-Wahab, M. F., Strickland, G. T., El Sahly, A., Ahmed, L., Zakaria, S., El Kady, N., and Mahmoud, S. (1980). *Schistosomiasis mansoni* in an Egyptian village in the Nile Delta. *Am. J. Trop. Med. Hyg.*, **29**, 868–74.

Abramowitz, M. and Stegun, I. A. (1964). *Handbook of mathematical functions*. Dover Publications, New York.

Abramson, P. R. and Rothschild, B. (1988). Sex, drugs and matrices: mathematical prediction of HIV infection. *J. Sex. Res.*, **25**, 106–22.

Acsadi, G. Y. and Nemeskeri, J. (1970). *History of human life span and mortality*. Ackademiai Kiado, Budapest.

Agadzi, V. K., Boatin, B. A., Appawa, M. A., Mingle, J. A. A., and Addy, P. A. (1984). Yellow fever in Ghana, 1977–80. *Bull. World Health Org.*, **62**, 577–83.

Albert, J. (1988). HIV isolation and antigen detection in infected individuals and their seronegative sexual partners. *AIDS*, **2**, 107–12.

Albrecht, P., Ennis, F. A., Saltzmann, E. J., and Krugman, S. (1977). Persistence of maternal antibody in infants beyond 12 months. Mechanisms of measles vaccine failure. *J. Paediatr.*, **91**, 715–18.

Allison, A. C. (1964). Polymorphism and natural selection in human populations. *Cold Spring Harbor Symp. Quant. Biol.*, **29**, 137–49.

Allison, A. C. (1982). Coevolution between hosts and infectious disease agents, and its effects on virulence. In *Population biology of infectious diseases*, (ed. R. M. Anderson and R. M. May), pp. 245–68. Springer-Verlag, New York.

Anderson, M. J., Higgins, P. J., Davis, L. R., *et al.* (1985). Experimental parvoviral infection in humans. *J. Infect. Dis.*, **56**, 257–65.

Anderson, R. M. (1974). Mathematical models of host–helminth parasite interactions. In *Ecological stability*, (ed. M. B. Usher and M. H. Williamson), pp. 43–70. Chapman and Hall, London.

Anderson, R. M. (1978a). Population dynamics of snail infection by miracidia. *Parasitology*, **77**, 201–24.

Anderson, R. M. (1978b). The regulation of host population growth by parasite species. *Parasitology*, **76**, 119–58.

Anderson, R. M. (1979). The influence of parasite infection on the dynamics of host population growth. In *Population dynamics*, (ed. R. M. Anderson, B. D. Turner, and L. R. Taylor), pp. 245–81. Blackwell, Oxford.

Anderson, R. M. (1980). The dynamics and control of direct life cycle helminth parasites. *Lect. Notes Biomath.*, **39**, 278–322.

Anderson, R. M. (1981a). The population dynamics of indirectly transmitted diseases: the vector component. In *Vectors of disease agents: interactions with plants, animals, and man*, (ed. J. J. McKelvey and B. E. Eldridge), pp. 13–43. Praeger, New York.

Anderson, R. M. (1981b). Population ecology of infectious disease agents. In *Theoretical ecology*, (ed. R. M. May), pp. 318–55. Blackwell Scientific, Oxford.

Anderson, R. M. (1982*a*). Epidemiology. In *Modern parasitology*, (ed. F. E. G. Cox), pp. 204–51. Blackwell, Oxford.

Anderson, R. M. (1982*b*). Transmission dynamics and control of infectious disease agents. In *Population biology of infectious diseases*, (ed. R. M. Anderson and R. M. May), pp. 149–76. Springer, Berlin.

Anderson, R. M. (1982*c*). Processes influencing the distribution of parasite numbers within host populations with special emphasis on parasite-induced host mortalities. *Parasitology*, **85**, 373–98.

Anderson, R. M. (ed.) (1982*d*). *Population dynamics of infectious diseases: theory and applications*. Chapman and Hall, London.

Anderson, R. M. (1985). Mathematical models in the study of the epidemiology and control of ascariasis in man. In *Ascariasis and its public health significance*, (ed. D. W. T. Crompton, M. C. Nesheim, and Z. S. Powlowski), pp. 39–68. Taylor and Francis, London.

Anderson, R. M. (1986). The population dynamics and epidemiology of intestinal nematode infections. *Trans. R. Soc. Trop. Med. Hyg.*, **80**, 686–96.

Anderson, R. M. (1987). Determinants of infection in human schistosomiasis. In *Baillière's clinical tropical medicine and communicable disease* (2nd edn), (ed. A. F. Mahmoud), pp. 279–300. Baillière Tindall, London.

Anderson, R. M. (1988*a*). The epidemiology of HIV infection: variable incubation plus infectious periods and heterogeneity in sexual activity. *J. R. Stat. Soc.*, **A1S1**, 66–98.

Anderson, R. M. (1988*b*). The role of mathematical models in the study of HIV transmission and the epidemiology of AIDS. *J. AIDS*, **1**, 241–56.

Anderson, R. M. (1989). Mathematical and statistical studies of the epidemiology of HIV. *AIDS*, **3**, 333–46.

Anderson, R. M. (1991). Populations and infectious diseases: ecology or epidemiology? *J. Anim. Ecol.* (In press.)

Anderson, R. M. and Crombie, J. (1984). Experimental studies of age prevalence curves for *Schistosoma mansoni* infections in populations of *Biomphalaria glabrata*. *Parasitology*, **89**, 79–105.

Anderson, R. M. and Crombie, J. A. (1985). Experimental studies of age–intensity and age–prevalence profiles of infection: *Schistosoma mansoni* in snails and mice. In *Ecology and genetics of host–parasite interactions*, (ed. D. Rollinson and R. M. Anderson), pp. 111–46. Academic Press, London.

Anderson, R. M. and Gordon, D. M. (1982). Processes influencing the distribution of parasite numbers within host populations with special emphasis on parasite-induced host mortalities. *Parasitology*, **85**, 373–98.

Anderson, R. M. and Grenfell, B. T. (1986). Quantitative investigation of different vaccination policies for the control of congenital rubella syndrome (CRS) in the U.K. *J. Hyg. Camb.*, **96**, 305–33.

Anderson, R. M. and Johnson, A. M. (1990). Rates of sexual partner change in homosexual and heterosexual populations in the United Kingdom. In *Kinsey Institute conference on sexual behaviour in relation to AIDS*, (ed. B. Voller). Oxford University Press, New York.

Anderson, R. M. and May, R. M. (1978). Regulation and stability of host–parasite population interactions. I. Regulatory processes. *J. Anim. Ecol.*, **47**, 219–47.

Anderson, R. M. and May, R. M. (1979*a*). Prevalence of schistosome infections within molluscan populations: observed patterns and theoretical predictions. *Parasitology*, **79**, 63–94.

Anderson, R. M. and May, R. M. (1979*b*). Population biology of infectious diseases: Part 1. *Nature*, **280**, 361–7.

Anderson, R. M. and May, R. M. (1981). The population dynamics of microparasites and their invertebrate hosts. *Phil. Trans. R. Soc.*, **291**, 451–524.

Anderson, R. M. and May, R. M. (1982*a*). The control of communicable diseases by age-specific immunization schedules. *The Lancet*, **i**, 160.

Anderson, R. M. and May, R. M. (1982*b*). The logic of vaccination. *New Sci.*, **96**, 410–15.

Anderson, R. M. and May, R. M. (1982*c*). Population dynamics of human helminth infections: control by chemotherapy. *Nature*, **297**, 557–63.

Anderson, R. M. and May, R. M. (1982*d*). Directly transmitted infectious diseases: control by vaccination. *Science*, **215**, 1053–60.

Anderson, R. M. and May, R. M. (1982*e*). Coevolution of hosts and parasites. *Parasitology*, **85**, 411–26.

Anderson, R. M. and May, R. M. (1983*a*). Vaccination against rubella and measles: quantitative investigations of different policies. *J. Hyg. Camb.*, **90**, 259–325.

Anderson, R. M. and May, R. M. (1983*b*). Two-stage vaccination programme against rubella. *The Lancet*, **iii**, 1416–17.

Anderson, R. M. and May, R. M. (1984). Spatial, temporal and genetic heterogeneity in host populations and the design of immunisation programmes. *IMA J. Math. Appl. Med. Biol.*, **1**, 233–66.

Anderson, R. M. and May, R. M. (1985*a*). Age-related changes in the rate of disease transmission: implications for the design of vaccination programmes. *J. Hyg. Camb.*, **94**, 365–436.

Anderson, R. M. and May, R. M. (1985*b*). Helminth infections of humans: mathematical models, population dynamics and control. *Adv. Parasitol.*, **24**, 1–101.

Anderson, R. M. and May, R. M. (1985*c*). Vaccination and herd immunity to infectious disease. *Nature*, **318**, 323–9.

Anderson, R. M. and May, R. M. (1985*d*). Herd immunity to helminth infection and implications for parasite control. *Nature*, **315**, 493–6.

Anderson, R. M. and May, R. M. (1986). The invasion, persistence and spread of infectious diseases within animal and plant communities. *Phil. Trans. R. Soc.*, **B314**, 533–70.

Anderson, R. M. and May, R. M. (1987). Directly transmitted infectious diseases: control by vaccination. *Science*, **215**, 1053–60.

Anderson, R. M. and May, R. M. (1988*a*). Epidemiological parameters of HIV transmission. *Nature*, **333**, 514–22.

Anderson, R. M. and May, R. M. (1988*b*). Complex dynamical behaviour in the interaction between HIV and the immune system. In *Cell to cell signalling*, (ed. A. Goldbeter), pp. 335–49. Academic Press, London.

Anderson, R. M. and Medley, G. F. (1985). Community control of helminth infections of man by mass and selective chemotherapy. *Parasitology*, **90**, 629–60.

Anderson, R. M. and Medley, G. F. (1988). Epidemiology of HIV infection and AIDS: incubation and infectious periods, survival and vertical transmission. *AIDS*, **2**, 857–64.

Anderson, R. M. and Schad, G. A. (1985). Hookworm burdens and faecal egg counts: an analysis of the biological basis of vaccination. *Trans. R. Soc. Trop. Med. Hyg.*, **79**, 812–25.

Anderson, R. M., Mercer, J. G., Wilson, R. A., and Carter, N. P. (1982). Transmission of *Schistosoma mansoni* from man to snail: experimental studies of miracidial survival and infectivity in relation to larval age, water temperature, host size and host age. *Parasitology*, **85**, 339–60.

Anderson, R. M., Grenfell, B. T., and May, R. M. (1984). Oscillatory fluctuations in the incidence of infectious disease and the impact of vaccination: time series analysis. *J. Hyg. Camb.*, **93**, 587–608.

Anderson, R. M., May, R. M., Medley, G. F., and Johnson, A. (1986). A preliminary study of the transmission dynamics of the human immunodeficiency virus (HIV), the causative agent of AIDS. *IMA J. Math. Appl. Med. Biol.*, **3**, 229–63.

Anderson, R. M., Crombie, J. A., and Grenfell, B. T. (1987a). The epidemiology of mumps in the U.K.: a preliminary study of virus transmission, herd immunity and the potential impact of immunisation. *Epidemiol. Infect.*, **99**, 65–84.

Anderson, R. M., Medley, G. F., Blythe, S. P., and Johnson, A. M. (1987b). Is it possible to predict the minimum size of the acquired immunodeficiency syndrome (AIDS) epidemic in the United Kingdom? *The Lancet*, **I**, 1073–6.

Anderson, R. M., May, R. M., and McLean, A. R. (1988a). Possible demographic consequences of AIDS in developing countries. *Nature*, **332**, 228–34.

Anderson, R. M., Gupta, S., and Ng, W. (1989a). The significance of sexual partner contact networks for the transmission dynamics of HIV. *J. AIDS*, **3**, 417–429.

Anderson, R. M., Ng, T. W., Boily, M.-C., and May, R. M. (1989b). The influence of different sexual-contact patterns between age classes on the predicted demographic impact of AIDS in developing countries. *Ann. N.Y. Acad. Sci.*, **569**, 240–74.

Anderson, R. M., May, R. M., and Ng, T. W. (1990). Age dependent choice of sexual partners and the transmission dynamics of HIV. *Phil. Trans. R. Soc.* (In press.)

Andreasen, V. (1989). Multiple time scales in the dynamics of infectious diseases. *Lect. Notes Biomath.*, **81**, 142–51.

APCO (1980). *Collected papers on the control of soil-transmitted helminthiases*. Asian Parasite Control Organisation, Tokyo.

APCO (1983). *Collected papers on the control of soil-transmitted helminthiases* (2nd edn). Asian Parasite Control Organisation, Tokyo.

Arita, I., Wickett, J., and Fenner, F. (1986). Impact of population density on immunization programmes. *J. Hyg.*, **96**, 459–66.

Armelagos, G. J. and McArdle, A. (1975). Population, disease and evolution. In *Population studies in archaeology and biological anthropology*, (ed. A. C. Swedlund), pp. 1–10. American Antiquity, Memoire 30.

Armstrong, J. C. (1978). Susceptibility to vivax malaria in Ethiopia. *Trans. R. Soc. Trop. Med. Hyg.*, **72**, 342–4.

Aron, J. L. (1982). Malaria epidemiology and detectability. *Trans. R. Soc. Trop. Med. Hyg.*, **76**, 595–601.

Aron, J. L. (1983). The dynamics of immunity boosted by exposure to infection. *Math. Biosci.*, **64**, 249–59

Aron, J. L. and May, R. M. (1982). The population dynamics of malaria. In *Population dynamics of infectious diseases*, (ed. R. M. Anderson), pp. 139–79. Chapman and Hall, London.

Aron, J. L. and Schwartz, I. B. (1984). Seasonality and period-doubling bifurcation in an epidemic model. *J. Theor. Biol.*, **100**, 665–79.

Bach, F., Bonourda, B., and Vitetta, E. (ed.) (1979). *T and B lymphocytes: recognition and function*. Academic Press, New York.

Bailey, N. J. T. (1956). On estimating the latent and infectious periods of measles. 1. Families with two susceptibles only. *Biometrika*, **43**, 15–22.

Bailey, N. J. T. (1975). *The mathematical theory of infectious diseases and its application*. Griffin, London.

Bailey, N. T. J. (1986). Use of simulation models to help control AIDS. In *Medinfo 86*, (ed. B. Blum and M. Jorgansen), pp. 741–4. Elsevier, Amsterdam.

Baker, J. R. (1966). *Parasitic protozoa.* Hutchinson, London.

Ball, F. (1983). The threshold behaviour of epidemic models. *J. Appl. Prob.*, **20**, 227–41.

Ballou, R. S., Hoffman, S. L., Sherwood, J. A. *et al.* (1987). Safety and efficacy of a recombinant DNA *Plasmodium falciparum* sporozoite vaccine. *The Lancet*, **i**, 1277–81.

Barbosa, E. S. (1962). Aspects of the ecology of the intermediate host of *Schistosoma mansoni* interfering with the transmission of bilharziasis in north-eastern Brazil. In *Bilharziasis: Ciba Foundation symposium*, (ed. G. E. Wolstenholme and M. O'Connor), pp. 23–35. Churchill, London.

Barbosa, E. S. and Oliver, L. (1958). Studies on the snail vectors of bilharziasis mansoni in north-eastern Brazil. *Bull. World Health Org.*, **18**, 895.

Barbour, A. D. (1978). Macdonald's model and the transmission of bilharzia. *Trans. R. Soc. Trop. Med. Hyg.*, **72**, 6–15.

Barbour, A. D. (1982). Schistosomiasis. In *Population dynamics of infectious disease: theory and applications*, (ed. R. M. Anderson), pp. 180–208. Chapman and Hall, London.

Barlow, C. H. and Muench, H. (1951). Life span and monthly mortality rate of *Bulinus truncatus* and *Planorbis boissyi*, the intermediate hosts of schistosomiasis in Egypt. *J. Parasitol.*, **37**. 165–73.

Barre-Sinoussi, F., Chermann, J. C., Rey, F., *et al.* (1983). Isolation of a T-lymphotropic retrovirus from a patient at risk for acquired immune deficiency syndrome (AIDS). *Science*, **220**, 868–70.

Barrett, J. A. (1983). Plant–fungus symbioses. In *Coevolution*, (ed. D. J. Futuyma and M. Slatkin), pp. 137–60. Sinauer, Sunderland, Massachusetts.

Barrett, J. (1985). The gene-for-gene hypothesis: parable or paradigm. In *Ecology and genetics of host–parasite interactions*, (ed. D. Rollinson and R. M. Anderson), pp. 215–25. Academic Press, London.

Bartholomew, R. K., Peters, P. A. S., and Jordan, P. (1989). *Schistosoma mansoni* in St. Lucian and Kenyan communities—a comparative study using the Kato stool examination technique. *Ann. Trop. Med. Parasit.*, **74**, 401–5.

Bartlett, M. S. (1955). *Stochastic processes.* Cambridge University Press.

Bartlett, M. S. (1956). Deterministic and stochastic models for recurrent epidemics. *Proc. of the Third Berkeley Symp. on Mathematical Stats. and Probability*, **4**, 81–108.

Bartlett, M. S. (1957). Measles periodicity and community size. *J. R. Statist. Soc.*, **A120**, 48–70.

Bartlett, M. S. (1960a). The critical community size for measles in the United States. *J. Roy. Statist. Soc.*, **123**, 37–44.

Bartlett, M. S. (1960b). *Stochastic population models in ecology and epidemiology.* Methuen, London.

Bauman, P. M., Bennett, H. J., and Ingalls, J. W. (1948). The molluscan intermediate host and *schistosomiasis aponicum*. II. Observations on the production and rate of emergence of cercariae of *schistosomiasis japonicum* from the molluscan intermediate host, *Oncomelania quadrasi. Am. J. Trop. Med.*, **28**, 567–75.

Beard, E. M., Benson, R. C. Jr., Kelalis, P. P., Elveback, L. R., and Kurland, L. T. (1977). The incidence and outcome of mumps orchitis in Rochester, Minnesota, 1935–1974. *Mao Clinic Proc.* **52**, 3–7.

Beck, K. (1984). Coevolution: mathematical analysis of host–parasite interactions. *J. Math. Biol.*, **19**, 63–78.

Beck, K., Keener, J. P., and Ricciardi, P. (1984). The effect of epidemics on genetic evolution. *J. Math. Biol.*, **19**, 79–94.

Becker, N. (1976). Estimation for an epidemic model, *Biometrics*, **32**, 769–77.

Becker, N. (1977). On a general epidemic model. *Theor. Pop. Biol.*, **13**, 23–36.

Becker, N. (1978). The use of epidemic models. *Biometrics*, **35**, 295–305.

Becker, N. and Angulo, J. (1981). On estimating the contagiousness of a disease transmitted from person to person. *Math. Biosci.*, **54**, 137–54.

Befus, A. D. (1975). Secondary infections of *Hymendepis diminuta* in mice: effects of varying worm burdens in primary and secondary infections. *Parasitology*, **71**, 61–75.

Begon, M. and Mortimer M. (1981). *Population ecology: a unified study of animals and plants.* Blackwell Scientific, Oxford.

Begon, M., Harper, J. L., and Townsend, C. R. (1986). *Ecology: individuals, populations and communities.* Blackwell Scientific, Oxford.

Behnke, J. M. (1987). Evasion of immunity by nematode parasites causing chronic infections. *Adv. Parasitol.*, **26**, 1–71.

Behnke, J. M. and Robinson, M. (1985). Genetic control of immunity to *Nematospiroides dubius*: a 9-day anti-helmintic abbreviated immunizing regime which separates weak and strong responder strains of mice. *Parasitol. Immunol.*, **7**, 235–53.

Bekessy, A., Molineaux, L., and Storey, J. (1976). Estimation of incidence and recovery rates of *Plasmodium falciparum* from longitudinal data. *Bull. World Health Org.*, **54**, 685–93.

Benenson, A. S. (1975). *Control of communicable diseases in man*, (12th edn). American Public Health Association, Washington, D.C.

Bensted-Smith, R., Anderson, R. M., Butterworth, A. E., *et al.* (1989). Evidence for predisposition of individual patients to reinfection with *Schistosoma mansoni* after treatment. *Trans. Roy. Soc. Trop. Med.*, **83**, 651–6.

Berding, C., Keymer, A. E., Murray, J. D., and Slater, A. F. G. (1986). The population dynamics of acquired immunity to helminth infection. *J. Theor. Biol.*, **122**, 459–71.

Berkley, S., Okware, S., and Naamora T. (1989). Surveillance for AIDS in Uganda. *AIDS*, **3**, 79–85.

Bernoulli, D. (1760). Essai d'une nouvelle analyse de la mortalité causée par la petite vérole et des advantages de l'inoculation pour la prévenir. *Mém. Math. Phys. Acad. Roy. Sci., Paris*, pp. 1–45.

Black, F. L. (1959). Measles antibodies in the population of New Haven, Connecticut. *J. Immunol.*, **82**, 74–83.

Black, F. L. (1966). Measles endemicity in insular populations: critical community size and its implications. *J. Theor. Biol.*, **11**, 207–11.

Black, F. L. (1982). The role of herd immunity in control of measles. *Yale J. Biol. Med.*, **55**, 351–60.

Blacklock, D. B. (1929). The development of *Onchocerca volvulus* in *Simulium damnosum*. *Ann. Trop. Med. Parasitol.*, **20**, 203–18.

Bliss, C. A. and Fisher, R. A. (1953). Fitting the negative binomial to biological data and a note on the efficient fitting of the negative binomial. *Biometrics*, **9**, 176–200.

Blythe, S. P. and Anderson, R. M. (1988a). Distributed incubation and infectious periods in models of the transmission dynamics of the human immunodeficiency virus (HIV). *IMA J. Math. Appl. Med. Biol.*, **5**, 1–19.

Blythe, S. P. and Anderson, R. M. (1988b). Variable infectiousness in HIV transmission models. *IMA J. Math. Appl. Med. Biol.*, **5**, 181–200.

Blythe, S. P. and Anderson, R. M. (1988c). Heterogeneous sexual activity models of HIV transmission in male homosexual populations. *IMA J. Math. Appl. Med. Biol.*, **5**, 237–60.

BMRB (1987). *Aids advertising campaign, report on four surveys during the first year of advertising, 1986–87.* British Market Research Bureau Limited.

Bodmer, W. F. (1980). The HLA system and diseases. *J. R. Coll. Phys. Lond.,* **14**, 43–59.

Boswell, M. T. and Patil, G. P. (1970). Chance mechanisms generating the negative binomial distribution. In *Random counts in models and structures,* (ed. G. P. Patil), pp. 3–32. Pennsylvania State University Press.

Bowen, D. L., Lane, H. C., and Fauci, A. S. (1985). Immunopathogenesis of the acquired immunodeficiency syndrome. *Ann. Intern. Med.,* **103**, 704–9.

Boyd, M. F. (1949a). Epidemiology of malaria: factors related to the intermediate host. In *Malariology,* (ed. M. F. Boyd). pp. 551–607. Saunders, Philadelphia.

Boyd, M. F. (1949b). Epidemiology: factors related to the definitive host. In *Malariology,* (ed. M. F. Boyd), pp. 608–97. Saunders, Philadelphia.

Boyd, M. F. (ed.) (1949c). *Malariology.* Saunders, Philadelphia.

Bradley, D. J. (1972). Regulation of parasite populations: a general theory of the epidemiology and control of parasite infections. *Trans. R. Soc. Trop. Med. Hyg.,* **66**, 697–708.

Bradley, D. J. and May, R. M. (1978). Consequences of helminth aggregation for the dynamics of schistosomiasis. *Trans. R. Soc. Trop. Med. Hyg.,* **72**, 262–73.

Bradley, D. J. and McCullough, F. S. (1973). Egg output stability and the epidemiology of *Schistosoma haematobium:* Part II. An analysis of the epidemiology of endemic *S. haematobium. Trans. R. Soc. Trop. Med. Hyg.,* **67**, 491–500.

Brayley, E. W. (ed.) (1722). *A journal of the plague year; or memorials of the great pestilence in London, in* 1665, *by Daniel Defoe.* Thomas Tegg, London.

Bremermann, H. J. and Pickering, J. (1983). A game-theoretical model of parasite virulence. *J. Theor. Biol.,* **100**, 411–26.

Broady, J. A., Sever, J. L., McAlister, R., Schuff, G. M., and Cutting, R. C. (1865). Rubella epidemic on St Paul island in the Pribilats, 1963. *J. Amer. Med. Assoc.,* **181**, 619–26.

Brookmeyer, R. and Gail, M. H. (1986). Minimum size of the acquired immunodeficiency syndrome (AIDS) epidemic in the United States. *The Lancet,* **II**, 1320–2.

Brouard, N. (1987). SIDA: Durée d'incubation taux de croissance, taux de reproduction nette. *Population,* **6**, 797–818.

Brown, A. W. A. and Pal, R. (1971). *Insecticide resistance in arthropods.* World Health Organisation, Geneva.

Brown, K. N. (1983). Host resistance to malaria. *Crit. Rev. Trop. Med.,* , 171–89.

Brownlee, J. (1906). Statistical studies in immunity: the theory of an epidemic. *Proc. Roy. Soc. Edn.,* **26**, 484–521.

Bruce-Chwatt, L. J. and Glanville, V. J. (1973). *Dynamics of tropical disease.* Oxford University Press.

Brun, L. O. (1973). Contribution a l'étude biologique et écologique des vecteurs majeurs de paludisme en Afrique de l'ouest. In *Contribution a l'etude biologique et ecologique des vecteurs majeurs de paludisme en Afrique de l'ouest.* Thesis. Universite de Rennes.

Bundy, D. A. P. (1986). Epidemiological aspects of *Trichuris* and trichuriasis in Caribbean communities. *Trans. R. Soc. Trop. Med. Hyg.,* **80**, 706–18.

Bundy, D. A. P. (1988). The population ecology of human helminth infections. *Phil. Trans. R. Soc.,* **B321**, 405–20.

Bundy, D. A. P. and Golden, M. H. N. (1987). The impact of host nutrition on gastrointestinal helminth populations. *Parasitology,* **95**, 623–35.

Bundy, D. A. P., Thompson, D. E., Cooper, E. S., Golden, M. H. N., and Anderson, R. M. (1985a). Population dynamics and chemotherapeutic control of *Trichuris trichuria* in children in Jamaica and St. Lucia. *Trans. R. Soc. Trop. Med, Hyg.,* **79**, 759–64.

Bundy, D. A. P., Thompson, D. E., Golden, M. H. N., Cooper, E. S., Anderson, R. M., and Harland, P. S. E. (1985b). Population distribution of *Trichuris trichuria* in a community of Jamaican children. *Trans. R. Soc. Trop. Med. Hyg.*, **79**, 232–7.

Bundy, D. A. P., Kan-Chua, S. P., and Rose, R. (1988a). Age-related prevalence, intensity and frequency distribution of gastrointestinal helminth infection in urban slum children from Kuala Lumpur, Malaysia. *Trans. R. Soc. Trop. Med. Hyg.*, **83**, 289–94.

Bundy, D. A. P., Wong, M. S., Lewis, L. L., and Horton, J. (1988b). Control of geohelminths by delivery of targetted chemotherapy through schools. *Trans. R. Soc. Trop. Med. Hug.*, **84**, 115–120.

Burnet, M. and White, D. O. (1972). *Natural history of infectious diseases.* Cambridge University Press.

Burnett, F. M. (1957). A modification of Jerne's theory of antibody production using the concept of clonal selection. *Aust. J. Sci.*, **20**, 67–71.

Busenberg, S. and Cooke, K. L. (1978). Periodic solutions of a non-linear delay differential equation. *SIAM J. Appl. Math.*, **35**, 704–21.

Butler, W. (1913). Measles. *Proc. R. Soc. Med.*, **6**, 704–21.

Butterworth, A. E., Taylor, D. W., Veith, M. C., Vadas, M. A., Dessein, A., Sturrock, R. F., and Wells, E. (1982). Studies on the mechanisms in human schistosomiasis. *Immun. Rev.*, **61**, 5–39.

Butterworth, A. E., Dalton, P. R., Dunne, D. W., et al. (1984). Immunity after treatment of human schistosomiasis mansoni. I. Study design, pretreatment observations and the results of treatment.*Trans. R. Soc. Trop. Med. Hyg.*, **78**, 108–23.

Butterworth, A. E., Capron, M., Cordingley, J. S., et al. (1985). Immunity after treatment of human schistosomiasis mansoni. II. Identification of resistant individuals and analysis of their immune responses. *Trans. R. Soc. Trop. Med. Hyg.*, **79**, 393–408.

Butterworth, A. E., Fulford, J. G., Dunne, D. W., Ouma, J. H., and Sturrock, R. F. (1988). Longitudinal studies on human schistosomiasis. *Phil. Trans. R. Soc.*, **B321**, 495–511.

Buxton, P. A. (1955). The natural history of tsetse flies. *Mem. Lond. Sch. Hyg. Trop. Med.* No. 10 Lewis, London.

Cabrera, B. D. (1980). Reinfection and infection studies of soil-transmitted helminthiases in Juban, Sarsogon. In *Collected papers on the control of soil-transmitted helminthiases*, pp. 181–92. Asian Parasite Control Organization, Tokyo.

Cabrera, B. D., Arambulo, P. V., and Partillo, G. P. (1975). Ascariasis control and/or eradication in a rural community in the Philippines. *South East Asian J. Trop. Med. Publ. Health*, **6**, 510–18.

Carne, C. A., Weller, I. V. D., Sutherland, S. et al. (1985). Rising prevalence of human T-lymphotropic virus type III (HTLV III) infection in homosexual men in London. *The Lancet*, **I**, 1261–2.

Carne, C. A., Johnson, A. M., Pearce, F., et al. (1987). Prevalence of antibodies to human immunodeficiency virus (HIV), gonorrhoea rates, and changed sexual behaviour in homosexual men in London. *The Lancet*, **I**, 656–8.

Carnevale, P., Frezil, J. L., Bosseno, M. F., Le Pont, F., and Lancien, J. (1978). Etude de l'agressivité d'*Anopheles gambiae* A en fonction de l'age et du sexe des sujets humains. *Bull. World Health Org.*, **56**, 147–54.

Castillo-Chavez, C., Cooke, K., Huang, W., and Levin, S. A. (1988a). The role of long periods of infectiousness in the dynamics of acquired immunodeficiency syndrome (AIDS). *J. Math. Biol.*, **27**, 373–98.

Castillo-Chavez, C., Hethcote, H. W., Andreasen, V., Levin, S. A., and Liu, W. M. (1988b). Cross immunity in the dynamics of homogeneous and heterogeneous populations. In

Mathematical ecology, (ed. L. J. Cross, T. G. Hallam, and S. A. Levin), pp. 303–16. World Scientific, Singapore.

CDC (1981*a*). Rubella—United States 1978–1981. *Morb. Mortal. Wkly. Rep.*, **30**, 513–15.

CDC (1981*b*). Measles encephalitis—United States 1962–1979. *Morb. Mortal. Wkly. Rep.*, **31**, 217–24.

CDC (1981*c*). Pneumocystis pneumonia—Los Angeles. *Morb. Mortal. Wkly. Rep.*, **30**, 250–2.

CDC (1981). Karposi's sarcoma and pneumocystis pneumonia among homosexual men—New York City and California. *Morb. Mortal. Wkly. Rep.*, **30**, 305–8.

CDC (1982). Update on acquired immunodeficiency syndrome (AIDS). United States. *Morb. Mortal. Wkly. Rep.*, **31**, 507–14.

CDC (1984). *Mumps surveillance, January, 1977–December, 1982. Atlanta, USA*. U.S. Department of Health and Human Services, CDC.

CDC (1985*a*). Acquired immunodeficiency syndrome in the San Francisco Cohort Study. *Morb. Mortal. Wkly. Rep.*, **34**, 573–5.

CDC (1985*b*). Revision of the case definition of Acquired Immunodeficiency Syndrome for national reporting—United States. *Morb. Mortal. Wkly. Rep.*, **34**, 373–5.

CDC (1986). Update: acquired immunodeficiency syndrome—Africa. *Morbid. Mortal. Wkly. Rep.*, **35**, 17–21.

CDC (1987). *A review of current knwledge and plans for expansion of HIV surveillance activities. A report to the domestic policy council*. U.S. Department of Health and Human Services, Public Health Service and Centres for Disease Control.

CDC (1988). *A review of current knowledge and plans for expansion of HIV surveillance activities*. U.S. Department of Health and Human Services, Public Health Service and Centres for Disease Control.

CDC (1989). Acquired immunodeficiency syndrome in the San Francisco cohort study, 1978–1985. *Morbid. Mortal. Wkly. Rep.*, **38**, 573–7..

Chamberlain, R. W., Sudia, W. D., and Gillett, J. D. (1959). St. Louis encephalitic virus in mosquitoes. *Am. J. Hyg.*, **70**, 221.

Chandra, R. K. and Newberne, P. M. (1977). *Nutrition, immunity and infection: mechanisms of interactions*. Plenum, New York.

Chapin, C. V. (1926). Measles in Providence, Rhode Island 1858–1923. *Am. J. Hyg.*, **5**, 635–55.

Chapman, H. D. (1984). Drug resistance in avian coccidia (a review). *Vet. Parasitol.* **15**, 11–27.

Chartres, J. C. (1955). Onchocerciasis. Incubation period, clinical course and treatment at first aid. *West Afr. Med. J.*, **4**, 130–4.

Cheever, A. W. (1968). A quantitative post mortem study of *Schistosomiasis mansoni* in man. *Am. J. Trop. Med. Hyg.*, **17**, 38–64.

Cheever, A. W., Kamel, I. A., *et al.* (1977). *Schistosoma mansoni* and *S. haematobium* infections in Egypt. II. Quantitative parasitological findings at necropsy. *Amer. J. Trop. Med. Hyg.*, **26, 702**, 702–16.

Cheke, R. A., Gorms, R., and Kerner, M. (1982). The fecundity of *Simulium damnosum* s.l. in northern Togo and infections with *Onchocerca* spp. *Ann. Trop. Med. Parasitol.*, **76**, 561–8.

Christensen, B. M. (1978). *Dirofilaria immitis*: effects on the longevity of *Aedes trivittatus*. *Exp. Parasit.*, **44**, 116–23.

Christensen, B. M. and Hollander, A. L. (1978). Effect of temperature on vector–parasite relationships of *Aedes trivittatus* and *Dirofilaria immitis*. *Proc. Helminth. Soc. Wash.*, **45**, 115–19.

Christensen, P. E., Schmidt, H., Bang, H. O., Anderson, V., Jadal, B., and Jensen, O. (1953). Measles in virgin soil, Greenland, 1951. *Danish Med. Bull.*, 1, 2–6.

Christie, A. B. (1974). *Infectious diseases: epidemiology and clinical practice.* Churchill Livingstone, London.

Christie, J. D. and Upatham, E. S. (1977). Control of *Schistosoma mansoni* transmission by chemotherapy in St. Lucia. II. Biological results. *Am. J. Trop. Med. Hyg.*, 26, 894–9.

Christophers, S. R. (1924). The mechanism of immunity against malaria in communities living under hyper-endemic conditions. *Indian J. Med. Res.*, 12, 273.

Christophers, S. R. (1949). Endemic and epidemic prevalence. In *Malariology*, (ed. M. F. Boyd), pp. 698–721. Saunders, Philadelphia.

Chu, K. Y., Massoud, J., and Sabbaghian, H. (1966a). Host–parasite relationship of *Bulinus truncatus* and *Schistosoma haematobium* in Iran. I. Effect of the age of *B. truncatus* on the development of *S. haematobium*. *Bull. World Health Org.*, 34, 113–19.

Chu, K. Y., Sabbaghian, H., and Massoud, J. (1966b). Host–parasite relationship of Bulinus truncatus and *Schistosoma haematobium* in Iran. 2. Effect of exposure dosage of miracidia on the biology of the snail host and the development of the parasites. *Bull. World Health Org.*, 34, 131–3.

Chunque, E., Marche, G., Plichart, R., Boutin, J. P., and Roux, J. (1989). Comparison of immunoglobulin-G enzyme-linked immunoabsorbent assay (IgG-ELISA) and haemagglutination inhibition (HI) test for the detection of dengue antibodies. Prevalence of dengue IgG-ELISA antibodies in Tahiti. *Trans. R. Soc. Trop. Med. Hyg.*, 83, 708–11.

Clark, C. W. (1976). *Mathematical bioeconomics.* Wiley, New York.

Clark, M., Schild, G. C., Boustred, J., McGregor, I. A., and Williams, K. (1980). Epidemiological studies of rubella virus in a tropical African community. *Bull. World Health Org.*, 58, 921–5.

Clarke, B. C. (1975). Frequency-dependent and density-dependent natural selection. In *The role of natural selection in human evolution*, (ed. F. M. Salzano), pp. 187–200. Amsterdam.

Clarkson, J. A. and Fine, P. E. M. (1985). The efficiency of measles and pertussis notifications in England and Wales. *Int. J. Epidemiol.*, 14, 153–68.

Cliff, A. P., Haggett, P., Ord, J. K., and Versey, G. R. (1981). *Spatial diffusion: an historical geography of epidemics in an island community.* Cambridge University Press.

Cliff, A. P., Haggett, P., and Ord, J. K. (1983). Forecasting epidemic pathways for measles in Iceland: the use of simultaneous equation and logic models. *Ecol. Disease*, 2, 377–96.

Cockburn, T. A. (1971). Infectious diseases in ancient populations. *Curr. Anthrop.*, 12, 45–62.

Cohen, J. E. (1973a). Heterologous immunity in human malaria. *Q. Rev. Biol.*, 48, 467–89.

Cohen, J. E. (1973b). Selective host mortality in a catalytic model applied to schistosomiasis. *Am. Nat.*, 197, 199–212.

Cohen, J. E. (1977). Mathematical models of schistosomiasis. *Ann. Rev. Ecol. Syst.*, 8, 209–33.

Cohen, J. E. (1987). Sexual behaviour and randomized responses. *Science*, 236, 1503.

Collins, S. D. (1929). Age incidence of the common communicable diseases of children. *U.S. Public Health Rep.* 44, 763–828.

Comins, H. N. (1977a). The management of pesticide resistance. *J. Theor. Biol.*, 65, 399–420.

Comins, H. N. (1977b). The development of insecticide resistance in the presence of migration. *J. Theor. Biol.*, 64, 177–97.

Comins, H. N. (1979). Analytical methods for the management of pesticide resistance. *J. Theor. Biol.*, **77**, 171–88.

Comins, H. N. (1984). The mathematical evaluation of options for managing pesticide resistance. In *Pest and pathogen control: strategic, tactical and policy models*, (ed. G. R. Conway), pp. 454–69. Wiley, New York.

Connor, E. M., Minnefor, A. B., and Oleske, J. M. (1987). Human Immunodeficiency virus infection in infants and children. In *Current Topics in AIDS*, (ed. M. S. Gottlieb, D. J. Jefferies, D. Mildvan, A. J. Pinching, T. C. Quinn, and R. A. Weiss), pp. 185–210. John Wiley and Sons, New York.

Cooke, K. L. (1982). Models for epidemic infections with asymptomatic cases, I: one group. *Math. Modelling*, **3**, 1–15.

Cooke, K. L. and Yorke, J. A. (1973). Some equations modelling growth processes and gonorrhea epidemics. *Math. Biosci.*, **16**, 75–101.

Cooper, D. A., Gould, J. Maclean, P., *et al.* (1985). Acute AIDS retrovirus infection. Definition of a clinical illness associated with seroconversion. *The Lancet*, **i**, 537–40.

Cooper, L. N. (1986). Theory of an immune system retrovirus. *Proc. Natl. Acad. Sci.*, **83**, 9159–63.

Cornille-Brögger, R., Matthews, H. M., Storey, J., Ashkar, T. S., Brogger, S., and Molineaux, L. (1978). Changing patterns in the humoral immune response to malaria before, during and after the application of control measures: a longitudinal study in the West African savanna. *Bull. World Health Org.*, **56**, 479–600.

Cox, F. E. G. (ed). (1982). *Modern parasitology*. Blackwell Scientific Publications, Oxford.

Cox, D. R. and Oates, D. (1984). *Analysis of survival data*. Chapman and Hall, London.

Cox, D. R. and Medley, G. F. (1989). A maximum likelihood method of prediction in the presence of reporting delays. *Phil. Trans. R. Soc.*, **B325**, 1350–450.

Creighton, C. (1894). *A history of epidemics in Britain*, Vols I and II. Cambridge University Press.

Crofton, H. D. (1971*a*). A model of host–parasite relationships. *Parasitology.*, **63**, 343–64.

Crofton, H. D. (1971*b*). A quantitative approach to parasitism. *Parasitology*, **63**, 111–20.

Croll, N. A., Anderson, R. M., Gyarkos, T. W., and Ghadirian, E. (1982). The population biology and control of *Ascaris lumbricoides* in a rural community in Iran. *Trans. R. Soc. Trop. Med. Hyg.*, **76**, 187–97.

Crombie, D. L. (1983). Whooping cough: what proportion of cases is notified in an epidemic. *Br. Med. J.*, **287**, 770–1..

Crombie, J. A. (1985). *Infection dynamics of Schistosoma mansoni in the laboratory mouse*. Ph.D. Thesis. London University.

Crombie, J. A. and Anderson, R. M. (1985). Population dynamics of *Schistosoma mansoni* in mice repeatedly exposed to infection. *Nature*, **315**, 491–3.

Crompton, D. W. T., Nesheim, M. C., and Pawlowski, Z. S. (ed.) (1985). *Ascariasis and its public health significance*. Taylor and Francis, London.

Crompton, D. W. T., Nesheim, M. C., and Pawlowski, Z. S. (ed.) (1989). *Ascariasis and its prevention and control*. Taylor and Francis, London.

Cross, G. A. M. (1978). Antigenic variation in trypanosomes. *Proc. R. Soc.*, **B202**, 55–72.

Cross, G. A. M. (1979). Immunological aspects of antigenic variation in trypanosomes. The Third Fleming Lecture. *J. Gen. Microbiol.*, **113**, 1–28.

Crow, J. F. and Kimura, M. (1970). *An introduction to the theory of population genetics*. Harper and Row, New York.

Curran, J. W., Lawrence, D. N., Jaffe, H., *et al.* (1984). Acquired Immunodeficiency Syndrome (AIDS) associated with transfusions. *New Engl. J. Med.*, **310 (2)**, 69–75.

Curran, J. W., Morgan, W. M., Hardy, A. M., *et al.* (1985). The epidemiology of AIDS: current status and future prospects. *Science*, **229**, 1352–7.

Curran, J. W., Jaffe, H. W., Hardy, A. M., *et al.* (1988). Epidemiology of HIV infection and AIDS in the United States, *Science*, **239**, 610–16.

Cvjetanovic, B., Grab, B., and Uemura, K. (1978). Dynamics of acute bacterial diseases, epidemiological models and their application to public health. *Bull. World Health Org.*, **56, suppl. no. 1**, 1–143.

Cvjetanovic, B., Grab, B., and Dixon, H. (1982). Epidemiological models of poliomyelitis and measles and their application in the planning of immunization programmes. *Bull. World Health Org.*, **60**, 405–22.

Dalmat, H. T. and Gibson, C. L. (1952). A study of flight range and longevity of blackflies infected with *Onchocerca volvulus*. *Ann. Entomol. Soc. Am.*, **45**, 605–12.

Dalton, P. (1976). A socio-ecological approach to the control of *Schistosoma mansoni* in St. Lucia. *Bull. World Health Org.*, **54**, 587–95.

Dalton, P. R. and Poole, D. (1978). Water contact patterns in relation to *Schistosoma haematobium* infection. *Bull. World Health Org.*, **56**, 417–26.

Davidson, G. and Draper, C. C. (1953). Field study of some of the basic factors concerned in the transmission of malaria. *Trans. R. Soc. Trop. Med. Hyg.*, **47**, 522–35.

Davis, A., Biles, J. E., and Ulrich, A. M. (1979). Initial experiences with praziquantel in the treatment of human infections due to *Schistosoma haematobium*. *Bull. World Health Org.*, **57**, 773–9.

Davis, J. W., Anderson, R. C., Karstad, L., and Trainer, D. O. (1971). *Infectious and parasitic infections of wild birds*. Iowa State University Press.

Davis, R. (1982). Measles in the tropics and public health practices. *Trans. R. Soc. Trop. Med. Hyg.*, **76**, 268–75.

Day, P. R. (1974). *Genetics of host–parasite interactions*. Freeman, San Francisco.

Dazo, B. C., Hairston, N. G., and Dawood, I. K. (1966). The ecology of *Bulinus truncatus* and *Biomphalaria alexandrina* and its implications for the control of bilharziasis in the Egypt-49 project area. *Bull. World Health Org.*, **35**, 339–56.

Dean, D. A. (1983). Schistosoma and related genera: acquired resistance in mice. *Exp. Parasitol.*, **55**, 1–104.

Deans, J. A. and Cohen, S. (1983). Immunology of malaria, *Ann. Rev. Microbiol.*, **37**, 25–49.

Deevey, E. S. (1960). The human population. *Sci. Am.*, **203**, 195–207.

DeGruttola, V. and Mayer, K. H. (1988). Assessing and modelling heterosexual spread of the human immunodeficiency virus in the United States. *Rev. Infect. Dis.*, **10**, 138–50.

Delyamure, S. L. (1955). The helminth fauna of marine animals in the light of their ecology and phylogeny. *Izd. Akad. Nauk SSSR, Moscow*, pp. 517. [Translation TT67-51202, US Dept of Commerce, Springfield, Va.]

Denham, D. A., Ponnadurai, G. S., Nelson, F., Rogers, R., and Guy, F. (1972). Studies with *Brugia pahangi*. II: The effect of repeated injection on parasite levels in cats. *Int. J. Parasit.*, **2**, 401–7.

De Quadros, C. A. (1980). More effective immunisation. *Proc. R. Soc.*, **B209**, 11–18.

Dietz, K. (1975). Transmission and control of arbovirus diseases. In *Epidemiology*, (ed. D. Ludwig and K. L. Cooke), pp. 104–21. SIAM, Philadelphia.

Dietz, K. (1976). The incidence of infectious diseases under the influence of seasonal fluctuations. *Lect. Notes Biomath.*, **11**, 1–15.

Dietz, K. (1980). Models for vector-borne parasitic diseases. *Lect. Notes Biomath.*, **39**, 264–77.

Dietz, K. (1981). The evaluation of rubella vaccination strategies. In *The mathematical theory of the dynamics of biological populations*, Vol II, (ed. R. W. Hiorns and D. Cooke), pp. 81–98. Academic, London.

Dietz, K. (1982a). The population dynamics of onchocerciasis. In *Population dynamics of infectious diseases*, (ed. R. M. Anderson), pp. 209–41. Chapman and Hall, London.

Dietz, K. (1982b). Overall population patterns in the transmission cycle of infectious agents. In *Population biology of infectious diseases*, (ed. R. M. Anderson and R. M. May), pp. 87–102. Springer, Berlin.

Dietz, K. (1988). Density-dependence in parasite transmission dynamics. *Parasitol. Today*, 4, 91–7.

Dietz, K. and Hadeler, K. P. (1988). Epidemiological models for sexually transmitted diseases. *J. Math. Biol.*, 26, 1–25.

Dietz, K. and Renner, H. (1985). Simulation of selective chemotherapy for the control of helminth diseases. In *Mathematics and computers in biomedical applications*, (ed. J. Eisenfield and C. Delisi), pp. 287–93. Elsevier, New York.

Dietz, K. and Schenzle, D. (1985). Mathematical models for infectious disease statistics. In *A celebration of statistics*, (ed. A. C. Atkinson and S. E. Fienberg), pp. 167–204. Springer Verlag, New York.

Dietz, K., Molineaux, L., and Thomas, A. (1974). A malaria model tested in African savanna. *Bull. Word Health Org.*, 50, 347–57.

Dobson, A. P. and May, R. M. (1986). Disease and conservation. In *Conservation Biology: the science of scarcity and diversity*, (ed. M. E. Soule), pp. 345–65. Sinauer, Sunderland, Mass.

Dobyns, H. F. (1966). Estimating aboriginal american population. *Current Anthropol.*, 7, 395–416.

Domingo, E. O., Tiu, E., Peters, P. A., Warren, K. S., Mahmoud, A. A. F., and Houser, H. B. (1980). Morbidity in schistosomiasis japonica in relation to intensity of infection: study of a community in Leyte, Philippines. *Am. J. Trop. Med. Hyg.*, 29, 858–67.

Dorf, M. E. (1981). *The role of the major histocompatibility complex in immunobiology*. Wiley, New York.

Downs, A. M., Ancelle, R. A., Jager, H. C., and Brunet, J. (1987). AIDS in Europe: current trends and short-term predictions estimated from surveillance data, January 1981–June 1986. *AIDS*, 1, 53–7.

Duke, B. O. L. (1970). Quantitative approach of the transmission of *Onchocerca volvulus*. *Trans. R. Soc. Trop. Med. Hyg.*, 64, 311–12.

Duke, B. O. L. (1980). Observations on *Onchocerca volvulus* in experimentally infected chimpanzees. *Troperimed-Parasitol.* 31, 41–54.

Duke, B. O. L., Lewis, D. J., and Moore, P. J. (1966). *Onchocerca–Simuliam* complexes. I. Transmission of forest and Sudan savanna strains of *Onchocerca volvulus* from Cameroon, by *Simuliam damnosum* from various West African bioclimatic zones. *Ann. Trop. Med. Parasit.*, 60, 318–36.

Duke, H. L. (1923). An inquiry into an outbreak of human trypanosomiasis in a *Glossina morsitans* belt to the east of Mwamza Territory, Tanganyika. *Proc. R. Soc.*, B94, 250–65.

Dye, C. (1988). The epidemiology of canine visceral leishmaniasis in Southern France: classical theory offers another explanation of the data. *Parasitology*, 96, 19–24.

Dye, C. M. and Hasibeder, G. (1986). Population dynamics of mosquito-borne disease: effects of flies which bite some people more frequently than others. *Trans. Roy. Soc. Trop. Med. Hyg.*, 83, 69–77.

Earle, W. C. (1939). The epidemiology of malaria with special reference to Puerto Rico. *Puerto Rico J. Public Health Trop. Med.*, **3**.

Earle, W. C., Perez, M., Del Rio, J., and Arzola, C. (1939). Observations on the course of naturally acquired malaria in Puerto Rico. *Puerto Rico J. Public Health Trop. Med.*, **14**, 391–406.

Edwards, M. A. and McDonnell, U. (eds.) (1982). *Animal disease in relation to animal conservation.* (Symposia of the Zoological Society of London, No. 50). Academic Press, London.

Eichmann, K. (1978). Expression and function of idiotypes on lymphocytes. *Adv. Immunol.*, **26**, 195–210.

El Alamy, M. A. and Cline, B. L. (1977). Prevalence and intensity of *Schistosoma haematobium* and *Schistosoma mansoni* infection in Qualyub, Egypt. *Am. J. Trop. Med. Hyg.*, **26**, 470–2.

Elderkin, R. H., Berkowitz, D. P., Farris, F. A., *et al.* (1977). On the steady state of an age-dependant model for malaria. In *Non-linear systems and applications*, (ed. V. Lakshmikantham), pp. 491–512. Academic, London.

Elkins, D. B., Haswell-Elkins, M., and Anderson, R. M. (1986). The epidemiology and control of intestinal helminths in the Publicat Lake region of Southern India. I. Study design and pre- and post-treatment observations on *Ascaris lumbricoides* infection. *Trans. R. Soc. Trop. Med. Hyg.*, **80**, 774–92.

Elkins, D. B., Haswell-Elkins, M., and Anderson, R. M. (1988). The importance of host age and sex to patterns of reinfection with *Ascaris lumbricoides* following mass antihelminthic treatment in a South Indian fishing community. *Parasitology*, **96**, 171–84.

Endler, J. A. (1977). *Geographic variation, speciation and clines.* Princeton University Press.

EPI (1986). EPI Global advising group. *Wkly Epidemiol. Rec.*, **61**, 13–16.

Esteban, J. I., Tai, C.-C., Kay, J. W. D., Sih, J. W.-K., Bodner, A. J., and Alter, H. J. (1985). Importance of western blot analysis in predicting infectivity of anti-HTLV-III/LAV positive blood. *The Lancet*, **ii**, 1083–6.

Evans, A. S. and Stirewalt, M. A. (1951). Variations in infectivity of cercariae of *Schistosoma mansoni. Exp. Parasitol.*, **1**, 19–33.

Evans, B. A. (1989). Trends in sexual behaviour and risk factors for HIV infection among homosexual men, 1984–1987. *Br. Med. J.*, **298**, 215–18.

Evered, D. and Clark, S. (ed.) (1987), *Filariasis. Ciba Foundation Symposium.* Wiley, Chichester.

Fain, A. (1963). Contribution to the study of the larval forms of helminths in the Belgian Congo, and especially of the larvae of *Schistosoma mansoni. Mem. Inst. R. Colon. Belg. Sect. Sci. Nat. Med.*, **22**, 1–312.

Fales, W. T. (1928). The age distribution of whooping cough, measles, chicken pox, scarlet fever and diphtheria in various areas of the United States. *Am. J. Hyg.*, **8**, 758–99.

Farr, W. (1840). Progress of epidemics. *Second report of the Registrar General of England*, pp. 91–8.

Fauci, A. S., Masur, H., and Gelman, E. P. (1985). The acquired immunodeficiency syndrome: An update. *Ann. Int. Med.*, **102**, 802–13.

Fay, R. E., Turner, C. F., Klassen, A. D., and Gagnon, J. H. (1989). Prevalence and patterns of same-gender sexual contact among men. *Science*, **243**, 338–48.

Fenner, F. (1948). The epizootic behaviour of mouse pox (infectious ectromelia of mice). II. The course of events in long-continued epidemics. *J. Hyg.*, **46**, 383–93.

Fenner, F. (1983). Biological control, as exemplified by smallpox eradication and myxomatosis. *Proc. R. Soc.*, **B218**, 259–85.

Fenner, F. and Myers, K. (1978). Myxoma virus and myxomatosis in retrospect: the first quarter century of a new disease. In *Viruses and environment*, (ed. E. Kurstak and K. Maramorosch), pp. 539–70. Academic, New York.

Fenner, F. and Ratcliffe, F. N. (1965). *Myxomatosis*. Cambridge University Press.

Fenner, F. and White, D. O. (1970). *Medical virology*. Academic, New York.

Fenwick, A. and Ligate, H. J. (1970). Attempts to eradicate snails from impounded water by the use of N-titrylmorpholine. *Bull. Wld. Hlth. Org.*, **42**, 581–8.

Ferrari, J. A. and Georghiou, G. P. (1981). Effects of insecticidal selection and treatment on reproductive potential of resistant, susceptible, and heterozygous strains of the southern house mosquito. *J. Econ. Entomol.*, **74**, 323–7.

Fine, P. E. M. (1975). Superinfection—A problem in formulating a problem (an historical critique of Macdonald's theory). *Trop. Dis. Bull.*, **72**, 475–88.

Fine, P. E. M. (1979). John Brownlee and the measurement of infectiousness: an historical study in epidemic theory. *J. R. Statist. Soc.*, **B142**, 347–62.

Fine, P. E. M. (1982). Control of infectious diseases (group report). In *Population biology of infectious diseases*, (ed. R. M. Anderson and R. M. May), pp. 121–48.

Fine, P. E. M. and Clarkson, J. A. (1982*a*). Measles in England and Wales. II. The impact of the measles vaccination programme on the distribution of immunity in the population. *Int. J. Epidemiol.*, **11**, 15–25.

Fine, P. E. M. and Clarkson, J. A. (1982*b*). Measles in England and Wales. I. An analysis of factors underlying seasonal patterns. *Int. J. Epidemiol.*, **11**, 5–14.

Fine, P. E. M. and Lehman, J. S. (1977). Mathematical models of schistosomiasis: Report of a workshop. *Am. J. Trop. Med. Hyg.*, **26**, 500–4.

Fischl, M. A., Dickinson, G. M., Scott, G. B. *et al.* (1987). Evaluation of heterosexual partners, children and household contacts of adults with AIDS. *J. Am. Med. Assoc.*, **257**, 640–4.

Fisher, R. A. (1930). *The genetical theory of natural selection*. Clarendon, Oxford.

Flint, J., Hill, A. V. S., Bowden, D. K., *et al.* (1986). High frequencies of α-thalassaemia are the result of natural selection by malaria. *Nature*, **321**, 744–50.

Forrester, D. J. (1971). Bighorn sheep lungworm—pneumonia complex. In *Parasitic diseases of wild mammals*, (ed. J. W. Davis and R. C. Anderson), pp. 158–73. Iowa State Univ. Press, Iowa.

Forsyth, K. P., Andes, R. F., Kemp, D. J., and Alpers, M. P. (1988). New approaches to the serotypic analysis of the epidemiology of *Plasmodium falciparum. Epidemiol. Ecol. Infect. Dis. Agents*, **1**, 159–65.

Forsyth, K. P., Grenfell, B., Spark, R., Kazura, J. W., and Alpers, M. P. (1990). Age-specific patterns of change in the dynamics of *Wuchereria bancrofti* infection in Papua New Guinea. *Am. J. Trop. Med. Hyg.* (In press.)

Francis, D. P. (1983). Selective primary health care: strategies for control of disease in the developing world. III. Hepatitis B virus and its related diseases. *Rev. Inf. Dis.*, **5**, 322–9.

Francis, H. L. and Quinn, T. C. (1987). AIDS in Africa. In *Current topics in AIDS*, (ed. M. S. Gottlieb, D. J. Jefferies, D. Mildvan, A. J. Pinching, T. C. Quinn, and R. A. Weiss), pp. 261–86. John Wiley and Sons, New York.

Fushimi, J. (1959). A consideration on the correlation between the so-called egg positive rate and the genuine infection rate of the unisexual parasitism on the mean number of infected worms in the case of ascarid infection. I. The examination of the fundamental materials for the construction of the theoretical models. *Japan. J. Parasitol.*, **8**, 108–14.

Gaines, H., Albert, J., von Sydow, M. *et al.* (1987). HIV antigenaemia and virus isolation from plasma during primary HIV infection. *The Lancet*, **i**, 1317–18.

Galbraith, N. S., Young, S. E. J., Pusey, J. J., Crombie, D. L., and Sparks, J. P. (1984). Mumps surveillance in England and Wales, 1962–1981. *The Lancet*, **1**, 91–4.

Gallo, R. C., Salahuddin, S. Z., Popovic, M. *et al.* (1984). Frequent detection and isolation of cytopathic retroviruses (HTLV-III) from patients with AIDS and at risk of AIDS. *Science*, **224**, 497–500.

Garnham, P. C. C. (1966). Immunity against the different stages of malarial parasites. *Bull. Soc. Pat. Exot.*, **59**, 549–57.

Garrett-Jones, C. (1964). The human blood index of malaria vectors in relation to epidemiological assessment. *Bull. World Health Org.*, **31**, 241–61.

Garrett-Jones, C. and Grab, B. (1964). The assessment of insecticidal impact on the malaria mosquito's vectorial capacity, from data on the population of parous females. *Bull. World Health Org.*, **31**, 71–86.

Garrett-Jones, C. and Shidrawi, G. R. (1969). Malaria vectorial capacity of a population of *Anopheles gambiae*. *Bull. World Health Org.*, **40**, 531–45.

Gellan, M. C. A. and Ison, C. A. (1986). Declining incidence of gonorrhea in London. A response to fear of AIDS. *The Lancet*, **II**, 920.

Getz, W. M. and Pickering, J. (1983). Epidemiological models: thresholds and population regulation. *Am. Nat.*, **121**, 892–8.

Gillespie, J. H. (1975). Natural selection for resistance to epidemics. *Ecology*, **56**, 493–5.

Gillies, M. T. and Wilkes, T. J. (1963). Observations on nulliparous and parous rates in a population of *A. funestus* in East Africa. *Ann. Trop. Med. Parasitol.*, **57**, 204–13.

Gillies, M. T. and Wilkes, T. J. (1965). A study of the age composition of populations of *Anopheles gambiae* Giles and *A. funestus* Giles in north-eastern Tanzania. *Bull. Entomol. Res.*, **56**, 237–62.

Ginzburg, H. M., Fleming, P. L., and Miller, K. D. (1988). Selected public health observations derived from Mullincenter AIDS cohort study. *J. AIDS*, **1**, 2–8.

Gleick, J. (1987). *Chaos: making a new science.* Viking, New York.

Goddard, M. J. (1978). On Macdonald's model for schistosomiasis. *Trans. R. Soc. Trop. Med. Hyg.*, **72**, 123–31.

Goddard, M. J. and Jordan, P. (1980). On the longevity of *Schistosoma mansoni* in man on St. Lucia, West Indies. *Trans. R. Soc. Trop. Med. Hyg.*, **74**, 185–91.

Goedert, J. J., Biggar, R. J., Winn, D. M. *et al.* (1984). Determinants of retrovirus (HTLV-III) antibody and immunodeficiency conditions in homosexual men. *The Lancet*, **ii**, 711–15.

Goedert, J. J., Biggar, R. J., Weiss, S. H. *et al.* (1986). Three year incidence of AIDS in five cohorts of HTLV III-infected risk group members. *Science*, **231**, 992–5.

Gordan, R. M., Davey, T. H., and Peaston, H. (1934). The transmission of human bilharziasis in Sierra Leone, with an account of the life-cycle of the schistosomes concerned. *Ann. Trop. Med. Parasitol.*, **28**, 323–419.

Gordon, J. E., Jansen, A. A. J., and Ascoli, W. (1965). Measles in rural Guatemala. *Trop. Paediatr.*, **66**, 779–86.

Gorms, R. (1983). Studies of the transmission of *Onchocerca–Simulium damnosum* complex occurring in Liberia. *Z. Angew. Zool.*, **70**, 101–11..

Goudsmit, J., Wolf, F., Paul, D. A. *et al.* (1986). Expression of human immunodeficiency virus antigens (HIV-Ag) in serum and cerebrospinal fluid during acute and chronic infection. *The Lancet*, **II**, 177–80.

Gough, K. J. (1977). The estimation of latent and infectious periods. *Biometrics*, **64**, 449–65.

Grant, R. M., Wiley, J. A., and Winkelstein, W. (1987). Infectivity of the human immunodeficiency virus: estimates from a prospective study of homosexual men. *J. Infect. Dis.*, **156**, 189–93.

Green, D. (1978). Self-oscillation for epidemic models. *Math. Biosci.*, **38**, 91–111.

Greenhalgh, D. (1987). Analytic results on the stability of age-structured epidemic models. *IMA J. Math. Appl. Med. Biol.*, **4**, 109–44.

Greenwood, M. (1949). The infectiousness of measles. *Biometrika*, **36**, 1–8.

Greenwood, M., Bradford-Hill, A., Topley, W. W. C., and Wilson, J. (1936). Experimental epidemiology. *Med. Res. Council. Spec. Rep.*, **209**, 204.

Gregg, N. M. (1941). Congenital cataract following German measles in the mother. *Trans. Ophthalmol. Soc. Aust.*, **3**, 35.

Grenfell, B. T. and Anderson, R. M. (1985). The estimation of age related rates of infection from case notifications and serological data. *J. Hyg.*, **95**, 419–36.

Gretillat, S. (1961). The epidemiology of vesical bilharziasis in eastern Senegal: observations on the ecology of *Bulinus guernei* and *Bulinus senegalensis*. *Bull. World Health Org.*, **25**, 459–66.

Griffiths, D. A. (1974). A catalytic model of infection for measles. *Appl. Stat.*, **23**, 330–9.

Gripenberg, G. (1980). Periodic solutions of an epidemic model. *J. Math. Biol.*, **271**, 280.

Groll, N. A., Anderson, R. M., Gyarkos, T. W., and Ghadirian, E. (1982). The population biology and control of *Ascaris lumbricoides* in a rural community in Iran. *Trans. R. Soc. Trop. Med. Hyg.*, **78**, 187–97.

Grossman, Z. (1980). Oscillatory phenomena in a model of infectious diseases. *Theor. Pop. Biol.*, **18**, 204–43.

Gryseels, B. and Nkulikyinka, L. (1989). Two-year follow-up of *Schistosoma mansoni* infection and morbidity after treatment with different regimens of oxamiquine and praziquantel. *Trans. R. Soc. Trop. Med. Hyg.*, **83**, 219–28.

Gupta, S., Anderson, R. M., and May, R. M. (1989). Networks of sexual contacts: implications for the pattern of spread of HIV. *AIDS*, **3**, 807–17.

Hadeler, K. P. and Dietz, K. (1983). Nonlinear hyperbolic partial differential equations for the dynamics of parasite populations. *Comp. Math. Appl.*, **9**, 415–30.

Hahn, B. H., Shaw, G. M., Taylor, M. E. *et al.* (1986). Genetic variation in HTLV-III/LAV over time in patients with AIDS or at risk for AIDS. *Science*, **232**, 1548–53.

Hairston, N. G. (1962). Population ecology and epidemiological problems. In *Proceedings of the CIBA Foundation symposium on bilharziasis*, pp. 36–80. Churchill, London.

Hairston, N. G. (1965a). On the mathematical analysis of schistosome populations. *Bull. World Health Org.*, **33**, 45–62.

Hairston, N. G. (1965b). An analysis of age–prevalence data by catalytic models. *Bull. World Health Org.*, **33**, 163–75.

Hairston, N. G. and Jackowski, L. A. (1968). Analysis of the *Wuchereria bancrofti* population in the people of American Samoa. *Bull. World. Health Org.*, **38**, 29–59.

Haldane, J. B. S. (1949). Disease and evolution. *La Ricerca Sci.*, **19, suppl.**, 68–76.

Halsey, N. A. (1983). *The optimal age for administering measles vaccine in developing countries*, Pan American Health Organisation, Scientific Publication No. **451**.

Halsey, N. A., Boulos, R., Mode, F., *et al.* (1985). Response to measles vaccine in Haitian infants 6 to 12 months old. Influence of maternal antibodies, malnutrition, and concurrent illnesses. *New Engl. J. Med.*, **313**, 544–9.

Halstead, S. B. (1984). Selective primary health care: strategies for control of disease in the developing world. XI. Dengue. *Rev. Infect. Dis.*, **6**, (**2**), 251–64.

Hamer, W. H. (1906). Epidemic disease in England. *The Lancet*, **i**, 733–9.

Hamilton, W. D. (1980). Sex versus non-sex versus parasite. *Oikos*, **35**, 282–90.

Hamis, J. E. (1987). The AIDS epidemic: looking into the 1990's. *Technol. Rev.*, **90**, 59–64.

Hanshaw, J. B. and Dudgeon, J. A. (1978). *Viral diseases of the foetus and newborn*. Saunders, London.

Harris, C., Small, C. B., Klein, R. S. *et al.* (1983). Immunodeficiency in female sexual partners of men with the acquired immunodeficiency syndrome. *New Engl. J. Med.*, **308**, 1181–4.

Harrison, G. (1978). *Mosquitoes, malaria and man*. Clarke, Irwin and Co., New York.

Harry, H. W. and Aldrich, D. V. (1958). The ecology of *Australorbis glabratus* in Puerto Rico. *Bull. World Health Org.*, **18**, 819–32.

Hassan, F. A. (1981). *Demographic Archaeology*. Academic Press, New York.

Hassell, M. P. (1978). *The dynamics of arthropod predator–prey systems*. Princeton University Press, Princeton.

Hassell, M. P. and May, R. M. (1984). From individual behaviour to population dynamics. In *Behaviourial ecology*, (ed. R. Sibly and R. Smith), pp. 3–32. Blackwell, Oxford.

Hassell, M. P., Anderson, R. C., Cohen, J. E., *et al.* (1982). Impact of diseases on host populations (group report). In *Population biology of infectious diseases*, (ed. R. M. Anderson and R. M. May), pp. 15–35. Springer Verlag, New York.

Haswell-Elkins, M., Elkins, D. B., and Anderson, R. M. (1987a). Evidence for predisposition in humans to infection with *Ascaris*, hookworm, *Enterobius* and *Trichuris* in a South Indian fishing community. *Parasitology*, **95**, 323–37.

Haswell-Elkins, M. R., Elkins, D. B., Manjuila, K., Michael, E., and Anderson, R. M. (1987b). The distribution and abundance of *Enterobius vermirularis* in a South Indian fishing community. *Parasitology*, **95**, 339–54.

Haswell-Elkins, M. R., Kennedy, M. W., Maizels, R. M., Elkins, D. B., and Anderson, R. M. (1989). The antibody recognition profiles of naturally infected humans against *Ascaris lumbricoides* larval excretory/secretory antigens. *Parasitol. Immunol.*, **11**, 615–27.

Hausermann, W. (1969). On the biology of *Simulium damnosum* (Theobald, 1903) the main vector of onchocerciasis in the Mahenge Mountains, Ulanga, Tanzania. *Acta Trop.*, **26**, 26–69.

Hawking, F. (1967). The 24 hours periodicity of microfilariae: biological mechanisms responsible for its production and control. *Proc. R. Soc.*, **B169**, 59–76.

Hayden, G. F., Modlin, J. F., and Wittle, J. J. (1977). Current status of rubella in the United States 1969–75. *J. Infect. Dis.*, **185**, 337–40.

Hedrich, A. W. (1933). Monthly estimates of the child population 'susceptible' to measles, 1900–1931, Baltimore, Md. *Am. J. Hyg.*, **17**, 613–36.

Henderson, E. C. (1916). A census of contagious diseases of 8,786 children. *Am. J. Public Health*, **6**, 871–91.

Henschen, F. (1965). *The history of diseases*. Longmans, London.

Hesselberg, C. A. and Andreassen, J. (1975). Some influences of population density on *Hymenlepis diminuta* in rats. *Parasitology*, **71**, 517–23.

Hethcote, H. W. (1976). Qualitative analyses of communicable disease models. *Math. Biosci.*, **28**, 335–56.

Hethcote, H. W. (1978). An immunization model for a heterogeneous population. *Theor. Pop. Biol.*, **14**, 338–49.

Hethcote, H. W. (1983). Measles and rubella in the United States. *Am. J. Epidemiol.*, **117**, 2–13.

Hethcote, H. W. and Tudor, D. W. (1980). Integral equation models for endemic infectious diseases. *J. Math. Biol.*, **9**, 37–47.

Hethcote, H. W. and Van Ark, J. W. (1986). Epidemiological models for heterogeneous populations: proportionate mixing, parameter estimation and immunization programs. *Math. Biosci.*, **84**, 84–118.

Hethcote, H. W. and Yorke, J. A. (1984). Gonorrhea: transmission dynamics and control. *Lect. Notes Biomath.*, **56**, 1–105.

Hethcote, H. W., Stech, H. W., and van der Driessche, P. (1981). Non-linear oscillations in epidemic models. *SIAM J. Appl. Math.*, **40**, 1–9.

Hethcote, H. W., Yorke, J. A., and Nold, A. (1982). Gonorrhoea modelling: a comparison of central methods. *Math. Biosci.*, **58**, 93–109.

Heymann, D. L., Kesseng Mayben, G., Murphy, K. R., Guyer, B., and Foster, S. O. (1983). Measles control in Yaounde: justification of a one dose, nine month minimum age vaccination policy in tropical Africa. *The Lancet*, **I**, 1470–1.

Hiatt, R. A. (1976). Morbidity from *Schistosoma mansoni* infections: an epidemiologic study based on quantitative analysis of egg excretion in two highland Ethiopian villages. *Am. J. Trop. Med. Hyg.*, **25**, 808–17.

Hiatt, R. A., Cline, B. L., Ruiz-Tiben, E., Knight, W. B., and Berrios-Duram, L. A. (1980). The Boqueron project after 5 years: a prospective community based study on infection with *Schistosoma mansoni* in Puerto-Rico. *Am. J. Trop. Med. Hyg.*, **29**, 1228–40.

Hinman, A. R. (1982). World eradication of measles. *Rev. Infect. Dis.*, **40**, 933–9.

Hirayama, K., Matsushita, S., Kikuchi, I., Iuchi, M., Ohta, N., and Sasazuki, T. (1987). HLA-DQ is epistatic to HLA-DR in controlling the immune response to schistosomal antigen in humans. *Nature*, **327**, 426–30.

HMSO (1981). *Whooping cough. Reports from the committee on safety in medicines and the joint committee on vaccination and immunisation.* HMSO, London.

HMSO (1988). *Short-term prediction of HIV infection and AIDS in England and Wales.* HMSO, London.

Ho, D. D., Sarngadharan, M. G., Resnick, L., *et al.* (1985). Primary human T-lymphotropic virus type III infection. *Ann. Intern. Med.*, **103**, 880–3.

Hoare, C. (1972). *The trypanosomes of mammals.* Blackwell Scientific, Oxford.

Hobsbawm, E. J. (1969). *Industry and Empire.* Penguin Books, Harmondsworth.

Hoffman, G. W. (1975). A theory of regulation and self–nonself discrimination in an immune network. *Eur. J. Immunol.*, **5**, 638–57.

Holden, A. V. (ed.) (1986). *Chaos.* Princeton University Press, Princeton.

Holford, T. R. and Hardy, R. J. (1976). A stochastic model for the analysis of age-specific prevalence curves in schistosomiasis. *J. Chron. Dis.*, **29**, 445–58.

Holmes, J. C. (1982). Impact of infectious disease agents on the population growth and geographical distribution of animals. In *Population biology of infectious diseases*, (ed. R. M. Anderson and R. M. May), pp. 37–51. Springer, Berlin.

Holstein, M. (1953). Enquetes sur l'onchocercose le long de la Volta Noire. *Bull. Soc. Pat. Exot.*, **46**, 329–34.

Hope Simpson, R. E. (1952). Infectiousness of communicable diseases in the household. *The Lancet*, **ii**, 549–54.

Hopkins, D. R., Hinman, A. R., Koplan, J. P., and Lare, J. M. (1982). The case for global measles eradication. *The Lancet*, **I**, 1145–55.

Hoppensteadt, F. C. (1974). An age dependent epidemic model. *J. Franklin Inst.*, **297**, 325–33.

Hoppensteadt, F. C. (1975). Mathematical theories of populations: demographics, genetics and epidemics. In *Regional conference series on applied mathematics*. SIAM, Philadelphia.

Horwitz, O., Grunfeld, K., Lysgaard-Hanson, B., and Kjeldsen, K. (1974). The epidemiology and natural history of measles in Denmark. *Am. J. Epidem.*, **100**, 136–49.

Hsieh, H. C. (1970). Studies on endemic hookworm. I. Survey and longitudinal observation in Taiwan. *Japan. J. Parasitol.*, **19**, 508–22.

Hsu, H. F., Hsu, S. Y. L., and Ritchie, L. S. (1955). Epidemiological study on schistosomiasis japonica in Formosa. *Am. J. Trop. Med. Hyg.*, **4**, 1042–8.

Hull, H. F., Williams, P. J., and Odfield, F. (1983). Measles mortality and vaccine efficiency in rural West Africa. *The Lancet*, **I**, 972–5.

Hunter, D. J. and De Gruttola, V. (1986). Estimation of risk outcomes in HTLV-III infection. *The Lancet*, **i**, 667–8.

Hutchinson, G. E. (1978). *An Introduction to population ecology.* Yale University Press, London.

Hyman, J. M. and Stanley, E. A. (1988*a*). Using mathematical models to understand the AIDS epidemic. *Math. Biosci.*, **90**, 415–74.

Hyman, J. M. and Stanley, E. A. (1988*b*). The effect of social mixing patterns on the spread of AIDS. *Math. Biosci.*, **90**, 415–73.

Isham, V. (1988). Mathematical modelling of the transmission dynamics of AIDS: a review. *J. R. Statist. Soc.*, **A151**, 5–49.

Jackson, C. H. N. (1948). The analysis of a tsetse fly population III. *Ann. Eugen. Camb.*, **14**, 91.

Jacobsen, R. H., Brooks, B. O., and Cypress, R. H. (1982). Immunity to *Nematospiroides dubius*: parasite stages responsible for and subject to resistance in high responder (LAF1/J) mice. *J. Parasitol.*, **68**, 1053–8.

Jacquez, J. A., Simon, C. P., Koopman, J., Sattenspiel, L., and Perry, T. (1988). Modelling and analysing HIV transmission: the effect of contact patterns. *Math. Biosci.*, **92**, 119–99.

James, S. P., Nicol, W. D., and Shute, P. G. (1932). A study of induced malignant tertian malaria. *Proc. Roy. Soc. Med.*, **25**, 1153–86.

Jansco, N. (1921). Experimentelle untersuchungen uner die malaria-infektion des Anopheles und des Menschen beeninflussenden umstande. *Beihefte z. Arch. f. Schiffs-u. Tropen-Hyg.*, **25**, 5.

Jenkins, D. C. and Phillipson, R. F. (1971). The kinetics of repeated low level infections of *Nippostrongylus brasiliensis* in the laboratory rat. *Parasitology*, **62**, 457–65.

Jenkins, G. M. and Watts, D. G. (1968). *Spectral analysis and its applications.* Holden-Day, San Francisco.

Jerne, N. K. (1974). Towards a network theory of the immune system. *Ann. Inst. Pasteur, Paris*, **125C**, 373–89.

John, T. J., Joseph, A., and Jessudos, J. (1980). Epidemiology and prevention of measles in rural South India. *Indian J. Med. Res.*, **72**, 153–8.

Johnson, A. M. and Gill, O. N. (1989). Evidence for recent changes in sexual behaviour in homosexual men in England and Wales. *Phil. Trans. R. Soc.*, **B325**, 153–61.

Johnson, A. M. and Laga, M. (1988). Heterosexual transmission of HIV. *AIDS*, **2 suppl. 1**, 548–56.

Johnson, K. S., Harrison, G. B. L., Lightowlers, M. W., *et al.* (1989). Vaccination against ovine cysticercosis using a defined recombinant antigen. *Nature*, **338**, 585–7.

Jones, R. M. (1981). A field study of the Morontel sustained release bolus in the seasonal control of parasite gastroenteritis in grazing calves. *Vet. Parasitol.*, **8**, 237–51.

Jordan, P. (1972). Epidemiology and control of schistosomiasis. *Br. Med. Bull.*, **28**, 55–9.

Jordan, P. (1977). Schistosomiasis—research to control. *Am. J. Trop. Med. Hyg.*, **26**, 877–86.

Jordan, P. and Webbe, G. (1982). *Schistosomiasis: epidemiology, treatment and control.* Heinemann, London.

Jordan, P., Christie, J. D., and Unrau, G. O. (1980). Schistosomiasis transmission with particular reference to possible ecological and biological methods of control. *Acta Trop.*, **37**, 95–138.

Kalbfleish, J. A. and Lawless, J. F. (1988). Estimation of the incubation period for AIDS patients. *Nature*, **33**, 504–5.

Kalen, A. E. and McLeod, D. A. (1977). Paramyxoviruses: comparative diagnosis of parainfluenza, mumps, measles, and respiratory syncytial infections. In *Comparative diagnosis of viral diseases. I. Human and related viruses part A*, (ed. E. Kurstak and C. Kurstak), pp. 503–607. Academic, New York.

Källén, A., Arcuri, P., and Murray, J. D. (1985). A simple model for the spatial spread and control of rabies. *J. Theor. Biol.*, **116**, 377–93.

Kanki, P. J., Alroy, J., and Essex, M. (1985). Isolation of a T-lymphotropic retrovirus related to HTLV-III isolated from wild caught African green monkeys. *Science*, **230**, 951–4.

Kanki, P. J., M'Boup, S. M., Ricard, D., *et al.* (1987). Human T-lymphotrophic virus type-4 and the human immunodeficiency virus in West Africa. *Science*, **236**, 827–31.

Kaplan, A. S. (1973). *The herpes viruses.* Academic, New York.

Kates, K. C., Colglazier, M. L., and Enzie, F. D. (1973). Experimental development of acambenadazole-resistant strain of *Haemonchus contortus* in sheep. *J. Parasitol.*, **59**, 169–74.

Kato, S., Muranaka, S., Takakura, I., Kimura, M., and Tsuji, J. (1982). HLA-DR antigens and the rubella-specific immune response in man. *Tissue Antigens*, **19**, 140–5.

Katz, S. L. (1983). International symposium on measles immunisation: summary and recommendations. *Paediatrics*, **71**, 653–4.

Katzman, W. and Dietz, K. (1985). Evaluation of age-specific vaccination strategies. *Theor. Pop. Biol.*, **23**, 125–37.

Keittivuti, B., D'Aynes, T., Keittivuti, A., and Viravaidya, M. (1983). The prevalence of parasite infections among Cambodian refugees residing in Ban-Kaeng Holding Center, Prachinburi Province, Thailand, In *Collected papers on the control of soil-transmitted helminthiases*, (2nd edn), pp. 59–65. Asian Parasite Control Organisation, Tokyo.

Kendall, D. G. (1949). Stochastic processes and population growth. *R. Statist. Soc.*, **B11**, 230–64.

Kennedy, C. R. (1975). *Ecological animal parasitology.* Blackwell Scientific, Oxford.

Kennedy, M. W., Qureshi, F., Haswell-Elkins, M., and Elkins, D. B. (1987). Homology and heterology between the secreted antigens of the parasite larval stages of *Ascaris lumbricoides* and *Ascaris suum*. *Clin. Exp. Immunol.*, **67**, 20–30.

Kermack, W. O. and McKendrick, A. G. (1927). A contribution to the mathematical theory of epidemics. *Proc. R. Soc.*, **A115**, 700–21.

Kershaw, W. E., Lavoipierre, M. M. J., and Chalmers, T. A. (1953). Studies on the intake of microfilariae by their insect vectors, and their effect on the survival of their vectors, I: *Dirofitana immitis* and *Aedes aegypti*. *Ann. Trop. Med. Parasitol.*, **47**, 207–24.

Keusch, G. T., Wilson, C. S., and Waksal, S. D. (1983). Nutrition, host defences and the lymphoid system. In *Advances in host defence mechanisms*, (ed. J. I. Gallin and A. S. Fauci), pp. 275–87. Plenum, New York.

Keyfitz, N. and Flieger, W. (1971). *Population: facts and methods of demography.* Freeman, San Francisco.

Keymer, A. (1981). Population dynamics of *Hymenolepsis diminuta* in the intermediate host. *J. Anim. Ecol.*, **50**, 941–50.

Keymer, A. E. (1985). Experimental epidemiology. *Nematospiroides dubius* and the laboratory mouse. In *Ecology and genetics of host–parasite interactions*, (ed. D. Rollinson and R. M. Anderson), pp. 55–76. Academic, London.

Keymer, A. E. and Hiorns, R. W. (1985). *Heligmosomoides polygyrus* (Nematoda): the dynamics of primary and repeated infection in outbred mice. *Proc. R. Soc.*, **B29**, 47–67.

Khan, A. Q. and Talibi, S. A. (1972). Epidemiological assessment of malaria transmission in an endemic area of Eastern Pakistan and the significance of congenital immunity. *Bull. World Health Org.*, **46**, 783–92.

King, W. V. (1029). On the development of malaria parasites in the mosquito. *Am. J. Hyg.*, **10**, 560.

Kliger, I. J. and Mer, G. (1937). Studies on the effect of various factors on the infection rate of *Anopheles elutus* with different species of *Plasmodium*. *Ann. Trop. Med.*, **31**, 71.

Kloos, H. and Lemma, A. (1980). The epidemiology of *Schistosoma mansoni* infection at Tensae Berhan: human water contact patterns. *Ethiop. Med. J.*, **18**, 91–8.

Knowles, T. and Basu, B. C. (1943). Laboratory studies on the infectivity of *Anopheles stephensi*. *J. Malar. Inst. India*, **5**, 1–29.

Knox, E. G. (1980). Strategy for rubella vaccination. *Int. J. Epidemiology.*, **9**, 13–23.

Knox, E. G. (1986). A transmission model for AIDS. *Eur. J. Epidemiol.*, **2**, 165–77.

Komiya, Y., Kozai, I., and Suzuki, R. (1962). The increase of the ratio of those expelling only unfertilized eggs of *Ascaris* as the rate of those positive for *Ascaris* eggs among the local social groups diminishes and the relationship of this observation to the eradication program of ascariasis in Japan. *Japan J. Parasitol.*, **11**, 45–52.

Konnings, E., Anderson, R. M., Morley, D., O'Riordon, T., and Meegan, M. (1988). Rates of sexual partner change among two pastoralist niolitic groups in East Africa. *AIDS*, **3**, 245–7.

Koopman, J., Simon, C., Jacquez, J., Sattenspiel, L., and Pork, T. (1988). Sexual partner selectiveness: effects on homosexual HIV transmission dynamics. *J. AIDS*, **1**, 486–504.

Kostitzin, V. A. (1934). *Symbiose, parasitisme et evolution*. Hermann, Paris.

Koura, M., Upathan, E. S., Awad, A. H., and Ahmed, M. D. (1981). Prevalence of *Schistosoma haematobium* in the Karyole and Merca districts of the Somali Democratic Republic. *Ann. Trop. Med. Parasit.*, **75**, 53–61.

Krafsur, E. S. and Armstrong, J. C. (1977). The bionomics and relative prevalence of *Anopheles* species with respect to the transmission of *Plasmodium* to man in Western Ethiopia. *J. Med. Entomol.*, **14**, 180–94.

Krafsur, E. S. and Garrett-Jones, C. (1977). The survival of *Wuchereria* infected *Anopheles funestus* Giles in north-eastern Tanzania. *Trans. R. Soc. Trop. Med. Hyg.*, **71**, 155–60.

Krebs, C. J. (1978). *Ecology: experimental analysis of distribution and abundance*. Harper and Row, New York.

Kreiss, J. K., Koech, D., Plummer, F. A., *et al.* (1986). AIDS virus infection in Nairobi prostitutes. *New Engl. J. Med.*, **314**, 414–18.

Krugman, S. and Katz, S. L. (1981). *Infectious diseases of children*. Mosby, St Louis.

Krupp, I. M. (1962). Effects of crowding and of superinfection on habitat selection and egg production in *Ancylostoma caninum*. *J. Parasitol.*, **47**, 957–61.

Kuntz, R. E. (1955). Biology of the schistosome complexes. *Am. J. Trop. Med. Hyg.*, **4**, 383–414.

Kurtak, D. C. (1986). Insecticide resistance in the onchocerciasis control programme. *Parasitol. Today*, **2**, 20–1.

Kvalsvig, J. D. and Schutte, C. H. J. (1986). The role of human water contact patterns in the transmission of schistosomiasis in an informal settlement near a major industrial area. *Ann. Trop. Med. Parasit.*, **80**, 13–26.

Lainson, R. Shaw, J. J. Fracha, H., Miles, M. A., and Draper, C. C. (1979). Chagas's disease in the Amazon basin: 1. *Trypanosoma cruzi* infections in silvatic mammals, triatomine bugs and man in the state of Para, North Brazil. *Trans. R. Soc. Trop. Med. Hyg.*, **73**, 193–204.

Lanciani, C. A. Parasite-induced alterations in host reproduction and survival. *Ecology*, **56**, 689–95.

Lange, J. M. A., Wolf, F., Danner, S. A., *et al.* (1986). Persistent HIV antigenaemia and decline of HIV core antibodies associated with transition to AIDS. *Br. Med. J.*, **293**, 1459–62.

Laurian, Y., Peynet, J., and Verroust, F. (1989). HIV infection in sexual partners of seropositive patients with hemophilia. *New Engl. J. Med.*, **320**, 183.

Lehman, J. S., Mott, K. E., Morrow, R. H., Muntz, T. M., and Boyer, M. H. (1976). The intensity and effects of infection with *Schistosoma mansoni* in a rural community in North East Brazil. *Am. J. Trop. Med. Hyg.*, **25**, 285–95.

LeJambre, L. F., Royal, W. M., and Martin, P. J. (1979). The inheritance of thiabendazole resistance in *Haemonchus contortus*. *Parasitology*, **78**, 107–19.

Levin, B. R. and Lenski, R. E. (1983). Coevolution in bacteria and their viruses and plasmids. In *Coevolution*, (ed. D. J. Futuyma and M. Slatkin), pp. 99–127. Sinauer, Sunderland, Massachusetts.

Levin, B. R., Allison, A. C., Bremermann, H. J., *et al.* (1982). Evolution of parasites and hosts (group report). In *Population biology of infectious diseases*, (ed. R. M. Anderson and R. M. May), pp. 212–43. Springer, New York.

Levin, S. A. (1983). Some approaches to the modelling of coevolutionary interactions. In *Coevolution*, (ed. M. Nitecki), pp. 21–65.

Levin, S. A. and Pimentel, D. (1981). Selection of intermediate rates of increase in parasite–host systems. *Am. Nat.*, **117**, 308–15.

Lewis, T. (1975a). A model for the parasitic disease bilharziasis. *Adv. Appl. Prob.*, **7**, 673–704.

Lewis, T. (1975b). Threshold results in the study of schistosomiasis. *Stat. Rep. Preprints*, **23**, 1–10.

Leyton, M. K. (1968). Stochastic models in populations of helminthic parasites in the definitive host. II. Sexual mating functions. *Math. Biosci.*, **3**, 413–19.

Lindenmann, J. (1964). Inheritance of resistance to influenza in mice. *Proc. Soc. Exp. Biol.*, **116**, 505–9.

Lloyd, M. and Dybas, H. S. (1966). The periodical cicada problem: I, population ecology. *Evolution*, **20**, 133–49.

London, W. P. and Yorke, J. A. (1973). Recurrent outbreaks of measles, chickenpox and mumps. I. Seasonal variation in contact rates. *Am. J. Epidemiol.*, **98**, 453–68.

Lorenz, E. N. (1963). Deterministic nonperiodic flow. *J. Atmos. Sci.*, **20**, 130–41.

Lotka, A. J. (1923). Contribution of the analysis of malaria epidemiology. *Am. J. Hyg.*, **3, suppl. 1**, 1–21.

Loveday, C. (1989). Human immunodeficiency viruses in patients attending a sexually transmitted disease clinic in London, 1982–87. *Br. Med. J.*, **298**, 419–22.

Lui, K. J. Lawrence, D. N., Morgan, W. M., Peterman, T. A., Hauerkos, H. W., and Bregman, D. J. (1986). A model based approach for estimating the mean incubation period of transfusion-associated acquired immunodeficiency syndrome. *Proc. Natl. Acad. Sci.*, **83**, 3051–5.

Lui, W. M., Hethcote, H. W., and Levin, S. A. (1987). Dynamical behaviour of epidemiological models with nonlinear incidence rates. *J. Math. Biol.*, **25**, 359–80.

Macdonald, G. (1926). Malaria in the children of Freetown, Sierra Leone. *Ann. Trop. Med. Parasit.*, **20**, 239–63.

Macdonald, G. (1950). The analysis of infection rates in diseases in which superinfections occur. *Trop. Dis. Bull.*, **47**, 907–15.

Macdonald, G. (1951). Community aspects of immunity to malaria. *Brit. Med. Bull.*, **8**, 33–6.

Macdonald, G. (1952). The analysis of equilibrium in malaria. *Trop. Dis. Bull.*, **49**, 813–29.

Macdonald, G. (1957). *The epidemiology and control of malaria.* Oxford University Press, London.

Macdonald, G. (1965). The dynamics of helminth infections, with special reference to schistosomes. *Trans. R. Soc. Trop. Med. Hyg.*, **59**, 489–506.

Macdonald, W. W. (1976). Mosquito genetics in relation to filarial infections. In *Genetic aspects of host–parasite relationships*, (ed. A. E. R. Taylor and R. Myller), pp. 1–24. Blackwell Scientific, Oxford.

MacGregor, J. D., MacDonald, J., Ingram, E. A., McDonnell, M., and Marshall, B. (1981). Epidemic measles in Shetland during 1977 and 1978. *Br. Med. J.*, **282**, 434–6.

Maema, M. M. (1986). *Dynamics of repeated infection of high and low responder inbred mice with Heligmosomoides polygyrus.* PhD thesis. London University.

Mahmoud, A. A. F. and Warren, K. S. (1980). Control of infection and disease in *Schistosomiasis mansoni* by targeted chemotherapy. *Clin. Res.*, **28**, 474.

Maizels, R. M., Meghj. M., and Ogilvie, B. M. (1983). Restricted sets of parasite antigens from the surʾace of different stages and sexes of the nematode parasite *Nippostrongylus brasiliensiʿ Immunol.*, **48**, 107–21.

Marasca, G. and McEvoy, M. (1986). Length of survival of patients with acquired immunodeficiency syndrome in the United Kingdom. *Brit. Med. J.*, **292**, 1727–9.

Martin, J. E. and Keymer, A. E. (1983). The prevalence and intensity of helminth infections in children from rural Bangladesh. *Trans. R. Soc. Trop. Med. Hyg.*, **77**, 702–6.

Martin, J. E., Lester, A., Price, E. V., and Schmale, J. D. (1970). Comparative study of gonococcal susceptibility to penicillin in the United States. *J. Infect. Dis.*, **122**, 459–61.

Martini, E. (1921). Berechnungen und Beobachtungen. In *Epiedemiologie und bekampfung der malaria.* Gente, Hamburg.

May, R. M. (1974). *Stability and complexity in model ecosystems* (second edition). Princeton University Press, Princeton.

May, R. M. (1976). Simple mathematical models with very complicated dynamics. *Nature*, **261**, 459–67.

May, R. M. (1977a). Togetherness among schistosomes: its effects on the dynamics of the infection. *Math. Biosci.*, **35**, 301–43.

May, R. M. (1977b). Dynamical aspects of host–parasite asociations—Crofton's model revisited. *Parasitology*, **75**, 259–76.

May, R. M. (1979). Bifurcations and dynamic complexity in ecological systems. *Ann. N.Y. Acad. Sci.*, **316**, 517–29.

May, R. M. (1984). Prehistory of Amazonian Indians. *Nature*, **312**, 19–20.

May, R. M. (1985). Regulation of populations with non-overlapping generations by microparasites: a purely chaotic system. *Amer. Natur.*, **125**, 573–84.

May, R. M. (1986). Population biology of microparasitic infections. In *Mathematical ecology: an introduction*, (ed. T. G. Hallam and S. W. Levin), pp. 405–42. Springer Verlag, New York.

May, R. M. (1987). Chaos and the dynamics of biological populations. *Proc. Roy. Soc.*, **A413**, 27–44.

May, R. M. (1988). HIV infection in heterosexuals. *Nature*, **331**, 655–6.

May, R. M. (1990). Population biology and population genetics of plant-pathogen associations. In *Pests, pathogens and plant communities*, (ed. J. J. Burdon and S. R. Leather), pp. 309–325. Blackwell Scientific, Oxford.

May, R. M. and Anderson, R. M. (1978). Regulation and stability of host–parasite population interactions: II. Destabilizing processes. *J. Anim. Ecol.*, **47**, 249–67.

May, R. M. and Anderson, R. M. (1979). Population biology of infectious diseases. Part II. *Nature*, **280**, 455–61.

May, R. M. and Anderson, R. M. (1983a). Epidemiology and genetics in the coevolution of parasites and hosts. *Proc. R. Soc.*, **B219**, 281–313.

May, R. M. and Anderson, R. M. (1983b). Parasite–host coevolution. In *Coevolution*, (ed. D. Futuyma and M. Slatkin), pp. 186–206. Sinauer, Sunderland, Massachusetts.

May, R. M. and Anderson, R. M. (1984). Spatial heterogeneity and the design of immunisation programmes. *Math. Biosci.*, **72**, 83–111.

May, R. M. and Anderson, R. M. (1985). Endemic infections in growing populations. *Math. Biosci.*, **76**, 1–16.

May, R. M. and Anderson, R. M. (1987). Transmission dynamics of HIV infection. *Nature*, **326**, 137–42.

May, R. M. and Anderson, R. M. (1988). The transmission dynamics of human immunodeficiency virus (HIV). *Phil. Trans. R. Soc.*, **B321**, 565–607.

May, R. M. and Anderson, R. M. (1990). Parasite-host coevolution. *Parasitology*, **100**, S89–S101.

May, R. M. and Dobson, A. P. (1986). Population dynamics and the rate of evolution of pesticide resistance. In *Pesticide resistance management*. NAS-NRC Publications, Washington.

May, R. M., Endler, J. A., and McMurtrie, R. E. (1975). Gene frequency clines in the presence of selection opposed by gene flow. *Am. Nat.*, **109**, 659–76.

May, R. M., Hassell, M. P., Anderson, R. M., and Tonkyn, D. W. (1981). Density-dependence in host–parasitoid models. *J. Anim. Ecol.*, **50**, 855–65.

May, R. M., Anderson, R. M., and Johnson, A. M. (1988a). The influence of temporal variation in the infectiousness of infected individuals on the transmission dynamics of HIV. In *AIDS*, AAAS Science Symposium Papers 1988, (ed. R. Kulstad), pp. 75–80.

May, R. M., Anderson, R. M., and McLean, A. R. (1988b). Possible demographic consequences of HIV/AIDS epidemics: II. Assuming HIV infection does not necessarily lead to AIDS. *Lecture Notes Biomath.*, **100**, 419–42.

May, R. M., Anderson, R. M., and McLean, A. R. (1988c). Possible demographic consequences of HIV/AIDS epidemics: I. Assuming HIV infection always leads to AIDS. *Math. Biosci.*, **90**, 475–505.

Mayr, E. (1963). *Animal species and evolution*. Harvard University Press, Cambridge, Massachusetts.

McClure, M. O. and Weiss, R. A. (1987). Human Immunodeficiency Virus and related viruses. In *Current topics in AIDS*, (ed. M. S. Gottlieb, D. J. Jeffries, D. Mildvan, A. J. Pinching, T. C. Quinn, and R. A. Weiss), pp. 95–117. Wiley, Chichester.

McEvoy, M. and Tillet, H. E. (1985). Some problems in the prediction of future numbers of cases of the acquired immunodeficiency syndrome in the U.K. *The Lancet*, **II**, 541–2.

McKeown, T. (1976). *The modern rise of population*. Edward Arnold, London.

McKeown, T. (1979). *The role of modern medicine: dream, mirage or nemesis?* Basil Blackwell, Oxford.

McKusick, L., Harlsman, W., and Coates, T. J. (1985*a*). AIDS and sexual behaviour reported by gay men in San Francisco. *Am. J. Public Health*, **75**, 493–6.

McKusick, L., Wiley, J. A., Coates, T. J., and Stall, G. (1985*b*). Reported changes in the sexual behaviour in men at risk from AIDS, San Francisco 1982–84: the AIDS Behavioural Research Project. *Public Health Rep.*, **100**, 622–9.

McLean, A. R. and Anderson, R. M. (1988*a*). Measles in developing countries. Part I. Epidemiological parameters and patterns. *Epidemiol. Infect.*, **100**, 111–33.

McLean, A. R. and Anderson, R. M. (1988*b*). Measles in developing countries. Part II. The predicted impact of mass vaccination. *Epidemiol. Infect.*, **100**, 419–42.

McManus, T. J. and McEvoy, M. (1987). Some aspects of male homosexual behaviour in the United Kingdom. *Brit. J. Sex. Med.*, **14**, 110–20.

McMullen, D. B. (1947). The control of schistosomiasis japonica. I. Observations on the habits, ecology, and life cycle of *Oncomelania quadrasi* the molluscan intermediate host of *Schistosoma japonicum* in the Philippine Islands. *Am. J. Hyg.*, **45**, 259–73.

McMullen, D. B., Endo-Itabashi, T., Sato, S., Komiyama, S., and Stone, P. R. (1951). Seasonal studies of *S. japonicum* in the intermediate host, *Oncomelania nosophora. Am. J. Hyg.*, **54**, 416–30.

McNeill, W. H. (1976). *Plagues and peoples.* Blackwell, Oxford.

Mears, J. G. and Lachman, H. M. (1981). Sickle gene: its origin and diffusion from West Africa. *J. Clin. Invest.*, **68**, 606–10.

Medley, G. F. and Anderson, R. M. (1985). Density-dependant fecundity in *Schistosoma mansoni* infections in man. *Trans. R. Soc. Trop. Med. Hyg.*, **79**, 532–4.

Medley, G. F. and Anderson, R. M. (1991). A stochastic simulation model of helminth parasite transmission and control in human communities. (*Manuscript in preparation.*)

Medley, G. F., Anderson, R. M., Cox, D. R., and Billard, L. (1987). Incubation period of AIDS in patients infected via blood transfusions. *Nature*, **328**, 719–21.

Medley, G. F., Billard, L., Cox, D. R., and Anderson, R. M. (1988). The distribution of the incubation period for the acquired immunodeficiency syndrome (AIDS). *Proc. R. Soc.*, **B233**, 367–77.

Meenan, P. N. (1958). Irish antibodies to poliomyelitus virus. *J. Irish Med. Assoc.*, **248**, 34–46.

Melbye, M., Madhok, R., Sarin, P. S., *et al.* (1984). HTLV-III seropositivity in European haemophiliacs exposed to factor VIII concentrate imported from the USA. *The Lancet*, **ii**, 1444–6.

Michael, E. and Bundy, D. A. P. (1989). Density-dependence in establishment, growth and worm fecundity in intestinal helminthiases; the population biology of *Trichuris trichuria* in CBA/Ca mice. *Parasitology*, **48**, 451–8.

Mildvan, D. and Solomon, S. L. (1987). The spectrum of disease due to human immunodeficiency virus infection. In *Current Topics in AIDS*, (ed. M. S. Gottlieb, D. J. Jeffries, D. Mildvan, A. J. Pinching, T. C. Quinn, and R. A. Weiss), pp. 31–56. John Wiley and Sons, New York.

Miller, M. J. (1958). Observations on the natural history of malaria in semi-resistant West Africans. *Trans. R. Soc. Trop. Med. Hyg.*, **52**, 152–68.

Milligan, P. J. M. and Baker, R. D. A. (1988). A model of tsetse-transmitted animal trypanosomiasis. *Parasitology*, **96**, 211–39.

Mimms, C. A. and White, D. O. (1984). *Viral pathogenesis and immunology.* Blackwell, Oxford.

Minchella, D. J. and Loverde, P. T. (1983). Laboratory comparison of the relative success of *Biomphalaria glabrata* stocks which are susceptible and insusceptible to infection with *Schistosoma mansoni. Parasitology*, **86**, 335–44.

Miner, J. R. (1923). The incubation period of typhoid fever. *Infect. Dis.*, **31**, 296–301.

Mitchell, G. F. (1979). Responses to infection with metazoan and protozoan parasites in mice. *Adv. Immunol.*, **28**, 451–511.

Mode, C. J. (1958). A mathematical model for the coevolution of obligate parasites and their hosts. *Evolution*. **12**, 158–65.

Molineaux, L. (1985). The pros and cons of modelling malaria transmission. *Trans. R. Soc. Trop. Med.*, **79**, 743–7.

Molineaux, L. and Gramiccia, G. (1980). *The Garki Project*. World Health Organization, Geneva.

Molineaux, L., Shidrawi, G. R., Clark, J. L., Boulzaguet, R., and Ashkar, T. S. (1979). Assessment of insecticidal impact on the malaria mosquito's vectorial capacity, from data on the man-biting range and age-composition. *Bull. World Health Org.*, **57**, 265–74.

Mollison, D. (1977). Spatial contact model for ecological and epidemic spread. *J. R. Statist. Soc.*, **B39**, 283–326.

Molvo, S. K., Steiger, R. F., Brun, R., and Boreham, P. F. L. (1971). Sleeping sickness survey in Musoma district, Tanzania. II. The role of *Glossina* in the transmission of sleeping sickness. *Acta Trop.*, **28**, 189–205.

Monath, T. P. (1985). Glad tidings from yellow fever. *Science*, **229**, 734–5.

Montagnier, L. (1985). Lymphadenopathy-associated virus: from molecular biology to pathogeneity. *Ann. Intern. Med.*, **103**, 689–93.

Moore, J. (1984). Parasites that change the behaviour of their host. *Sci. Amer.*, **250(5)**, 108–15.

Morgan, W. M. and Curran, J. W. (1986). Acquired immunodeficiency syndrome: current and future trends. *Public Health Rep.*, **101**, 459–65.

Morley, D. C. (1969*a*). Severe measles in the tropics. I. *Br. Med. J.*, **1**, 293–300.

Morley, D. (1969*b*). Severe measles in the tropics. II. *Br. Med. J.*, **1**, 363–5.

Morley, D., Woodland, M., and Martin, W. J. (1963). Measles in Nigerian children. *J. Hyg.*, **61**, 115–35.

Mortimer, P. P. (1978). Mumps prophylaxis in the light of a new test for antibody. *Br. Med. J.*, **2**, 1523–4.

Mortimer, P. P., Vandervelde, E. M., Jesson, W. J., and Pereira, M. S. (1985). HTLV-III antibody in Swiss and English intravenous drug abusers. *The Lancet*, **ii**, 449–50.

Mochkovskii, Sh. D. (1950). *Basic laws of the epidemiology of malaria*. AMN, Moscow. (In Russian.)

Moss, A. R., Osmond, D., Bacchetti, P., Chermann, J.-C., Barre-Sinoussi, F., and Carlson, J. (1987). Risk factors for AIDS and HIV seropositivity in homosexual men. *Am. J. Epidemiol.*, **125 (6)**, 1035–47.

Muench, H. (1959). *Catalytic models in epidemiology*. Harvard University Press. Cambridge, Massachusetts.

Muirhead-Thomson, R. C. (1954). Factors determining the reservoir of infection of *Plasmodium falciparum* and *Wuchereria bancrofti* in a West African village. *Trans. R. Soc. Trop. Med. Hyg.*, **48**, 208–25.

Muller, A. S., Voorhoeve, A. M., Mannetje, W., and Schulpen, T. W. J. (1977). The impact of measles in a rural area of Kenya. *E. Afr. Med. J.*, **54**, 364–72.

Muller, R. (1972). *Worms and disease: a manual of medical helminthology*. William Heinemann, London.

Muller, R. (1975). *Worms and disease: a manual of medical helminthology*, (2nd edn). William Heinemann, London.

Mulligan, H. W. (1970). *The African trypanosomiases*. George Allen and Unwin, London.

Murray, G. D. and Cliff, A. D. (1975). A stochastic model for measles epidemics in a multi-region setting. *Inst. Br. Geog.*, **2**, 158–74.

Myers, T. (1974). Spanish contacts and social change on the Ueayali River, Peru. *Ethnohistory*, **21**, 135–57.

Myers, T. (1981). Aboriginal trade networks in Amazonia. In *Networks of the past: regional interaction in archaeology*, (ed. P. D. Francis, F. J. Kense, and P. G. Duke), pp. 84–99. Chacmool, Calgary.

Nakajima, N., Desselberger, U., and Palese, P. (1978). Recent human influenza A(H1N1) viruses are closely related genetically to strains isolated in 1950. *Nature*, **274**, 334–9.

Nasell, I. (1976a). On eradication of schistosomiasis. *Theor. Pop. Biol.*, **10**, 133–44.

Nasell, I. (1976b). A hybrid model of schistosomiasis. *Theor. Pop. Biol.*, **10**, 47–69.

Nasell, I. (1977). On transmission and control of schistosomiasis, with comments on Macdonald's model. *Theor. Pop. Biol.*, **12**, 335–65.

Nasell, I. and Hirsch, W. M. (1972a). The transmission dynamics of schistosomiasis. *Comm. Pure Appl. Math.*, **26**, 395–453.

Nasell, I. and Hirsch, W. M. (1972b). A mathematical model of some helminthic infections. *Comm. Pure Appl. Math.*, **25**, 459–77.

Nathanson, N. and Martin, J. R. (1979). The epidemiology of poliomyelitis: enigmas surrounding its appearance, epidemicity, and disappearance. *Am. J. Epidemiol.*, **110**, 672–92.

Nawalinski, T., Schad, G. A., and Chowdhury, A. D. (1978). Population biology of hookworms in children in rural West Bengal. II. Acquisition and loss of hookworms. *Am. J. Trop. Med. Hyg.*, **27**, 1162–73.

Nesheim, M. C. (1989). Ascariasis and human nutrition. In *Ascariasis and its prevention and control*, (ed. D. W. T. Crompton, M. C. Nesheim, and Z. S. Paulowski), pp. 87–100. Taylor and Francis, London.

Nicholson, A. J. and Bailey, V. A. (1935). The balance of animal populations, part I. *Proc. Zoo. Soc. Lond.*, **1**, 551–98.

Noah, N. (1985). The strategy of immunisation. *Comm. Med.*, **5**, 140–7.

Nokes, D. J. (1987). *Seroepidemiology of rubella virus in England and the design of control programmes based on mass vaccination*. PhD thesis, University of London.

Nokes, D. J. and Anderson, R. M. (1987). Rubella vaccination policy: a note of caution. *The Lancet*, **i**, 1441–2.

Nokes, D. J. and Anderson, R. M. (1988). The use of mathematical models in the epidemiological study of infectious diseases and in the design of mass immunisation programmes. *Epidemiol. Infect.*, **101**, 1–20.

Nokes, D. J., Anderson, R. M., and Anderson, M. J. (1986). Rubella epidemiology in South East England. *J. Hyg.*, **86**, 291–304.

Nokes, D. J., Anderson, R. M., and Jennings, R. (1987). Longitudinal serological study of rubella in South Yorkshire. *The Lancet*, **ii**, 1156–7.

Nold, A. (1980). Heterogeneity in disease transmission modelling. *Math. Biosci.*, **52**, 227–40.

Norman, C. (1985). AIDS trends: projections from limited data. *Science*, **230**, 1020–1.

O'Donnell, I. J. and Mitchell, G. F. (1980). An investigation of the antigens of *Ascaris lumbricoides* using a radioimmunoassay and sera of naturally infected humans. *Int. Arch. Allergy Appl. Immunol.*, **61**, 213–19.

Olsen, L. F. (1987). Low dimensional strange attractors in epidemics of childhood diseases in Copenhagen, Denmark. In *Chaos in biological systems*, (ed. H. Degn, A. V. Holden, and L. F. Olsen), pp. 249–54. Plenum Press, London.

Olveda, R. M., Tiu, E., Fevidal, P., deVeyra, F., Icatto, F. C., and Domingo, E. O. (1983).

Relationship of prevalence and intensity of infection to morbidity in *Schistosomiasis japonica*: a study of three communities in Leyte, Philippines. *Am. J. Trop. Med. Hyg.*, **32**, 1312–21.

Oomen, A. P. (1969). The epidemiology of onchocerciasis in S.W. Ethiopia. *Trop. Geogr. Med.*, **21**, 105–37.

Pan, C. T. (1965). Studies on the host–parasite relationship between *Schistosoma mansoni* and the snail *Australorbic glabratus*. *Am. J. Trop. Med. Hyg.*, **14**, 931–76.

Park, T. (1948). Experimental studies of interspecies competition. *Ecol. Monogr.*, **18**, 267–307.

Paul, J. R. (1955). Epidemiology of poliomyelitis. *World Health Org. Monogr.*, **26**, 9–30.

Pederson, C., Nielson, C. M., Vestergaard, B. F., *et al.* (1987). Temporal relation of antigenaemia and loss of antibodies to core antigens to development of clinical disease in HIV infection. *Br. Med. J.*, **295**, 567–9.

Pellegrino, J. and de Maria, M. (1966). Results of exposing mice to natural pond water harbouring a colony of *Australorbis glabratus* highly infected with *Schistosoma mansoni*. *Am. J. Trop. Med. Hyg.*, **15**, 333–6.

Pereira, M. S. (1979). Global surveillance of influenza. *Brit. Med. Bull.*, **35**, 9–14.

Perrin, W. F. and Powers, J. E. (1980). Role of a nematode in natural mortality of spotted dolphins. *J. Wildl. Mgmt.*, **44**, 960–3.

Pesigan, T. P., Forooq, M., Hairston, N. G., *et al.* (1958a). Studies on *Schistosoma japonicum* infection in the Philippines. 1. General considerations and epidemiology. *Bull. World Health Org.*, **18**, 345–455.

Pesigan, T. P., Hairston, N. G., Jaurequi, J. J., Garcia, E. G., Santos, B. C., and Besa, A. A. (1958b). Studies on *Schistosoma japonicum* infection in the Philippines. 2. The molluscan host. *Bull. World Health Org.*, **18**, 481–578.

Peterman, T. A., Drotman, D. P., and Curran, J. W. (1985). Epidemiology of the Acquired Immunodeficiency Syndrome (AIDS). *Epidemiol. Rev.*, **7**, 1–21.

Peterman, T. A., Stoneburner, R. L., Allen, J. R., Jaffe, H. W. and Curran, J. W. (1988). Risk of human immunodeficiency: virus transmission from heterosexual adults with transfusion-associated infection. *J. Am. Med. Assoc.*, **259**, 55–7.

Peters, W. (1985). The problem of drug resistance in malaria. *Parasitology*, **90**, 705–16.

Peters, W. and Standfast, H. A. (1960). Studies on the epidemiology of malaria in New Guinea. II. Holoendemic malaria, the entomological picture. *Trans. R. Soc. Trop. Med. Hyg.*, **54**, 249–60.

Phillip, M., Parkhouse, R. M. E., and Ogilvie, B. M. (1980). Changing proteins on the surface of a parasitic nematode. *Nature*, **538**, 538–40.

Pickering, J., Wiley, J. A., Lieb, L. E., *et al.* (1986). Modelling the incidence of acquired immunodeficiency syndrome in San Francisco, Los Angeles and New York. *Math. Model.*, **7**, 661–88.

Pielou, E. C. (1969). *An introduction to mathematical ecology*. Wiley, New York.

Piot, P., Quinn, T. C., and Taelman, H. (1984). Acquired immunodeficiency syndrome in a heterosexual population in Zaire. *The Lancet*, **ii**, 65–9.

Piot, P., Plummer, F. A., Mhalu, F. S., Lamboray, J., Chin, J., and Mann, J. M. (1988). AIDS: an international perspective. *Science*, **239**, 573–9.

Polderman, A. M. and Mahshande, J. P. (1981). Failure of targeted mass treatment to control schistosomiasis. *The Lancet*, **1**, 27–8.

Pollard, J. H. (1973). *Mathematical models for the growth of human populations*. Cambridge University Press.

Post, W. M., DeAngelis, D. L., and Travis, C. C. (1983). Endemic disease in environments with spatially heterogeneous host populations. *Math. Biosci.*, **63**, 289–302.

Preblud, S. R., Serdula, M. K., Frank, J. A. Jr., Brandling-Bennett, A. D., and Hinman, A. R. (1980). Rubella vaccination in the United States: a ten year review. *Epidemiol. Rev.*, **2**, 171–94.

Pringle, G. and Avery-Jones, S. (1966). Observations on the early course of untreated falciparum malaria in semi-immune African children following a short period of protection. *Bull. World Health Org.*, **34**, 269–72.

Pritchard, D. I., Maizels, R. M., Behnke, J. M., and Appleby, P. (1984). Stage specific antigens of *Nematospiroides dubius*. *Immunology*, **53**, 325–35.

Pritchard, D. I., Quinnell, R. J., Slater, A. F. G., *et al.* (1989). The epidemiological significance of acquired immunity to *Necator americanus*: humoral responses to parasite collagen and excretory–secretory antigens. *Parasitology*, **100**, 317–26.

Prost, A. and Prescott, N. (1984). Cost-effectiveness of blindness prevention by the Onchocerciasis Control Programme in Upper Volta. *Bull. World Health Org.*, **5**, 795–802.

Pull, J. H. and Grab, B. (1974). A simple epidemiological model for evaluating the malaria inoculation rate and the risk of infection in infants. *Bull. World Health Org.*, **51**, 507–15.

Putnam, P. (1931). Statistical analysis of intensity of malaria infection (Appendix in Studies on malaria in Southern Nigeria by M. A. Barber and M. T. Olinger). *Ann. Trop. Med.*, **25**, 461–501.

Quinn, T. C., Mann, J. M., Curran, J. W., and Piot, P. (1986). AIDS in Africa: an epidemiologic paradigm. *Science*, **234**, 955–63.

Rabo, E. and Taranger, J. (1984). Scandinavian model for eliminating measles, mumps and rubella. *Br. Med. J.*, **289**, 1402–4.

Ranki, A., Valle, S. L., Krohn, M., *et al.* (1987). Long latency precedes overt seroconversion in sexually transmitted human immunodeficiency virus infection. *The Lancet*, **II**, 589–93.

Rayendran, S. and Jayewickreme, S. H. (1951a). Malaria in Ceylon. Part I, The control and prevention of epidemic malaria by the residual spraying of houses with DDT. *Indian J. Malaria*, **5**, 1–73.

Rayendran, S. and Jayewickreme, S. H. (1951b). Malaria in Ceylon. Part II, The control of endemic malaria at Anuradhapura by the residual spraying of houses with DDT. *Indian J. Malaria*, **5**, 75–124.

Razzell, P. E. (1974). 'An interpretation of the modern rise of population in Europe'—a critique. *Pop. Studies*, **28**, 5–17.

RCGP (1974). A retrospective study of the complications of mumps. *J. R. Coll. Gen. Pract.*, **24**, 552–5.

Read, C. P. (1950). The crowding effect in tapeworm infections. *J. Parasitol.*, **37**, 174–8.

Redfield, R. R., Markham, P. D., Salahuddin, S. Z., Wright, D. C., Sarngadharan, M. G., and Gallo, R. C. (1985). Heterosexually acquired HTLV-III/LAV disease (AIDS-related complex and AIDS). *J. Am. Med. Assoc.*, **254**, (15), 2094–6.

Reeves, G. K. and Overton, S. E. (1988). Preliminary survival analysis of U.K. AIDS data. *The Lancet*, **I**, 880.

Regniere, J. (1984). Vertical transmission of diseases and population dynamics of insects with discrete generations: a model. *J. Theor. Biol.*, **287**, 301.

Remme, J. H. F. (1989). *The epidemiology and control of onchocerciasis in West Africa*, pp. 3–195. University of Rotterdam.

Reynolds, G. H. and Chan, Y. K. (1975). A control model for gonorrhea. *Bull. Inst. Int. Stat.*, **106**, (2), 264–79.

Riordan, K. (1977). Long term variations in trypanosome infection rates in highly infected tsetse flies on a cattle route in southern-western Nigeria. *Ann. Trop. Med. Parasitol.*, **71**, 9–20.

Ritchie, L. S., Radke, M. G., and Ferguson, F. F. (1962). Population dynamics of *Australorbis glabratus* in Puerto Rico. *Bull. World Health Org.*, **27**, 171–81.

Roberts, J. M. D., Neumann, E., Gockel, C. W., and Highton, R. B. (1967). Onchocerciasis in Kenya, 9, 11, and 18 years after elimination of the vector. *Bull. World Health Org.*, **37**, 195–212.

Rogers, D. J. and Boreham, P. F. L. (1973). Sleeping sickness survey in the Serengeti area (Tanzania) 1971. II. The vector role of *Glossina swynnertoni* Austen. *Acta Trop.*, **30**, 24–35.

Rogers, D. J. (1988). The dynamics of vector-transmitted diseases in human communities. *Phil. Trans. R. Soc.*, **B321**, 513–37.

Roitt, I. (1988). *Essential immunology*, (6th edn). Blackwell Scientific, Oxford.

Roitt, I., Brostoff, J., and Male, D. (1985). *Immunology*. Gower, London.

Rosen, L. (1955). Observations on the epidemiology of human filariasis in French Oceania. *Am. J. Hyg.*, **61**, 219–48.

Ross, R. (1908). *Report on the prevention of malaria in Mauritius*. London.

Ross, R. (1911). *The prevention of malaria*, (2nd edn). Murray, London.

Ross, R. (1915). Some *a priori* pathometric equations. *Br. Med. J.*, **1**, 546–7.

Ross, R. (1916). An application of the theory of probabilities to the study of *a priori* pathometry, I. *Proc. R. Soc.*, **A92**, 204–30.

Ross, R. (1917). An application of the theory of probabilities to the study of *a priori* pathometry, II. *Proc. R. Soc.*, **A93**, 212–25.

Ross, R. and Hudson, H. P.(1917). An application of the theory of probabilities to the study of *a priori* pathometry, III. *Proc. R. Soc.*, **A93**, 225–40.

Ross, R. and Thomson, D. (1910). A case of sleeping sickness studied by precise enumerative methods: regular periodical increase of the parasite described. *Proc. R. Soc.*, **B82**, 411–15.

Rothenberg, R., Woelfe, M., Stoneburner, R., *et al.* (1988). Survival with the acquired immunodeficiency syndrome. *New Engl. J. Med.*, **317**, 1297–302.

Roush, R. T. and Croft, B. A. (1986). Experimental population genetics and ecological studies of pesticide resistance in insects and mites. In *Pesticide resistance: strategies and tactics for management*, pp. 257–70. National Academy Press, Washington, D.C.

Rowley, J. T., Anderson, R. M., and Ng, T. W. (1990). Reducing the spread of HIV infection in sub-Saharan Africa: some demographic and economic implications. *AIDS*, **4**, 47–56.

Samarawickrema, W. A. and Laurence, B. R. (1978). Loss of filarial larvae in a natural mosquito population. *Ann. Trop. Med. Parasitol.*, **72**, 561–5.

Sartwell, P. E. (1950). The distribution of incubation periods of infectious disease. *Am. J. Hyg.*, **51**, 310–18.

Sartwell, P. E. (1966). The incubation period and the dynamics of infectious disease. *Am. J. Epidemiol.*, **83**, 204–16.

Sasa, M., Kanda, T., Mitsui, G., Shirasaka, A., Ishii, A., and Chinzei, H. (1970). The filariasis control programmes in Japan and their evaluation by means of epidemiological analysis of microfilaria survey data. In *Recent advances in researches on filariasis and schistosomiasis in Japan*, pp. 3–72. University of Tokyo Press.

Schad, G. A. and Anderson, R. M. (1985). Predisposition to hookworm in man. *Science*, **228**, 1537–40.

Schad, G. A., Nawalinski, T. A., and Kochar, V. K. (1984). Human behaviour and the regulation of hookworm population. In *Human ecology and infectious diseases*, (ed. J. Cross), pp. 187–223. Academic Press, New York.

Schaffer, W. M. and Kot, M. (1986). Differential systems in ecology and epidemiology. In *Chaos*, (ed. A. V. Holden), pp. 158–78. Princeton University Press, Princeton.

Schapira, A., Suleimanov, G. E., and Halloran, M. E. (1990). Longitudinal study of malaria in Maputo, Mozambique. (Unpublished.)

Schenzle, D. (1984). An age-structured model of pre- and post-vaccination measles transmission. *IMA J. Math. Appl. Med. Biol.*, 1, 169–91.

Schiff, C. J., Evans, A., Yiannakis, C., and Eardley, M. (1975). Seasonal influence on the production of *Schistosoma haematobium* and *S. mansoni* cercariae in Rhodesia. *J. Parasitol.*, 5, 119–23.

Schmidt, G. D. and Roberts, L. S. (1977). *Foundations of parasitology*. Mosby, St Louis.

Schreiber, F. G. and Schubert, M. (1949). Experimental infections of the snail *Australorbis glabratus* with the trematode *Schistosoma mansoni* and the production of cercariae. *J. Parasitol.*, 35, 91–100.

Schuffner, W. A. P. (1938). Two subjects relating to the epidemiology of malaria. Part I. The importance of determining the spleen rate and the limits of its usefulness. *J. Malaria Inst. India*, 1, 221–56.

Schwartz, I. B. (1985). Multiple recurrent outbreaks and predictability in seasonally forced nonlinear epidemic models. *J. Math. Biol.*, 21, 347–61.

Schwartz, I. B. and Smith, H. L. (1984). Infinite subharmonic bifurcation in an SEIR epidemic model. *J. Math. Biol.*, 18, 233–53.

Scorza Smeraldi, R., Lazzarin, A., Moroni, M., Fabio, G., Eisera, N. B., and Zanussi, C. (1986). HLA-associated susceptibility to acquired immunodeficiency syndrome in Italian patients with human-immunodeficiency-virus infection. *The Lancet*, ii, 1187–9.

Scott, D., Senker, K., and England, E. C. (1982). Epidemiology of human *Schistosoma haematobium* infection around Volta Lake, Ghana, 1973–1975. *Bull. World Health Org.*, 60, 89–100.

Scott, J. A. (1942). The epidemiology of schistosomiasis in Venezuela. *Am. J. Hyg.*, 35, 337–66.

Scott, M. E. (1988). The impact of infection and disease on animal populations: implications for conservation biology. *J. Consv. Biol.*, 2, 40–56.

Scott, M. E. and Anderson, R. M. (1984). The population dynamics of *Gyrodactylus bullatarudis* (Monogenea) within laboratory populations of the fish host *Poecilia reticulata*. *Parasitology*, 89, 159–94.

Scrimshaw, N. S., Taylor, C. E., and Gordan, J. E. (1968). Interactions of nutrition and infection. *WHO Monogr. Ser.*, 57, 329.

Seger, J. (1988). Dynamics of some simple host-parasite models with more than two genotypes in each species. *Phil. Trans. R. Soc.*, B319, 541–55.

Seo, B. (1980). The third report on research (1979)—study on the control programmes of Ascariasis in Korea. In *Collected papers on the control of soil-transmitted helminthiases*, pp. 197–212. Asian Parasite Control Organisation, Tokyo.

Seo, B. S., Cho, S. Y., Chai, J. Y., and Hang, S. T. (1980). Comparative efficiency of various interval mass treatment on *Ascaris lumbricoides* infection in Korea. *Korean J. Parasitol.*, 18, 145–51.

Seo, B. S., Cho, S. Y., and Chai, J. Y. (1979). Frequency distribution of *Ascaris lumbricoides* in rural Koreans with special reference on the effect of changing endemicity. *Korean J. Parasitol.*, 17, 105–13.

Seo, B. S., Lee, S. H., and Chai, J. Y. (1983). An evaluation of the student directed mass control programme against ascariasis in Korea. In *Collected papers on the control of soil-transmitted helminthiases*, (2nd edn), pp. 238–53. Asian Parasite Control Organisation, Tokyo.

Sergent, E. and Poncet, A. (1956). Etude expérimentale du paludisme des rongeurs à *P. bhergei*, IV. Résistance acquise. *Arch. Inst. Pasteur d'Algérie*, **34**, 1–51.

Serwadda, D., Mugerwa, R. D., Sewankambo, N. K., et al. (1985). Slim disease: a new disease in Uganda and its association with HTLV-III infection. *The Lancet*, **ii**, 849–52.

Sethi, S. P. (1974). Quantitative guidelines for communicable disease control program: a complete synthesis. *Biometrics*, **30**, 681–91.

Siddons, L. B. (1944). Observations on the influence of atmospheric temperature and humidity on the infectivity of *Anopheles culicifacies* Giles. *J. Malaria Inst. India*, **5**, 375.

Sinniah, B., Kan-Chua, S. P., and Subramaniam, K. (1983). Evaluating the reliability of egg counts in determining intensity of *Ascaris* infections. In *Collected papers on the control of soil-transmitted helminthiases*, (2nd edn), pp. 5–10. Asian Parasite Control Organisation, Tokyo.

Siongok, T. K. A., Mahmoud, A. A. F., Ouma, J. H., et al. (1976). Morbidity in schistosomiasis mansoni in relation to intensity of infection: study of a community in Machakos, Kenya. *Am. J. Trop. Med. Hyg.*, **25**, 273–84.

Sithithaworn, P. (1986). *Population dynamics of Schistosoma mansoni in laboratory mice exposed to repeated infection.* PhD thesis, London University.

Slater, A. F. G. (1988). The influence of dietary protein on the experimental epidemiology of *Heligmosomoides polygyrus* (Nematoda) in the laboratory mouse. *Proc. R. Soc.*, **B234**, 239–54.

Slater, A. F. G. and Keymer, A. E. (1986). *Heligmosomoides polygyrus* (Nematoda): the influence of dietary protein on the dynamics of repeated infection. *Proc. R. Soc.*, **B229**, 69–83.

Slatkin, M. (1973). Gene flow and selection in a cline. *Genetics*, **75**, 733–56.

Sleigh, A. C., Mott, K. E., Hoff, R., et al. (1985). Three-year prospective study of the evolution of Manson's schistosomiasis in north-east Brazil. *The Lancet*, **II**, 63–66.

Sloof, R. and Verdrager, J. (1972). *Anopheles balabacensis* (Baisas, 1963) and malaria transmission in southern-eastern areas of Asia. Unpublished document WHO/MAL/72.765. World Health Organisation, Geneva.

Smillie, W. G. (1924). Control of hookworm disease in Southern Alabama. *Southern Med. J.*, **17**, 494–502.

Smith, H. L. (1978). Periodic solutions for a class of epidemic equations. *Math. Anal. Appl.*, **64**, 467–79.

Smith, K. M. (1976). *Virus–insect relationships.* Longman, London.

Smithers, S. R. (1956). On the ecology of schistosome vectors in The Gambia, with evidence of their role in transmission. *Trans. R. Soc. Trop. Med. Hyg.*, **50**, 354–65.

Smithers, S. R. and Terry, R. J. (1969). Immunity in schistosomiasis. *Ann. N.Y. Acad. Sci.*, **160**, 826–40.

Sobeslavsky, O. (1980). Prevalence of markers for hepatitis B virus infection in various countries: a WHO collaboration study. *Bull. World Health Org.*, **58**, 621–8.

Soper, M. A. (1929). The interpretation of periodicity in disease prevalence. *J. R. Stat. Soc.*, **A92**, 34–61.

South, M. A. and Sever, J. L. (1985). Teratogen update: the congenital rubella syndrome. *Teratology*, **31**, 297–307.

Southwood, T. R. E. (1981). Bionomic strategies and population parameters. In *Theoretical ecology*, (ed. R. M. May), pp. 30–52. Blackwell Scientific, London.

Spencer, M. J., Cherry, J. D., Powell, K. R., *et al.* (1977). Antibody responses following rubella immunisation analysed by HLA and ABO types. *Immunology*, **4**, 365–72.

Standen, O. D. (1949). Experimental schistosomiasis. II. Maintenance of *Schistosoma mansoni* in the laboratory, with some notes on experimental infection with *S. haematobium*. *Ann. Trop. Med. Parasitol.*, **43**, 268–83.

Stech, H. and Williams, M. (1981). Stability for a class of cyclic epidemic models with delay. *J. Math. Biol.*, **11**, 95–103.

Stewart, G. J., Cunningham, A. L., Driscoll, G. L., *et al.* (1985). Transmission of human T-cell lymphotropic virus type III (HTLV-III) by artificial insemination by donor. *The Lancet*, **ii**, 581–4.

Stiven, A. E. (1962). Experimental studies on the epidemiology of the host parasite system hydra and *Hydramoeba hydroxena* (Entz), I: The effect of the parasites on the individual host. *Physiological Zoology*, **35**, 166–78.

Stirewalt, M. A. (1954). Effect of snail maintenance temperature on development of *Schistosoma mansoni*. *Exp. Parasitol.*, **3**, 504–16.

Stone, B. F. (1972). The genetics of resistance by ticks to ascaricides. *Aust. Vet. J.*, **48**, 345–50.

Stratman-Thomas, W. K. (1940). The influence of temperature on *Plasmodium vivax*. *Am. J. Trop. Med.*, **20**, 703–6.

Strong, R. P. (1937). Onchocerciasis in Central America and Africa. *Trans. R. Soc. Trop. Med. Hyg.*, **18**, 1–57.

Stuart-Harris, C. H. (1982). The epidemiology of influenza: key facts and remaining problems. In *Influenza models*, (ed. P. Selby), pp. 87–103. MTP, Boston.

Sturrock, B. M. (1967). The effect of infection with *Schistosoma haematobium* on the growth and reproductive rates of *Bulinus* (*Physopsis*) *nasutus productus*. *Ann. Trop. Med. Parasitol.*, **62**, 321–5.

Sturrock, B. M. and Sturrock, R. F. (1970). Laboratory studies of the host–parasite relationship of *Schistosome mansoni* and *Biomphalaria. glabrata* from St. Lucia, West Indies. *Ann. Trop. Med. Parasitol.*, **64**, 357–63.

Sturrock, R. F. (1973). Field studies on the transmission of *Schistosoma mansoni* and on the bionomics of its intermediate host *Biomphalaria glabrata* on St. Lucia, West Indies. *Int. J. Parasitol.*, **3**, 175–94.

Sturrock, R. F. and Webbe, G. (1971). The application of catalytic models to schistosomiasis in snails. *J. Helminth.*, **45**, 189–200.

Sturrock, R. F., Cohen, J. E., and Webbe, G. (1975). Catalytic curve analysis of schistosomiasis in snails. *Ann. Trop. Med. Parasitol.*, **69**, 133–4.

Sturrock, R. F., Kimani, R., Cottrell, B. J., *et al.* (1983). Observations on possible immunity to reinfection among Kenyan school children after treatment for *Schistosoma mansoni*. *Trans. R. Soc. Trop. Med. Hyg.*, **77**, 366–71.

Sturrock, R. F., Cottrell, B. J., and Kimani, R. (1984). Observations on the ability of repeated light exposure to *Schistosoma mansoni* cercaria to induce resistance to reinfection in Kenyan baboons (*Papio anubis*). *Parasitology*, **88**, 515–14.

Sturrock, R. F., Bensted-Smith, R., Butterworth, A. E., *et al.* (1987). Immunity after treatment of human schistosomiasis mansoni. III. Long term effects of treatment and retreatment. *Trans. R. Soc. Trop. Med. Hyg.*, **81**, 303–14.

Sugihara, G. and May, R. M. (1990). Nonlinear forecasting as a way of distinguishing chaos from measurement error in time series. *Nature*, **344**, 734–41.

Sugihara, G., Grenfell, B. and May, R. M. (1990). Distinguishing error from chaos in ecological time series. *Phil. Trans. R. Soc.*, **B330**, 235–51.

Sugiura, S. (1933). Studies on the biology of *Oncomelania nosphora* (Robson), an intermediate host of schistosomiasis japonicum. *Niigata Ika Daigaku Byorigaku Kyoshitsu Kenkyu Hokoku*, **31**, 1–18.

Sweet, W. C. (1925). Average egg count per gm faeces per female hookworm in Ceylon. *J. Parasitol.*, **12**, 39–42.

Sydenstricker, E. and Hedrich, A. W. (1929). Completeness of reporting of measles, whooping cough and chickenpox at different ages. *U.S. Public Health Rep.*, **44**, 1537–43.

Tahori, A. S. (1978). Resistance of ticks to ascaricides. *Refu. Vet.*, **35**, 177–9.

Tallis, G. M. and Leyton, M. (1966). A stochastic approach to the study of parasite populations. *J. Theor. Biol.*, **13**, 251–60.

Taylor, J. M. G., Schwartz, K., and Detels, R. (1986). The time from infection with human immunodeficiency virus (HIV) to the onset of AIDS. *J. Infect. Dis.*, **154**, 694–7.

Tayo, M. A., Pugh, R. N. H., and Bradley, A. K. (1980). Malumfashi Endemic Diseases Project, XI. Water contact activities in the schistosomiasis study area. *Ann. Trop. Med. Parasitol.*, **74**, 347–54.

Teesdale, C. (1962). Ecological observations on the molluscs of significance in the transmission of bilharziasis in Kenya. *Bull. World Health Org.*, **27**, 759–82.

Theiler, M. and Smith, H. H. (1973). The use of yellow fever virus modified by *in vitro* cultivations for human immunization. *J. Exp. Med.*, **65**, 787–800.

Thein-Hliang (1985). *Ascaris lumbricoides* infections in Burma. In *Ascaris and its public health significance*, (ed. D. W. T. Crompton, M. C. Nesheim, and Z. S. Paulowski), pp. 83–112. Taylor and Francis, London.

Thein-Hliang (1989). Epidemiological basis of survey design, methodology and data analysis for *Ascaris*. In *Ascariasis and its prevention and control*, (ed. D. W. T. Crompton, M. C. Nesheim, and Z. S. Paulowski), pp. 351–68. Taylor and Francis, London.

Thein-Hliang, Than Saur, Myint Lwin, Htay Htay Aye, and Thein Maung Myint (1984). Epidemiology and transmission dynamics of *Ascaris lumbricoides* in Okpo village in rural Burma. *Trans. R. Soc. Trop. Med. Hyg.*, **78**, 497–504.

Tiglao, T. V. and Camacho, A. C. (1983). Water contact behaviour among humans in Leyte, Philippines. *S.E. Asian J. Trop. Med. Public Health*, **14**, 18–24.

Tingley, G. A., Butterworth, A. E., Anderson, R. M., et al. (1980). Water contact as a measure of exposure to infection in human schistosomiasis: the relationship to faecal egg counts. *Trans. R. Soc. Trop. Med. Hyg.*, **82**, 448–52.

Tocher, K. D. (1963). *The art of simulation*. English Universities Press, London.

Tyrell, D. A. J. (1980). Approaches to the control of infectious diseases. *Proc. R. Soc. Med.*, **63**, 1181–9.

Ukkonen, P. and von Bronsdorff, C. (1988). Rubella immunity and morbidity: effects of vaccination in Finland. *Scand. J. Infect. Dis.*, **20**, 255–9.

Unhanand, M., Srinophakun, S., Seedonrushimi, T., Jeradit, C., Nilapan, S., and Sathiloyathai, A. (1980). Study on the efficacy of an alcoholic extract substance from Ma-Klua (*Diospyros mollis*) against hookworm, *Ascaris* and *Trichuris* infections. In *Collected papers on the control of soil-transmitted helminthiases*, pp. 289–300. Asian Parasite Control Organisation, Tokyo.

Urbain, J. (1986). Idiotypic networks: a noisy background or a breakthrough in immunological thinking? The broken mirror hypothesis. *Ann. Immunol. (Inst. Pasteur)*, **137C**, 57–64.

Urquhart, G. E. D. (1980). *Communicable Diseases Scotland Weekly Report*, **24**, 7–8.

van der Perre, P., Carael, M., Robert-Guroff, M., et al. (1985). Female prostitutes, a risk group for infection with human T-cell lymphotrophic virus type III. *The Lancet*, **ii**, 524–7.

Van der Plank, J. E. (1975). *Principles of plant infection*. Academic Press, New York.

van Griensuen, G. J. P., de Vroome, E. M. M., Goudsmit, J., and Coutinho, R. A. (1989). Changes in sexual behaviour and the fall of incidence of HIV infection among homosexual men. *Br. Med. J.*, **298**, 218–21.

Van Pruten, J. A. M., Boo, Th., Jager, H. C., *et al.* (1986). AIDS prediction and intervention. *The Lancet*, **I**, 852–3.

Vermund, S. H., Bradley, D. J., and Ruiz-Tiben, E. R. (1988). Survival of *Schistosoma mansoni* in the human host: estimate from a community-based prospective study in Puerto Rico. *Am. J. Trop. Med. Hyg.*, **32**, 1040–8.

Vickerman, K. (1978). Antigenic variation in trypanosomes. *Nature*, **273**, 613–17.

Vogel, H. (1948). Maintenance of *Oncomelania hupensis* and experimental infection of it with *Bilharzia japonicum*. *Z. Parasitol.*, **14**, 70–91.

Vogt, M. W., Craven, D. E., Crawford, D. F., *et al.* (1986). Isolation of HTLV-III/LAV from cervical secretions of women at risk for AIDS. *The Lancet*, **i**, 525–7.

Wagenvoort, J. H., Harmsden, M., Boutahar-Trouw, B. J. K., Kraaijeveld, C. A., and Winkler, K. C. (1980). Epidemiology of mumps in the Netherlands. *J. Hyg.*, **85**, 313–26.

Wakelin, D. (1978). Genetic control of susceptibility and resistance to parasitic infection. *Adv. Parasitol.*, **169**, 219–308.

Wakelin, D. (1984). *Immunity to parasites*. Edward Arnold, London.

Wakelin, D. (1985). Genetic control of immunity to helminth infections. *Parasitol. Today*, **1**, 17–23.

Wakelin, D. (1986*a*). Genetics, immunity and parasite survival. In *Ecology and genetics of host–parasite interactions*, (ed. D. Rollinson and R. M. Anderson), pp. 39–54. Academic, London.

Wakelin, D. (1986*b*). Genetic and other constraints on resistance to infection with gastrointestinal nematodes. *Trans. R. Soc. Trop. Med. Hyg.*, **80**, 742–7.

Wakelin, D. and Blackwell, J. M. (ed.) (1988). *Genetics of resistance to bacterial and parasitic infection*. Taylor and Francis, London.

Wall, R. A., Denning, D. W., and Amos, A. (1987). HIV antigenaemia in acute HIV infection. *The Lancet*, **i**, 566.

Walliker, D., Quakyi, I. A., Wellons, T. E., *et al.* (1987). Genetic analysis of the human malaria parasite *Plasmodium falciparum*, **236**, 1661–5.

Walsh, J. A. (1983). Selective primary health care: strategies for control of disease in the developing world. IV. Measles. *Rev. Infect. Dis.*, **5**, 330–40.

Walsh, J. A. and Warren, K. S. (1979). Selective primary health care: an interim strategy for disease control in developing countries. *New Engl. J. Med.*, **301**, 967–74.

Waltman, P. (1974). Deterministic threshold models in the theory of epidemics. In *Lecture notes in biomathematics*, pp. 19–64. Springer-Verlag, New York.

Ward, R. A. (1963). Genetic susceptibility of mosquitoes to malarial infection. *Exp. Parasitol.*, **13**, 328–41.

Warren, K. S. (1973). Regulation of the prevalence and intensity of schistosomiasis in man: immunology or ecology. *J. Infect. Dis.*, **127**, 595–609.

Warren, K. S. (1979). Diseases due to helminths. In *Principles and practice of infectious diseases*, (ed. G. L. Mondel, R. G. Douglas, and J. E. Bennet), pp. 1562–68. Wiley, New York.

Warren, K. S. (1981). The control of helminths: nonreplicating infectious agents of man. *Ann. Rev. Public Health*, **2**, 101–15.

Warren, K. S. (1984). Selective primary health care: strategies for control of disease in the developing world. 1. Schistosomiasis. *Rev. Infect. Dis.*, **4**, 715–26.

Warren, K. S. and Mahmoud, A. F. (1976). Targeted mass treatment: a new approach to the control of schistosomiasis. *Trans. Assoc. Am. Phys.*, **89**, 195–203.

Warren, K. S. and Mahmoud, A. A. F. (1980). Targeted mass treatment: a new approach to the control of schistosomiasis. *Clin. Res.*, **28**, 195–204.

Warren, K. S. and Mahmoud, A. A. F. (1984). *Tropical and geographical medicine.* McGraw-Hill, New York.

Warren, K. S., Mahmoud, A. A. F., Cummings, P., Murphy, D. J., and Houser, H. B. (1974). Schistosomiasis mansoni in Yemeni in California: duration of infection, presence of disease, and therapeutic management. *Am. J. Trop. Med. Hyg.*, **23**, 902–9.

Warren, K. S., Arap Siongok, T. K., Houser, H. B., Ouma, J. H., and Peters, P. A. (1978). Quantification of infection with *Schistosoma haematobium* in relation to epidemiology and selective chemotherapy. I. Minimal number of daily egg counts in urine necessary to establish intensity of infection. *J. Infect. Dis.*, **138**, 849–55.

Weatherall, D. J., Bell, J. I., Clegg, J. B., *et al.* (1988). Genetic factors as determinants of infectious disease transmission in human communities. *Phil. Trans. R. Soc.*, **B321**, 327–48.

Webbe, G. (1962*a*). Population studies on intermediate hosts in relation to transmission of bilharziasis in East Africa. In *Bilharziasis: Ciba Foundation symposium*, (ed. G. E. Wolstenholme and M. O'Connor), pp. 7–22. Churchill, London.

Webbe, G. (1962*b*). The transmission of *Schistosoma haematobium* in an area of Lake Province, Tanganyika. *Bull. World Health Org.*, **27**, 59–85.

Webber, R. H. (1975). Theoretical considerations in the vector control of filariasis. *S.E. Asian J. Trop. Med. Public Health*, **4**, 544–8.

Weinbaum, F. I., Evans, C. B., and Tigelaar, R. E. (1976). An *in vitro* assay for T-cell immunity to malaria in mice. *J. Immunol.*, **116**, 1280–3.

Weiss, R. A. (1982). The persistence of retroviruses. In *Virus persistence*, (ed. B. W. J. Mahy, A. C. Minson and G. K. Darby), pp. 267–88. Cambridge University Press, London.

Weiss, R. A. (1985). Human T-cell retroviruses. In *RNA tumour viruses*, (ed. R. A. Weiss, N. M. Teich, H. E. Varmus, and J. Coffin), pp. 406–85. Cold Spring Harbor Laboratory, New York.

Weller, I. V. D., Hindley, D. J., Adler, M. W., and Melchum, J. T. (1984). Gonorrhoea in homosexual man and media coverage of the acquired immune deficiency syndrome in London, 1982–3. *Br. Med. J.*, **289**, 1041–2.

Wenyon, C. M. (1921). The incidence and aetiology of malaria in Macedonia, 1915–1919. *J. R. Army Med. Corps*, **37**, 172.

Whittle, P. (1955). The outcome of a stochastic epidemic—a note on Bailey's paper. *Biometrika*, **42**, 154–62.

WHO (1975). *Manual on practical entomology in malaria.* WHO offset publication, No. 13.

WHO (1980). Influenza nomenclature. *Wkly. Epidem. Rec.*, **55**, 294–5.

WHO (1985*a*). *Ten years of onchocerciasis control*, World Health Organisation Report, No. OCP/GVA/85.1B. World Health Organisation, Geneva.

WHO (1985*b*). The control of schistosomiasis—report of a WHO expert committee. *WHO Tech. Rep. Ser.*, **728**.

Wickwire, K. (1977). Mathematical models for the control of pests and infectious diseases: a survey. *Theor. Pop. Biol.*, **11**, 182–238.

Wilkins, H. A. (1987). *Schistosoma haematobium* in a Gambian community. I. The intensity and prevalence of infection. *Ann. Trop. Med. Parasitol.*, **71**, 53–8.

Wilkins, H. A. and Scott, A. (1978). Variation and stability in *Schistosoma haematobium* egg counts: a four year study of Gambian children. *Trans. R. Soc. Trop. Med. Hyg.*, **72**, 397–404.

Wilkins, H. A., Goll, P. H., Marshall, T. F. de C., and Moore, P. J. (1984*a*). Dynamics of *Schistosoma haematobium* infection in a Gambian community. I. The pattern of infection in the study area. *Trans. R. Soc. Trop. Med. Hyg.*, **78**, 216–21.

Wilkins, H. A., Goll, P. H., Marshall, T. F. de C., and Moore, P. J. (1984*b*). Dynamics of *Schistosoma haematobium* infection in a Gambian community. III. Acquisition and loss of infection. *Trans. R. Soc. Trop. Med. Hyg.*, **78**, 227–32.

Wilkins, H. A., Blumenthal, U. J., Hagan, P., Hayes, R. J., and Tulloch, S. (1987). Resistance to reinfection after treatment for urinary schistosomiasis. *Trans. R. Soc. Trop. Med. Hyg.*, **81**, 29–35.

Williams, P. and Kershaw, W. E. (1961). Studies on the intake of microfilaria by their insect vectors, their survival, and their effect on the survival of their vectors. X. The survival of the tropical rat mite, the vector of filariasis in the cotton rat. *Ann. Trop. Med. Parasitol.*, **55**, 274–83.

Wilson, E. B. and Worcester, J. (1941). Contact with measles. *Proc. Natl. Acad. Sci., Wash.*, **27**, 7–13.

Wilson, G. N. (1904). Measles: its prevalence and mortality in Aberdeen. *Report of the Medical Office of Health, Aberdeen*, 41–51.

Winkelstein, W. (1987). The San Francisco men's health study: III. Reduction in human immunodeficiency virus transmission among homosexual/bisexual men, 1982–1986. *Am. J. Public Health*, **76**, 685–9.

Winkelstein, W., Lyman, D. M., Padian, N., *et al.* (1987). Sexual practices and risk of infection by the human immunodeficiency virus: the San Francisco Men's Health Study. *J. Am. Med. Assoc.*, **257**, 321–5.

Wolda, H. and Foster, R. (1978). *Zunacetha annulata* (Lepidoptera: Dioptidae), outbreak insect in a neotropical forest. *Geo. Eco. Trop.*, **2**, 443–54.

Wong-Staal, F. and Gallo, R. C. (1985). Human T-lymphotropic retrovirus. *Nature*, **317**, 395–403.

Wright, W. H. (1973). Geographical distribution of schistosomes and their intermediate hosts. In *Epidemiology and control of schistosomiasis (bilharziasis)*, (ed. N. Ansari), pp. 32–249. S. Karger, London.

Wright, W. H., McMullen, D. B., Bennett, H. J., Bauman, P. M., and Ingalls, J. W. (1947). The epidemiology of *Schistosomiasis japonica* in the Philippine Islands and Japan. III. Surveys of endemic areas of *Schistosomiasis japonica* in Japan. *Am. J. Trop. Med.*, **27**, 417–47.

Wrigley, E. A. and Schofield, R. S. (1981). *The population history of England, 1541–1871*. Harvard University Press, Cambridge, Mass.

Yekutiel, P. (1980). *Eradication of infectious diseases*. S. Karger, Basel.

Yihao, Z. and Wannian, S. (1983). A review of the current impact of measles in the People's Republic of China. *Rev. Infect. Dis.*, **5**, 411–16.

Yokogawa, M. (1985). JOICEP's experience in the control of ascariasis within an integrated programme. In *Ascariasis and its public health significance*, (ed. D. W. T. Crompton, M. C. Nesheim, and Z. S. Paulowski), pp. 265–78. Taylor and Francis, London.

Yorke, J. A. and London, W. P. (1973). Recurrent outbreaks of measles, chickenpox and mumps; II systematic differences in contact rates and stochastic effects. *Am. J. Epidemiol.*, **98**, 469–82.

Yorke, J. A., Hethcote, H. W., and Nold, A. (1978). Dynamics and control of the transmission of gonorrhea. *Sex. Transm. Dis.*, **5**, 51–6.

Yorke, J. A., Nathanson, N., Pianingiani, G., and Martin, J. (1979). Seasonality and the requirements for perpetuation and eradication of viruses. *Am. J. Epidemiol.*, **109**, 103–23.

Zahar, A. R. (1974). Review of the ecology of malaria vectors in the WHO Eastern Mediterranean region. *Bull. World Health Org.*, **50**, 427–40.

Zavala, F., Tam, J. P., Hollingdale, M., Cochrane, A. H., Quakyi, I., and Nussenzweig, R. S. (1985). Rationale for development of a synthetic vaccine against *Plasmodium falciparum* malaria. *Science*, **228**, 1436–40.

Zuckerman, A. (1974). Functional aspects of immunity in malarial rats. In *Basic research on malaria*, Technical Report ERO-5-74, (ed. J. B. Bateman), pp. 87–102. US Army European Research Office, London.

Author index

References to the publications of R. M. Anderson and of R. M. May are not indexed. Authors subsumed under *et al.* in the text are indexed under their individual names.

Subject index

HIV 236–9
  antibody detection 243
  basic reproductive rate 297
  identification 236
  origin 262–3
  pathogenic mechanism 237–8
  primary infection 243–4
  research 238
  see also AIDS
homogeneous mixing, empirical testing 155–71
  age-dependence in force of infection 160–70
    epidemics in 'virgin' populations 165–8
    measles data 160–3
    pertussis 163, 165
    serological evidence 168–70
  after immunization
    age at infection 155–7
    fraction susceptible 155
    interepidemic period 156–60
hookworm
  density dependence 451
  predisposition to infection 459
host population regulation 627–41
  coevolution of hosts/parasites 648–53
    avirulence tendency 648–9
    and infection with more than one strain 652
    myxoma virus example 649–52
  human evolution and 653–6
  macroparasites
    continuously overlapping generations 638–9
    discrete generations 636–8
  microparasites
    continuously overlapping generations 630–4
    discrete generations 627–30
    laboratory mice studies 634–6
  natural populations 639–41
  population biology, and agricultural revolution 654
  population genetics 641–8
    epidemiological analysis 643–8
    gene-for-gene interactions 642
    selective forces 641–2
  see also infection processes, macroparasites; infection processes, microparasites, basic models
human parvovirus (HPV), immune response to 29, 30
hunter-gatherer populations
  and host threshold densities 653–4
  mortality patterns 653

immunity
  and age 50–1
  to bacteria 38
  loss, as infection model complication 61–2

to macroparasites
  acquired 451–3
  protozoa 38–9
  response 433–4, 599–605
to malaria 38–9, 409–19
to viruses 27–37
  antigen-driven systems 32–5
  immune response 28–9
  immunological memory 31–2, 34
  network-regulated systems 35–7
  parvovirus 29, 30
  phases in infection 29–31
  see also acquired immunity; herd immunity; maternal antibody protection
  against malaria, and strain variability 624–5
immunization
  and age at infection 92–7, 155–7, 172
  age-dependent 671–2
    schedule, static aspects 660–2
  age-specific susceptibility 146–8
  'age window' in developing countries
    measles 327–8
    rubella 78
  analytical results 148–9
  basic reproductive rate, microparasite, and 91–2
  critical coverage for heterogeneous populations 219
  direct/indirect effects 87
  equilibrium changes 90–2
  fraction susceptible after 155
  and increase of serious illness 99–121
    criterion for 118–21
    measles encephalitis 110–14
    mumps 116–18
    poliomyelitis 99–100, 114–15
    risk of, and age 100–2
    rubella 100, 102–10
  interepidemic period after 157–60
  against macroparasites 494–6
    acquired immunity and 539–40
    and host heterogeneity 544–5, 547–8
  for malaria
    age 421–2
    and genetic variability 624–5
    for eradication 421
  for measles
    and age at infection 156–7
    age window effect 327–8
    in developing countries 329–30, 336–9, 340–1, 343–3
    dynamics 153
    eradication criteria 88, 90, 96, 98–9
    and fraction susceptible 155
    impact 186–7
    interepidemic period after 157–59
    as measles/mumps/rubella vaccine 109
    short-term dynamics 184–6
    steady state 181–3